Essentials of Dental Radiography

for Dental Assistants and Hygienists

Essentials of Dental Radiography

for Dental Assistants and Hygienists

NINTH EDITION

Evelyn M. Thomson, BSDH, MS

Adjunct Assistant Professor
Gene W. Hirschfeld School of Dental Hygiene
Old Dominion University
Norfolk, Virginia

Orlen N. Johnson, BS, DDS, MS

College of Dentistry
University of Nebraska Medical Center
Lincoln, Nebraska

Pearson

Boston   Columbus   Indianapolis   New York   San Francisco   Upper Saddle River
Amsterdam   Cape Town   Dubai   London   Madrid   Milan   Munich   Paris   Montreal   Toronto
Delhi   Mexico City   Sao Paulo   Sydney   Hong Kong   Seoul   Singapore   Taipei   Tokyo

Library of Congress Cataloging-in-Publication Data

Cataloging-in-Publication data on file with the Library of Congress.

Notice: The authors and the publisher of this volume have taken care that the information and technical recommendations contained herein are based on research and expert consultation and are accurate and compatible with the standards generally accepted at the time of publication. Nevertheless, as new information becomes available, changes in clinical and technical practices become necessary. The reader is advised to carefully consult manufacturers' instructions and information material for all supplies and equipment before use and to consult with a health care professional as necessary. This advice is especially important when using new supplies or equipment for clinical purposes. The authors and publisher disclaim all responsibility for any liability, loss, injury, or damage incurred as a consequence, directly or indirectly, of the use and application of any of the contents of this volume.

Publisher: Julie Levin Alexander
Assistant to Publisher: Regina Bruno
Editor-in-Chief: Mark Cohen
Executive Editor: John Goucher
Development Editor: Melissa Kerian
Assistant Editor: Nicole Ragonese
Editorial Assistant: Rosalie Hawley
Media Editor: Amy Peltier
Media Product Manager: Lorena Cerisano
Managing Production Editor: Patrick Walsh
Production Liaison: Christina Zingone

Production Editor: Sunitha Arun Bhaskar, Laserwords
Manufacturing Manager: Alan Fischer
Design Director: Jayne Conte
Cover Designer: Suzanne Behnke
Director of Marketing: David Gesell
Executive Marketing Manager: Katrin Beacom
Marketing Specialist: Michael Sirinides
Composition: Laserwords
Printer/Binder: RR Donnelley
Cover Printer: RR Donnelley
Cover Image: Dental X-Rays, Ocean Photography/Veer.

10 16

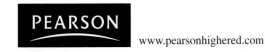

www.pearsonhighered.com

ISBN-13: 978-0-13-801939-6
ISBN-10:   0-13-801939-8

To my husband, Hu Odom, once again your loving patience, support, and encouragement gets me through.

—Evie

Contents

Preface

The study of oral radiological principles and the practice of oral radiography techniques require an understanding of theoretical concepts and a mastery of the skills needed to apply these concepts. *Essentials of Dental Radiography for Dental Assistants and Hygienists* provides the student with a clear link between theory and practice. Straightforward and well balanced, *Essentials of Dental Radiography for Dental Assistants and Hygienists* provides in-depth, comprehensive information that is appropriate for an introductory course in dental radiography, without overwhelming the student with nonessential information. It is comprehensive to prepare students for board and licensing examinations and, at the same time, practical, with practice points, procedure boxes, and suggested lab activities that prepare students to apply theory to clinical practice and patient management.

True to its title, *Essentials of Dental Radiography for Dental Assistants and Hygienists* clearly demonstrates its ability to explain concepts that both dental assistants and dental hygienists must know. The examples and case studies used throughout the book include situations that pertain to the roles of both dental assistants and dental hygienists as members of the oral health care team.

Essentials of Dental Radiography for Dental Assistants and Hygienists is student-friendly, beginning each chapter with learning objectives from both the knowledge and the application levels. Each objective is tested by study questions presented at the end of the chapter, allowing the student to assess learning outcomes. The objectives and study questions are written in the same order that the material appears in the chapter, guiding the student through assimilation of the chapter content. Key words are listed at the beginning of each chapter and bolded within the text with their definitions, and realistic rationales for learning the material are presented in each chapter introduction. The chapter outline provides a ready reference to locate the topics covered. Meaningful case studies relate directly to radiological applications presented in the chapter and challenge students to apply the knowledge learned in the reading to real-life situations through decision-making activities.

The thirty chapters of the ninth edition are organized into nine topic sections.

- Historical Perspective and Radiation Basics
- Biological Effects of Radiation and Radiation Protection
- Dental X-ray Image Receptors and Processing Techniques
- Dental Radiographer Fundamentals
- Intraoral Techniques
- Radiographic Errors and Quality Assurance
- Mounting and Viewing Dental Radiographs
- Patient Management and Supplemental Techniques
- Extraoral Techniques

Educators can easily utilize the chapters and topic sections in any order and have the option to tailor what material is covered in their courses. The sequencing of material for presentation in this text begins with the basics of radiation physics, biological effects, and protection to give the student the necessary background to operate safely, followed by a description of the radiographic equipment, film and film processing, and digital image receptors to help the student understand how radiation is utilized for diagnostic purposes. Prior to learning radiographic techniques, the student will study the fundamentals of infection control, legal and ethical responsibilities, and patient relations. The student will then be prepared to begin to practice the intraoral technique skills necessary to produce diagnostic-quality periapical, bitewing, and occlusal radiographs and learn to mount, evaluate, and interpret the images. Following the interpretation chapters, the student will now possess the basic skills of intraoral radiography and is ready to grasp supplemental techniques and alterations of these basic skills by studying management of special patients and extraoral and panoramic techniques.

Changes made to this ninth edition represent educators' requests for an up-to-date book that speaks to both dental assisting and dental hygiene students, provides comprehensive information without overwhelming the student with nonessential details, and is student centered. Outstanding features of this edition include the following:

- Integration of digital imaging where appropriate throughout the text. Film-based imaging is an established standard of care, and licensing board examinations continue to require oral health care professionals to demonstrate a working knowledge of the use of film-based radiography. However, digital imaging has become an integral part of oral health care practice. For this reason, the all-encompassing term *image receptor* is used to allow educators the option to teach the use of film, solid-state digital sensors, or photostimuable phosphor plate technology. Additionally the chapter on digital imaging has been moved from the section on supplemental techniques to a position earlier in the book to assist with integration of this technology as the student learns the basics of radiography.

- The paralleling and bisecting techniques have been separated into their own chapters to provide distinct lessons for the student. Teaching strategies suggest that introducing two similar, but difficult, concepts together may impede learning either technique well. Placing these two important radiographic techniques into their own chapters will allow the educator to assign one or the other in any order and at distinctly different times in the curriculum.

- The addition of the chapter on safety and environmental responsibilities in radiography is in response to the awareness of the ecological impact of oral health practice today. Students should be trained in the safe handling and environmentally sound disposal of potentially hazardous materials and chemicals used in radiography.

- Update on extraoral radiography and alternate imaging modalities. It is beyond the scope of this book to teach extraoral maxillofacial imaging to competency, and many oral health care professionals who may be called on to utilize these techniques will most likely require additional training. Therefore, the information on the seven common techniques was condensed to key points and placed into a table that enhances learning without overwhelming the student. This chapter now builds on the students' knowledge of digital imaging with an introduction to cone beam computed tomography (CBCT), purported to become the standard of care for periodontal implant assessment in the future.

- Each chapter was critically evaluated to update material, add new study questions, redraw complex illustrations, and include new images, all to enhance student comprehension.

- Each of the 30 chapters in the ninth edition continues to provide Procedure Boxes, which highlight and simplify critical steps of radiographic procedures and serve as a handy reference when providing radiographic services in a clinical setting; Practice Points, which call student attention to possible use of theory in real-life situations, providing a "mental break" from studying theory by illustrating how that theory is applied; and Case Studies and activities for possible lab exercises, research outside class time, essay writing, and investigation using the Internet.

The focus of the ninth edition of *Essentials of Dental Radiography for Dental Assistants and Hygienists* is on the individual responsibility of the oral radiographer and conveys to the reader the importance of understanding what ionizing radiation is and what it is not; protecting oneself, the patient, and the oral health care team from unnecessary radiation exposure; practicing within the scope of the law and ethically treating all patients; producing diagnostic-quality radiographs and appropriately correcting errors that diminish radiographic quality; knowing when and how to apply supplemental techniques; and assisting in the interpretation of radiographs for the benefit of the patient.

Whereas *Essentials of Dental Radiography for Dental Assistants and Hygienists* is written primarily for dental assisting and dental hygiene students, practicing dental assistants, dental hygienists, and dentists may also find this book to be a helpful reference, particularly when preparing for a relicensing examination in another jurisdiction. Additionally, *Essentials of Dental Radiography for Dental Assistants and Hygienists* may be a valuable study guide for on-the-job-trained oral health care professionals who may be seeking radiation safety certification credentials.

Acknowledgments

Thank you to Dr. Orlen Johnson for his continued confidence in allowing me to coauthor this ninth edition of *Essentials of Dental Radiography for Dental Assistants and Hygienists.* It is a privilege to be associated with a textbook with this long-standing history. Thank you to everyone at Pearson for their guidance and patience. I particularly want to express appreciation to Mark Cohen, editor-in-chief, who 14 years ago guided my first efforts at textbook writing; Melissa Kerian, associate editor, who has worked patiently with me on several book editions now; and John Goucher, executive editor, who has kindly encouraged me and listened to my ideas. The quality of this edition is the direct result of the assistance and support of the students, faculty, and staff at the Gene W. Hirschfeld School of Dental Hygiene at Old Dominion University, Norfolk, Virginia. I would like to express my special appreciation to the class of 2011 for helping me to remember why I so enjoy teaching oral radiology.

Evie Thomson

Reviewers

Roberta Albano, CDA, RDH
Springfield Technical College
Springfield, Massachusetts

Dr. Robert Bennett
Texas State Technical College
Harlingen, Texas

Joanna Campbell, RDH, MA
Bergen Community College
Paramus, New Jersey

Armine Leila Derdiarian, DDS
Oxnard College
Oxnard, California

Barbara R. Ellis, RDH, MA
Monroe Community College
Rochester, New York

Mary Emmons, RDH, MSEd
Parkland College
Champaign, Illinois

Joy L. Evans, RDA, EFDA, BS
IntelliTec College
Grand Junction, Colorado

Ann Gallerie, AAS, RDA
Hudson Valley Community College
Troy, New York

Carol Anne Giaquinto, CDA, RDH, MEd
Springfield Technical College
Springfield, Massachusetts

Martha L McCaslin, MA
Dona Ana Community College
Las Cruces, New Mexico

Frances McConaughy RDH, MS
Weber State University
Ogden, Utah

Jean Magee, RDH, Med
NHTI Community College
Concord, New Hampshire

Jennifer Meyer, RDH, BSDH
Southern Illinois University
Carbondale, Illinois

Ann Prey RDH, MS
Milwaukee Area Technical College
Milwaukee, Wisconsin

Judith E. Romano, RDH, MA
Hudson Valley Community College
Troy, New York

Jennifer S. Sherry, RDH
Southern Illinois University
Carbondale, Illinois

Jane H. Slach BA
Kirkwood Community College
Cedar Rapids, Iowa

Gail Renee St. Pierre-Piper, RDH, MA
Iowa Central Community College
Fort Dodge, Iowa

Desiree Sutphen, BA
Volunteer State Community College
Gallatin, Tennessee

Victoria Viera CDA, RDA
Missouri College
Saint Louis, Missouri

Darlene Walsh, RDH, EdM
State University of New York—Orange
Middletown, New York

Janice M. Williams, BSDH, MS
Tennessee State University
Nashville, Tennessee

Essentials of Dental Radiography

for Dental Assistants and Hygienists

History of Dental Radiography

OBJECTIVES

Following successful completion of this chapter, you should be able to:

1. Define the key words.
2. State when x-rays were discovered and by whom.
3. Trace the history of radiography, noting the prominent contributors.
4. List two historical developments that made dental x-ray machines safer.
5. Explain how rectangular PIDs reduce patient radiation exposure.
6. Identify the two techniques used to expose dental radiographs.
7. List five uses of dental radiographs.
8. Become aware of other imaging modalities available for use in the detection and evaluation of oral conditions.

KEY WORDS

Bisecting technique
Computed tomography (CT)
Cone
Cone beam computed tomography (CBCT)
Cone beam volumetric imaging (CBVI)
Digital imaging
Dosage
Oral radiography
Panoramic radiography
Paralleling technique

Position indicating device (PID)
Radiograph
Radiography
Radiology
Roentgen ray
Roentgenograph
Sensor
Tomography
X-ray
X-ray film

Introduction

Technological advancements continue to affect the way we deliver oral health care. Although new methods for diagnosing disease and treatment planning comprehensive care have been introduced, dental radiographs, the images produced by x-rays, remain the basis for many diagnostic procedures and play an essential role in oral health care. **Radiography** is the making of radiographs by exposing an image receptor, either film or digital sensor. The purpose of dental radiography is to provide the oral health care team with radiographic images of the best possible diagnostic quality. The goal of dental radiography is to obtain the highest quality radiographs while maintaining the lowest possible radiation exposure risk for the patient.

Dental assistants and dental hygienists meet an important need through their ability to produce diagnostic quality radiographs. The basis for development of the skills needed to expose, process, mount, and evaluate radiographic images is a thorough understanding of radiology concepts. All individuals working with radiographic equipment should be educated and trained in the theory of x-ray production. The concepts and theories regarding x-ray production that emerged during the early days of x-radiation discovery are responsible for the quality health care available today. The purpose of this chapter is to present a historical perspective that recognizes the contributions of the early scientists and researchers who supplied us with the fundamentals on which we practice today and advance toward the future.

Discovery of the X-ray

Oral **radiology** is the study of x-rays and the techniques used to produce radiographic images. We begin that study with the history of dental radiography and the discovery of the x-ray. The x-ray revolutionized the methods of practicing medicine and dentistry by making it possible to visualize internal body structures noninvasively. Professor Wilhelm Conrad Roentgen's (pronounced "rent'gun"; Figure 1-1) experiment in Bavaria (Germany) on November 8, 1895, produced a tremendous advance in science. Professor Roentgen's curiosity was aroused during an experiment with a vacuum tube called a Crookes tube (named after William Crookes, an English chemist). Roentgen observed that a fluorescent screen near the tube began to glow when the tube was activated by passing an electric current through it. Examining this strange phenomenon further, he noticed that shadows could be cast on the screen by interposing objects between it and the tube. Further experimentation showed that such shadow images could be permanently recorded on photographic film (Figure 1-2). For his work, Dr. Roentgen was awarded the first Nobel Prize for physics in 1901.

In the beginning, Roentgen was uncertain of the nature of this invisible ray that he had discovered. When he later reported his finding at a scientific meeting, he spoke of it as an **x-ray** because the symbol x represented the unknown. After his findings were reported and published, fellow scientists honored him by calling the invisible ray the **roentgen ray** and the image produced on photosensitive film a **roentgenograph**. Because a photographic negative and an x-ray film have basic similarity and

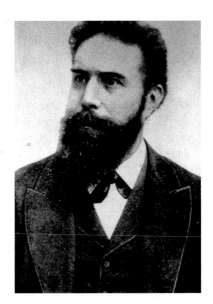

FIGURE 1-1 Wilhelm Conrad Roentgen (1845–1923). (Reprinted with permission from Radiology Centennial, Inc., Copyright 1993)

the x-ray closely resembles the radio wave, the prefix *radio-* and the suffix *-graph* have been combined into **radiograph.** The latter term is used by oral health care professionals because it is more descriptive than x-ray and easier to pronounce than roentgenograph.

Important Scientists and Researchers

A few weeks after Professor Roentgen announced his discovery, Dr. Otto Walkhoff, a German physicist, was the first to expose a prototype of a dental radiograph. This was accomplished by covering a small, glass photographic plate with

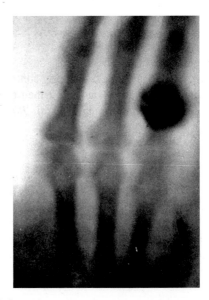

FIGURE 1-2 This famous radiograph, purported to be Mrs. Bertha Roentgen's hand, was taken on December 22, 1895. (Reprinted with permission from Radiology Centennial, Inc., Copyright 1993)

black paper to protect it from light and then wrapping it in a sheath of thin rubber to prevent moisture damage during the 25 minutes that he held the film in his mouth. A similar exposure can now be made in 1/10th of a second. The resulting radiograph was experimental and had little diagnostic value because it was impossible to prevent film movement, but it did prove that the x-ray would have a role in dentistry. The length of the exposure made the experiment a dangerous one for Dr. Walkhoff. The dangers of overexposure to radiation were not known at that time.

We will probably never know who made the first dental radiograph in the United States. It was either Dr. William Herbert Rollins, a Boston dentist and physician, Dr. William James Morton, a New York physician, or Dr. C. Edmund Kells, a New Orleans dentist. Dr. Rollins was one of the first to alert the profession to the need for radiation hygiene and protection and is considered by many to be the first advocate for the science of radiation protection. Unfortunately, his advice was not taken seriously by many of his fellow practitioners for a long time.

Dr. Morton is known to have taken radiographs on skulls very early. He gave a lecture on April 24, 1896, before the New York Odontological Society calling attention to the possible usefulness of roentgen rays in dental practice. One of Dr. Morton's radiographs revealed an impacted tooth, which was otherwise undetectable clinically.

Most people claim Dr. Kells took the first dental radiograph on a living subject in the United States. He was the first to put the radiograph to practical use in dentistry. Dr. Kells made numerous presentations to organized dental groups and was instrumental in convincing many dentists that they should use **oral radiography** as a diagnostic tool. At that time, it was customary to send the patient to a hospital or physician's office on those rare occasions when dental radiographs were prescribed.

Two other dental x-ray pioneers who should be mentioned are William David Coolidge and Howard Riley Raper. The most significant advancement in radiology came in 1913 when Dr. Coolidge, working for the General Electric Company, introduced the hot cathode tube. The x-ray output of the Coolidge tube could be predetermined and accurately controlled. Professor Raper, at Indiana Dental College, wrote the first dental radiology textbook, *Elementary and Dental Radiology,* and introduced bitewing radiographs in 1925.

Because x-rays are invisible, scientists and researchers working in the field of radiography were not aware that continued exposure produced accumulations of radiation effects in the body and, therefore, could be dangerous to both patient and radiographer. When radiography was in its infancy, it was common practice for the dentist or dental assistant to help the patient hold the film in place while making the exposure. These oral health care professionals were exposed to unnecessary radiation. Frequent repetition of this practice endangered their health and occasionally led to permanent injury or death. Fortunately, although the hazards of prolonged exposure to radiation are not completely understood, scientists have learned how to reduce them drastically by proper use of fast film and digital sensors, safer x-ray machines, and strict adherence to safety protocol.

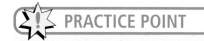

PRACTICE POINT

Never hold the film packet or digital sensor in the patient's oral cavity during the exposure. If the patient cannot tolerate placement of the image receptor or hold still throughout the exposure, the patient's parent or guardian may have to assist or an extraoral radiograph may have to be substituted. The parent or guardian should be protected with lead or lead equivalent barriers such as an apron or gloves when they will be in the path of the beam.

Today, it can be assumed that every dental office in the United States that offers comprehensive oral health care to patients will have x-ray equipment. It is worth noting that initially few hospitals and only the most progressive physicians and dentists possessed x-ray equipment. This limited use of dental radiography can be attributed to the fact that the early equipment was primitive and sometimes dangerous. Also, x-rays were used for entertainment purposes by charlatans at fairgrounds, so people often associated them with quackery. Resistance to change, ignorance, apathy, and fear delayed the widespread acceptance of radiography in dentistry for years.

Table 1-1 lists noteworthy scientists and researchers and their contributions to dental radiology.

Dental X-ray Machines

Dental x-ray machines manufactured before 1920 were an electrical hazard to oral health care professionals because of the open, uninsulated high-voltage supply wires. In 1919, William David Coolidge and General Electric introduced the Victor CDX shockproof dental x-ray machine. The x-ray tube and high-voltage transformer were placed in an oil-filled compartment that acted as a radiation shield and electrical insulator. Modern x-ray machines use this same basic construction. Variable, high-kilovoltage machines were introduced in the middle 1950s, allowing increased target–image receptor distances to be used, which in turn increased the use of the paralleling technique.

Within the last 30 years, major progress has been made in restricting the size of the x-ray beam. One such development is the replacement of the pointed **cone** through which x-rays pass from the tube head toward the patient by open cylinders. When the pointed cones were first used, it was not realized that the x-rays were scattered through contact with the material of the cones. Because cones were used for so many years, many still refer to the open cylinders or rectangular tubes as cones. The term **position indicating device (PID)** is more descriptive of its function of directing the x-rays, rather than of its shape. A further improvement has been the introduction of rectangular

TABLE 1-1	Noteworthy Scientists and Researchers in Dental Radiography	
NAME	EVENT	YEAR
W. C. Roentgen	Discovered x-rays	1895
C. E. Kells	May have taken first dental radiograph in U.S.	1896
W. J. Morton	May have taken first dental radiograph in U.S.	1896
W. H. Rollins	May have taken first dental radiograph in U.S.	1896
	Published "X Light Kills," warning of x-ray dangers	1901
O. Walkhoff	First to make a dental radiograph	1896
W. A. Price	Suggested basics for both bisecting and paralleling techniques	1904
A. Cieszynski	Applied "rule of isometry" to bisecting technique	1907
W. D. Coolidge	Introduced the hot cathode tube	1913
H. R. Raper	Wrote first dental x-ray textbook	1913
	Introduced bitewing radiographs	1924
F. W. McCormack	Developed paralleling technique	1920
G. M. Fitzgerald	Designed a "long-cone" to use with the paralleling technique	1947
Francis Mouyen	Developed the first digital imaging system called RadioVisioGraphy	1987

lead-lined PIDs. This shape limits the size of the x-ray beam that strikes the patient to the actual size of the image receptor (Figure 1-3).

Panoramic radiography became popular in the 1960s with the introduction of the panoramic x-ray machine. Panoramic units are capable of exposing the entire dentition and surrounding structures on a single image. Today, many oral health care practices have a panoramic x-ray machine.

As **digital imaging** continues to develop, exciting advances in the development of imaging systems that allow for enhanced two- and three-dimensional images are being used in the diagnosis and treatment of dental conditions, particularly implant evaluation and orthodontic interventions. Medical imaging modalities such as **tomography** and **computed tomography (CT scans)**, a method of imaging a single selected plane of tissues has been used to assist dentists with complex diagnosis and treatment planning since the early 1970s. Because these medical imaging modalities deliver high radiation doses, sometimes up to 600 times more than a panoramic radiograph, the development of **cone beam volumetric imaging (CBVI)** or **cone beam computed tomography (CBCT)** with lower radiation doses (4 to 15 times that required for a panoramic radiograph) for dental application is purported to become the gold standard of diagnosis for certain dental applications in the very near future.

Dental X-ray Film

Although today it is increasingly common to see paperless dental practices equipped with computers and image receptors that allow for the digital capture of radiographic images, film has been the standard for producing dental radiographs since 1896. Early dental **x-ray film** packets consisted of glass photographic plates wrapped in black paper and rubber. In 1913, the Eastman Kodak Company marketed the first hand-wrapped, moisture-proof dental x-ray film packet. It was not until 1919 that the first machine-wrapped dental x-ray film packet became commercially available (also from Kodak).

Early film had emulsion on only one side and required long exposure times. Today, both sides of the dental x-ray film are coated with emulsion and require only about 1/16th the amount of exposure required 50 years ago.

Digital Image Receptors

Digital imaging systems (see Chapter 9) replace film as the image receptor with a **sensor**. In 1987, Francis Mouyen, a French dentist, introduced the use of a digital radiography

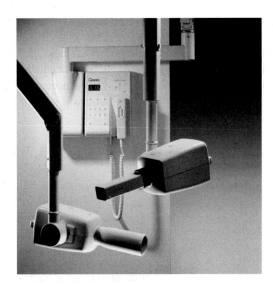

FIGURE 1-3 Comparison of circular and rectangular PIDs.
(Image courtesy of Gendex Dental Corporation)

system marketed for dental imaging, called RadioVisioGraphy. The first digital sensor was bulky and had limitations. Since that time image sensors have been improved and are now comparable to film in dimensions of the exposed field of view and approach film in overall radiographic quality. Their advantages include a reduction in radiation **dosage**, the elimination of film and processing chemistry, and the subsequent disposal of film packaging materials such as lead foils and spent processing chemicals, both potentially hazardous to the environment.

Dental X-ray Techniques

Two basic techniques are used in intraoral radiography. The first and earliest technique is called the **bisecting technique**. The second and newer technique is referred to as the **paralleling technique**. The paralleling method is the technique of choice and is taught in all dental assisting, dental hygiene, and dental schools.

In 1904, Dr. Weston A. Price suggested the basics of both the bisecting and paralleling techniques. As others were working on the same problems and were unaware of Price's contributions, the credit for developing the techniques went to others.

In 1907, A. Cieszynski, a Polish engineer, applied the *rule of isometry* to dental radiology and is credited for suggesting the bisecting technique. The bisecting technique was the only method used for many years.

The search for a less-complicated technique that would produce better radiographs more consistently resulted in the development of the paralleling technique by Dr. Franklin McCormack in 1920. Dr. G. M. Fitzgerald, Dr. McCormack's son-in-law, designed a long "cone" PID and made the paralleling technique more practical in 1947.

Advances in Dental Radiographic Imaging

Radiography, aided by the introduction first of transistors and then computers, has allowed for significant radiation reduction in modern x-ray machines. Advances in two-dimensional and three-dimension imaging systems are predicted to move radiography away from static interpretation of pictures of images and toward representations of real-life conditions. This introduction of a computed approach with its almost instantaneous images is sure to benefit the quality of oral health care.

Today, an oral health care practice would find it impossible to provide patients with comprehensive dental care without dental radiographs (Figure 1-4). Many practices have multiple intraoral dental x-ray machines (one in each operatory) and supplement these with a panoramic x-ray machine. Although no diagnosis can be based solely on radiographic evidence without a visual and physical examination, many conditions might go undetected if not for radiographic examinations (Box 1-1).

The discovery of x-radiation revolutionized the practice of preventive oral health care. Future technological advances undoubtedly will improve both the diagnostic use and the safety of radiography in the years ahead.

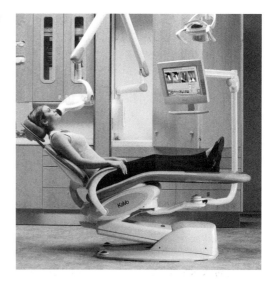

FIGURE 1-4 Radiography in a modern oral health care practice. (Image courtesy of Gendex Dental Corporation)

BOX 1-1   Uses of Dental Radiographs

- To detect, confirm, and classify oral diseases and lesions
- To detect and evaluate trauma
- To evaluate growth and development
- To detect missing and supernumerary (extra) teeth
- To document the oral condition of a patient
- To educate patients about their oral health

REVIEW—Chapter summary

Professor Wilhelm Conrad Roentgen's discovery of the x-ray on November 8, 1895, revolutionized the methods of practicing medicine and dentistry by making it possible to visualize internal body structures noninvasively. The usefulness of the x-ray as a diagnostic tool was recognized almost immediately as scientists and researchers contributed to its advancement. The use of radiographs in medical and dental diagnostic procedures is now essential.

In the early 1900s, scientists and researchers working in the field of radiography were not aware that radiation could be dangerous, resulting in exposure to unnecessary radiation. Early x-ray equipment was primitive and sometimes dangerous. Today improved equipment, advanced techniques, and educated personnel make it possible to obtain radiographs with high diagnostic value and minimal risk of unnecessary radiation to patient or operator.

Although film has been the standard image receptor since the discovery of the x-ray, dental practices continue to adopt the computer and digital sensor as the method of acquiring a dental radiographic image. Digital imaging reduces patient radiation dose, eliminates the need to maintain an inventory of film and processing chemistry, and avoids disposal of the potentially environmental hazards of lead foils and spent processing chemicals.

The two basic techniques for acquiring a dental radiographic image are the bisecting technique and the paralleling technique.

Cone beam volumetric or computed tomography (CBVT or CBCT) produces two- and three-dimension images for dental diagnosis. This technology may become the gold standard for diagnosing certain dental conditions.

RECALL—Study questions

For questions 1–5, match each term with its definition.

    a. Radiograph
    b. Radiography
    c. Radiology
    d. Roentgen ray
    e. X-ray

    _____ **1.** The study of x-radiation

    _____ **2.** Image or picture produced by x-rays

    _____ **3.** An older term given to x-radiation in honor of its discoverer

    _____ **4.** The original term Roentgen applied to the invisible ray he discovered

    _____ **5.** The making of radiographs by exposing and processing x-ray film

6. Who discovered the x-ray?
    a. C. Edmund Kells
    b. William Rollins
    c. Franklin McCormack
    d. Wilhelm Conrad Roentgen

7. When were x-rays discovered?
    a. 1695
    b. 1795
    c. 1895
    d. 1995

8. Who is believed to have exposed the prototype of the first dental x-ray film?
    a. A. Cieszynski
    b. Otto Walkhoff
    c. Wilhelm Conrad Roentgen
    d. C. Edmund Kells

9. Who is considered by many to be the first advocate for the science of radiation protection?
    a. Weston Price
    b. William Morton
    c. William Herbert Rollins
    d. Franklin McCormack

10. Replacing the pointed "cone" position indicating device (PID) with an open-cylinder PID reduced the radiation dose to the patient *because* open-cylinder PIDs eliminate scattered x-rays through contact with the cone material.
    a. Both the statement and reason are correct and related.
    b. Both the statement and reason are correct but NOT related.
    c. The statement is correct, but the reason is NOT.
    d. The statement is NOT correct, but the reason is correct.
    e. NEITHER the statement NOR the reason is correct.

11. Which imaging modality will most likely become the gold standard for imaging certain dental conditions in the near future?
    a. Cone beam volumetric tomography
    b. Computed tomography
    c. Digital imaging
    d. Tomography

12. Who is given credit for applying the rule of isometry to the bisecting technique?
    a. William Rollins
    b. A. Cieszynski
    c. G. M. Fitzgerald
    d. Otto Walkhoff

13. Who is given credit for developing the paralleling technique?
    a. W. D. Coolidge
    b. H. R. Raper
    c. William Morton
    d. Franklin McCormack

14. List five uses of dental radiographs.
    a. _____
    b. _____
    c. _____
    d. _____
    e. _____

REFLECT—Case study

Your patient today tells you that she recently watched a television documentary on the dangers of excess radiation exposure. Based on your reading in this chapter, develop a brief conversation between you and this patient explaining how historical developments have increased dental radiation safety to put the patient at ease.

RELATE—Laboratory application

Perform an inventory of the x-ray machine used in your facility. Using the historical lessons learned in this chapter, identify the parts of the x-ray machine, type of film or digital sensor used, and the safety protocol and posted exposure factors in place. Specifically list the following:

a. Unit manufacturer

Using the Internet, research the manufacturer's Web site to determine the company origin. How old is the company? Are they a descendant of an original manufacturer? Who developed the design for the x-ray unit produced today? Do they offer different unit designs? What is the reason your facility chose this model?

b. Shape and length of the PID

Does the machine you are observing reduce radiation exposure? Why or why not? Why was the PID you are observing chosen over other shapes and lengths?

c. Names of the dials on the control panel.

How does this differ from the dental x-ray machines used in dental practices in the early 1900s? What exposure factors are inherent to the unit, and what factors may be varied by the radiographer? What are the advantages and disadvantages to using an x-ray machine where the exposure settings are fixed? Variable?

d. What are the recommended exposure settings for various types of radiographs? How do these differ from the settings used by the first dentists to use x-rays in practice in the early 1900s?

e. Describe the film or digital sensor used to produce a radiographic image.

What is the film size and speed, and how is it packaged? Does the film or sensor used in your facility allow you to produce a quality radiograph using the least amount of radiation possible? What is the rationale for using this film type in your facility?

f. Are the safety protocols regarding x-ray machine operation known to all operators? How is this made evident? List the safety protocols in place in your facility.

REFERENCES

Carestream Health, Inc. (2007). *Kodak dental systems: Radiation safety in dental radiography.* Pub. N-414, Rochester, NY: Author.

Horner, K., Drage, N., & Brettle, D. (2008). *21st century imaging.* London: Quintessence Publishing.

Langland, O. E., Langlais, R. P., & Preece, J. W. (2002). *Principles of Dental Imaging* (2nd ed.). Philadelphia: Williams & Wilkins.

Miles, D. A. (2008). *Color atlas of cone beam volumetric imaging for dental applications.* Chicago: Quintessence Publishing.

Scarfe, W. C., Farnam, A. G., & Sukovic, P. (2006). Clinical applications of cone-beam computed tomography in dental practice. *Journal of the Canadian Dental Association, 72,1.*

White, S. C., & Pharoah, M. J. (2008). *Oral radiology. Principles and interpretation* (6th ed.). St. Louis: Elsevier.

Characteristics and Measurement of Radiation

CHAPTER OUTLINE

OBJECTIVES

Following successful completion of this chapter, you should be able to:

1. Define the key words.

2. Draw and label a typical atom.

3. Describe the process of ionization.

4. Differentiate between radiation and radioactivity.

5. List the properties shared by all energies of the electromagnetic spectrum.

6. Explain the relationship between wavelength and frequency.

7. Explain the inverse relationship between wavelength and penetrating power of x-rays.

8. List the properties of x-rays.

9. Identify and describe the two processes by which kinetic energy is converted to electromagnetic energy within the dental x-ray tube.

10. List and describe the four possible interactions of dental x-rays with matter.

11. Define the terms used to measure x-radiation.

12. Match the Système Internationale (SI) units of x-radiation measurement to the corresponding traditional terms.

13. Identify three sources of naturally occurring background radiation.

KEY WORDS

Absorbed dose

Absorption

Alpha particle

Angstrom (Å)

Atom

Atomic number

Atomic weight

Background radiation

Beta particle

Binding energy

Characteristic radiation

Coherent scattering

Compton effect (scattering)

Coulombs per kilogram (C/kg)

Decay

Dose	Hard radiation	Rad
Dose equivalent	Ion	Radiation
Effective dose equivalent	Ion pair	Radioactivity
Electromagnetic radiation	Ionization	Radiolucent
Electromagnetic spectrum	Ionizing radiation	Radiopaque
Electron	Isotope	Rem
Element	Kinetic energy	Roentgen (R)
Energy	Microsievert (µSv)	Secondary radiation
Energy levels	Molecule	Sievert (Sv)
Exposure	Neutron	Soft radiation
Frequency	Particulate radiation	Système Internationale (SI)
Gamma rays	Photoelectric effect	Velocity
General/bremsstrahlung radiation	Photon	Wavelength
Gray (Gy)	Proton	Weighting factor

Introduction

The word *radiation* is attention grabbing. When news head-lines incorporate words such as *radiation, radio-activity,* and *exposure,* the reader pays attention to what follows. Patients often link dental x-rays with other types of radiation exposure they read about or see on TV. Patients assume that oral health care professionals who are responsible for taking dental x-rays are knowledgeable regarding all types of ionizing radiation exposures and can adequately answer their questions. Although the study of quantum physics is beyond the scope of this book, it is important that dental assistants and dental hygienists understand what dental radiation is, what it can do, and what it cannot do. In this chapter we will explore the characteristics of x-radiation and look at where dental x-rays fit in relation to other types and sources of radiations.

Prior to studying the production of x-rays, the radiographer should have a base knowledge of atomic structure. The scientist understands that the world consists of matter and energy. Matter is defined as anything that occupies space and has mass. Things that we see and recognize are forms of matter. **Energy** is defined as the ability to do work and overcome resistance. Heat, light, electricity, and x-radiation are forms of energy. Matter and energy are closely related. Energy is produced whenever the state of matter is altered by natural or artificial means. The difference between water, steam, and ice is the amount of energy associated with the molecules. Such an energy exchange is produced within the x-ray machine and will be discussed later.

Atomic Structure

To understand radiation, we must understand atomic structure. Currently we know of 118 basic **elements** that occur either singly or in combination in natural forms. Each element is made up of atoms. An **atom** is the smallest particle of an element that still retains the properties of the element. If any given atom is split, the resulting components no longer retain the properties of the element. Atoms are generally combined with other atoms to form molecules. A **molecule** is the smallest particle of a substance that retains the properties of that substance. A simple molecule such as sodium chloride (table salt) contains only two atoms, whereas a complex molecule like DNA (deoxyribonucleic acid) may contain hundreds of atoms.

Atoms are extremely minute and are composed of three basic building blocks: electrons, protons, and neutrons.

- **Electrons** have a negative charge and are constantly in motion orbiting the nucleus.
- **Protons** have a postitive charge. The number of protons in the nucleus of an element determines its **atomic number.**
- **Neutrons** have no charge.

The atom's arrangement in some ways resembles the solar system (Figure 2-1). The atom has a nucleus as its center or sun, and the electrons revolve around it like planets. The protons and neutrons form the central core or nucleus of the atom. The electrons orbit around the nucleus in paths called shells or energy levels. Normally, the atom is electrically neutral, having equal numbers of protons in its nucleus and electrons in orbit.

The nucleus of all atoms except hydrogen contains at least one proton and one neutron (hydrogen in its simplest form has only a proton). Some atoms contain a very high number of each. The electrons and the nucleus normally remain in the same position relative to one another. To accommodate the electrons revolving about the nucleus, the larger atoms have several concentric orbits at various distances from the nucleus. These are referred to as electron shells, which some chemists call **energy levels.** The innermost level is referred to as the K shell, the next as the L shell, and so on, up to 7 shells (Figure 2-1).

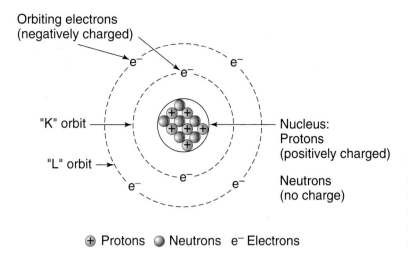

Orbiting electrons
(negatively charged)

"K" orbit

"L" orbit

Nucleus:
Protons
(positively charged)

Neutrons
(no charge)

⊕ Protons ◯ Neutrons e⁻ Electrons

FIGURE 2-1 **Diagram of carbon atom.** In the neutral atom, the number of positively charged protons in the nucleus is equal to the number of negatively charged orbiting electrons. The innermost orbit or energy level is the K shell, the next is the L shell, and so on.

Electrons are maintained in their orbits by the positive attraction of the protons, known as **binding energy.** The binding energy of an electron is strongest in the intermost K shell and becomes weaker in the outer shells.

Ionization

Atoms that have gained or lost electrons are electrically unstable and are called ions. An **ion** is defined as a charged particle. The formation of ions is easier to understand if we review the normal structural arrangement of the atom. The atom normally has the same number of protons (positive charges) in the nucleus as it has electrons (negative charges) in the orbital levels. When one of these electrons is removed from its orbital level in a neutral atom, the remainder of the atom loses its electrical neutrality.

An atom from which an electron has been removed has more protons than electrons, is positively charged, and is called a positive ion. The negatively charged electron that has been separated from the atom is a negative ion. The positively charged atom ion and the negatively charged electron ion are called an **ion pair. Ionization** is the formation of ion pairs. When an atom is struck by an x-ray photon, an electron may be dislodged and an ion pair created (Figure 2-2). As high-energy electrons travel on, they push out (like charges repel) electrons from the orbits of other atoms, creating additional ion pairs. These unstable ions attempt to regain electrical stability by combining with another oppositely charged ion.

Ionizing Radiation

Radiation is defined as the emission and movement of **energy** through space in the form of electromagnetic radiation (x- and **gamma rays**) or **particulate radiation** (**alpha** and **beta particles**). Any radiation that produces ions is called **ionizing radiation.** Only a portion of the radiation portrayed on the electromagnetic spectrum, the x-rays and the gamma

and cosmic rays, are of the ionizing type. In dental radiography, our concern is limited to the changes that may occur in the cellular structures of the tissues as the ions are produced by the passage of x-rays through the cells. The mechanics of biologic tissue damage are explained in Chapter 5.

Radioactivity

Radioactivity is defined as the process whereby certain unstable elements undergo spontaneous disintegration (decay) in an effort to attain a stable nuclear state. Unstable **isotopes** are radioactive and attempt to regain stability through the release of energy, by a process known as **decay.** Dental x-rays do not involve the use of radioactivity.

Scientists have learned to produce several types of radiations that are identical to natural radiations. Ultraviolet

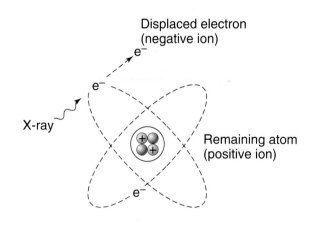

Displaced electron
(negative ion)

X-ray

Remaining atom
(positive ion)

⊕ Protons ◯ Neutrons e⁻ Electrons

FIGURE 2-2 **Ionization is the formation of ion pairs.** When an atom is struck by an x-ray, an electron may be dislodged, and an ion pair results.

waves are produced artificially for sunlamps or fluorescent lights and for numerous other uses. Another man-made radiation is the laser beam, whose potential impact on oral health is still being explored.

Electromagnetic Radiation

Electromagnetic radiation is the movement of wavelike energy through space as a combination of electric and magnetic fields. Electromagnetic radiations are arranged in an orderly fashion according to their energies in what is called the **electromagnetic spectrum** (Figure 2-3). The electromagnetic spectrum consists of an orderly arrangement of all known radiant energies. X-radiation is a part of the electromagnetic spectrum, which also includes cosmic rays, gamma rays, ultraviolet rays, visible light, infrared, television, radar, microwave, and radio waves. All energies of the electromagnetic spectrum share the following properties:

- Travel at the speed of light
- Have no electrical charge
- No weight

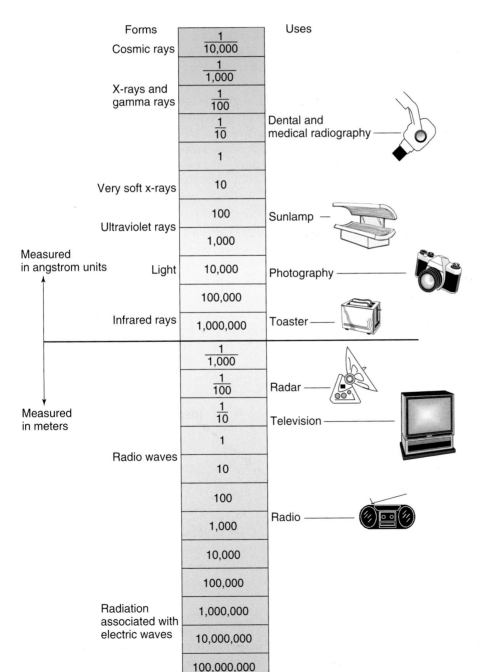

FIGURE 2-3 The electromagnetic spectrum. Electromagnetic radiations are arranged in an orderly fashion according to their energies.

- Have no mass or weight
- Pass through space as particles and in a wavelike motion
- Give off an electrical field at right angles to their path of travel and a magnetic field at right angles to the electric field
- Have energies that are measurable and different

Electromagnetic radiations display two seemingly contradictory properties. They are believed to move through space as both a particle and a wave. Particle or quantum theory assumes the electromagnetic radiations are particles, or quanta. These particles are called photons. **Photons** are bundles of energy that travel through space at the speed of light. Wave theory assumes that electromagnetic radiation is propagated in the form of waves similar to waves resulting from a disturbance in water. Electromagnetic waves exhibit the properties of wavelength, frequency, and velocity.

- **Wavelength** is the distance between two similar points on two successive waves, as illustrated in Figure 2-4. The symbol for wavelength is the Greek letter lambda (λ). Wavelength may be measured in the metric system or in **angstrom (Å)** units (1 Å is about 1/250,000,000 in. or 1/100,000,000 cm). The shorter the wavelength, the more penetrating the radiation.
- **Frequency** is a measure of the number of waves that pass a given point per unit of time. The symbol for frequency is the Greek letter nu (ν). The special unit of frequency is the hertz (Hz). One hertz equals 1 cycle per second. The higher the frequency, the more penetrating the radiation.
- **Velocity** refers to the speed of the wave. In a vacuum, all electromagnetic radiations travel at the speed of light (186,000 miles/sec or 3×10^8 m/sec).

No clear-cut separation exists between the various radiations represented on the electromagnetic spectrum; consequently, overlapping of the wavelengths is common. Each form

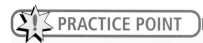

PRACTICE POINT

Wavelength and frequency are inversely related. When the wavelength is long, the frequency is low, resulting in low-energy, less penetrating x-rays (Figure 2-4). When the wavelength is short, the frequency is high, resulting in high-energy, more penetrating x-rays.

of radiation has a range of wavelengths. This accounts for some of the longer infrared waves being measured in meters, whereas the shorter infrared waves are measured in angstrom units. It therefore follows that all x-radiations are not the same wavelength. The longest of these are the Grenz rays, also called **soft radiation,** that have only limited penetrating power and are unsuitable for exposing dental radiographs. The wavelengths used in diagnostic dental radiography range from about 0.1 to 0.5 Å and are classified as **hard radiation,** a term meaning radiation with great penetrating power. Still shorter wavelengths are produced by super-voltage machines when greater penetration is required, as in some forms of medical therapy and industrial radiography.

Properties of X-rays

X-rays are believed to consist of minute bundles (or quanta) of pure electromagnetic energy called photons. These have no mass or weight, are invisible, and cannot be sensed. Because they travel at the speed of light (186,000 miles/sec

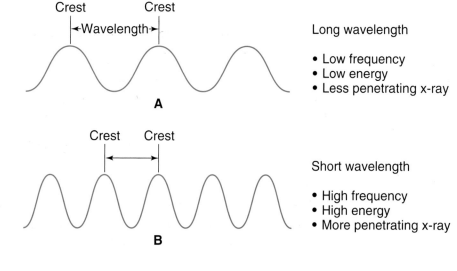

Long wavelength

- Low frequency
- Low energy
- Less penetrating x-ray

Short wavelength

- High frequency
- High energy
- More penetrating x-ray

FIGURE 2-4 Differences in wavelengths and frequencies. Only the shortest wavelengths with extremely high frequency and energy are used to expose dental radiographs Wavelength is determined by the distances between the crests. Observe that this distance is much shorter in (**B**) than in (**A**). The photons that comprise the dental x-ray beam are estimated to have over 250 million such crests per inch. Frequency is the number of crests of a wavelength passing a given point per second.

or 3×10^8 meters/sec), these x-ray photons are often referred to as "bullets of energy." X-rays have the following properties. They

- Are invisible
- Travel in straight lines
- Travel at speed of light
- Have no mass or weight
- Have no charge
- Interact with matter causing ionization
- Can penetrate opaque tissues and structures
- Can affect photographic film emulsion (causing a latent image)
- Can affect biological tissue

X-ray photons have the ability to pass through gases, liquids, and solids. The ability to penetrate materials or tissues depends on the wavelength of the x-ray and the thickness and density of the object. The composition of the object or the tissues determines whether the x-rays will penetrate and pass through it or whether they will be absorbed in it. Materials that are extremely dense and have a high **atomic weight** will absorb more x-rays than thin materials with low atomic numbers. This partially explains why dense structures such as bone and enamel appear **radiopaque** (white or light gray) on the radiograph, whereas the less dense pulp chamber, muscles, and skin appear **radiolucent** (dark gray or black).

Production of X-rays

X-rays are generated inside an x-ray tube located in the tube head of a dental x-ray machine (Chapter 3). X-rays are produced whenever high-speed electrons are abruptly stopped or slowed down. Bodies in motion are believed to have **kinetic energy** (from the Greek word *kineticos*, "pertaining to motion"). In a dental x-ray tube, the kinetic energy of electrons is converted to electromagnetic energy by the formation of general or *bremsstrahlung* radiation (German for "braking") and characteristic radiation.

- **General/bremsstrahlung radiation** is produced when high-speed electrons are stopped or slowed down by the tungsten atoms of the dental x-ray tube. Referring to Figure 2-5, observe that the impact from both (A) and (B) electrons produce general/bremsstrahlung. When a high-speed electron collides with the nucleus of an atom in the target metal, as in (A), all its kinetic energy is transferred into a single x-ray photon. In (B), a high-speed electron is slowed down and bent off its course by the positive pull of the nucleus. The kinetic energy lost is converted into an x-ray. The majority of x-rays produced by dental x-ray machines are formed by general/bremsstrahlung radiation.
- **Characteristic radiation** is produced when a bombarding electron from the tube filament collides with an orbiting K electron of the tungsten target as shown in Figure 2-5 (C). The K-shell electron is dislodged from the atom. Another

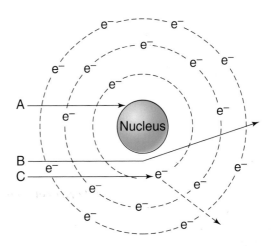

FIGURE 2-5 **General/bremsstrahlung and characteristic radiation.** High-speed electron (**A**) collides with the nucleus, and all its kinetic energy is converted into a single x-ray. High-speed electron (**B**) is slowed down and bent off its course by the positive pull of the nucleus. The kinetic energy lost is converted into an x-ray. The impact from both A and B electrons produce general radiation. Characteristic radiation is produced when a high-speed electron (**C**) hits and dislodges a K shell (orbiting) electron. Another electron in an outer shell quickly fills the void, and x-ray energy is emitted. Characteristic radiation only occurs above 70 kVp with a tungsten target.

electron in an outer shell quickly fills the void, and an x-ray is emitted. The x-rays produced in this manner are called characteristic x-rays. Characteristic radiation can only be produced when the x-ray machine is operated at or above 70 kilovolts (kVp) because a minimum force of 69 kVp is required to dislodge a K electron from a tungsten atom. Characteristic radiation is of minor importance because it accounts for only a very small part of the x-rays produced in a dental x-ray machine.

Interaction of X-rays with Matter

A beam of x-rays passing through matter is weakened and gradually disappears. Such a disappearance is referred to as **absorption** of x-rays. When so defined, absorption does not imply an occurrence such as a sponge soaking up water, but instead refers to the process of transferring the energy of the x-rays to the atoms of the material through which the x-ray beam passes. The basic method of absorption is ionization.

When a beam of x-rays pass through matter, four possibilities exist:

1. **No interaction.** The x-ray can pass through an atom unchanged and no interaction occurs (Figure 2-6).

   - In dental radiography about 9 percent of the x-rays pass through the patient's tissues without interaction.

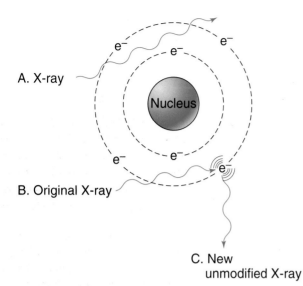

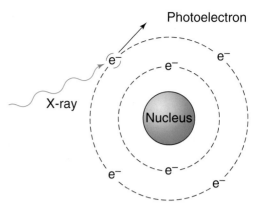

FIGURE 2-7 **Photoelectric effect.** The incoming x-ray gives up all its energy to an orbital electron of the atom. The x-ray is absorbed and simply vanishes. The electromagnetic energy of the x-ray is imparted to the electron in the form of kinetic energy of motion and causes the electron to fly from its orbit, creating an ion pair. The high-speed electron (called a photoelectron) knocks other electrons from the orbits of other atoms forming secondary ion pairs.

FIGURE 2-6 **X-rays interacting with atom.** X-ray (**A**) passes through an atom unchanged and no interaction occurs. Incoming x-ray (**B**) interacts with the electron by causing the electron to vibrate at the same frequency as the incoming x-ray. The incoming x-ray ceases to exist. The vibrating electron radiates new x-ray (**C**) energy with the same frequency and energy as the original incoming x-ray. The new x-ray is scattered in a different direction than the original x-ray.

- Photoelectric effect accounts for about 30 percent of the interactions of matter with the dental x-ray beam.

4. **Compton effect.** The Compton effect (often called Compton scattering) is similar to the photoelectric effect in that the dental x-ray interacts with an orbital electron and ejects it. But in the case of Compton interaction, only a part of the dental x-ray energy is transferred to the electron, and a new, weaker x-ray is formed and scattered in some new direction (Figure 2-8). This **secondary radiation** may travel in a direction opposite that of the original x-ray. The new x-ray may undergo another Compton scattering or it may be

2. **Coherent scattering** (unmodified scattering, also known as Thompson scattering). When a low-energy x-ray passes near an atom's outer electron, it may be scattered without loss of energy (Figure 2-6). The incoming x-ray interacts with the electron by causing the electron to vibrate at the same frequency as the incoming x-ray. The incoming x-ray ceases to exist. The vibrating electron radiates another x-ray of the same frequency and energy as the original incoming x-ray. The new x-ray is scattered in a different direction than the original x-ray. Essentially, the x-ray is scattered unchanged.

- Coherent scattering accounts for about 8 percent of the interactions of matter with the dental x-ray beam.

3. **Photoelectric effect.** The photoelectric effect is an all-or-nothing energy loss. The x-ray imparts all its energy to an orbital electron of some atom. This dental x-ray, because it consisted only of energy in the first place, simply vanishes. The electromagnetic energy of the x-ray is imparted to the electron in the form of kinetic energy of motion and causes the electron to fly from its orbit with considerable speed. Thus, an ion pair is created (Figure 2-7). Remember, the basic method of the interaction of x-rays with matter is the formation of ion pairs. The high-speed electron (called a photoelectron) knocks other electrons from the orbits of other atoms (forming secondary ion pairs) until all its energy is used up. The positive ion atom combines with a free electron, and the absorbing material is restored to its original condition.

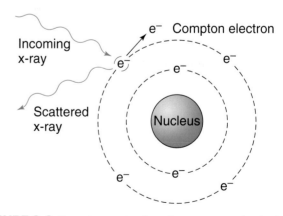

FIGURE 2-8 **Compton scattering.** Compton scattering is similar to the photoelectric effect in that the incoming x-ray interacts with an orbital electron and ejects it. But in the case of Compton interaction, only a part of the x-ray energy is transferred to the electron, and a new, weaker x-ray is formed and scattered in a new direction. The new x-ray may undergo another Compton scattering or it may be absorbed by a photoelectric effect interaction.

absorbed by a photoelectric effect interaction. The positive ion atom combines with a free electron, and the absorbing material is restored to its original condition. It is important to remember that the Compton effect causes x-rays to be scattered in all directions.

- Compton effect accounts for about 60 percent of the interactions of matter with the dental x-ray beam.

A question often asked is, "Do x-rays make the material they pass through radioactive?" The answer is no. Dental x-rays have no effect on the nucleus of the atoms they interact with. Therefore, equipment, walls, and patients do not become radioactive after exposure to x-rays.

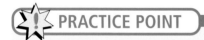 **PRACTICE POINT**

"How long should you wait after exposure before entering the room where the radiation was?"

X-rays travel at the speed of light and cease to exist within a fraction of a second. This question is similar to asking, "How long will it take for the room to get dark after turning off the light switch?"

Units of Radiation

The terms used to measure x-radiation are based on the ability of the x-ray to deposit its energy in air, soft tissues, bone, or other substances. The International Commission on Radiation Units and Measurements (ICRU) has established standards that clearly define radiation units and radiation quantities (Table 2-1). The most widely accepted terms used for radiation units of measurement come from the **Système Internationale (SI),** a modern version of the metric system. The Système Internationale (SI) units are

1. Coulombs per kilogram (C/kg)
2. Gray (Gy)
3. Sievert (Sv)

Older traditional units of radiation measurement are now considered obsolete, although they may be observed in some older documents, especially those dealing with health and safety. The traditional units are

1. Roentgen (R)
2. Rad (radiation absorbed dose)
3. Rem (roentgen equivalent [in] man)

The American Dental Association requires the use of SI terminology on national board examinations, and following the guidelines established by the National Institute of Standards and Technology, this book will use SI units first, followed by the traditional units in parentheses. It is important to note that numerical amounts of radiation expressed using SI terminology do not equal the numerical amounts of radiation expressed using the traditional terms. For example, consider the metric system of measurement adopted by most of the world with the traditional units of measurement used in the United States. Whereas the global community uses the term kilometers to measure distance, in the United States distance is more commonly measured in miles. One kilometer does not equal 1 mile. Instead, 1 kilometer equals approximately 0.62 miles. When comparing measurements of radiation, it is important to remember that SI units and traditional units, although measuring the same thing, are not equal numerically.

A "quantity" may be thought of as a description of a physical concept such as time, distance, or weight. The measure of the quantity is a "unit" such as minutes, miles (kilometers), or pounds (kilograms).

For practical x-ray protection measurement the following are used:

1. Exposure
2. Absorbed dose
3. Dose equivalent
4. Effective dose equivalent

Exposure

Exposure can be defined as the measurement of ionization in air produced by x- or gamma rays. The unit for measuring exposure is **coulombs per kilogram (C/kg) (roentgen (R))**. A coulomb is a unit of electrical charge. Therefore, the unit C/kg measures electrical charges (ion pairs) in a kilogram of air. Coulombs per kilogram (roentgen) only applies to x- or gamma radiation and only measures ion pairs in air. It does not measure the radiation absorbed by tissues or other materials. Therefore, it is not a measurement of **dose.** An exposure does not become a dose until the radiation is absorbed in the tissues.

TABLE 2-1 Radiation Measurement Terminology		
QUANTITY	SYSTÈME INTERNATIONAL (SI) UNIT	TRADITIONAL UNIT
Exposure	coulombs per kilogram (C/kg)	roentgen (R)
Absorbed dose	gray (Gy)	rad
Dose equivalent	sievert (Sv)	rem

Absorbed Dose

Absorbed dose is defined as the amount of energy deposited in any form of matter (such as teeth, soft tissues, treatment chair, and so on), by any type of radiation (alpha or beta particles, gamma or x-rays). The unit for measuring the absorbed dose is the **gray (Gy) (rad).**

One gray equals 1 joule (J; a unit of energy) per kilogram of tissue. One gray equals 100 rads.

Dose Equivalent

Dose equivalent is a term used for radiation protection purposes to compare the biological effects of the various types of radiation. Dose equivalent is defined as the product of the absorbed dose times a biological-effect qualifying or **weighting factor.** Because the weighting factor for x-rays is 1, the absorbed dose and the dose equivalent are numerically equal. The unit for measuring the dose equivalent is the **sievert (Sv) (rem).** One sievert is the product of 1 Gy times a biological-effect weighting factor. Because the weighting factor for x- and gamma radiation equals 1, the number of sieverts is identical to the absorbed dose in grays for these radiations. One sievert equals 100 rem.

In dental radiology, gray (rad) and sievert (rem) are equal, and it should be pointed out that only x-rays and gamma rays are measured in coulombs per kilogram (roentgens). Gray (rad) and sievert (rem) are used to measure all radiations: gamma and x-rays, alpha and beta particles, neutrons, and high-energy protons.

When pertaining to exposures from dental radiation, smaller multiples of these units are commonly used. For example, milligray (mGy), where the prefix *milli* means "one-thousandth of," would more likely be used to express the smaller dose of radiation used in most dental applications.

Effective Dose Equivalent

To aid in making more accurate comparisons between different radiographic exposures, the **effective dose equivalent** is used to compare the risk of the radiation exposure producing a biological response. The effective dose equivalent is expressed using the term **microsievert (μSv),** meaning 1/1,000,000 of a sievert. The effective dose equivalent compensates for the differences in area exposed and the tissues, critical or less critical, that may be in the path of the x-ray beam. For example, comparing the skin dose of a chest x-ray (approximately 0.2 mSv) and a single periapical radiograph (approximately 2.5 mSv) does not take into consideration that the chest x-ray delivers its dose to a larger area and to more tissues than the single periapical radiograph. Using the measurement for effective dose equivalent, the chest x-ray is approximately 80 μSv, and the effective dose equivalent for the single periapical using F-speed film and a round PID is approximately 1.3 μSv.

Background Radiation

Dental x-rays are artificially produced, and when grouped with medical x-rays they account for approximately 5 percent of the total radiation exposure to the population. In fact, the total radiation exposure to the U.S. population from all medical applications of ionizing radiation including x-rays, computed tomography (CT scans), and nuclear medication is approximately 48 percent. Consumer products and activities such as smoking, building materials, and combustion of fossil fuels make up another approximately 2 percent of exposure to the population. However, it is important to note 50 percent of total exposure to the population comes from naturally occurring, background sources of radiation (Figure 2-9). **Background**

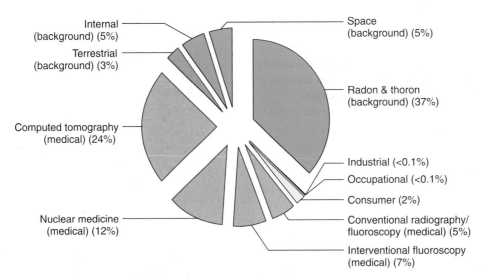

FIGURE 2-9 Annual effective dose equivalent of ionizing radiations. This chart illustrates the approximate percentage of exposure of the U.S. population to background and artificial radiations.(Reprinted with permission of the National Council on Radiation Protection and Measurements, http://NCRPonline.org)

radiation is defined as ionizing radiation that is always present in our environment. The human race has always been subjected to exposure from natural background radiations originating from the following sources:

- Cosmic radiations from outer space
- Terrestrial radiations from the earth and its environments including radon gas
- Background radiations from naturally occurring radionuclides (unstable atoms that emit radiations) that are deposited in our bodies by inhalation and ingestion

The average natural background radiation levels for the U.S. population is estimated to be about 3.1 mSv (millisievert) or 310 mrem (millirem) per year or about 0.9 mrem per day. The exact amount varies according to locality, the amount of radioactive material present, and the intensity of the cosmic rays—this intensity varies according to altitude and latitude. For example, persons living on the Colorado plateau receive an increased dose of background radiation because of the increased cosmic radiation at the higher altitude and more terrestrial radiation from soils enriched in naturally occurring uranium that raise the levels of terrestrial radionuclides located there.

REVIEW—Chapter summary

The three basic building blocks of an atom are protons, neutrons, and electrons. Protons and neutrons make up the central nucleus, which is orbited by the electrons revolving in the energy levels. Binding energy between the positive protons and negative electrons maintains the electrons in their orbits.

Ionization is the formation of charged particles called ions. A positive ion and a negative ion are called an ion pair. Ionizing radiation is defined as any radiation that produces ions.

Electromagnetic radiation is the movement of wavelike energy through space. Electromagnetic radiation exhibits the properties of wavelength, frequency, and velocity. Short-wavelength x-rays, called hard radiation, are very penetrating. Long-wavelength x-rays, called soft radiation, have limited penetrating power. The electromagnetic spectrum consists of an orderly arrangement of all known radiant energies.

X-rays are invisible, travel in straight lines at the speed of light, interact with matter causing ionization, affect photographic film, and affect living tissue. X-rays are produced whenever high-speed electrons are abruptly stopped or slowed down. They may pass through a patient with no interaction, or they may be absorbed by the photoelectric effect or scattered by either Compton scattering or coherent scattering.

Four x-ray measurement quantities are exposure (C/kg; roentgen), absorbed dose (gray/Gy; rad), dose equivalent (sievert/Sv; rem), and effective dose equivalent (microsievert/μSv).

Dental and medical x-rays make up approximately 5 percent of the total radiation exposure to the U.S. population. All medical uses of ionizing radiations including CT scans and nuclear medicine account for 48 percent of the total ionizing radiation exposure. Background radiation consisting of cosmic radiation, terrestrial radiations and radon gas, and naturally occurring radionuclides that are deposited in our bodies by inhalation and ingestion accounts for 50 percent of the total radiation exposure. The average natural background radiation levels for the U.S. population is estimated to be about 3.1 mSv (millisievert) or 310 mrem (millirem) per year or 0.9 mrem per day.

RECALL—Study questions

1. What term describes the smallest particle of an element that retains the properties of that element?
   a. Atom
   b. Molecule
   c. Photon
   d. Isotope

2. Draw and label a typical atom.

3. Which of these subatomic particles carries a negative electric charge?
   a. Proton
   b. Neutron
   c. Nucleus
   d. Electron

4. Radiant energy sufficient to remove an electron from its orbital level of an atom is called
   a. atomic.
   b. electronic.
   c. ionizing.
   d. ultrasonic.

5. What term describes the process by which unstable atoms undergo decay in an effort to obtain nuclear stability?
   a. Absorption
   b. Radioactivity
   c. Radiolucent
   d. Ionization

6. Which of the following is NOT a property shared by all energies of the electromagnetic spectrum?
   a. Have energy that is measurable and different
   b. Travel in a pulsating motion at the speed of sound
   c. Have no electrical charge, mass, or weight
   d. Emit an electrical field at right angles to the path of travel

7. What is the distance between two similar points on two successive waves called?
   a. Wavelength
   b. Frequency
   c. Velocity
   d. Energy level

8. Which of these electromagnetic radiations has the shortest wavelength?
   a. Radar
   b. Ultraviolet rays
   c. Infrared rays
   d. X-rays

9. Which of these forms of radiation has the greatest penetrating power?
   a. Visible light
   b. X-rays
   c. Sunlamp
   d. Radio waves

10. Which of these forms of radiation is least capable of causing ionization of body tissue cells?
    a. Cosmic rays
    b. Gamma rays
    c. X-rays
    d. Infrared light

11. List five properties of x-rays.
    a. _____
    b. _____
    c. _____
    d. _____
    e. _____

12. Radiation produced when high-speed electrons are stopped or slowed down by the tungsten atoms of the dental x-ray tube is called
    a. general/bremsstrahlung.
    b. characteristic.
    c. coherent.
    d. Compton.

13. What term best describes the process of transferring x-ray energy to the atoms of the material through which the x-ray beam passes?
    a. Compton scattering
    b. Photoelectric effect
    c. Absorption
    d. Bremsstrahlung

14. Which of these terms is the unit used to measure radiation exposure?
    a. Angstrom (Å)
    b. Gray (rad)
    c. Sievert (rem)
    d. Coulombs per kilogram (roentgen)

15. The Système Internationale (SI) unit that has replaced the traditional unit rem is
    a. gray.
    b. sievert.
    c. rad.
    d. coulomb/kilogram.

16. Dental and medical x-rays account for what percentage of the overall total exposure to ionizing radiation to an individual in the United States?
    a. 5
    b. 10
    c. 25
    d. 50

17. List three sources of background radiation.
    a. _____
    b. _____
    c. _____

18. What is the average amount of background radiation to an individual in the United States?
    a. 2.2 mSv (220 millirem) per year
    b. 4.2 mSv (420 millirem) per year
    c. 3.1 mSv (310 millirem) per year
    d. 8.2 mSv (820 millirem) per year

REFLECT—Case study

While taking a full mouth series of dental radiographs on your patient, he begins to consider the number of radiographs that are exposed in this operatory on a daily basis. He decides to ask you questions such as, "How long do you have to wait after each exposure before you can re-enter the room?" and "Are the walls and equipment in this room becoming radioactive from all the exposures taken in here?" Prepare a conversation with this patient addressing these two questions based on what you learned in this chapter on radiation physics.

RELATE—Laboratory application

Research recent media (magazine or journal articles, newspaper reports, or the Web) for stories on radiation exposure. Select an article for review, and critique the article for clarity and readability. Summarize how many different types of radiation are mentioned in the article. What units of radiation measurement does the author use? Does the article use these terms in a manner that is appropriate for what is being measured? Consider the type of radiation described in this article. Is it naturally occuring/background radiation or a radiation generated by an artificial or man-made source? How many key words from this chapter can you find in the article? Anticipate what questions your patient may have for you after reading this article.

REFERENCES

Bushberg, J. T., Seibert, J. A., Leidholdt, E. M., Jr., & Boone, J. M. (2001). *The essential physics of medical imaging* (2nd ed.). Baltimore: Lippincott Williams & Wilkins.

National Council on Radiation Protection and Measurements. (2009). *Report No 160: Ionizing radiation exposure of the population of the United States.* Bethesda, MD: Author.

Taylor, B. N., & Thompson, A. (Eds.). (2008). *The international system of units.* Washington, DC: National Institute of Standards and Technology, U. S. Dept. of Commerce, Special Publication 330.

Thompson, A., & Taylor, B. N. (2008). *Guide to the SI, with a focus on usage and unit conversions. Guide for the use of the international system of units (SI).* National Institute of Standards and Technology Special Publication 811.Gaithersburg, MD: National Institute of Standards and Technology.

United States Nuclear Regulatory Commission, Office of Public Affairs. (2003). *Fact sheet.* Washington, DC: Author.

United States Nuclear Regulatory Commission. (2007, December 4). Standards for protection against radiation, Title 10, Part 20, of the *Code of Federal Regulations.* Retrieved April 11, 2010, from http://www.nrc.gov/reading-rm/doc-collections/cfr/part020/part020-1201.html

White, S. C., & Pharoah, M. J. (2008). *Oral radiology. Principles and interpretation* (6th ed.). St. Louis, MO: Mosby Elsevier.

3

The Dental X-ray Machine: Components and Functions

CHAPTER OUTLINE

OBJECTIVES

Following successful completion of this chapter, you should be able to:

1. Define the key words.
2. Identify the three major components of a dental x-ray machine.
3. Identify and explain the function of the five controls on the control panel.
4. State the three conditions necessary for the production of x-rays.
5. Draw and label a dental x-ray tube.
6. Identify the parts of the cathode and explain its function in the production of x-rays.
7. Identify the parts of the anode and explain its function in the production of x-rays.
8. Trace the production of x-rays from the time the exposure button is activated until x-rays are released from the tube.
9. Demonstrate, in sequence, steps in operating the dental x-ray machine.

KEY WORDS

Alternating current (AC)
Amperage
Ampere (A)
Anode
Autotransformer
Cathode
Central ray
Collimator
Control panel
"Dead-man" exposure switch
Direct current (DC)
Electrical circuit
Electric current

Electrode
Electron cloud
Exposure button
Extension arm
Filament
Filter
Focal spot
Focusing cup
Impulse
Incandescence
Intensity
Kilovolt (kV)
Kilovolt peak (kVp)

Introduction

At the time of exposure, the radiographer who activates the exposure button is responsible for the radiation dose the patient incurs. The role of exposing dental radiographs is an important one for the dental assistant and dental hygienist, making it essential that these professionals understand how the x-ray machine works to produce ionizing radiation. To operate dental x-ray equipment safely and competently, the radiographer needs to develop a base knowledge of the components of the dental x-ray machine and possess an understanding of how these components work together to produce ionizing radiation. The purpose of this chapter is to discuss the conventional dental x-ray machine, its components, and its functions.

Evolution of the Dental X-ray Machine

Improvements in early x-ray generating machines began to occur after the dangers of radiation exposure became evident. The Coolidge hot cathode vacuum tube, invented by Dr. W. D. Coolidge in 1913, improved the previous erratic radiation output of earlier machines. Then during the mid-1950s, variable kilovoltage machines were introduced that allow for different penetrating abilities of the x-beam. In 1966, the recessed PID was introduced (Figure 3-1). On x-ray machines of conventional design, the x-ray tube is located in the front section of the tube head; on those using a recessed design, the x-ray tube is located in the back of the tube head. This configuration allows for a sharper image. (The role a longer x-ray tube-to-object distance plays in producing sharp images will be discussed in Chapter 4.)

In 1974, the federal government began regulating the manufacture and installation of all dental x-ray machines. State and local governing agencies also set guidelines on the safe installation and use of dental x-ray equipment. New technology employing miniaturized solid-state transformers and rare-earth materials for filtration of the x-ray beam have also contributed to the development of a modern dental x-ray machine that is safe, compact, easy to position, and simple to operate.

Dental X-ray Machine Components

Although dental x-ray machines vary in size and appearance, they have similar structural components (Figure 3-2). The dental x-ray machine typically consists of three parts:

1. The **control panel,** which contains the regulating devices
2. The **extension arm** or bracket, which enables the tube head to be positioned
3. The **tube head,** which contains the x-ray tube from which x-rays are generated

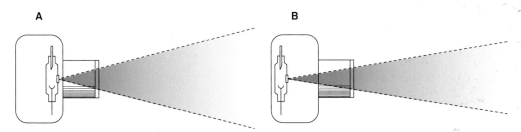

FIGURE 3-1 Comparison of conventional and recessed tube position within the tube head. (**A**) Conventional position with tube in front of tube head. Note how quickly the x-ray beam pattern flares out. (**B**) With a recessed tube a relatively more parallel x-ray beam is produced. This will produce a sharper radiographic image.

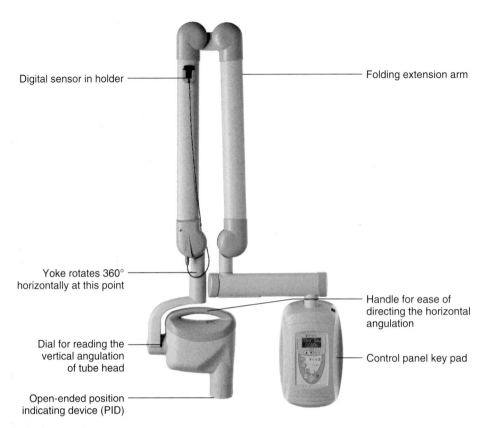

Digital sensor in holder

Folding extension arm

Yoke rotates 360° horizontally at this point

Handle for ease of directing the horizontal angulation

Dial for reading the vertical angulation of tube head

Control panel key pad

Open-ended position indicating device (PID)

FIGURE 3-2 **Typical wall-mounted dental x-ray machine.** (Image courtesy of Progeny, A Midmark Company)

Control Panel

The **electric current** enters the control panel either through a cord plugged into a grounded outlet in the wall or through a direct connection to a power line in the wall. The control panel may be integrated with the extension arm and tube head for ease of access during exposures (Figure 3-3), or it may be remote

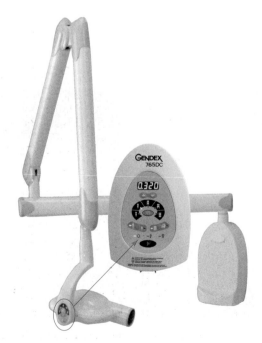

FIGURE 3-3 **Control panel integrated with tube head support.** (Image courtesy of Gendex Dental Corporation)

from the unit, mounted on a shelf or wall (Figure 3-4). One control panel may serve two or more tube heads. In the past dental x-ray machines were readily available with variable milliamperage and kilovoltage controls of the incoming electricity that the operator would manually adjust (Figure 3-5). Increasingly more common are dental x-ray machines with these controls preset by the manufacturer (Figure 3-6). If the milliamperage and the kilovoltage are preset by the manufacturer, the control panel will indicate at what variables these units are preset. Five major controls may be operated or will be preset on dental x-ray machines: (1) the line switch to the electrical outlet, (2) the milliampere selector, (3) the kilovoltage selector, (4) the timer, and (5) the exposure button. The function of each of these is discussed next.

LINE SWITCH The **line switch** on the control panel of the dental x-ray machine may be a toggle switch that can be flicked on or off with light finger pressure, or it may be an ON/OFF push button or a keypad (Figure 3-5). It is generally located on the side or face of the cabinet or control panel. In the ON position, this switch energizes the circuits in the control panel, but not the low- or high-voltage circuits to the transformers. An indicator light turns on, indicating the machine is operational.

MILLIAMPERE (mA) SELECTOR The **milliampere** measures the amount of current passing through the wires of the circuit. The **amperage** is set by turning a selector knob, depressing the marked push button, or touching a keypad. (Figure 3-5). On a dental x-ray machine with the amperage preset, its activation is connected

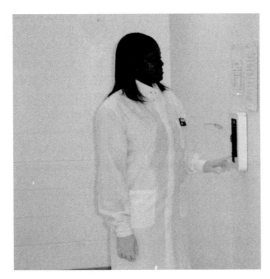
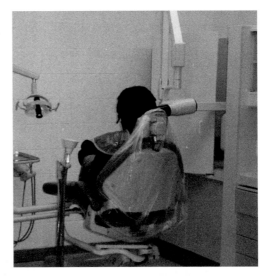

FIGURE 3-4 Control panel mounted in protected area.

directly to the ON/OFF switch. The amperage determines the available number of free electrons at the cathode filament and, therefore, the amount of x-rays that will be produced.

KILOVOLT PEAK (kVp) SELECTOR   The **voltmeter** measures the difference in potential or voltage across the x-ray tube. A **kilovolt peak (kVp)** selector in the form of a dial, push button, knob, or keypad (Figure 3-5) enables the operator to change the peak kilovoltage (Figure 3-5). On a dental x-ray machine with the kVp preset, its activation is connected directly to the ON/OFF switch. The kVp determines the speed of electrons traveling toward the target on the anode and, therefore, the penetrating ability of the x-rays produced.

TIMER   The timer is set by turning the selector knob, depressing the marked push button, or touching a keypad (Figure 3-6). The **timer** serves to regulate the duration of the interval that the current will pass through the x-ray tube. Dental x-ray machines are equipped with accurate electronic timers. Timer settings may be in fractions of a second or **impulses.** There are 60 impulses in a second. For example, a 1/10th of a second exposure lasts 6 impulses, 1/5th of a second lasts 12 impulses, and so forth. X-ray machines with electronic digital timers are accurate to 1/100th of a second intervals and work well with digital radiography systems. The time selected determines the duration of the exposure.

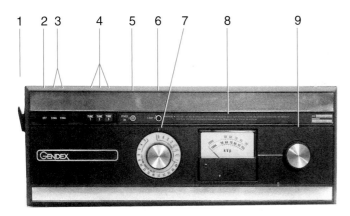

FIGURE 3-5 Control panel of a dental x-ray machine that allows for manual adjustment of exposure variables. (**1**) Exposure button holder, (**2**) main ON/OFF switch, (**3**) mA control, (**4**) x-ray tube selector (this master control accommodates three remote tube heads), (**5**) power ON light, (**6**) x-ray emission indicator light, (**7**) timer control, (**8**) kVp meter, (**9**) kVp control. This control panel allows the operator to choose settings of 50 kVp to 90 kVp at 15 mA, and 50 kVp to 100 kVp at 10 mA.

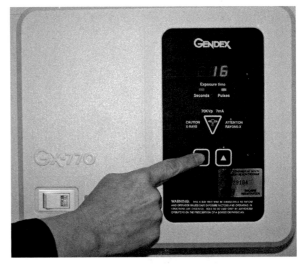

FIGURE 3-6 Operator setting the exposure time. The display indicates 16 impulses. Note the preset milliamperage and kilovoltage values.

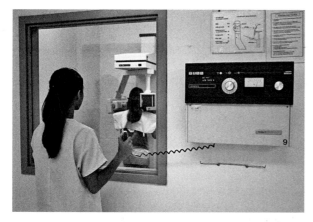

FIGURE 3-7 Exposure button on the handle of the timer cord. Operator is exposing a panoramic radiograph from behind a lead-lined glass window.

EXPOSURE BUTTON Depressing the **exposure button** or keypad activates the x-ray production process. The exposure button may be located on the handle of the timer cord (Figure 3-7) or at a remote location in a protected area (Figure 3-4). If the exposure button is located on the end of the timer cord, the cord must be sufficiently long to enable the operator to step into an area of protection from radiation, usually at least 6 ft (1.83 m) from the source of the x-ray beam. Because the possibility exists that the operator may not utilize the full length of the timer cord to be safely protected from the x-rays generated, an exposure switch permanently mounted to the control panel or wall in a protected area is preferred. In fact, many state regulations now require that the exposure button be permanently mounted in a protected area. Older x-ray machines equipped with exposure buttons on timer cords must be modified to attach the exposure button to an unmovable, permanent mount to meet this requirement.

All dental x-ray machines are required to be equipped with a **"dead-man" exposure switch** that automatically terminates the exposure when the operator's finger ceases to press on the timer button. This makes it necessary to maintain firm pressure on the button during the entire exposure. Failure to do so results in the formation of an insufficient number of x-rays to properly expose the image receptor (film or digital sensor). When the exposure button is activated, the operator will hear an audible beep (required by law) that indicates x-rays are being generated. Additionally, exposure buttons installed directly on the control panel allow the operator to observe a light indicating that x-rays are being generated.

The manufacturing trend is toward simpler and automated controls. In addition to preset milliamperage and kilovoltage, many dental x-ray machines now have a default timer that automatically resets itself and does not have to be altered unless a change in the exposure time is desired. Also available are programmable preset exposure settings that the operator can select directly from the tube head for quickly changing the settings chairside (Figure 3-3).

Extension Arm

The folding extension arm is a support from which the tube housing is suspended (Figure 3-2). The extension arm allows for moving and positioning the tube head. The extension arm is

hollow to permit the passage of electrical wires from the control panel to the tube head from one or both sides at a point where the tube head attaches to the yoke. The tube head is attached to the extension arm by means of a **yoke** that can revolve 360 degrees horizontally where it is connected. In addition, the tube head can be rotated vertically within the yoke. All sections of the extension arm and yoke are heavily insulated to protect the patient and the operator from electrical shock.

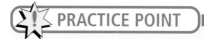

After use, the extension arm bracket should be folded into a neutral, closed position. The tube head is finely counterbalanced in its suspension from the extension arm. This balance can be disturbed if the tube head is left suspended for prolonged time periods with the extension arm stretched out. This may lead to instability and tube head drifting.

Tube Head (Tube Housing)

The tube head (sometimes called tube housing; Figure 3-8) is a tightly sealed heavy metal (usually cast aluminum), lead-lined housing that contains the dental x-ray tube, insulating oil, and step-up and step-down transformers. The metal housing performs several important functions:

1. Protects the x-ray tube from accidental damage
2. Increases the safety of the x-ray machine by grounding its high-voltage components (the x-ray tube and the transformers) to prevent electrical shock
3. Prevents overheating of the x-ray tube by providing a space filled with oil, gas, or air to absorb the heat created during the production of x-rays
4. Lined with lead to absorb any x-rays produced that do not contribute to the primary beam that exits through the port in the direction of the position indicating device (PID)

Older dental x-ray machine tube heads are heavy and bulky. The trend is toward using lighter weight materials and miniaturized solid-state components. Reducing the size and the weight of the tube head helps make it easier for the operator to position.

Electricity

Because electricity is needed to produce dental x-rays, an understanding of basic electrical concepts is necessary. Electricity can be defined as electrons in motion. An electric current is a movement of electrons through a conducting medium (such as copper wire). Electric current can flow in either direction along a wire or conductor. It can flow steadily in one direction (direct current) or flow in pulses and change directions (alternating current).

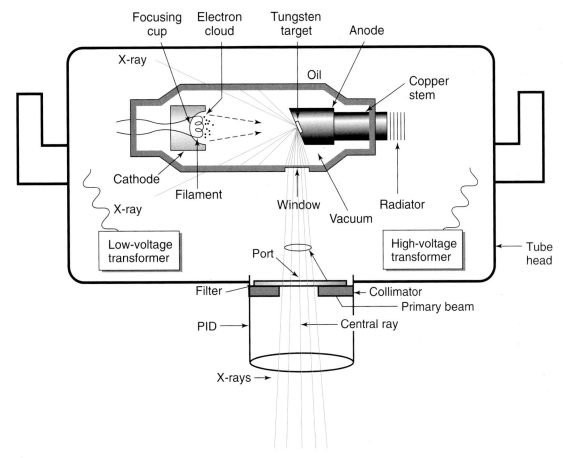

FIGURE 3-8 Dental x-ray tube head, containing x-ray tube, transformers, and oil. When an electric current is applied to the high-voltage circuit (between the cathode and the anode), the boiled off electrons are propelled from the cathode to the target on the anode, producing heat and x-rays. Although x-rays are emitted in all directions, because of the 20-degree angle of the anode target most of the x-rays travel through the window toward the port opening. These x-rays make up the primary x-ray beam. The central ray is the x-ray in the center of the primary beam.

Direct Current

Direct current (DC) flows continuously in one direction. The unidirectional current is similar to that used in flashlight batteries. Direct current dental x-ray machines are well suited for use with digital imaging (see Chapter 9).

Alternating Current

The household current used in the United States is a 110-V or 220-V, 60-cycle **alternating current (AC),** which changes its direction of flow 60 times per second (Figure 3-9). The alternating current has two phases—one positive and the other negative—and alternates between these phases.

Electrical Circuit

The path the electricity flows is called an **electrical circuit.** Two electrical circuits are used in producing dental x-rays.

1. A filament circuit provides low voltage (3–8 V) to the filament of the x-ray tube to generate a source of electrons needed for the production of x-rays.
2. A high-voltage circuit provides the high voltage (60–100 kV) necessary to accelerate the electrons from the cathode filament to the anode target.

Transformers

A **transformer** is an electromagnetic device for changing the current coming into the dental x-ray machine. Transformers are required to decrease (step down) or increase (step up) the ordinary 110-V or 220-V current that enters the x-ray machine. The step-down and step-up transformers are located in the tube head.

Step-down Transformer

A **step-down** (low-voltage) **transformer** decreases the voltage from the wall outlet to approximately 5 V, just enough to heat the filament and form an electron cloud.

Step-up Transformer

A **step-up** (high-voltage) **transformer** increases the voltage from the wall outlet to approximately 60–100 kVp to propel the electrons toward the target. The high-voltage current begins to flow through the cathode–anode circuit when the exposure button on the line switch is depressed.

Autotransformer

An **autotransformer,** located in the control panel, is a voltage compensator that corrects minor fluctuations in the current flowing through the wires.

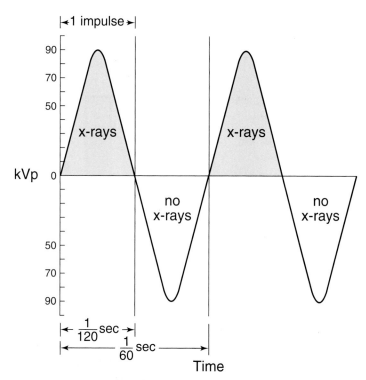

FIGURE 3-9 **Sine wave of 60-cycle alternating current operating at 90,000 V (90 kVp).** Ordinary household electric current is called 60-cycle alternating current because the current changes its direction of flow 60 times a second. During the time that the x-ray tube is producing x-rays, the cathode and the anode each change from negative to positive 60 times per second. The crest of the wave represents the maximum voltage when the current is moving in one direction, while the trough of the wave represents the maximum voltage when the current is moving in the other direction. The total cycle takes place in 1/60 sec. This alternation in current direction occurs every 1/120 sec (twice during each full cycle) on x-ray machines using alternating current, producing x-rays in a series of bursts, or impulses, rather than in a continuous flow.

The electrical terms **amperage**, the measurement of the number of electrons moving through a wire conductor, and voltage, the measurement of electrical force that causes electrons to flow through a conductor, will be used to describe the x-rays generated.

Amperage

Amperage measures the number of electrons that move through a conductor. The **ampere (A)** is the unit of quantity of electric current. An increase in amperage results in an increase in the number of electrons that is available to travel from the cathode to anode when the tube is activated. This results in a production of more x-rays. Only a small current is required to generate a number of electrons necessary to produce dental x-rays; therefore, the term *milliampere* (mA), denoting 1/1,000th of an ampere, is used. Dental x-ray machines typically operate in ranges from 4 to 15 mA. The setting will vary by manufacturer and is usually preset, although some x-ray machines allow the operator to choose the setting best suited for the exposure.

Voltage

Voltage or **volt (V)** is the electrical pressure (sometimes called potential difference) between two electrical charges. In the production of x-rays the voltage determines the speed of the electrons when traveling from cathode to anode. This speed of the electrons, in turn, determines the energy (penetrating power) of the x-rays produced. When the voltage is increased, the electrons travel faster and produce a harder type of radiation. Because dental x-ray machines operate at very high voltages, it is customary to express voltage in terms of **kilovolts.**

A kilovolt equals 1,000 V and is abbreviated **kV.** The voltage varies during an exposure, producing a **polychromatic** beam (x-rays of many different energies) containing high-energy rays and also containing soft rays that have barely enough energy to escape from the tube. The highest voltage to which the current in the tube rises during an exposure is called the kilovolt peak (kVp). So if the x-ray machine controls are set at 75 kVp (75,000 V), the maximum x-ray energy that can be produced during this exposure is 75 kVp. Dental x-ray machines typically operate within a range of 60 kVp to 100 kVp. The setting will vary by manufacturer and is usually preset, although some x-ray machines allow the operator to choose the setting best suited for the exposure.

The X-ray Tube

X-rays are produced when a stream of high-speed electrons are suddenly stopped or slowed down and diverted off course. Three conditions must exist for x-rays to be produced:

1. An available source of free electrons
2. High voltage to impart speed to the electrons
3. A target that is capable of stopping/slowing the electrons

The x-ray tube and the circuits within the machine are designed to create these conditions. The **x-ray tube,** located inside the tube head, is a glass bulb from which the air has been pumped to create a vacuum. A **cathode** (the negative **electrode**) and an **anode** (the positive electrode) are sealed within the vacuum tube, and the two protruding arms of the electrodes permit the passage of the current through the tube with minimum resistance.

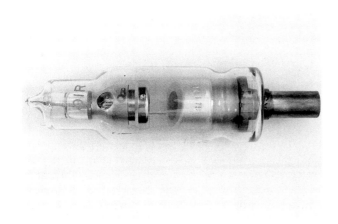

FIGURE 3-10 Dental x-ray tube.

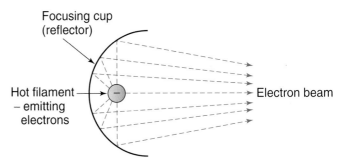

FIGURE 3-12 Formation of electron beam by focusing cup. A focusing cup, within the cathode structure into which the filament is placed, focuses the electron beam in a similar manner as light is focused by a flashlight reflector. When the high-voltage circuit is activated, the free electrons are accelerated toward the focal spot on the anode target.

In most dental x-ray tubes, the space between the electrodes is less than 1 in. (25.4 mm; Figure 3-10).

Cathode

The purpose of the cathode is to supply the electrons necessary to produce x-rays. The cathode, or negative electrode, consists of a thin, spiral filament of **tungsten** wire. This **filament** wire, when heated to **incandescence** (red hot and glowing), produces the electrons (Figure 3-11). This process is known as **thermionic emission.** A familiar example of this phenomenon is the tungsten electric lightbulb. Tungsten's high atomic number makes it possible to liberate electrons, through thermionic emission, from their orbital shells when the metal is heated. The released electrons form an **electron cloud** around the wire. The wire filament is recessed into a molybdenum **focusing cup,** which directs the electrons toward the target on the anode (Figure 3-12). The milliamperage setting accurately controls the thermionic emission and therefore controls the quantity of free electrons available.

Anode

The kilovoltage imparts speed to the electrons sending them flying across the tube from cathode to anode. The purpose of the anode is to provide the target to stop or significantly slow the high-velocity electrons, converting their kinetic energy into x-rays (electromagnetic energy). The anode, or positive electrode, consists of a copper bar with a tungsten plate imbedded in the end that faces the focusing cup of the cathode. This tungsten plate, called the **target,** is set into the copper at an angle of 20 degrees to the cathode. This angle directs most of the x-rays produced in one direction to become the **primary beam.** The **focal spot** is a small rectangular area on the target of the anode to which the focusing cup directs the electron beam. In Chapter 4 we will see that the smaller the focal spot, the sharper the radiographic image.

In summary, when the tube is in operation, a cloud of electrons first forms around the filament wire of the cathode as the tube warms. Then, when the high-voltage current is applied, these electrons are attracted and electrically charged to propel toward the focal spot on the target.

A Summary of the Principles of X-ray Tube Operation

Before x-ray production can begin, the machine must be turned on. If not preset by the manufacturer, the radiographer must set the correct mA and kVp by adjusting the dials on the control panel. The radiographer will then set the correct exposure time. The process of x-ray production is initiated by firmly pressing the exposure button. This permits the current to enter the filament circuit of the x-ray machine. A step-down transformer reduces the voltage before it enters the filament circuit and heats the filament of the cathode to incandescence, separating electrons from their atoms. The degree to which the filament is heated depends on the milliamperage setting: The higher the mA, the more electrons in the electron cloud. These electrons are now in a state of excitation as they hover around the tungsten filament recessed in the molybdenum focusing cup. After just a

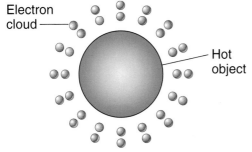

Electron emission from hot object

FIGURE 3-11 Cross section of a filament wire. The filament wire in the cathode is heated to incandescence. The attached electrons are literally boiled out of the wire and become available as a source of free electrons necessary for x-ray production. The milliamperage setting determines the number of electrons available to be accelerated across to the target of the anode.

fraction of a second time delay, the line current enters the cathode–anode high-voltage circuit. A step-up transformer then increases the voltage to impart sufficient force to propel the free electrons toward the focal spot on the target at the anode. These high-velocity electrons are stopped or slowed when they collide with the tungsten atoms in the target resulting in the production of general radiation (bremsstrahlung) and/or characteristic radiation. (This process is explained fully in Chapter 2.) The **kinetic energy** (the high-velocity electrons) is converted into approximately 1 percent x-ray energy. The other 99 percent of the kinetic energy generated is lost as heat energy.

The metal tungsten (symbol W and atomic number 74; also known as wolfram) is ideally suited for use in the filament and target because it can withstand extremely high temperatures (melting point 3370°C). Because it is subjected to such extreme heat and has low thermal conductivity, the tungsten plate is imbedded in a core of copper. Copper is highly conductive and carries the heat generated off to the **radiator,** which is just outside the tube (refer to the tube diagram in Figure 3-8). The large mass of copper conducts the heat out of the tube into a radiator that transfers the heat to the oil, gas, or air that surrounds the tube.

Although the target is set into the copper at an angle to direct most of the x-rays toward the window (a thin area in the glass tube) located at a point where the emission of x-rays is most intense, some x-rays are emitted out in all directions within the tube housing. These x-rays are absorbed by the glass tube, oil, air, wires, transformers, and the tube head lining. If the tube head is properly sealed, the **port** (an opening in the tube housing) is the only place through which the x-rays can escape the tube head (Figure 3-8). The port is covered by a permanent seal of glass, beryllium, or aluminum. The PID (position indicating device) fits over the port and can be moved to aim the primary beam of x-rays in the desired direction. After completion of the predetermined exposure, the high-voltage current is automatically shut off, and x-ray production stops.

The X-ray Beam

X-rays are produced in 360-degree direction at the focal spot of the target. However, because of the angle of the anode, a high concentration of x-rays travels toward the port opening of the tube head. Only a beam of radiation the size of the port seal is allowed to exit the tube head. The other x-rays are stopped (absorbed) by the contents and walls of the tube head. After the beam exits through the port, the lead **collimator** (explained in Chapter 6) further restricts the x-ray beam to the desired size.

The x-ray beam is cone shaped because x-rays travel in diverging straight lines as they radiate from the focal spot. This beam of x-rays is called the primary beam or the **useful beam.** The primary beam is the original useful beam of x-rays that originates at the focal spot and emerges through the port of the tube head. The **central ray** is the x-ray in the center of the primary beam.

The x-ray beam formed at the focal spot is polychromatic, consisting of x-rays of various wavelengths. Only x-rays with sufficient energy to penetrate oral structures are useful for diagnostic dental radiographs. X-rays of low penetrating power

(long wavelength) add to the patient dose but not to the information recorded on the image receptor. To remove the soft x-rays, a thin sheet of aluminum called a **filter** is placed in the path of the x-ray beam (explained in Chapter 6).

The **intensity** of the x-ray beam refers to the quantity and quality of the x-rays. **Quantity** refers to the number of x-rays in the beam. **Quality** refers to the energy strength or penetrating ability of the x-ray beam (see Chapter 4). Intensity is defined as the product of the number of x-rays (quantity) and the energy strength of the x-rays (quality) per unit of area per unit of time. Intensity of the x-ray beam is affected by milliamperage (mA), kilovoltage (kVp), exposure time, and distance.

Operation of the Dental X-ray Machine

The specific steps to safe and effective use of a dental x-ray machine are outlined in the operating manual provided by the manufacturer. All persons operating an x-ray machine should study the manual until they are thoroughly familiar with the operational capability and maintenance requirements of the machine. To achieve consistent results, the radiographer should follow a systematic and orderly procedure (Procedure Box 3-1). Additionally, whenever x-ray exposures are made on patients, it is assumed here and in all subsequent instructions that:

- The radiographer is competent and can follow radiation safety protocol. (Some states require anyone placing and exposing dental radiographs to successfully complete a training course in radiation safety and protection protocols.)
- The radiographer performs all radiographic procedures in accordance with federal, state, and local regulations and recommendations.
- Infection control is maintained throughout the procedure (see Chapter 10).
- The procedure has been explained, and the patient has given consent.
- The patient has received verbal instructions and is able to cooperate with the procedure.
- Image receptor holding devices are utilized for all intraoral radiographs.

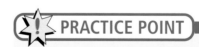

PRACTICE POINT

For maximum effectiveness in exposing dental radiographs, prepare the patient and the x-ray equipment and set the controls on the x-ray unit prior to positioning the image receptor in the oral cavity. Following an orderly sequence reduces the likelihood of errors and retakes.

PROCEDURE 3-1
Operation of the dental x-ray machine

1. Turn power on. A light on the control panel will indicate that the machine is ready to operate.
2. Unless preset by the manufacturer, select mA and kVp best suited for the exposure to be made.
3. Set timer for the desired exposure time.
4. Place the image receptor into the holding device and position in the patient's oral cavity.
5. Utilizing the extension arm and yoke, adjust the tube head by aligning the PID so that the central beam of radiation is directed toward the center of the image receptor at the appropriate horizontal and vertical angulations.
6. Establish appropriate protected location from the tube head.
7. Depress exposure button and hold it down firmly until the exposure is completed. The audible signal and x-ray exposure indicator light will activate for the duration of the exposure.
8. Remove the image receptor and holder from the patient's oral cavity after the exposure.
9. When the procedure is complete, fold the tube head support extension arm into the closed, neutral position.
10. Turn off the power to the x-ray machine.

REVIEW—Chapter summary

All x-ray machines, regardless of size and voltage range, operate similarly and have the same components (control panel, extension arm, and tube head) and electrical parts (x-ray tube, low- and high-voltage circuits, and a timing device).

The control panel may be integrated with the x-ray machine tube head support, or it may be remote from the unit, mounted on a shelf or wall. There are five major controls, some of which will be preset by the manufacturer or may be selected by the operator: (1) the line switch to the electrical outlet, (2) the milliampere selector, (3) the kilovoltage selector, (4) the timer, and (5) the exposure button.

A folding extension arm is a support from which the tube housing is suspended. The tube head is a tightly sealed heavy metal housing that contains the dental x-ray tube, insulating oil, and step-up and step-down transformers.

Three conditions must exist to produce x-rays: (1) a source of free electrons, (2) high voltage to accelerate them, and (3) a target to stop them. The dental x-ray tube creates these conditions. X-rays are produced only when the unit is turned on and a firm pressure is maintained on the exposure button.

Electric current flows into the x-ray machine and proceeds either through the step-down transformer or the step-up transformer. The step-down transformer reduces the electric current from the wall outlet to heat up the filament inside the focusing cup of the cathode (negative) side of the tube. Thermionic emission results in freed electrons available to make x-rays. The step-up transformer increases the electric current to impart kinetic energy to the freed electrons to cause them to propel across the tube to strike the target (at the focal spot) on the anode (positive) side of the tube.

The degree to which the filament is heated and, therefore, the quantity of electrons made available depends on the milliamperage setting. Quantity refers to the number of x-rays in the beam. The higher the mA, the more electrons available. The penetrating ability or quality of the resultant x-rays is determined by the kilovoltage setting. The higher the kVp, the more penetrating the x-rays.

The beam of radiation that exits the port seal of the tube head is the primary or useful beam. The polychromatic beam must be filtered to allow only x-rays with sufficient energy to reach the oral structures.

The radiographer must be familiar with the operation of the machine, and the patient must understand the procedure and provide consent. To achieve consistent results, the radiographer should follow a systematic and orderly procedure.

RECALL—Study questions

1. Each of the following may be located on the control panel EXCEPT one. Which one is the EXCEPTION?
   a. mA selector
   b. kVp selector
   c. Focusing cup
   d. Line switch

2. Which of the following activates the x-ray production process?
   a. Exposure button
   b. Milliamperage
   c. Voltmeter
   d. Timer selector

3. The x-ray machine component that allows the operator to position the tube head is called the
   a. timer cord.
   b. control panel.
   c. dead-man switch.
   d. extension arm.

4. Fill in the blanks.
   a. 30 impulses = _____ second.
   b. 45 impulses = _____ second.
   c. 1/3 second = _____ impulses.
   d. 1/10 second = _____ impulses.

5. To produce a larger quantity of electrons available to produce x-rays, increase the
   a. mA (milliamperage).
   b. kVp (kilovoltage).
   c. PID (position indicating device).
   d. DC (direct current).

6. What term describes the electrical pressure (difference in potential) between two electrical charges?
   a. Amperage
   b. Voltage
   c. Ionization
   d. Incandescence

7. Which term best describes an x-ray beam that is composed of a variety of energy wavelengths?
   a. Collimated
   b. Short-scale
   c. Filtered
   d. Polychromatic

8. List the three conditions that must exist for x-rays to be produced.
   a. _____
   b. _____
   c. _____

9. Draw and label the parts of the dental x-ray tube.

10. The process of heating the cathode wire filament until red hot and electrons boil off is called
    a. autotransformation.
    b. self-rectification.
    c. thermionic emission.
    d. kilovoltage peak.

11. What metal is used for the target in the x-ray tube?
    a. Copper
    b. Tungsten
    c. Aluminum
    d. Molybdenum

12. Which of these must be charged negatively during the time that the x-ray tube is operating to produce x-rays?
    a. Radiator
    b. Target
    c. Anode
    d. Cathode

13. Which of these changes the current coming into the x-ray machine?
    a. Transformer
    b. Collimator
    c. Radiator
    d. Rectifier

14. What percent of the kinetic energy inside the x-ray tube is converted into x-rays?
    a. 1%
    b. 50%
    c. 75%
    d. 99%

15. What term describes the opening in the tube housing that allows the primary beam to exit?
    a. Yoke
    b. Filament
    c. Port
    d. Focusing cup

16. Which of the following removes the low-energy, long-wavelength energy from the beam?
    a. Transformer
    b. Collimator
    c. Filter
    d. Radiator

17. After depressing the exposure button the radiographer will hear an audible beep sound indicating that the
    a. x-rays are being generated.
    b. kilovoltage has reached the peak.
    c. cathode and anode are reversing polarity.
    d. alternating current has been transformed into direct current.

REFLECT—Case study

To help you understand the practical use of altering exposure variables on a dental x-ray machine, consider the following patients with these characteristics:

- A 9-year-old female, height 4' 8" and weight 85 pounds, who has been assessed for bitewing radiographs to determine the evidence of caries.

- A 21-year-old male college football player, height 6' 1", 280 pounds, who has been assessed for periapical radiographs of suspected impacted third molars.
- A 58-year-old female, diagnosed with Bell's palsy with slight head and neck tremors, who has been assessed for a full mouth series for the evaluation of periodontal disease.

1. Would you select an increased or decreased amount of radiation to produce diagnostic quality radiographic images for each of these patients?
2. Which of these three exposure variables—milliamperage, kilovoltage, or time—control(s) the amount of radiation produced?
3. Which exposure variable would be the *best* choice to alter to increase or decrease the amount of radiation produced for each of these patients?
4. Would you select an increased or decreased penetrating ability of the x-ray beam to produce diagnostic quality radiographic images for each of these patients?
5. Which of the three exposure variables—milliamperage, kilovoltage, or time—control(s) the penetrating ability of the x-ray beam?
6. Which exposure variable would be the *best* choice to alter to increase or decrease the penetrating ability of the x-ray beam?
7. Suppose that you wanted to decrease the amount of time of the exposure, as may be needed when patient movement is anticipated (as in the case of patient 3), but still wanted to produce enough radiation to achieve a diagnostic quality radiographic image. Which variable—milliamperage or kilovoltage—would you adjust? Would you increase or decrease this variable?

Think of other characteristics patients may present with that would require you to adjust these x-ray machine variables. Keep in mind that increasing one factor may necessitate decreasing an opposing factor. Discuss the rationale for your choices.

RELATE—Laboratory application

For a comprehensive laboratory practice exercise on this topic, see Thomson, E. M. (2012). *Exercises in oral radiography techniques: A laboratory manual* 3rd ed.). Upper Saddle River, NJ: Pearson Prentice Hall. Chapter 1, "Introduction to Radiation Safety and Dental Radiographic Equipment"

REFERENCES

Bushberg, J. T., Seibert, J. A., Leidholdt, E. M., Jr., & Boone, J. M. (2001). *The essential physics of medical imaging* (2nd ed.). Baltimore: Lippincott Williams & Wilkins.

Carestream Health Inc. (2007). *Exposure and processing for dental film radiography.* Rochester, NY: Author.

White, S. C., & Pharoah, M. J. (2008). *Oral radiology. Principles and interpretation* (6th ed.). St. Louis, MO: Mosby Elsevier

Producing Quality Radiographs

OBJECTIVES

Following successful completion of this chapter, you should be able to:

1. Define the key words.

2. Evaluate a radiographic image identifying the basic requirements of acceptability.

3. Differentiate between radiolucent and radiopaque areas on a dental radiograph.

4. Define radiographic density and contrast.

5. List the rules for casting a shadow image.

6. Differentiate between subject contrast and film contrast.

7. List the factors that influence magnification and distortion.

8. List the geometric factors that affect image sharpness.

9. Summarize the factors affecting the radiographic image.

10. Describe how mA, kVp, and exposure time affect image density.

11. Discuss how kVp affects the image contrast.

12. Explain target–surface, object–image receptor, and target–image receptor distances.

13. Demonstrate the practical use of the inverse square law.

KEY WORDS

Contrast

Crystal

Definition

Density

Distortion

Exposure chart

Exposure factors

Exposure time

Extraoral radiography

Film contrast

Focal spot

Geometric factors

Grid

Intensifying screen

Intraoral radiography

Inverse square law

Kilovoltage peak (kVp)

Long-scale contrast

Magnification

Milliampere (mA)

Milliampere/second (mAs)

Motion

Object–image receptor distance

Penumbra

Position indicating device (PID)

Radiographic contrast

Radiolucent

Radiopaque

Introduction

Each patient presents with a unique set of characteristics for which a customized approach to exposure settings is needed. The dental radiographer has an ethical responsibility to produce the highest diagnostic quality radiographs for patients who agreed to be exposed to ionizing radiation. To consistently produce diagnostic quality radiographs at the lowest possible radiation dose, the dental radiographer needs to understand the interrelationships of the components of the dental x-ray machine.

There are three basic requirements for an acceptable diagnostic radiograph (Figure 4-1).

1. All parts of the structures recorded must be imaged as close to their natural shapes and sizes as the patient's oral anatomy will permit. Distortion and superimposition of structures should be kept to a minimum.
2. The area examined must be imaged completely, with enough surrounding tissue to distinguish between the structures.
3. The radiograph should be free of errors and show proper density, contrast, and definition.

The quality of a radiograph depends on both the physical factors and the subjective opinion of the individual who reads it. The purpose of this chapter is to describe the physical attributes of a quality radiographic image and to study the factors that affect these attributes.

Terminology

The following terms should be used when describing radiographic images: radiolucent, radiopaque, density, contrast, and sharpness.

When a film-based dental radiograph is viewed on a light source and digital images are viewed on a computer monitor, the image appears black and white, with various shades of gray in between. The terms used to describe the black and white areas are radiolucent and radiopaque, respectively.

Radiolucent

Radiolucent refers to that portion of the image that is dark or black (Figure 4-1). Structures that appear radiolucent permit the passage of x-rays with little or no resistance. Soft tissues and air spaces are examples of structures that appear radiolucent on a radiograph.

Radiopaque

Radiopaque refers to that portion of the image that is light or white (Figure 4-1). Structures that appear radiopaque are dense and absorb or resist the passage of x-rays. Enamel, dentin, and bone are examples of structures that appear radiopaque on the radiograph.

Radiolucent and radiopaque are relative terms. For instance, even though both enamel and dentin are radiopaque, enamel is more radiopaque (appears lighter) than dentin.

Three visual image characteristics that directly influence the quality of the radiographic image are density, contrast, and sharpness.

Density

Density is the degree of darkness or image blackening (Figure 4-2). A radiographic image that appears light is said to have little density. A radiographic image that appears dark is said to be more dense. The blackness results when x-rays strike sensitive crystals in the film emulsion, and subsequent processing causes the crystals to darken. When using a digital sensor, sensitive pixels capture the radiation, and "processing" by computer software produces darker pixels. The degree of darkening of the radiograph is increased when the milliamperage or the exposure time is increased and more x-rays are produced to reach the film emulsion or digital sensor.

Radiographs need just the right amount of density to be viewed properly. If the density is too light or too dark, the images

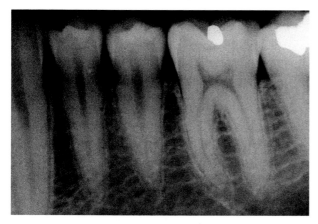

FIGURE 4-1 An acceptable diagnostic radiograph.

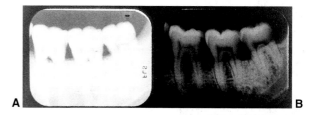

FIGURE 4-2 **Radiographic density.** Radiograph (**A**) is underexposed and appears too light (less dense). Radiograph (**B**) is overexposed and appears too dark (more dense).

of the teeth and supporting tissues cannot be visually separated from each other. The ideal radiograph has the proper amount of density for the interpreter to view black areas (radiolucent), white areas (radiopaque), and gray areas.

Contrast

Contrast refers to the many shades of gray that separate the dark and light areas (Figure 4-3). An image with good contrast will contain black, white, and enough shades of gray to differentiate between structures and their conditions. A radiograph that shows just a few shades is said to have short-scale or high contrast, whereas one that shows many variations in shade is said to possess long-scale or low contrast.

The term **short-scale contrast** (also called high contrast; Figure 4-4) describes a radiograph in which the density differences between adjacent areas are large. The contrast is high because there are fewer shades of gray and more black against white. The gray tones indicate the differences in absorption of the x-ray photons by the various tissues of the oral cavity or the head and neck region. The radiograph is radiolucent (dark) where the tissues are soft or thin and radiopaque (white) where the tissues are hard or thick. Such radiographs result when low (60–70) kVp is applied.

The term **long-scale contrast** (also called low contrast; Figure 4-4) describes a radiograph in which the density differences between adjacent areas are small. The contrast is low and very gradual because there are many shades of gray. Such radiographs result when high (80–100) kVp is applied.

Sharpness

Sharpness/definition is a geometric factor that refers to the detail and clarity of the outline of the structures shown on the radiograph. Unsharpness is generally caused by movement of the patient, image receptor, or tube head during exposure. Digital imaging sharpness can be affected by pixel size and distribution and will be discussed in Chapter 9.

Shadow Casting

A radiograph is a two-dimensional image of three-dimensional objects. Therefore, it is necessary to apply the rules for creating a shadow image to produce a quality radiographic image. The following rules for casting a shadow image will help to reproduce the size and shape of the objects of the oral cavity accurately.

Rules for Casting a Shadow Image

1. Small focal spot: to reduce the size of the **penumbra** (partial shadow around the objects of interest) resulting in a sharper image and slightly less magnification

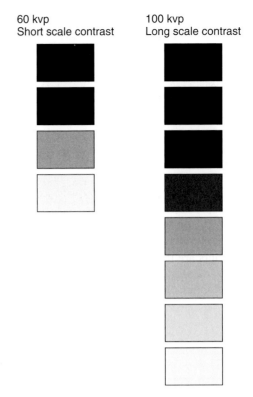

60 kvp
Short scale contrast

100 kvp
Long scale contrast

FIGURE 4-3 Penetrometer tests demonstrate radiographically that a longer contrast scale results from the use of 100-kilovolt exposures. Dental radiographs exposed at 100 kVp have long-scale contrast. Radiographs exposed at 60 kVp have short-scale contrast.

2. Long target-object distance: to reduce the penumbra and magnification
3. Short object-image receptor distance: to reduce penumbra and magnification
4. Parallel relationship between object and image receptor: to prevent distortion of the image
5. Perpendicular relationship between the central ray of the x-ray beam and both the object and the image receptor: to prevent distortion of the image

Because x-rays belong to the same electromagnetic spectrum as light (see Chapter 2), these two energies share many of the same characteristics. Therefore, when considering the application of shadow cast rules, it is helpful to compare the shadows cast by light with the shadows that x-rays will cast of the structures of the oral cavity. For example, if you were outside during the morning hours when the sun was low on the horizon, the

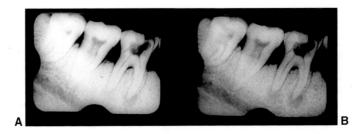

FIGURE 4-4 Radiographic contrast. Radiograph (**A**), exposed at 60 kVp, has high contrast. Radiograph (**B**), exposed at 90 kVp, has low contrast.

sun's rays would be directed at your body at a low angle, casting a shadow that was elongated, or longer than your actual height. If you were outside at midday, when the sun was directly overhead, the sun's rays would be directed at your body at a steep angle, casting a shadow that was foreshortened, or shorter than your actual height. At some time during the day, the sun's light would be cast at the precise angle to your body that your shadow on the ground would be at the same length as your actual height. Directing a flashlight at an object, such as the child's game of producing hand puppet shadows, is another example of shadow casting. Depending on the direction of the flashlight beam alignment and the distance the light must travel to reach the object, accurate or distorted shadow images result.

Shadow cast rules are often referred to as the **geometric factors** that contribute to the quality of the radiographic image. Geometric factors are those factors that relate to the relationships of angles, lines, points, or surfaces. Each of the shadow cast rules will be discussed in detail as to its role in producing quality radiographic images.

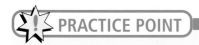

PRACTICE POINT

Some clinicians prefer the short-scale contrast radiographs that result from a low kVp setting to diagnose caries and long-scale contrast radiographs that result from a high kVp setting to diagnose periodontal disease. In theory, short-scale contrast images should be better at showing a radiolucency (depicting evidence of decalcification indicating caries) against radiopaque tooth enamel, whereas long-scale contrast radiographs are purported to be better at showing subtle changes (gray areas) indicating alveolar bone changes. However, research indicates that both short- and long-scale contrast images perform equally well in providing the clinician with the necessary information for interpretation and diagnosis. The ideal level of contrast is often a matter of individual preference.

Factors Affecting the Radiographic Image

The dental radiographer must have a working knowledge of the factors that affect the radiographic image. Although density is important for producing the detail and visibility of a radiograph, it is the radiographic contrast and sharpness/definition that interpretation and diagnosis of oral conditions depend on (Table 4-1).

Radiographic Contrast

Radiographic contrast defined as the visible difference between densities depends on the following variables.

1. **Subject (types of tissues being imaged).** The **subject contrast** is the result of differences in absorption of the x-rays by the tissues under examination. The subject to be imaged must have contrast. A radiograph of a 1-inch-thick sheet of plastic would show no contrast because the plastic is of uniform thickness and composition. Patients have contrast because human tissues vary in size, thickness, and density.

2. **Kilovoltage peak (kVp).** There is an inverse relationship between kVp and contrast (Figure 4-4). In relative terms, higher kilovoltages produce lower contrast. The blacks are grayer, the whites are grayer, and there are many shades (or steps) of gray in between. Lower kilovoltages produce higher contrast. The blacks are blacker, the whites are whiter, and there are fewer shades (or steps) of gray in between.

3. **Scatter radiation.** In Chapter 2 we learned that Compton scattering occurs whenever dental x-rays interact with matter such as the tissues of the patient's head. These scattered x-rays add a uniform exposure to the radiograph, thereby decreasing the contrast. For **intraoral radiography** (inside the mouth), a collimator (lead diaphragm) is used to keep the beam size as small as possible to help reduce scatter radiation. For **extraoral radiography** (outside the mouth), grids are sometimes used to absorb scattered x-rays. A **grid** is a mechanical device composed of thin strips of lead alternating with a radiolucent material (plastic). The grid is placed between the patient and the image receptor to absorb scattered x-rays (see Figure 29-10).

4. **Film/digital sensor type.** Each film has its own inherent (built-in) contrast that may vary by manufacturer. Digital sensor pixel size and the effects on the image contrast and density will be discussed in detail in Chapter 9.

5. **Exposure.** An underexposed or an overexposed radiograph will result in diminished or poor contrast. Accidental exposure of the film to stray radiation or other conditions such as heat and humidity will create film fog (Chapter 18). Fog is the formation of a thin, cloudy layer that reduces the image contrast. A radiograph that is too light, too dark, or fogged will not have significantly different shades of gray to provide optimal contrast.

6. **Processing.** Maximum **film contrast** can only be obtained through meticulous film processing procedures (Chapter 8). If improper development time or temperature is used, the radiograph will not have the ideal contrast the manufacturer built into it.

film based

Sharpness/Definition

Sharpness, also known as definition, refers to the clarity of the outline of the structures on the radiograph. Radiographic image sharpness depends on the following variables (see Table 4-2).

1. **Focal spot size.** As explained in Chapter 3, the **focal spot** is the small area on the target where bombarding electrons are

TABLE 4-1 Summary of Factors Influencing Radiographic Image Contrast

FACTORS	VARIABLES	IMAGE CONTRAST
Subject thickness (different tissues of the body)	Region with tissues of different densities (enamel, dentin, pulp of the tooth)	Higher contrast between these different tissues
	Region with tissues of similar densities (supporting alveolar bone)	Lower contrast between the different areas of bone
kVp (kilovoltage peak)	High kVp	Lower contrast
	Low kVp	Higher contrast
Scatter radiation	Increased scatter radiation (large beam diameter used for intraoral radiographs/no grid used for extraoral radiographs)	Lower contrast
	Decreased scatter radiation (beam diameter narrowed with collimation for intraoral radiographs/grid used for extraoral radiographs)	Higher contrast
Image receptor type	Different manufacturers	Higher or lower contrast is inherent and depends on the manufacturer
Exposure	Under- or overexposure and film fog	Each will lower contrast
Processing	Accurate time-temperature processing followed	Adequate contrast
	Inaccurate time-temperature processing followed	Lower or poor contrast

converted into x-rays. The smaller the focal spot area, the sharper the image appears (Figure 4-5). A large focal spot creates more penumbra (partial shadows) and therefore loss of image sharpness (Figure 4-6). Ideally, the focal spot should be a point source, then no penumbra would be present. However, a single point source would create extreme heat and burn out the x-ray tube. Focal spot size is determined by the manufacturer of the x-ray machine. To ensure that the focal spot remains small, the tube head must remain perfectly still during the exposure. Even slight vibration of the tube head increases the size of the focal spot (Figure 4-7).

2. **Target–image receptor distance.** The **target–image receptor distance** is the distance between the source of x-ray production (which is at the target on the anode inside the tube head) and the image receptor. PIDs are used to establish the target–image receptor distance. PIDs are classified as being short or long and come in standard lengths of 8 inches (20.5 cm), 12 inches (30 cm), and 16 inches (41 cm) for

TABLE 4-2 Summary of Factors Influencing Radiographic Image Sharpness

FACTORS	VARIABLES	IMAGE SHARPNESS
Focal spot size	Small focal spot	Increase sharpness
	Large focal spot	Decrease sharpness
Target–image receptor distance	Long target–image receptor distance	Increase sharpness
	Short target–image receptor distance	Decrease sharpness
Object–image receptor distance	Short object–image receptor distance	Increase sharpness
	Long object–image receptor distance	Decrease sharpness
Motion	No movement	Sharp image
	Movement	Fuzzy image
Screen thickness	Thin screen	Increase sharpness
	Thick screen	Decrease sharpness
Screen–film contact	Close contact	Increase sharpness
	Poor contact	Decrease sharpness
Film crystal/pixel size	Small crystals/pixels	Increase sharpness
	Large crystals/pixels	Decrease sharpness

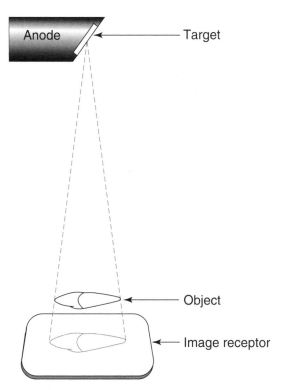

FIGURE 4-5 Using a small focal spot on the target, a long target–image receptor distance, and a short object–image receptor distance will result in a sharp image.

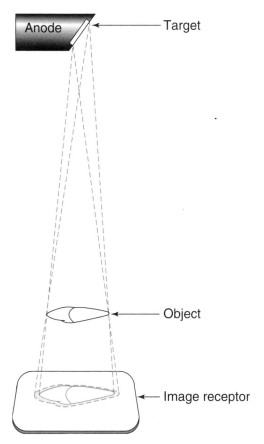

FIGURE 4-6 Large focal spot on the target and long object–image receptor distance results in more penumbra and loss of image sharpness.

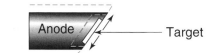

FIGURE 4-7 Movement of the tube head. Motion, even slight, of the tube head will effectively create a larger surface area of the focal spot, resulting in penumbra.

intraoral projections. The shorter the target–image receptor distance, the more divergent the x-ray beam (Figure 4-8). A long target–image receptor distance has x-rays in the center of the beam that are nearly parallel. Therefore, the image on the radiograph will be sharper. Also a longer target–image receptor distance will result in less image magnification (explained later in this chapter).

3. **Object–image receptor distance.** The **object–image receptor distance** is the distance between the object being radiographed (the teeth) and the dental x-ray image receptor (film or digital sensor.) The image receptor should always be placed as close to the teeth as possible. The closer the proximity of the image receptor to the teeth, the sharper the image and the less magnification (image enlargement). The image will become fuzzy (more penumbra) and magnified as the object–image receptor distance is increased (Figure 4-6).

4. **Motion.** Movement of the patient and/or the image receptor in addition to the tube head results in a loss of image sharpness (Figure 4-9).

5. **Screen thickness. Intensifying screens** (often referred to as screens), used in extraoral radiography, are made of crystals that emit light when struck by x-rays. The light, in turn, exposes the film and helps to produce the image. Intensifying screens require less radiation to produce a radiographic image than direct exposure film, resulting in less radiation exposure to the patient. However, the use of intensifying screens decreases the sharpness of the radiographic image (Figure 4-10). The thicker the screen, the less radiation required to expose the film. However, these thicker screens produce a less sharp radiographic image. Generally, the radiographer should use the highest speed screen and film combination, determined by the thickness of the phosphor

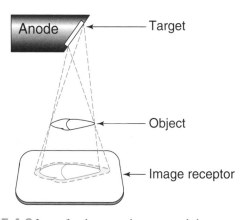

FIGURE 4-8 Large focal spot on the target and short target–image receptor distance results in more penumbra and loss of image sharpness.

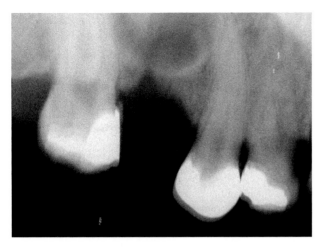

FIGURE 4-9 Blurry, unsharp image caused by movement of the patient, the image receptor, or the tube head.

layer, that is consistent with good diagnostic results. Intensifying screens are explained in detail in Chapter 29.

6. **Screen–film contact.** The film should be in close physical contact with the intensifying screen. Poor screen–film contact results in the wider spread of light and fuzziness (penumbra) of the image. Intensifying screens should be examined periodically for proper functioning. Additionally, only one film should be placed in contact with the screen. Attempting to make a duplicate image by placing two films into one cassette is not acceptable practice unless using a film type made especially for this purpose.

7. **Crystal/pixel size of intraoral image receptors.** X-ray film emulsion contains crystals that are struck by x-rays when exposed and in turn will produce the radiographic image. Image sharpness is influenced by the size of these **crystals.** Similar to the crystal size of intensifying screens, the smaller the size of the crystals within the film emulsion, the sharper the radiographic image. However, small crystal size contributes to a slow speed film, requiring the patient to receive a larger dose of radiation. Film manufacturers strive to produce film with the smallest sized crystals

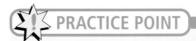

to avoid loss of image sharpness and yet maintain the maximum reduction in radiation exposure. Dental x-ray film is explained in detail in Chapter 7.

Digital sensors (Chapter 9) use pixels (short for *picture element*) that capture discrete units of information that the computer then combines into a radiographic image. The smaller the pixel size, the sharper the resultant image.

Magnification/Enlargement *appears bigger*

Magnification or enlargement is the increase in size of the image on the radiograph compared to the actual size of the object. In Chapter 3, we learned that x-rays travel in diverging straight lines as they radiate from the focal spot of the target. Because of these diverging x-rays, there is some magnification present in every radiograph.

Magnification is mostly influenced by the **target–object distance** and the object–image receptor distance. The target–object distance is determined by the length of the PID. When a long PID is used, the x-rays in the center of the beam are more parallel, resulting in less image magnification (Figure 4-11). The object–image receptor distance should be kept to a minimum. Always place the film/sensor as close to the teeth as possible, while maintaining a parallel relationship between the long axes of the teeth and the plane of the image receptor, to decrease magnification.

Increasing the target–object distance and decreasing the object–image receptor distance will minimize image

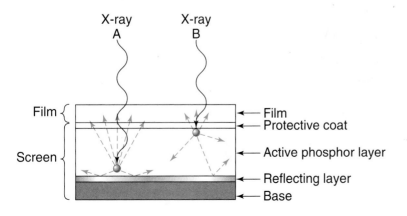

FIGURE 4-10 Screen thickness. X-ray A strikes a crystal far from the film and the divergent light exposes a wide area of the film, resulting in unsharpness. X-ray B strikes a crystal close to the film, resulting in less divergence of the light that exposes the film and therefore a sharper image. The thicker the screen, the less sharp the image.

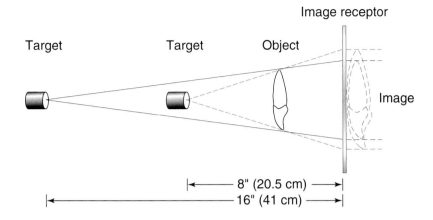

FIGURE 4-11 **Magnification.** Comparison of 8-in. (20.5-cm) and 16-in. (41-cm) target-object and target–image receptor distances. The image is magnified (enlarged) when these distances are shortened.

magnification. Note that these two shadow cast rules for reducing magnification also increase image sharpness.

Distortion

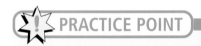

Distortion is the result of unequal magnification of different parts of the same object. Distortion results when the image receptor is not parallel to the object (Figure 4-13) and/or when the central ray of the x-ray beam is not perpendicular to the object and the plane of the image receptor (Figure 4-14). To minimize image distortion, the two shadow cast rules for placement of the image receptor and x-ray beam positioning must be followed. Rules 4 and 5 state that the plane of the image receptor must be positioned parallel to the long axes of the teeth, and the central ray of the x-ray beam must be aligned perpendicular to both the image receptor and the teeth.

Effects of Varying the Exposure Factors

Density and contrast have a tremendous influence on the diagnostic quality of the radiograph. The x-ray machine exposure settings can affect both density and contrast (Table 4-3).

PRACTICE POINT

When positioning the PID for intraoral exposures, it is important to place the open end of the PID as close as possible to (without touching) the skin surface of the patient's face. Image quality is improved when the target–surface distance is increased. However, it is important to note that increasing the distance between the target and the skin surface of the patient is determined by the length of the PID and not by positioning the PID a greater distance away from the patient (Figure 4-12). Positioning the open end of the PID away from the skin surface of the patient's face will result in a larger diameter of radiation exposure and an underexposed image.

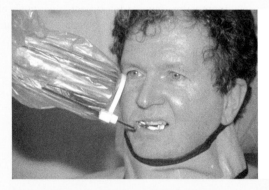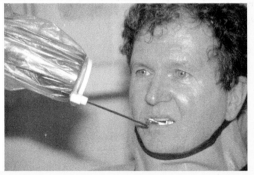

FIGURE 4-12 **Correct and incorrect PID positioning.** Left image illustrates the correct position of the open end of the PID as close to the patient's skin as possible. Right image illustrates an incorrect position of the PID. This PID position will result in a greater beam diameter of exposure to the patient and will produce an underexposed image.

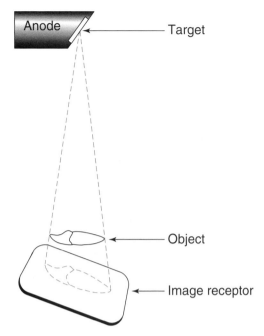

FIGURE 4-13 Object and image receptor are not parallel, resulting in distortion.

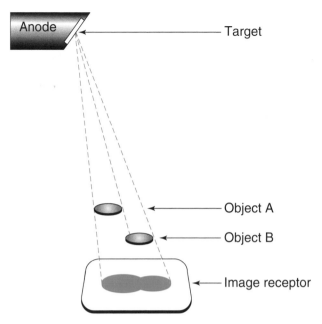

FIGURE 4-14 **Central ray of x-ray beam is not perpendicular to the objects and image receptor,** resulting in distortion and overlapping of object A and object B. Note that object A is magnified larger than object B because object A is a greater distance from the image receptor than object B.

The milliamperage, exposure time, and kilovoltage are known as the **exposure,** control, or radiation **factors.** Whenever one of the exposure factors is altered, one or a combination of the other factors must be altered proportionally to maintain radiographic density. For example, exposure time will need to be decreased when milliamperage or kilovoltage is increased to maintain optimal image density.

Variations in Milliamperage (mA)

The amount of electric current used in the x-ray machine is expressed in **milliamperes (mA).** The mA selected by the operator, or preset by the unit manufacturer, determines the quantity or number of x-rays that are generated within the tube. The density of the radiograph is affected whenever the milliamperage is changed. Increasing the mA increases (darkens) the density of the radiograph, whereas decreasing the mA decreases (lightens) the density of the radiograph.

Variations in Exposure Time

Exposure time is the interval that the x-ray machine is fully activated and x-rays are produced. The principal effect of changes in exposure time is on the density of the radiograph. Increasing the exposure time darkens the radiograph, whereas decreasing exposure time lightens it. Opinions differ on optimum density and contrast because visual perception varies from person to person; some practitioners may prefer lighter radiographs, whereas others may prefer darker radiographs. Of the three controls, exposure time is easiest to change. In fact, many x-ray machines today have preset fixed milliamperage and kilovoltage, so that time is the only exposure factor that can be changed by the operator.

TABLE 4-3 Effect of Varying Exposure Factors on Image Density	
EXPOSURE ADJUSTMENT[a]	IMAGE DENSITY
Increase mA	Darker
Decrease mA	Lighter
Increase time	Darker
Decrease time	Lighter
Increase kVp	Darker[b]
Decrease kVp	Lighter[b]

[a]When any exposure factor is increased, or decreased, one or more of the other exposure factors must be adjusted to maintain optimum image density.
[b]Varying kVp primarily affects the image contrast, but it will also (secondarily) affect the image density. Increase kVp for less contrast and decrease kVp for more contrast.

Milliampere/seconds (mAs)

Because both milliamperage and exposure time are used to regulate the number of x-rays generated and have the same effect on radiographic density, they are often combined into a common factor called **milliampere/seconds (mAs).** Combining the milliamperage with the exposure time is an effective way to determine the total radiation generated.

A simple formula for determining this total is: mA multiplied by the exposure time (in seconds or impulses) equals mAs.

$$mA \times s = mAs$$

PROBLEM. Consider a practical problem using this formula. Assume the following exposure factors are in use: 10 mA, 0.6 sec, 90 kVp, and 12-in. (30-cm) target–image receptor distance. If the mA is increased to 15, but the kVp and target–image receptor distance remain constant, what should the new exposure time be to maintain image density?

SOLUTION. The only exposure factor that was changed is the mA, which was increased from 10 mA to 15 mA. We need to compensate for the increase in mA by decreasing the exposure time.

$$mA \times s = mAs$$
$$10\,mA \times 0.6\,sec. = 6\,mAs$$
$$15\,mA \times ?\,sec. = 6\,mAs$$
$$?\,sec. = \frac{6\,mAs}{15\,mAs}$$
$$?\,sec. = 0.4\,sec$$

ANSWER. The new exposure time is 0.4 sec.

When the mA is increased, the exposure time must be decreased to produce identical radiographic image density between the first and second radiographs. A practical use for applying this formula would be when patient movement is anticipated—in this case, increasing the amount of radiation produced, so that the duration of exposure could be shortened.

Variations in Kilovoltage (kVp)

The quality of the radiation (wavelength or energy of the x-ray photons) generated by the x-ray machine is determined by the kilovoltage peak (kVp). The more the kVp is increased, the shorter the wavelength and the higher the energy and penetrating power of the x-rays produced. Kilovoltage is the only exposure factor that directly influences the contrast of a dental radiograph. However, increasing the kVp will also increase the number (quantity) of x-rays produced and therefore, increase the density of the radiograph. As the kVp of the x-ray beam is increased for the purpose of producing a lower contrast image, the density of the radiograph is held constant by reducing the milliampere-seconds (mAs) or exposure time. Because the exposure time is usually the easiest exposure factor to change, the following rule applies: When increasing the kVp by 15, for example from 70 kVp to 85 kVp, decrease the exposure time by dividing by 2; when decreasing the kVp by 15, increase the exposure time by multiplying by 2. One exposure factor balances the other to produce a radiographic image of acceptable density.

Effects of Variations in Distances

The operator must take into account several distances to produce the ideal diagnostic quality image:

• The distance between the x-ray source (at the focal spot on the target) and the surface of the patient's skin
• The distance between the object to be x-rayed (usually the teeth) and the image receptor
• The distance between the x-ray source and the recording plane of the image receptor

Various terms are used to describe these distances. The terms target–surface (skin), anode–surface, tube–surface, and source–surface are synonymous, as are target–image receptor, anode–image receptor, and source–image receptor. In this text, the terms target–surface distance, object–image receptor distance, target–object distance, and target–image receptor distance are used (Figure 4-15).

Target–Surface Distance

Generally, whenever the image receptor is positioned intraorally, the length of the **target–surface distance** depends on the length of the **position indicating device (PID)** used. All intraoral techniques require the open end of the PID be positioned to almost touch the patient's skin to standardize the distance used and the image density.

Object–Image Receptor Distance

The object–image receptor distance depends largely on the method that is employed to hold the receptor in position next to the teeth. When the bisecting technique is used (see Chapter 15), the image receptor is pressed against the palatal or lingual tissues as close as the oral anatomy will permit. This results in the object–image receptor distance being shorter in the area of the crown where the tooth and image receptor touch than in the area of the root, where the thickness of the bone and gingiva may cause a divergence between the long axis of the tooth and the image receptor (Figure 4-16). The least divergence occurs in the mandibular molar areas. The greatest divergence is in the maxillary anterior areas, where the palatal structures may curve sharply.

With the paralleling technique, most image receptor holders are designed so that the receptor is held parallel to the long axis of the tooth of interest. This necessitates positioning the receptor sufficiently into the middle of the oral cavity, away from the teeth, to avoid impinging on the supporting bone and gingival structures. This technique results in object–image receptor distances that are often more than 1 in. (25 mm). The paralleling technique compensates for this increased object–image receptor distance by recommending an increase in the target–image receptor distance (use a longer PID) to help offset the distortion, explained next.

Target–Image Receptor Distance

The target–image receptor distance is the sum of the target–object and the object–image receptor distance (Figure 4-15). The quality of the radiographic image improves whenever the target–image receptor distance is increased. Magnification

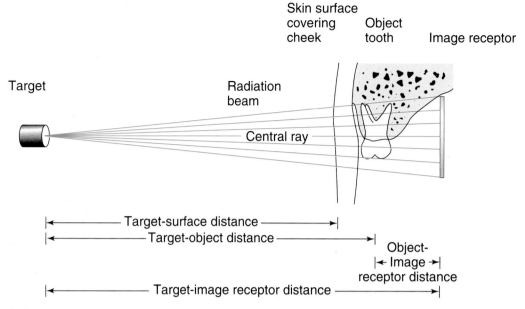

FIGURE 4-15 Distances. Relationship among target, skin surface, object (tooth), and image receptor distance.

is reduced, and sharpness of detail (definition) is increased. Increasing the target-image receptor distance reduces the fuzzy outline (penumbra) that is seen around the radiographic images. Therefore, positioning the image receptor far enough from the teeth to enable it to be held parallel and using a long 12-in. (30-cm) or 16-in. (41-cm) PID will increase the quality of the image definition. These techniques are described in detail in Chapter 13.

The location of the x-ray tube within the tube housing can affect the target–image receptor distance. In the conventional dental x-ray machine, the target (located on the anode within the tube) is situated in the tube head in front of the transformers. The attached PID length can be visibly determined. When the tube is recessed within the tube head, located behind the transformers, enough space is gained within the tube head so that a long target–image receptor distance is achieved even though a short PID is in place (see Figure 3-1).

Inverse Square Law

The x-ray photons, traveling in straight lines, spread out (diverge) as they radiate away from the source (target). It follows that the intensity of the beam is reduced as this occurs (Figure 4-17). How much the beam intensity decreases is based on the **inverse square law,** which states that the intensity of radiation varies inversely as the square of the distance from its source.

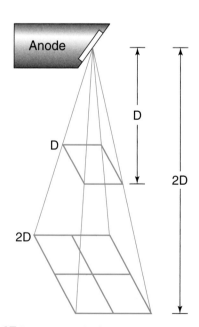

FIGURE 4-17 Inverse square law. Relationship of distance (D) to the area covered by x-rays emitted from the x-ray tube. X-rays emerging from the tube travel in straight lines and diverge from each other. The areas covered by the x-rays at any two points are proportional to each other as the square of the distances measured from the source of radiation.

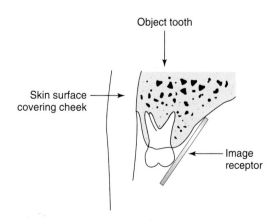

FIGURE 4-16 Object–image receptor distance. This placement of the image receptor places the crown of the tooth closer to the receptor than the root.

The inverse square law may be written as:

$$\frac{I_1}{I_2} = \frac{(D_2)^2}{(D_1)^2}$$

where:

    I_1 is the original intensity

    I_2 is the new intensity

    D_1 is the original distance

    D_2 is the new distance

The inverse square law is applied when considering the distance between the source of radiation and the image receptor, as in the length of the PID, and when considering the distance between the source of radiation and the operator, as in where the operator stands to maintain radiation protection during exposure. The distance between the source of radiation and the image receptor will have an affect on the image quality. When changing the PID length, a corresponding change must occur in the exposure time to maintain image density. It is important to understand that the intensity of the radiation decreases by the square of the distance increased.

Consider the following problem where distance is considered as a means of operator protection.

PROBLEM. A dental radiographer stands 3 feet (0.9 m) from the source of radiation where the measured intensity is 100 milliroentgens (mR) per minute. The radiographer then moves to a new location 6 ft (1.8 m) from the source of radiation. What is the radiation intensity at the new location?

SOLUTION.

$$I_1 = 100 \text{ mR/min}$$
$$D_1 = 3 \text{ ft}$$
$$D_2 = 6 \text{ ft}$$

Find I_2.

$$\frac{100}{I_1} = \frac{6^2}{3^2}$$

$$\frac{100}{I_2} = \frac{2^2}{1^2}$$

$$\frac{100}{I_2} = \frac{4}{1}$$

$$\left(\frac{1}{4}\right)\frac{100}{I_2} = \frac{4}{1}\left(\frac{1}{4}\right)$$

$$I_2 = 25 \text{ mR per minute}$$

ANSWER. The intensity at the new location is 25 mR/min.

In this case, the radiographer's new location is a safer place to stand during exposure because this new location at 6 ft away from the source of radiation receives only one-fourth the exposure of the old location at 3 ft away for the source of radiation.

Consider the following problem where distance is considered when changing the length of the PID.

PROBLEM. A quality dental radiograph is obtained using an 8-in. (20.5-cm) PID and an exposure time of 3 impulses. The 8-in. (20.5-cm) PID is removed from the tube head and replaced with a 16-in. (41 cm) PID. What should the new exposure time be to maintain image density of radiographs exposed at this new target–image receptor distance?

We know that the radiation intensity at a distance of 16 inches (41 cm) will be less than the intensity at the old distance of 8 inches (20.5-cm). Applying the inverse square law formula we would see that the intensity of the radiation will have decreased by the square of the distance, producing a radiographic image that would be less dense (lighter) than the original radiograph produced using an 8-in. (20.5-cm) PID. To produce a radiograph of equal density using a 16-in. (41-cm) PID, use the following modification of the inverse square law formula to determine the new exposure setting:

$$\frac{I_1}{I_2} = \frac{(D_1)^2}{(D_2)^2}$$

where:

    I_1 is the original exposure time (in impulses)

    I_2 is the new exposure time (in impulses)

    D_1 is the original distance

    D_2 is the new distance

SOLUTION.

$$I_1 = 3 \text{ impulses}$$
$$D_1 = 8 \text{ inches}$$
$$D_2 = 16 \text{ inches}$$

Find I_2.

$$\frac{3}{I_2} = \frac{8^2}{16^2}$$

$$\frac{3}{I_2} = \frac{1^2}{2^2}$$

$$\frac{3}{I_2} = \frac{1}{4}$$

$$\frac{(4)3}{I_2} = \frac{1(4)}{4}$$

$$I_2 = 12 \text{ impulses}$$

ANSWER. The impulse setting required to maintain image density at the new 16-in. (41-cm) source-to-image receptor distance is 12 impulses.

Because the x-rays emerging from the tube travel in straight lines and diverge from one another, it follows that the intensity of the beam is reduced unless a corresponding increase is made in one or a combination of the target–image receptor distance exposure factors. Such changes in exposure factors are essential to maintaining optimum image density. Usually time is the easiest exposure factor to change. This formula is useful for obtaining the appropriate exposure time when only the target–image receptor distance is altered.

Exposure Charts

Operators may memorize exposure factors needed for a particular technique; however, safety protocol dictates that **exposure charts,** available commercially or custom made by the practice, be posted at the x-ray unit control panel for easy reference. In fact, in some locations regulations require that exposure charts be posted. These charts show at a glance how much exposure time is required for a film of any given speed or a digital sensor when used with all possible combinations of exposure time, milliamperage, and peak kilovoltage.

Some dental x-ray machine manufacturers have incorporated the commonly used exposure factors into the dial of the control panel. With these units, the operator only has to set the pointer to the desired region to be examined, and the unit automatically sets the required exposure factors.

REVIEW—Chapter summary

An acceptable diagnostic radiograph must show the areas of interest—the designated teeth and surrounding bone structures—completely and with minimum distortion and maximum sharpness. When evaluating a radiographic image, the oral health care professional should utilize appropriate scientific terminology such as density, contrast, sharpness, magnification, and distortion. The term *radiolucent* refers to the dark or black portion of the image, whereas the term *radiopaque* refers to the light or white portion of the image. High-contrast images, those with black and white and few shades of gray, are called short-scale, whereas low-contrast images, those with grayer whites and grayer blacks with many shades of gray, are called long-scale.

The detail and visibility of a radiograph depends on two factors—radiographic contrast and sharpness/definition. Radiographic contrast depends on: the subject (types of tissues being imaged), kilovoltage peak (kVp) setting, scatter radiation, film/digital sensor type, exposure, and processing. Sharpness is determined by the geometric factors: focal spot size, target–image receptor distance, object–image receptor distance, motion, screen thickness, and screen–film contact, and by the crystal/pixel size of the image receptor.

To create a sharp image, the radiographer must follow the rules for casting a shadow image: small focal spot, long target–image receptor distance, short object–image receptor distance, parallel relationship between object and image receptor, and perpendicular relationship between central ray of the x-ray beam and the object and image receptor. Image magnification and loss of sharpness is further reduced by limiting movement of the tube head and PID, the patient, and the image receptor during exposure.

Although not all dental x-ray units allow the operator to manually alter all exposure factors, when available, the radiographer should take advantage of the ability to vary the exposure factors to produce radiographs that have the desired image qualities. When altering one exposure factor, a corresponding change must be made to another factor to produce identical radiographic image density. The formula for altering

exposure time and milliamperage is mA × s = mAs, where the mA is multiplied by the exposure time to determine the millimaperage seconds. The formula for altering kilovoltage is if increasing the kVp by 15, decrease the exposure time by dividing by 2; if decreasing the kVp by 15, increase the exposure time by multiplying by 2.

When changing the PID length, the inverse square law is used to adjust the exposure time to produce identical radiographic image density. This inverse square law states that the intensity of radiation varies inversely as the square of the distance from its source. The inverse square law formula is

$$\frac{I_1}{I_2} = \frac{(D_1)^2}{(D_2)^2}$$

RECALL—Study questions

1. List the three criteria for acceptable radiographs.
   a. _____
   b. _____
   c. _____

2. Dense objects appear radiolucent *because* dense objects absorb the passage of x-rays.
   a. Both the statement and reason are correct and related.
   b. Both the statement and reason are correct but NOT related.
   c. The statement is correct, but the reason is NOT.
   d. The statement is NOT correct, but the reason is correct.
   e. NEITHER the statement NOR the reason is correct.

3. The degree of darkening of the radiographic image is referred to as
   a. contrast.
   b. definition.
   c. density.
   d. penumbra.

4. Which of the following describes the radiographic image produced with a kVp exposure setting of 100?
   a. Short scale
   b. Long scale
   c. High contrast
   d. Low density

5. Image contrast is NOT affected by
   a. processing procedures.
   b. type of film.
   c. scatter radiation.
   d. milliamperage.

6. What factor has the greatest effect on image sharpness?
   a. Movement
   b. Filtration
   c. Kilovoltage
   d. Amperage

7. As crystals in the film emulsion increase in size, the radiographic image sharpness increases *because* the amount of radiation needed to expose the film at an acceptable density decreases.
   a. Both the statement and reason are correct and related.
   b. Both the statement and reason are correct but NOT related.
   c. The statement is correct, but the reason is NOT.
   d. The statement is NOT correct, but the reason is correct.
   e. NEITHER the statement NOR the reason is correct.

8. What term best describes a fuzzy shadow around the outline of the radiographic image?
   a. Magnification
   b. Distortion
   c. Detail
   d. Penumbra

9. Distortion results when
   a. object and image receptor are not parallel.
   b. x-ray beam is perpendicular to the object and image receptor.
   c. using a short object–image receptor distance.
   d. using a small focal spot.

10. The dental radiograph will appear less dense (lighter) if one increases the
    a. mA.
    b. kVp.
    c. exposure time.
    d. target–image receptor distance.

11. The exposure factors used at an oral health care facility are: 10 mA, 0.9 sec, 70 kVp, and 16-in. (41-cm) target–image receptor distance. The radiographer increases the mA to 15, but leaves the kVp and target–image receptor distance constant. To maintain identical image density, what should the new exposure time be?
    a. 0.3
    b. 0.6
    c. 1.2
    d. 1.8

12. Which of the following is appropriate to increase radiographic contrast while maintaining image density?
    a. Increase the kVp and increase the exposure time.
    b. Increase the kVp and decrease the exposure time.
    c. Decrease the kVp and increase the exposure time.
    d. Decrease the kVp and decrease the exposure time.

13. Based on the inverse square law, what happens to the intensity of the x-ray beam when the target–image receptor distance is doubled?
    a. Intensity is doubled.
    b. Intensity is not affected.
    c. Intensity is one-half as great.
    d. Intensity is one-fourth as great.

14. A radiographer stands 4 ft (1.22 m) from the head of the patient while exposing a dental radiograph. Her personnel monitoring device measures the radiation dose at that position to be 0.04 millisievert (mSv). The radiographer decides to move to a new location 8 ft (2.44 m) from the head of the patient. What is the dose at the new location?
    a. 0.01 mSv
    b. 0.02 mSv
    c. 0.08 mSv
    d. 0.16 mSv

15. A patient presents whose radiographs must be taken utilizing the bisecting technique. The radiographer decides to replace the 16-in. (41-cm) PID with an 8-in. (20.5-cm) PID to better accommodate the bisecting technique. Currently the impulse setting, with the 16-in. (41-cm) PID, is 12. To maintain image density, what will the new impulse setting be with the 8-in. (20.5-cm) PID?
    a. 3
    b. 6
    c. 24
    d. 48

REFLECT—Case study

You have just been hired to work in a new oral health care facility. Prior to providing patient services, you are asked to help develop exposure settings and equipment recommendations for the practice. The equipment and image receptor manufacturers' suggestions are as follows:

F Speed Film   8-in. (20.5-cm) PID   85 kVp

| | Impulses | |
Bitewings	Adult	Child
Posterior	10	8
Anterior	6	4
Periapicals		
Maxillary anterior	8	6
Maxillary premolar	12	8
Maxillary molar	14	10
Mandibular anterior	6	4
Mandibular premolar	8	6
Mandibular molar	10	8

1. You recommend that the facility replace the 8-in. (20.5-cm) PID with a 16-in. (41-cm) PID. Develop a new exposure chart for using the new 16-in. (41-cm) PID.

2. You recommend using a kVp setting of 70 when exposing radiographs for the purpose of detecting caries. Develop a new exposure chart for 70 kVp.

3. You recommend using a kVp setting of 100 when exposing radiographs for the purpose of evaluating supporting bone and periodontal disease. Develop a new exposure chart for 100 kVp.

RELATE—Laboratory application

Obtain an inanimate object of varying densities that can be exposed at different exposure variables and compare the results. For example expose a seashell placed on a size #2 intraoral film at the following exposure settings: 7 mA, 70 kVp, 10 impulses. Expose subsequent films varying one or more of the exposure settings and process normally. Using a view box, analyze the resultant radiographic images. Identify which settings produced darker or lighter images, and which settings produced low or high contrast images.

REFERENCES

Carestream Health Inc. (2007). *Exposure and processing for dental film radiography.* Rochester, NY: Author.

Thomson, E. M., & Tolle, S. L. (1994). A practical guide for using radiographs in the assessment of periodontal disease, Part I. *Practical Hygiene, 3*(1):11–16.

White, S. C., & Pharoah, M. J. (2008). *Oral radiology: Principles and interpretation* (6th ed.). St. Louis, MO: Mosby Elsevier.

PART II • BIOLOGICAL EFFECTS OF RADIATION AND RADIATION PROTECTION

Effects of Radiation Exposure

OBJECTIVES

Following successful completion of this chapter, you should be able to:

1. Define the key words.
2. Explain the difference between the direct and indirect theories of biological damage.
3. Determine the relative radiosensitivity or radioresistance of various kinds of cells in the body.
4. Explain the difference between somatic and genetic effects.
5. Explain the difference between a threshold dose–response curve and a nonthreshold dose–response curve.
6. Identify the factors that determine radiation injuries.
7. List the sequence of events that may follow exposure to radiation.
8. Explain the difference between deterministic and stochastic effects.
9. List the possible short- and long-term effects of irradiation.
10. Identify critical tissues for dental radiography in the head and neck region.
11. Discuss the risks versus benefits of dental radiographs.
12. Utilize effective dose equivalent to make radiation exposure comparisons.
13. Adopt an ethical responsibility to follow ALARA.

KEY WORDS

Acute radiation syndrome (ARS)
ALARA (as low as reasonably achievable)
Cumulative effect
Deterministic effect
Direct theory
Dose–response curve
Genetic cells
Genetic effect
Genetic mutation
Indirect theory

Ionization
Irradiation
Irreparable injury
Latent period
Law of B and T
Lethal dose (LD)
Nonthreshold dose–response curve
Period of injury
Radiolysis of water
Radioresistant

KEY WORDS (*Continued*)		
Radiosensitive	Somatic cells	Stochastic effect
Recovery period	Somatic effect	Threshold dose–response curve
Risk		

Introduction

Patients are often concerned with the safety of dental x-ray procedures. Such concerns are shared by oral health care professionals. The fact that ionizing radiation produces biological damage has been known for many years. The first x-ray burn was reported just a few months following Roentgen's discovery of x-rays in 1895. As early as 1902, the first case of x-ray-induced skin cancer was reported in the literature. Events such as the 1945 bombing of Hiroshima and the 1986 Chernobyl nuclear power plant accident continued to generate unfavorable attitudes toward ionizing radiation and concern over the use of x-rays in dentistry and medicine as well. Although public concern is warranted, there are also some sensational and unsubstantiated articles appearing in newspapers and magazines, on television, and on the Internet. Much of what we know about the effects of radiation exposure comes from data that is extrapolated from high doses and high dose rates. Studies of occupational workers exposed to chronic low levels of radiation have shown no adverse biological effect (U.S. Nuclear Regulatory Commission, http://www.nrc.gov). However, even the radiation experts have not been able to determine whether or not a threshold level exists below which radiation effects would not be a risk. Because even the experts cannot always predict a specific outcome from an amount of radiation exposure, the radiation protection community conservatively assumes that any amount of radiation may pose a risk. The purpose of this chapter is to explain the theories of radiation injury and to identify factors that increase the risk of producing a biological response.

Theories of Biological Effect Mechanisms

As pointed out in Chapter 2, x-rays belong to the ionizing portion of the electromagnetic spectrum. X-rays have the ability to detach and remove electric charges from the complex atoms that make up the molecules of body tissues. This process, known as

ionization, creates an electrical imbalance within the normally stable cells. Because disturbed cellular atoms or molecules generally attempt to regain electrical stability, they often accept the first available opposite electrical charge. In such cases, the undesirable chemical changes become incompatible with the surrounding body tissues. During ionization, the delicate balance of the cell structure is altered, and the cell may be damaged or destroyed.

There are two generally accepted theories on how radiation damages biological tissues: (1) the direct theory and (2) the indirect (radiolysis of water) theory (Figure 5-1).

- **Direct theory:** According to the direct theory, x-ray photons collide with important cell chemicals and break them apart by ionization, causing critical damage to large molecules. One-third of biological alterations from x-radiation exposure result from a direct effect. However, most dental x-ray photons probably pass through the cell with little or no damage. A healthy cell can repair any minor damage that might occur. Moreover, the body contains so many cells that the destruction of a single cell or a small group of cells will have no observable effect.

- **Indirect theory** (**Radiolysis of water**): This theory is based on the assumption that radiation can cause chemical damage to the cell by ionizing the water within it (Figure 5-2). Because about 80 percent of body weight is water and ionization can dissociate water into hydrogen and hydroxyl radicals, the theory proposes that new chemicals such as hydrogen peroxide could be formed under certain conditions. These chemicals act as toxins (poisons) to the body, causing cellular dysfunction. Two-thirds of biological alterations from x-radiation exposure result from indirect effects. Fortunately, when the water is broken down during irradiation, the ions have a strong tendency to recombine immediately to form water again instead of seeking out new combinations, keeping cellular damage to a minimum. Under ordinary circumstances, even when a new chemical such as
(poison water theory)
H_2O_2

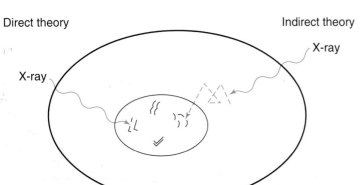

Direct theory | Indirect theory

X-ray

X-ray

FIGURE 5-1 Direct theory and indirect theory. In the direct theory, x-ray photons collide with large molecules and break them apart by ionization. The indirect theory is based on the assumption that radiation can cause chemical damage to the cell by ionizing the water within it.

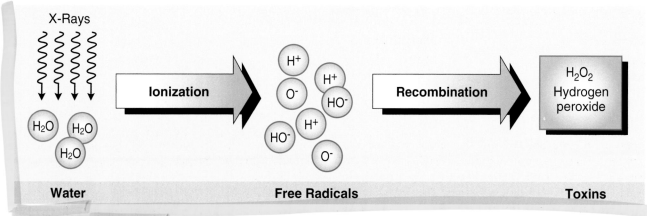

FIGURE 5-2 **Indirect theory.** X-rays ionize water, resulting in the formation of free radicals, which recombine to form toxins.

hydrogen peroxide is formed, other cells that are not affected can take over the functions of the damaged cells until recovery takes place. Only in extreme instances, where massive irradiation has taken place, will entire body tissues be destroyed or death result. However, it should be remembered that cellular destruction is not the only biological effect; the potential exists for the cell to become malignant.

Cell Sensitivity to Radiation Exposure

The terms **radiosensitive** and **radioresistant** are used to describe the degree of susceptibility of various cells and body tissues to radiation. All cells are not equally sensitive to radiation. The relative sensitivity of cells to radiation was first described in 1906 by two French scientists, Bergonie and Tribondeau, and is known as the **law of B and T.** The first half of the law of B and T states that actively dividing cells, such as red blood cells, are more sensitive than slowly dividing cells. The cell is most susceptible to radiation injury during mitosis (cell division). Embryonic and immature cells are more sensitive than mature cells of the same tissue. The second half of the law of B and T states that the more specialized a cell is, the more radioresistant it is. The exceptions to this law are white blood cells (lymphocytes) and reproductive cells (oocytes), which do not divide and are very specialized and yet are radiosensitive.

Based on these factors, it is possible to rank various kinds of cells in descending order of radiosensitivity:

- White blood cells (lymphocytes)   High sensitivity
- Red blood cells (erythrocytes)
- Immature reproductive cells
- Epithelial cells
- Endothelial cells
- Connective tissue cells
- Bone cells
- Nerve cells
- Brain cells
- Muscle cells   Low sensitivity

more sensitive = less resistant

Additionally, a distinction should be made between irradiation of somatic cells and reproductive cells. Somatic cells are all the cells of the body, except the reproductive cells. A **somatic effect** occurs when the biological change or damage occurs in the irradiated individual, but is not passed along to offspring. A **genetic effect** describes the changes in hereditary material that do not manifest in the irradiated individual, but in future generations.

The experts do not fully understand all these effects or their future consequences. Scientists believe that some of these effects are **cumulative,** especially if exposure is too great and the intervals between exposures too frequent for the body cells to repair themselves. Unless the damage is too severe or the subject is in extremely poor health, many body cells (somatic cells) have a recovery rate of almost 75 percent during the first 24 hours; after that, repair continues at the same rate.

In determining whether or not an exposure is potentially harmful, the radiographer should consider the quantity and the duration of the exposure and which body area is to be **irradiated.** Continued exposure over prolonged periods alters the ability of the **genetic cells** (eggs and sperm) to reproduce normally. Current evidence indicates that chromosome damage is cumulative, increasing in effect by each successive additional radiation exposure, and genetic cells cannot repair themselves. Radiation may alter the genetic material in the reproductive cells so that mutations (abnormalities) may be produced in future generations.

The Dose–Response Curve

Radiation doses, like doses of drugs or other biologically harmful agents, can be plotted with response or damage produced, in an attempt to establish acceptable levels of exposure. In plotting these two variables, a **dose–response curve** is produced. A **threshold dose–response curve** indicates that there is a "threshold" amount of radiation, below which no biological response would be expected; a **nonthreshold dose–response curve** indicates that any amount of radiation, no matter how small, has the potential to cause a biological response. These two possibilities are illustrated in Figure 5-3.

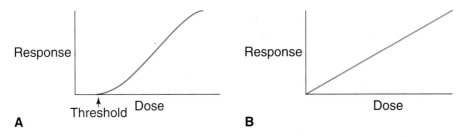

FIGURE 5-3 Diagram of dose–response curve. (**A**) A typical "threshold" curve. The point at which the curve intersects the base line (horizontal line) is the threshold dose that is the dose below which there is no response. If an easily observable radiation effect, such as erythema (reddening of the skin) is taken as "response," then this type of curve is applicable. (**B**) A linear "nonthreshold" curve, in which the curve intersects the base line at its origin. Here it is assumed that any dose, no matter how small, causes some response.

Unfortunately, radiobiologists have been unable to determine radiation effects at very low levels of exposure (for example, doses below 100 mSv) and cannot be certain whether or not a threshold dose exists. (To help put 100 mSv into perspective, a full mouth series of 18 F-speed films, at 90 kVp with 16-in. [41-cm] length PID is approximately 30 mSv skin exposure.) Therefore, the radiation protection community takes the conservative approach and considers any amount of ionizing radiation exposure as being nonthreshold. This assumption has been made in the establishment of radiation protection guidelines and in radiation control activities. The concept that every dose of radiation produces damage and should be kept to the minimum necessary to meet diagnostic requirements is known as the **ALARA** concept, where ALARA stands for **as low as reasonably achievable.** ALARA is explained in detail in Chapter 6.

Factors That Determine Radiation Injury

Biological responses to low doses of radiation exposure are often too small to be detected. The body's defense mechanisms and ability to repair molecular damage often result in no residual effects. In fact, the following five outcomes are possible: (1) nothing—the cell is unaffected by the exposure; (2) the cell is injured or damaged but repairs itself and functions at preexposure levels; (3) the cell dies, but is replaced through normal biological processes; (4) the cell is injured or damaged, repairs itself, but now functions at a reduced level; or (5) the cell is injured or damaged and repairs itself incorrectly or abnormally, resulting in a biophysical change (tumor or malignacy). Determining which of these five outcomes might occur depends on all the following.

Total dose: The total dose of radiation depends on the type, energy, and duration of the radiation. The greater the dose, the more severe the probable biological effect.

Dose rate: The rate at which the radiation is administered or absorbed is very important in the determination of what effects will occur. Because a considerable degree of recovery occurs from the radiation damage, a given dose will produce less effect if it is divided (thus allowing time for recovery between dose increments) than if it is given in a single exposure. For instance, an exposure of 1 R/week for 100 weeks would result in less injury than a single exposure of 100 R.

Area exposed: The amount of injury to the individual depends on the area or volume of tissue irradiated. The larger the area exposed, other factors being equal, the greater the injury to the organism. Intraoral dental radiographic exposures use a very small (2.75 in. or 7 cm) beam diameter (or less if using rectangular collimation, see Figure 6-4) to limit the area of radiation exposure to the area of diagnostic concern.

- **Variation in species:** Various species have a wide range of radiosensitivity. Lethal doses for plants and microorganisms are usually hundreds of times higher than those for mammals.

- **Individual sensitivity:** Individuals vary in sensitivity within the same species. The genetic makeup of some individuals may pre-dispose them to ionizing radiation damage. For this reason the **lethal dose (LD)** for each species is expressed in statistical terms, usually as the LD 50/30 for that species, or the dose required to kill 50% of the individuals in a large population in a 30-day period. For humans, the LD 50/30 is estimated to be 4.5 gray (Gy) or 450 rad (gray and rad are units of absorbed dose; see Chapter 2).

- **Variation in cell sensitivity:** Within the same individual, a wide variation in susceptibility to radiation damage exists among different types of cells and tissues. As the law of B and T points out, cells with a potential for rapid division are more sensitive to radiation than those that do not divide. Furthermore, primitive or nonspecialized cells are more sensitive than those that are highly specialized. Within the same cell families, then, the immature forms, which are generally primitive and rapidly dividing, are more radiosensitive than the older, mature cells, which have specialized function and have ceased to divide.

- **Variation in tissue sensitivity:** Some tissues (organs) of the body are more radiosensitive than others. For instance, blood-forming organs such as the spleen and red bone marrow are more sensitive than the highly specialized heart muscle. *Thyroid, eyes, + mandible are very susceptible.*

☆ Frequency

mutation = alteration of a cell

- **Age:** Younger, more rapidly dividing cells are more radiosensitive than older, mature cells, so it follows that children may be more susceptible to injury than adults from an equal dose of radiation. Also, in children the distance from the oral cavity to the reproductive and other sensitive organs is less than for adults. Therefore the dental doses to the critical organs may be higher than they would be for an adult. Additionally, an increase in radiation sensitivity is observed again in old age. As the body ages, the cells may begin to lose the ability to repair damage.

Sequence of Events Following Radiation Exposure

The sequence of events following radiation exposure are latent period, period of injury, and recovery period, assuming, of course, that the dose received was nonlethal.

- **Latent period:** Following the initial radiation exposure, and before the first detectable effect occurs, a time lag called the latent period occurs. The latent period may be very short or extremely long, depending on the initial dose and other factors described earlier. Effects that appear within a matter of minutes, days, or weeks are called short-term effects, and those that appear years, decades, and even generations later are called long-term effects. Again, this relates to the types of cells involved and their corresponding rates of mitosis (cell division).

- **Period of injury:** Following the latent period, certain effects can be observed. One of the effects seen most frequently in growing tissues exposed to radiation is the stoppage of mitosis, or cell divisions. This may be temporary or permanent, depending on the radiation dosage. Other effects include breaking or clumping of chromosomes, abnormal mitosis, and formation of giant cells (multinucleated cells) associated with cancer.

- **Recovery period:** Following exposure to radiation, some recovery can take place. This is particularly apparent in the case of short-term effects. Nevertheless, there may be a certain amount of damage from which no recovery occurs, and it is this **irreparable injury** that can give rise to later long-term effects (Figure 5-4).

Radiation Effects on Tissues of the Body

Low levels of radiation exposure do not usually produce an observable adverse biological effect. As the dose of radiation increases and enough cells are destroyed, the affected tissue will begin to exhibit clinical signs of damage. The severity of these clinical manifestations is dependent on the dose and dose rate. For example, erythema (redness of the skin) would not be expected from exposing the skin to sunlight for a few seconds. However, as the time of exposure to sunlight increased, the erythema would be expected to increase proportionally. When the severity of the change is dependent on the dose, the effect is called a **deterministic effect.**

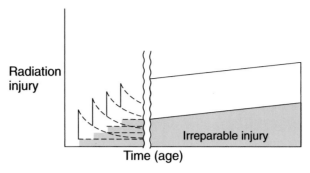

FIGURE 5-4 **Concept of accumulated irreparable injury.** After exposure to radiation cell recovery can take place. However, there may be a certain amount of damage from which no recovery occurs, and it is this irreparable injury that can give rise to later long-term effects.

When a biological response is based on the probability of occurrence rather than the severity of the change, it is called a **stochastic effect.** The occurrence of cancer is a stochastic effect of radiation exposure; it is an "all-or-nothing" occurrence. When the dose of radiation is increased, the "probability" of the stochastic effect (cancer) occurring increases, but not its severity.

Short- and Long-term Effects of Radiation

The effects of radiation are classified as either short term or long term. Short-term effects of radiation are those seen minutes, days, or months after exposure. When a very large dose of radiation is delivered in a very short period of time, the latent period is short. If the dose of radiation is large enough (generally over 1.0 Gy or 100 rads, whole-body), the resultant signs and symptoms that comprise these short-term effects are collectively known as **acute radiation syndrome (ARS).** ARS symptoms include erythema (redness of the skin), nausea, vomiting, diarrhea, hemorrhage, and hair loss. ARS is not a concern in dentistry because dental x-ray machines cannot produce the very large exposures necessary to cause it.

Long-term effects of radiation are those that are seen years after the original exposure. The latent period is much longer (years) than that associated with the acute radiation syndrome (hours or days). Delayed radiation effects may result from a previous acute, high exposure that the individual has survived or from chronic low-level exposures delivered over many years.

No unique disease associated with the long-term effects of radiation has been established. Instead, there can be a statistical increase in the incidence of certain conditions that can have causes other than radiation exposure such as cancer, embryological defects, low birth weights, cataracts, (somatic effects), and genetic mutations (genetic effect). Because of the low normal incidence of these conditions, one must observe large numbers of exposed persons to evaluate the increases as an effect of long-term radiation exposure.

The long-term effects observed have been somatic damage, which may result in an increased incidence of the following.

- **Cancer:** Anything that is capable of causing cancer is called a *carcinogen.* X-rays, like certain drugs, chemicals, and viruses, have been shown to have carcinogenic effects. Carcinogenic mechanisms are not clearly understood. Moreover, cancer is probably "caused" by the simultaneous interaction of several factors, and the presence of some of these factors without the others may not be sufficient to cause the disease.

  Some explanations for the carcinogenic action of x-rays include the following: x-rays activate viruses already present in cells; x-rays damage chromosomes, and certain diseases (such as leukemia) are associated with chromosomal injury; x-rays cause mutations in somatic cells, which may result in uncontrolled growth of cells; and x-rays ionize water, which results in chemical "free radicals" that may cause cancer.

  Any one or a combination of these theories may explain how cancer is caused. X-radiation is only one of a number of possible carcinogens involved, and the precise mechanism is not yet understood. Much of the evidence that x-radiation is carcinogenic comes from studies of early radiation workers, including dentists, who were exposed to large amounts of radiation (Figures 5-5 and 5-6).

- **Embryological defects:** The immature, undifferentiated, rapidly growing cells of the embryo are highly sensitive to radiation. The first trimester of a pregnancy when the fetus undergoes the period of major organogenesis (formation of organs) is especially critical. High doses of radiation may cause birth abnormalities, stunting of growth, and mental retardation. It is important to note that the dose from a dental x-ray examination is less than 0.0003 to 0.003 milligray (0.03 to 0.3 millirad), and the use of a lead or lead-equivalent barrier apron reduces this potential dose to zero.

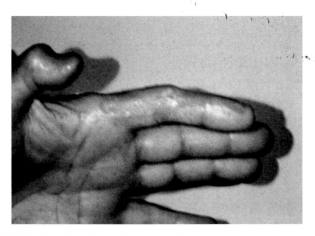

FIGURE 5-6 Radiation injury on the finger of a dentist caused by holding films in the patient's oral cavity during exposure. A lesion of this type would be likely to result in squamous cell carcinoma (cancer).

- **Low birth weight:** Medical (not dental) x-radiation exposure of pregnant females has been associated with an increase in the incidence of full-term pregnancies resulting in below-normal-birth-weight infants. Because the reproductive organs are not located in a critical area, exposure of necessary dental radiographs has not been contraindicated during pregnancy. In 2004 the American Medical Association published research that investigated the effect on pregnancy outcomes of radiation exposure of the pregnant female's hypothalamus and the pituitary and thyroid glands. This research suggests that dental radiation exposure may be associated with full-term low-birth-weight infants. More research in this area may lead to altered guidelines on the assessment of pregnant females for dental radiographs. (Discussed further in Chapter 27.)

- **Cataracts:** When the lens of the eye becomes opaque, it is called a cataract. Various agents, including x-rays, have been known to cause cataracts. It takes at least 2 Gy (200 rads) of x-radiation to cause cataract formation. The dose to the eye from dental radiographic procedures is in the order of milligray (millirad). Dental x-rays have never been reported to cause cataracts.

- **Genetic mutations:** The genetic material is the means by which hereditary traits are passed from one generation to another. In addition to x-radiation, drugs, chemicals, and even elevated body temperatures are also capable of causing mutations. Genetic effects are especially important because it is unknown what size dose of radiation, whether naturally occurring or from man-made sources, may be capable of producing a change in the genetic material of cells.

  Because the scatter radiation reaching the gonads from dental radiography is less than 0.0001 that of the exposure to the surface of the face (ranging from 0.0 to about 0.002 milligrays [0.2 millirad] per radiograph), the risk of genetic mutations is extremely small. Furthermore, by using a lead or lead-equivalent barrier apron and thyroid collar, the dose is essentially reduced to zero.

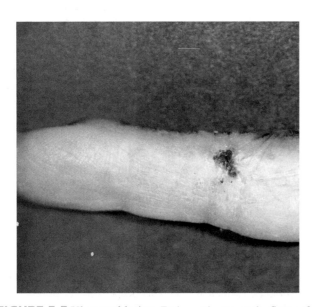

FIGURE 5-5 Ulcerated lesion. Early carcinoma on the finger of a dentist who admitted holding films in the patient's oral cavity during exposure.

Quantity
~~Duraction~~ Duration
Area Irradiated
⊕ Frequency

TABLE 5-1   Critical Organs and Doses for Dental Radiography

CRITICAL ORGAN	EFFECT	MINIMUM DOSE REQUIRED TO PRODUCE EFFECT	DENTAL DOSE FROM A FMS
Eye	cataract	2,000 mSv	0.4 mSv
Hematopoietic	leukemia	50 mSv	8.0 mSv
Skin	cancer	250 mSv	12.6 mSv
Thyroid gland	cancer	65 mSv	0.4 mSv
Gonads	sterility	4,000 to 6,000 mSv	0.005 mSv *(no lead apron)* to 0.0003 mSv *(lead apron)*

Risk Estimates

A **risk** may be defined as the likelihood of injury or death from some hazard. The primary risk from dental radiography is radiation-induced cancer and, possibly, the potential to affect pregnancy outcomes. Otherwise, the facial and oral structures, composed largely of bone, nerve, and muscle tissue, are fairly radioresistant (Table 5-1).

Risk estimates vary, depending on several factors, such as speed of film, collimation, and the technique used. In dental radiography, the most critical tissues of the head and neck are the mandible (red bone marrow), the lens of the eye, the thyroid gland, and possibly the hypothalamus-pituitary-thyroid combination.

The mandible contains an estimated 15 grams of red bone marrow. However, it should be noted that this is only about 1 percent of the total amount of red bone marrow in the adult body. Although x-radiation can cause cataracts, the dental radiation exposure to the lens of the eye during some maxillary exposures is well below the dose needed to produce cataracts. The thyroid gland is relatively radiosensitive. Until recently the focus has been on radiation exposure causing cancer of the thyroid gland. A study published in the Journal of the American Medical Association (2004) has demonstrated a possible link between radiation exposure to the thyroid gland and/or to the hypothalamus-pituitary-thyroid combination of a pregnant female and low-birth-weight infants delivered after the full 9-month term. Until more is documented regarding this phenomenon, the focus is on radiation-induced cancer as the primary risk from dental radiography.

The potential risk of a full mouth dental x-ray examination inducing cancer in a patient has been estimated to be 2.5 per 1,000,000 examinations. It should be noted that every day we assume hundreds of risks such as climbing stairs, crossing the

TABLE 5-2   One in One Million Fatality Risk

RISK	NATURE
Smoking 1.4 cigarettes/day	Cancer
Riding 10 miles on a bicycle	Accident
Travel 300 miles by auto	Accident
Travel 1,000 miles by airplane	Accident

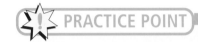

PRACTICE POINT

Dental radiographs should be prescribed only when necessary. Consider the following case: If a female patient is assessed for bitewing radiographs, and then she reveals that she may be pregnant, would the need for the bitewing radiographs change? Would she still need the radiographs? Or would these once-needed radiographs now be radiographs that can wait? If radiographs can wait, they are not necessary radiographs.

street, riding a bicycle, and driving a car. Activities with a fatality risk of 1 in 1,000,000 include riding 300 miles in an automobile, traveling 1,000 miles in an airplane, or smoking 1.4 cigarettes a day (Table 5-2). People accept these risks every day because we perceive a benefit from them.

- **Risk versus benefit:** Dental radiographs should be taken only when the benefit outweighs the risk of biologic injury to the patient. When dental radiographs are properly prescribed (see Chapter 6), exposed, and processed, the health benefits to the patient far outweigh any risk of injury. There have been no reports of radiation injuries caused by normal dental procedures since safety protocols have been adopted.

Radiation Exposure Comparisons

Patients often have questions regarding the amount of radiation dental radiographs are adding to their accumulated lifetime exposure. The exact amount of radiation exposure produced when taking dental radiographs varies, depending on many factors, such as the film speed, technique used, and collimation type (circular or rectangular). Additionally, dental exposures are often quoted as skin surface amounts rather than amounts to the more important bone marrow and other deeper structures

The effective dose equivalent (Chapter 2) can be used to compare dental radiation exposures with days of natural background exposure. The average effective dose equivalent from naturally

TABLE 5-3   Effective Dose Equivalent[a]

EXAMINATION	EFFECTIVE DOSE	DAYS OF NATURAL EXPOSURE[b]
Single intraoral exposure[c]	1.3 μSv	0.2
Bitewing radiographs[c] (4 films)	5.2 μSv	0.7
Full mouth series[c] (18 films)	23.4 μSv	2.9
Panoramic radiograph	7 μSv	0.9
CT scan of the maxilla	240–1200 μSv	40–200
CT scan of the mandible	480–3324 μSv	80–547.5
Cone beam CT mandible	75 μSv	12.5
Cone beam CT maxilla	42 μSv	7
Chest x-ray	80 μSv	10
Upper GI	2440 μSv	305
Lower GI	4060 μSv	507.5

[a]References: White, S. C., & Pharoah, M. (2008). *Oral radiology: Principles and interpretation* (6th ed.). St. Louis, MO: Elsevier, and Horner, K., Drage, N., & Brettle, D. (2008). *21st century imaging.* London: Quintessence Publishing Co Ltd.
[b]Fractions rounded up.
[c]F-speed, round PID.

occuring background radiation to the population of the United States is approximately 8 μSv (microseiverts) per day. A full mouth series of radiographs using F-speed film and a round PID has an effective dose equivalent of approximately 23.4 μSv. Therefore, the full mouth series is equal to approximately 2.9 days of naturally occurring background radiation exposure (Table 5-3).

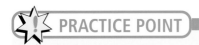

PRACTICE POINT

Be careful not to tell the patient that a full mouth series is equal to 2.9 days "in the sun." Naturally occurring background radiation includes not only the sun, or cosmic energy, but also terrestrial and internal sources of background radiation (see Chapter 2). Additionally, most patients are aware that exposure to the sun's rays is harmful and many take precautions against putting themselves at risk for skin damage. To compare dental x-rays to sun exposure may provoke a response from the patient to avoid dental x-rays as well.

Much about radiation effects remains to be discovered. Future research may demonstrate that human beings are not as sensitive to radiation damage as we now believe. But until we have such evidence, common sense dictates improving radiographic safety techniques in every way possible.

REVIEW—Chapter summary

Ionizing radiation has the potential to produce biological damage because x-rays can detach subatomic particles from larger molecules and create an imbalance within a normally stable cell. The two generally accepted theories on how radiation may cause damage to cellular tissues are: (1) the direct theory, and (2) the indirect theory or the radiolysis of water. Whether cell damage from radiation is physical or chemical, it has been established that minor damage is soon repaired by a healthy body.

The terms *radiosensitive* and *radioresistant* are used to describe the degree of susceptibility of various cells and body tissues to radiation. According to the law of B and T, cells that are highly specialized and have a lesser reproductive capacity are considered to be radioresistant, and cells that are undifferentiated and have a greater capacity for reproduction are considered to be radiosensitive.

Biological changes or damage that occur in somatic cells will affect the irradiated individual but will not be passed along to offspring. Biological changes or damage that do not affect the irradiated individual but are passed to future generations are called genetic effects.

The cumulative effect of irradiation is defined as an amount of radiation damage from which no recovery occurs, giving rise to later long-term effects.

The dose–response curve is a method used to plot the dosage of radiation administered with the response produced to establish responsible levels of radiation exposure. The conservative view that every dose of radiation potentially produces damage and should be kept to a minimum is expressed by the ALARA concept—as low as reasonably achievable.

Factors that influence a biological response to irradiation include dose amount, dose rate, area exposed, species exposed, individual sensitivity, cell sensitivity, tissue sensitivity, and age. Assuming that the dose received is not lethal, the sequence of events following radiation exposure are (1) a latent period, (2) a period of injury, and (3) a recovery period.

The term *deterministic* is used when referring to a tissue response, such as erythema, whose severity is directly related to the radiation dose. The term *stochastic effect* is used when referring to a tissue response, such as cancer, that is based on the probability of occurrence rather then the severity of the response.

The effects of radiation exposure may be short or longterm. Short-term effects include erythema and general discomfort. Long-term effects may result in an increased incidence of cancer, embryological defects, poor pregnancy outcomes, cataracts, and genetic mutations.

The potential benefits of dental radiographs outweigh the risk. With proper radiation safety protocol, there is minimal risk of injury caused by necessary dental radiographic procedures. The critical tissues in the head and neck are (1) the red bone marrow in the mandible, (2) lens of the eye, and (3) thyroid gland, but most facial tissues are fairly radioresistant.

The effective dose equivalent can be used to compare the risks of different radiation exposures and to compare dental radiation exposures with days of natural background exposure.

RECALL—Study questions

1. The primary cause of biological damage from radiation is
   a. ionization.
   b. direct effect.
   c. indirect effect.
   d. genetic effect.

2. Direct injury from radiation occurs when the x-ray photons
   a. ionize water and form toxins.
   b. pass through the cell.
   c. strike critical cell molecules.
   d. All of the above.

3. Indirect injury from radiation occurs when the x-ray photons
   a. ionize water and form toxins.
   b. pass through the cell.
   c. strike critical cell molecules.
   d. All of the above.

4. According to the law of B and T, cells with a high reproductive rate are described as
   a. radiopaque.
   b. radiolucent.
   c. radioresistant.
   d. radiosensitive.

5. Which of these cells are most radiosensitive?
   a. Brain cells
   b. Nerve cells
   c. White blood cells
   d. Mature bone cells

6. Which of these cells are most radioresistant?
   a. Endothelial cells
   b. Muscle cells
   c. Epithelial cells
   d. Red blood cells

7. When the effect of a radiation exposure is observed in the offspring of an irradiated person, but not in the irradiated person, this is called the
   a. somatic effect.
   b. genetic effect.
   c. direct effect.
   d. indirect effect.

8. A dose–response curve indicating that any amount of radiation, no matter how small, has the potential to cause a biological response is called
   a. stochastic
   b. deterministic
   c. threshold
   d. nonthreshold

9. ALARA stands for _____.

10. List the five possible biological responses of an irradiated cell.
    a. _____
    b. _____
    c. _____
    d. _____
    e. _____

11. Each of the following is a factor that determines radiation injury EXCEPT one. Which one is the EXCEPTION?
    a. Size of the irradiated area
    b. Amount of radiation
    c. Patient gender
    d. Dose rate

12. According to the factors that determine radiation injury, based on age, who is the most radiosensitive?
    a. a 6-year-old
    b. a 16-year-old
    c. a 26-year-old
    d. a 46-year-old

13. Which of the following is the correct sequence of events following radiation exposure?
    a. Period of injury, latent period, recovery period
    b. Latent period, period of injury, recovery period
    c. Latent period, recovery period, period of injury
    d. Recovery period, latent period, period of injury

14. When a biological response is based on the probability of occurrence rather than the severity of the change, it is called a

    a. short-term effect.
    b. long-term effect.
    c. deterministic effect.
    d. stochastic effect.

15. Which of these is considered a short-term outcome following radiation exposure?

    a. Embryological defects
    b. Cataracts
    c. Acute radiation syndrome
    d. Cancer

16. Full-term, low birth weight is possibly associated with radiation exposure to which of the following?

    a. Thyroid gland
    b. Hypothalamus
    c. Pituitary gland
    d. All of the above

17. During exposure of an intraoral dental radiograph, approximately how much smaller is the dose of radiation in the gonadal area than at the surface of the face?

    a. 0.10
    b. 0.01
    c. 0.001
    d. 0.0001

18. Each of the following is in the path of the x-ray beam during exposure of an intraoral dental radiograph on an adult patient. Which one, because of its relative radioresistancy is NOT considered critical for dental radiography?

    a. Mandible
    b. Lens of the eye
    c. Spinal cord
    d. Thyroid gland

19. The potential risk of a full mouth dental x-ray examination inducing cancer in a patient has been estimated to be

    a. 2.5 per 1,000 examinations.
    b. 2.5 per 10,000 examinations.
    c. 2.5 per 100,000 examinations.
    d. 2.5 per 1,000,000 examinations.

20. What term best expresses comparisons between dental radiation exposures and natural background exposure?

    a. Absorbed dose
    b. Effective dose equivalent
    c. Accumulated dose
    d. Lethal dose

REFLECT—Case study

Retaking a radiograph because of a technique or processing error causes an increase in radiation exposure for the patient. Discuss ways a retake radiograph affects the factors that determine radiation injury.

RELATE—Laboratory application

Calculate your radiation dose. Visit the United States Environmental Protection Agency at http://www.epa.gov/radiation/understand/calculate.html, where you can estimate your average annual radiation dose. Based on the questions posed by this calculator, what conclusions can you draw about (1) the source of radiation exposure, (2) the region in which people live, (3) sources of internal radiation exposure, and (4) situations and/or products with the ability to increase your dose of radiation exposure?

REFERENCES

American Dental Association Council on Scientific Affairs. (2006). The use of dental radiographs: Update and recommendations. *Journal of the American Dental Association, 137*(9), 1304–1312.

Carestream Health Inc. (2007). *Kodak Dental Systems. Radiation safety in dental radiography.,* Rochester NY: Author.

Hujoel, P. P., Bollen, A., Noonan, C. J., & del Aguila, M. A. (2004). Antepartum dental radiography and infant low birth weight. *JAMA, 291*(16), 1987–1993.

National Council on Radiation Protection and Measurements. (2009). *Report No 160: Ionizing radiation exposure of the population of the United States.* Bethesda, MD: Author.

National Council on Radiation Protection and Measurements. (1991). *Implementation of the principle of as low as reasonably achievable (ALARA) for medical and dental personnel.* NCRP report no. 107. Washington, DC: Author.

United States Nuclear Regulatory Commission. (2007, December 4). Standards for protection against radiation, Title 10, Part 20, of the *Code of Federal Regulations.* Retrieved April 11, 2010, from http://www.nrc.gov/reading-rm/doc-collections/cfr/part020/part020-1201.html

U.S. Nuclear Regulatory Commission. (2010). *Radiation protection.* Retrieved April 16, 2010, from http://www.nrc.gov/about-nrc/radiation.html

White, S. C., & Pharoah, M. J. (2008) *Oral radiology: Principles and interpretation* (6th ed.). St. Louis, MO: Mosby Elsevier.

Radiation Protection

OBJECTIVES

Following successful completion of this chapter, you should be able to:

1. Define the key words.
2. Adopt the ALARA concept.
3. Use the selection criteria guidelines to explain the need for prescribed radiographs.
4. Explain the roles communication, working knowledge of quality radiographs, and education play in preventing unnecessary radiation exposure.
5. Explain the roles technique and exposure choices play in preventing unnecessary radiation exposure.
6. Explain the function of the filter.
7. State the filtration requirements for an intraoral dental x-ray unit that operates above and below 70 kVp.
8. Compare inherent, added, and total filtration.
9. State the federally mandated diameter of the intraoral dental x-ray beam at the patient's skin.
10. Explain the difference between round and rectangular collimation.
11. List the two functions of a collimator.
12. Explain how PID shape and length contribute to reducing patient radiation exposure.
13. Identify film speeds currently available for dental radiography use.
14. Explain the role image receptor holders play in reducing patient radiation exposure.
15. Advocate the use of the lead/lead equivalent thyroid collar and apron.
16. Explain the role darkroom protocol and film handling play in reducing patient radiation exposure.
17. Summarize the radiation protection methods for the patient.
18. Explain the roles time, shielding, and distance play in protecting the radiographer from unnecessary radiation exposure.
19. Utilize distance and location to take a position the appropriate distance and angle from the x-ray source at the patient's head during an exposure.
20. Describe monitoring devices used to detect radiation.
21. Summarize the radiation protection methods for the radiographer.
22. List the organizations responsible for recommending and setting exposure limits.
23. State the maximum permissible dose (MPD) for radiation workers and for the general public.

Introduction

In Chapter 5 we learned that radiation exposure in sufficient doses may produce harmful biological changes in humans. Although it is the consensus of radiobiologists that the dose received from a dental x-ray exposure is not likely to be harmful, even the experts do not know what risk a small dose carries. Therefore, it must be assumed that any dose may be capable of potential risk. The patient has agreed to be subjected to the risks of radiation exposure because he/she believes that the oral health care practitioner will follow safety protocols that protect the patient from excess exposure.

In this chapter we discuss radiation safety protocols, including selection criteria used in prescribing dental radiographs and methods to minimize x-ray exposure to both the dental patient and the radiographer.

ALARA

The oral health care team has an ethical responsibility to embrace the **ALARA (as low as reasonably achievable)** concept, recommended by the International Commission on Radiological Protection to minimize radiation risks. The ALARA concept implies that "any radiation dose that can be reduced without major difficulty, great expense, or inconvenience should be reduced or eliminated." ALARA is not simply a phrase, but a culture of professional excellence. ALARA should guide practice principles. In an ideal world, the oral health care team would like to get the diagnostic benefits of dental radiographs with a zero dose radiation exposure to the patient. In reality, this is not possible; all dental radiographs will result in a small but acceptable level of risk. The best way to prevent this risk from increasing is to keep the exposure ALARA.

Protection Measures for the Patient

Professional Judgment

The benefits of radiographs in dentistry outweigh the risks when proper safety procedures are followed. The most important way to ensure that the patient receives a reasonably low dose of radiation is to use evidence-based **selection criteria** when determining which patients need radiographs. Guidelines developed by an expert panel of health care professionals convened by the Public Health Service and adopted by the American Dental Association have been published to assist in deciding when, what type, and how many radiographs should be taken (Table 6-1). These guidelines allow the dentist to base the decision regarding x-rays for the patient on expert recommendations. Although the dentist prescribes the radiographic exam for the patient based on these guidelines, these recommendations are subject to clinical judgment and may not apply to every patient.

Evidence-based selection criteria guidelines are applied only after reviewing the patient's health history and completing a clinical examination. The time frames suggested in the guidelines are used in the absence of positive historical findings and signs and symptoms presented by the patient. For example, a patient who presents with a toothache would most likely be assessed for a radiographic exam of this symptom even if the patient had radiographs within the suggested time frame for this patient's category. Additionally, a radiographic examination should not wait until a patient presents with pain or other symptom of pathology. The time frames suggested by the selection criteria guidelines are preventive measures that are evidence-based effective. The dentist uses these guidelines to prescribe the radiographic exam for the patient, but the dental hygienist may use the guidelines during initial examination of the patient to make a preliminary assessment for the recommendation of radiographic need; the dental hygienist and the dental assistant rely on the selection criteria guidelines to assist with explaining radiographic need to the patient. Once the decision to expose radiographs is made, every reasonable effort must be made to minimize exposure to the patient and to the operator and to those who may be in the area of the x-ray machine.

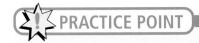

Technical Ability of the Operator

- **Communication.** Reduction of radiation exposure begins with communication skills. The patient's cooperation must be secured to perform radiographic examinations accurately and safely. Patient protection during a radiographic procedure should begin with clear, concise instructions. When responsibilities are adequately defined through effective communication, the patient understands what must be done and can more fully cooperate with the radiographer and avoid retake mistakes.

- **Working knowledge of quality radiographs.** The radiographer should understand what a quality dental radiograph should image. Based on this knowledge, the radiographer needs to take every precaution against retaking radiographs. **Retake radiographs** are necessary when the first exposure results in errors that compromise image quality. When a radiograph is retaken, the second exposure doubles the dose and dose rate of radiation for the patient. The best way to avoid retake radiographs is to develop an understanding of common technique and processing errors (see Chapter 18). Armed with this knowledge, the radiographer can better avoid mistakes that lead to an increase in patient radiation exposure.

- **Education.** Continuing education is the cornerstone of all health care professions. Rapidly advancing technology is constantly changing the scope of oral health care

practice. Some of the methods and procedures learned for the practice of oral health care just a few years ago may be obsolete in today's world. For example, we are currently witnessing the possible elimination of film-based dental radiography. With the increasing use of computers and the advancement of digital imaging, new technology will surely contribute to the reduction of dental radiation exposure. The radiographer who continues to learn about and adopt these new practices will further help decrease radiation exposure for the patient and the radiographer.

Technique Standards

- **Intraoral technique choice.** The paralleling technique should be the operator's first choice when exposing periapical radiographs. The paralleling technique yields more accurate and precisely sized radiographic images (see Chapter 14). However, consideration should also be given to which technique, paralleling or bisecting, will produce the best results for the patient. The more efficient and convenient the technique, the less likely there will be retake radiographs. The radiographer should be skilled at both techniques and should possess the knowledge on which to base the decision regarding which one to use.

- **Exposure factors.** Operating the dental x-ray machine includes selecting the appropriate **exposure factors**—kilovoltage (kVp), milliamperage (mA), and time—for the patient and the area to be imaged. The radiographer should possess a working knowledge of appropriate exposure factors to avoid overexposing the patient unnecessarily. Underexposures can also lead to additional exposures for the patient if a retake is necessary. A working knowledge of the exposure factors includes the ability to adjust each of the variables—kilovoltage (kVp), milliamperage (mA), and time—in relation to each other. In Chapter 4, we learned that an adjustment in one variable usually leads to a necessary counteradjustment in another variable to maintain exposure control. To assist in radiation safety, exposure charts should be posted near the control panel for easy reference.

Equipment Standards

Using proper equipment is the next step in reducing radiation exposure to the patient. All dental x-ray machines in the United States are safe from a radiological health point of view. The Federal Performance Standard for Diagnostic X-Ray Equipment became effective on August 1, 1974. The provisions of the standard require that all x-ray equipment manufactured after that date meet certain radiation safety requirements including filtration, collimation, and PID (position indicating device).

- **Filtration** is the absorption of the long wavelength, less penetrating, x-rays of the polychromatic x-ray beam by

TABLE 6-1 Guidelines for Prescribing Dental Radiographs

TYPE OF ENCOUNTER	CHILDREN		ADOLESCENT	ADULT	
	Primary Dentition (*prior to eruption of first permanent tooth*)	Transitional Dentition (*after eruption of first permanent tooth*)	Permanent Dentition (*prior to eruption of third molars*)	Dentate or Partially Edentulous	Edentulous
New Patient* Being evaluated for dental disease and dental development	Individualized radiographic exam consisting of selected periapical/occlusal views and/or posterior bitewings if proximal surfaces cannot be visualized or probed. Patients without evidence of disease and with open proximal contacts may not require a radiographic exam at this time.	Individualized radiographic exam consisting of posterior bitewings with panoramic exam or posterior bitewings and selected periapical images.	Individualized radiographic exam consisting of posterior bitewings with panoramic exam or posterior bitewings and selected periapical images. A full mouth intraoral radiographic exam is preferred when the patient has clinical evidence of generalized dental disease or a history of extensive dental treatment.		Individualized radiographic exam, based on clinical signs and symptoms.
Recall Patient* With clinical caries or at increased risk for caries**	Posterior bitewing exam at 6- to 12-month intervals if proximal surfaces cannot be examined visually or with a probe.			Posterior bitewing exam at 6- to 18-month intervals.	Not applicable.
Recall Patient* With no clinical caries and not at risk for caries**	Posterior bitewing exam at 12- to 24-month intervals if proximal surfaces cannot be examined visually or with a probe.		Posterior bitewing exam at 18- to 36-month intervals.	Posterior bitewing exam at 24- to 36-month intervals.	Not applicable.
Recall Patient* With periodontal disease	Clinical judgment as to the need for and type of radiographic images for the evaluation of periodontal disease. Imaging may consist of, but is not limited to, selected bitewing and/or periapical images of areas where periodontal disease (other than nonspecific gingivitis) can be identified clinically.				Not applicable.
Patient* For monitoring of growth and development	Clinical judgment as to the need for and type of radiographic images for the evaluation and/or monitoring of dentofacial growth and development.		Clinical judgment as to the need for and type of radiographic images for evaluation and/or monitoring of dentofacial growth and development. Panoramic or periapical exam to assess developing third molars.	Not usually indicated.	

Patient

With other circumstances including, but not limited to, proposed or existing implants, pathology, restorative/endodontic needs, treated periodontal disease and caries remineralization.

Clinical judgment as to the need for and type of radiographic images for the evaluation and/or monitoring in these circumstances.

*Clinical situations for which radiographs may be indicated include but are not limited to:

A. Positive historical findings
1. Previous periodontal or endodontic treatment
2. History of pain or trauma
3. Familial history of dental anomalies
4. Postoperative evaluation of healing
5. Remineralization monitoring
6. Presence of implants or evaluation for impact placement

B. Positive clinical signs/symptoms
1. Clinical evidence of periodontal disease
2. Large or deep restorations
3. Deep carious lesions
4. Malposed or clinically impacted teeth
5. Swelling
6. Evidence of dental/facial trauma
7. Mobility of teeth
8. Sinus tract ("fistula")
9. Clinically suspected sinus pathology
10. Growth abnormalities
11. Oral involvement in known or suspected systemic disease
12. Positive neurologic findings in the head and neck
13. Evidence of foreign objects
14. Pain and/or dysfunction of the temporomandibular joint
15. Facial asymmetry
16. Abutment teeth for fixed or removable partial prosthesis
17. Unexplained bleeding
18. Unexplained sensitivity of teeth
19. Unusual eruption, spacing, or migration of teeth
20. Unusual tooth morphology, calcification, or color
21. Unexplained absence of teeth
22. Clinical erosion

**Factors increasing risk for caries may include but are not limited to:
1. High level of caries experience or demineralization
2. History of recurrent caries
3. High titers of cariogenic bacteria
4. Existing restoration(s) of poor quality
5. Poor oral hygiene
6. Inadequate fluoride exposure
7. Prolonged nursing (bottle or breast)
8. High-sucrose frequency diet
9. Poor family oral health
10. Developmental or acquired enamel defects
11. Developmental or acquired disability
12. Xerostomia
13. Genetic abnormality of teeth
14. Many multisurface restorations
15. Chemo/radiation therapy
16. Eating disorders
17. Drug/alcohol abuse
18. Irregular dental care

Data from U.S. Dept. of Health and Human Services: *The Selection of Patients for Dental Radiographic Examinations.* Revised 2004 by the American Dental Association: Council on Dental Practice, Council on Dental Benefit Program, Council on Scientific Affairs.

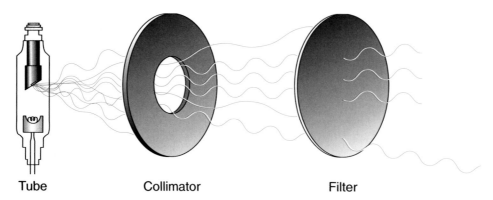

Tube   Collimator   Filter

FIGURE 6-1 Collimator and filter. The collimator is a lead washer that restricts the size of the x-ray beam. The filter is an aluminum disc that filters (removes) the long wavelength x-rays.

passage of the beam through a sheet of material called a **filter** (Figure 6-1). A filter is an absorbing material (usually aluminum) placed in the path of the x-ray beam to remove a high percentage of the soft x-rays (the longer wavelengths) and reduce patient radiation dose.

In the dental x-ray machine, these aluminum filter disks vary in thickness. The **half-value layer (HVL)** of an x-ray beam is the thickness (measured in millimeters) of aluminum that will reduce the intensity of the beam by one-half. Measuring the HVL determines the penetrating quality of the x-ray beam. The HVL is more accurate than kilovoltage to describe the x-ray beam quality and penetration. Two similar x-ray machines operating at the same kilovoltage may not produce x-rays of the same quality and penetration. The half-value layer is used by radiological health personnel when determining filtration requirements.

Filters may be sealed into the tube head or inserted into the port where the PID attaches. Pure aluminum or its equivalent will not hinder the passage of high-energy

x-rays, but will absorb a high percentage of the low-energy x-rays. The latter do not contribute to the radiographic image. Low-energy x-rays are harmful to the patient because they are absorbed by the skin, increasing the patient's dose (Figure 6-2).

Any material the x-ray beam passes through filters the beam. Filtration may be built into the tube head (inherent), or it may be added.

Inherent filtration is the filtration built into the machine by the manufacturer. This includes the glass of the x-ray tube, the insulating oil, and the material that seals the port. All x-ray units have some built-in filtration. Usually the inherent filtration is not sufficient to meet state and federal standards, requiring that filtration be added.

Added filtration is the placement of aluminum discs in the path of the x-ray beam between the port seal of the tube head and the PID. When the inherent filtration is not sufficient to meet safety standards, a disk of aluminum of the appropriate thickness (usually 0.5 mm) can be inserted between the port of the tube head and the PID. Several manufacturers have introduced x-ray units in which the traditional aluminum filter is replaced with samarium, a rare-earth metal.

Total filtration is the sum of the inherent and added filtration expressed in millimeters of **aluminum equivalent.** Beam **filtration** must comply with state and federal laws. Present safety standards require an equivalent of 1.5 mm aluminum for x-ray machines operating in ranges below 70 kVp and a minimum of 2.5 mm aluminum for machines operating at or above 70 kVp.

- **Collimation** controls the size and shape of the useful beam.

  Collimation of the beam is accomplished by using a lead diaphragm or washer. The lead diaphragm collimator is placed in the path of the **primary beam** as it exits the tube housing at the port (Figure 6-3). Rectangular collimation may also be achieved through the use of external collimators that attach to the PID (Figure 6-4.) The function of the

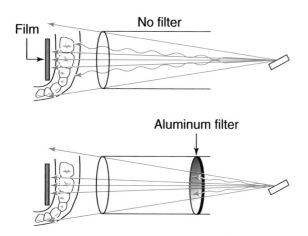

FIGURE 6-2 Effect of filtration on skin exposure. Aluminum filters selectively absorb the long wavelength x-rays.

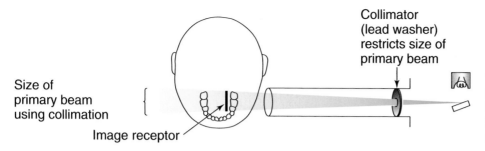

Size of
primary beam
using collimation

Image receptor

Collimator
(lead washer)
restricts size of
primary beam

FIGURE 6-3 Effect of collimation on primary beam. Lead collimators control the shape and size of the primary beam. The beam is limited to the approximate size of the image receptor.

collimator is to reduce the size of the x-ray beam and the amount of scattered radiation. Collimators may have either a round or a rectangular opening and are matched with a round or rectangular PID. Federal regulations require that round opening collimators restrict the x-ray beam to 2.75 in. (7 cm) at the patient end of the PID (Figure 6-5). Rectangular collimators restrict the beam to the approximate size of the image receptor. Figure 6-6 shows the excess radiation the patient receives with a round collimator when exposing a

#2-sized image receptor. Rectangular collimation reduces patient radiation exposure by up to 70 percent (Figure 6-7).

Collimation also reduces **scatter radiation** (sometimes called **secondary radiation**). Scatter radiation is radiation that has been deflected from its path by impact during its passage through matter. In addition to increasing patient radiation dose, scattered radiation decreases the quality of the radiographic image through fogging. In summary, the two important functions of collimation are

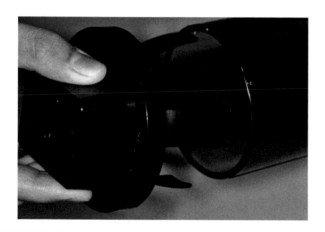

FIGURE 6-4 External collimator attaches to the PID to reduce the area of radiation exposure.

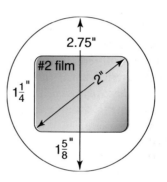

FIGURE 6-6 Although circular collimation provides a large enough area of exposure to adequately cover a size #2 image receptor, the patient also receives excess radiation not needed for the exposure of this receptor.

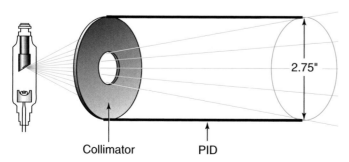

Collimator   PID

FIGURE 6-5 The collimator restricts the size of the primary beam to 2.75 in. (7 cm) at the end of the PID.

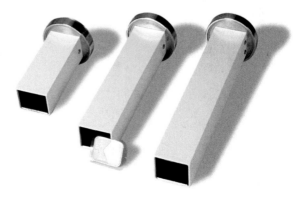

FIGURE 6-7 Rectangular PIDs restrict the x-ray beam to the approximate size of a #2 intraoral image receptor. Rectangular PIDs are available in 8, 12, and 16 inches (20.5, 30, and 41 cm). (Courtesy of Margraf Dental Manufacturing Inc.)

- Reduces the radiation dose to the patient by reducing the volume of tissue exposed
- Reduces scatter radiation that causes poor contrast of the radiograph (see Chapter 4)

- The **position indicating device (PID)** (or **beam indicating device [BID]**) is an extension of the tube housing and is used to direct the primary x-ray beam. The shape of the PID indicates the shape of the collimator. Although rectangular collimation reduces patient radiation exposure by up to 70 percent over a round-collimated beam, most dental x-ray machines are sold with round PIDs attached. Rectangular PIDs can be purchased to replace the round PIDs and reduce patient radiation exposure (Figure 6-7).

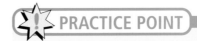

PRACTICE POINT

Pointed, closed-end cones, originally designed to aid in aiming the x-ray beam at the center of the film packet, are no longer used (Figure 6-8). Pointed cones cause the deflection or scattering of x-rays through contact with the material of the cones. Because these pointed cones were used for so many years, many still refer to the PID as a "cone." The term *position indicating device (PID)* is more descriptive of its function of directing the x-rays, rather than of its shape.

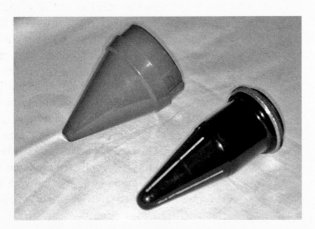

FIGURE 6-8 Plastic closed-ended, pointed "cones" are no longer used.

(20.5 cm), 12 in. (30 cm), and 16 in. (41 cm). (See Figures 6-7 and 6-9.) The longer the PID (12-in. or 16-in. length), the less radiation dose to the patient and the better quality radiographic image (see Figure 4-11). With a longer PID, there is less divergence of the beam, creating a smaller diameter of exposure (Figure 6-10).

It is important to note that the dental x-ray machine may appear to have a short PID when it actually may be long. Some dental x-ray machines feature a recessed PID, where the tube is recessed back in the tubehead behind the transformers, therefore creating a longer target–surface distance (see Figure 3-1).

PRACTICE POINT

All intraoral techniques require that the end of the PID be placed as close to the patient's skin as possible, without touching, during the exposure. This is necessary to establish the desired target–surface distance. Increasing the distance between the open end of the PID and the patient's skin will not establish the desired target–surface distance. For example, positioning the open end of an 8-in. (20.5-cm) PID an additional 4 inches (10.2 cm) away from the patient's face is not the same as using a 12-in. (30-cm) PID. See Figure 4-12.

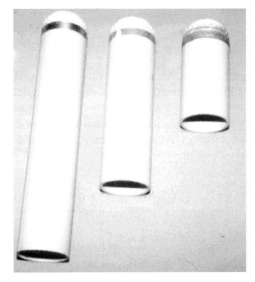

FIGURE 6-9 **Round PIDs** are available in 16, 12, and 8 inches (41, 30, and 20.5 cm).

The length of the PID also has an effect on the radiation dose the patient receives. The length of the PID helps to establish the desired target-surface distance. Both round and rectangular PIDs are available in three lengths: 8 in.

- **Fast film and digital image sensors** require less radiation for exposure and are essential for exposure reduction. In fact, after rectangular collimation, high-speed film is the most effective equipment for reducing radiation to the

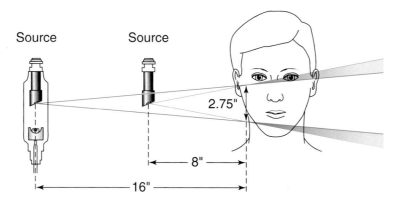

FIGURE 6-10 Target-surface distance. The longer the target-surface distance, the more parallel the x-rays and the less tissue exposed. Note that the beam size at the patient's skin entrance is 2.75 in. (7 cm) for both target-surface distances. It is the exit beam size that increases to expose a larger area when using the shorter target-surface distance.

patient. Currently, intraoral dental x-ray film is available in three speed groups, D, E and F. E-speed film, when compared to D-speed film, is twice as fast and therefore requires only one-half the exposure time. F-speed film can reduce radiation exposure 20 percent compared to E-speed film. The American Dental Association and the American Academy of Oral and Maxillofacial Radiology recommend the use of the fastest speed film currently available. Digital image sensors can further reduce the amount radiation required to produce a diagnostic image and will be discussed in Chapter 9.

- **Image receptor holding devices** that position the film packet or digital sensor intraorally are recommended. The use of a **film** or **image receptor holder** eliminates having the patient hold the receptor in the oral cavity with the fingers (Figure 6-11). Unnecessarily exposing the patient's fingers is not ethical practice in keeping with ALARA. The use of image receptor holders with external aiming devices will assist the operator in aligning the x-ray beam, which may afford the patient additional protection by reducing the number of retakes that may result from alignment

errors. These devices also stabilize the image receptor in the mouth and reduce the possibility of movement and of film bending that often result when the patient uses a finger to hold the receptor in position.

- **The lead apron** made of at least 0.25-mm lead or **lead-equivalent** materials is placed over the patient's abdomen to protect the reproductive organs and other radiosensitive tissues from potential scatter radiation during radiographic procedures (Figure 6-12). The use of a **lead apron** was recommended for protecting patients during exposure of dental radiographs many years ago when dental x-ray machine output was less reliable and film speeds were slower than today's standards. Using a fast-speed film or digital image sensor and a dental x-ray machine that is appropriately collimated and filtered essentially eliminates the requirement for covering the patient's abdomen with a lead apron. The National Council on Radiation Protection and Measurements has determined that lead aprons do not significantly reduce doses from intraoral dental exposures. Nevertheless some states still have laws requiring the use of a lead apron over the abdominal area, and patients have come to expect it. Even if it is not legally required, the use of a lead or lead-equivalent apron is in keeping with the ALARA concept and remains a prudent if not essential practice.

Lead and lead-equivalent aprons should be stored flat or hung unbent. Folding the apron may cause the material inside to crack. This is most likely to occur when aprons are repeatedly folded in the same place day after day. Cracks in the material allow radiation to penetrate and render the apron less effective.

- **Thyroid collar.** Lead and lead-equivalent aprons are available with or without an attached thyroid collar (Figure 6-13). The **thyroid collar,** when in place around the patient's neck, protects the thyroid gland and other radiosensitive tissues in the neck region during exposure of intraoral radiographs. Because of the direction of the dental x-ray

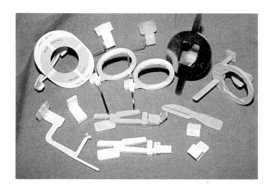

FIGURE 6-11 Many image receptor holding devices are available to fit most situations. The use of a holder prevents asking patients to put their fingers in the path of the primary beam.

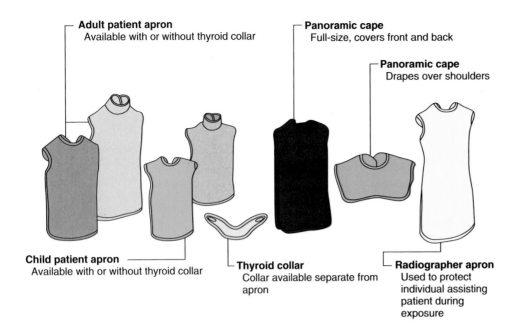

Adult patient apron
Available with or without thyroid collar

Panoramic cape
Full-size, covers front and back

Panoramic cape
Drapes over shoulders

Child patient apron
Available with or without thyroid collar

Thyroid collar
Collar available separate from apron

Radiographer apron
Used to protect individual assisting patient during exposure

FIGURE 6-12 Lead aprons and thyroid collars are available in a wide range of sizes. Aprons are available with an attached thyroid collar, or the thyroid collar may be a separate part.

beam in this region, lead or lead-equivalent thyroid collars are recommended for all patients, and especially for children and pregnant females and women of child-bearing age. (This topic is discussed further in Chapter 27.)

PRACTICE POINT

The use of a thyroid collar is contraindicated when exposing panoramic radiographs using rotational panoramic equipment because the collar or upper part of the apron to which it is attached may obscure diagnostic information or interfere with the rotation of the panoramic unit. This is one of the reasons lead aprons are available without thyroid collars.

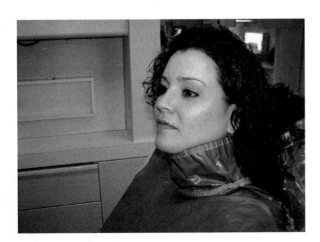

FIGURE 6-13 Patient protected with lead apron with thyroid collar in place.

Optimum Film Processing

An often-overlooked step in producing diagnostic radiographs is film processing. Processing errors increase patient radiation exposure by resulting in retake radiographs. The patient deserves the attention that must be paid to meticulous processing procedures and careful film handling to produce ideal diagnostic quality radiographs. Darkroom procedures should be outlined and followed carefully (see Chapter 8).

Careful attention to chemical replenishment and following the time–temperature method of processing produces radiographs of ideal quality and avoids retakes. There are ethical considerations to proper processing protocols as well. In the past, it was sometimes observed that an unethical practitioner would call for overexposing (increasing the radiation dose to the patient) and underdeveloping the film in an attempt to save time during certain procedures. Another unethical practice noted in history has been to let processing chemicals go too long between replenishment or solution change. As the processing chemistry weakens, the resultant images appear less dense (lighter). Unethical practitioners would increase the dose of radiation to compensate for the weakening processing solutions. It was the patient who bore the brunt of this practice by enduring the additional radiation burden. Patient protection techniques should be used at all times to keep radiation exposures as low as possible (Box 6-1).

Protection Measures for the Radiographer

All measures taken to protect the patient from radiation also benefit the radiographer (Box 6-2). Specific radiation protection methods for the radiographer include time, shielding, and distance. The radiographer should spend a minimal amount of time, protected by shielding, at the greatest distance from the source of radiation to avoid unnecessary exposure.

BOX 6-1 Summary of Protection Methods for the Patient

- Evidence-based prescribing
- Communication
- Working knowledge of quality radiographs
- Education
- Selection of technique
- Posted exposure factors
- Filtration
- Collimation
- Open-ended, 16-in. (41-cm) rectangular PID
- F-speed film/digital image receptors
- Image receptor holders
- Lead/lead-equivalent thyroid collar/apron
- Darkroom protocol

BOX 6-2 Summary of Methods to Protect the Radiographer

- Follow all patient protection measures.
- Do not contact the tubehead during exposure.
- Avoid retakes.
- Do not hold the image receptor for the patient.
- Use a protective barrier/shield.
- Use leaded protective clothing when necessary.
- Remain 6 ft (1.82 m) away and at a 45° angle from the exiting primary beam.
- Use radiation monitoring.

Time

When careful attention is focused on producing the highest quality radiographs, the need for retake radiographs is decreased, which in turn decreases the time the radiographer spends near the x-ray machine. Additionally, the dental radiographer should avoid the pitfalls that may lure movement into the path of the primary beam. For example, a drifting tube head should never be held during the exposure. **Radiation leakage** from the tube head can expose the operator to a significant amount of radiation. If the tube head drifts, it should be serviced to stabilize it.

If a patient must be stabilized during the procedure, as is sometimes the case with a small child, a parent or guardian may have to be asked to assist with the procedure. The parent or guardian should be protected with lead, or lead-equivalent barriers such as an apron or gloves, when they will be in the path of the x-ray beam. The radiographer must never place him/herself in the primary beam.

Image receptor holding devices should be used to stabilize the receptor in the patient's oral cavity. If placement with an image receptor holding device is difficult to achieve, as is the case with a patient with a small mouth, low and/or sensitive palatal vault, or an exaggerated gag reflex, the radiographer should experiment with other holders, smaller-sized films, or the bisecting technique. The radiographer must not hold the image receptor in the patient's mouth. Additionally, another member of the oral health care team must not be allowed to

place themselves in the path of the primary beam while the radiographer presses the exposure button.

Shielding

Structural shielding provides the radiographer with protection from potential scattered radiation. Safe installation of dental x-ray machines will provide an exposure button permanently mounted behind a **protective barrier,** providing protection for the operator (see Figure 3-4). Most oral health care practices are located in buildings that have incorporated adequate shielding in walls such as these regularly used construction materials: plaster, cinderblock, $2\frac{1}{2}$ to 3 inches of drywall, 3/16 inch steel, or 1 millimeter of lead. Additionally, lead-lined walls or windows, thick or specially constructed partitions between the rooms, or specially constructed lead screens offer excellent protection for the operator during exposure (see Figure 3-7.)

Distance

If a protective barrier is not present, as may be the case in an open-bay designed practice setting, distance plays an important role in safeguarding the radiographer during patient exposures. The operator should always stand as far away as practical—at least 6 ft (1.8 m)—from the head of the patient (the source of scatter radiation) while making the exposure. The intensity of the x-radiation diminishes the farther the x-rays travel (Figure 6-14). In addition to distance, it is important to remain in a position 45 degrees to the primary x-ray beam as it exits the patient, as this is the area of minimum scatter when the patient is seated upright. Maximum scatter is most likely to occur back in the direction of the tube head. (Figure 6-15). If exposing radiographs while the patient is in a supine position (lying prone in the dental chair), the radiographer should take a position at an angle of 135 to 180 degrees behind the patient's head where the least scatter radiation occurs.

All persons, whether other oral health care team members or other patients not directly involved with the x-ray exposure, must be protected by shielding and/or distance.

Radiation Monitoring

The only way to be sure that x-ray equipment is not emitting too much radiation and that operators are not receiving more than the maximum permissible dose is to use radiation measuring devices to monitor equipment and personnel. In radiography, **monitoring** is defined as periodic or continuing measurement to determine the exposure rate in a given area or the dose received by an operator.

Area Monitoring

Area monitoring involves making an on-site survey to measure the output of the dental x-ray unit, to check for possible high-level radiation areas in the operatory, and to determine if any radiation is passing through walls. Special equipment is needed to detect the exact amount of ionizing radiation at any given area. Numerous companies specialize in area monitoring. In some regions, this service may be performed by qualified state inspectors.

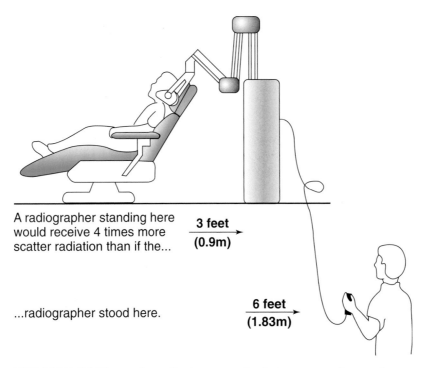

FIGURE 6-14 Distance is an effective means of reducing exposure from scatter radiation.

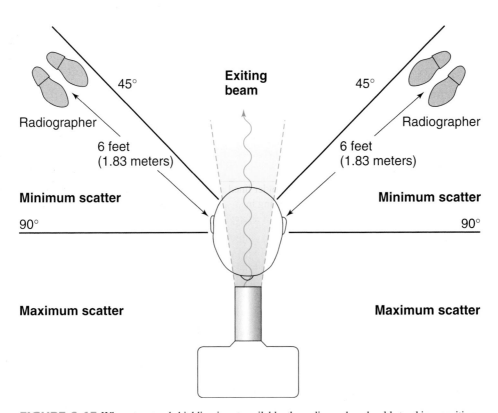

FIGURE 6-15 When structural shielding is not available, the radiographer should stand in a position at least 6 ft (1.83 m) from the head of the patient at an angle of 45° to the exiting primary beam.

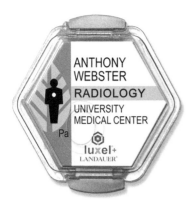

FIGURE 6-16 OSL **radiation monitor** worn by the radiographer to monitor radiation exposure. (http:/www.landauerinc.com)

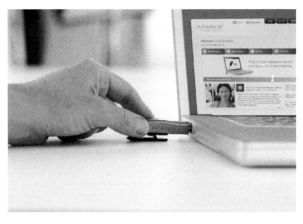

FIGURE 6-17 DIS radiation monitor. Sized and shaped similar to a thumb drive, this device has a clip to allow the radiographer to wear the monitor while working with ionizing radiation. The device uses a USB connector to plug into a computer with Internet access. When logged on to the manufacturer's Web site, real-time radiation exposure readings may be downloaded from the device. (Courtesy of Quantum Products.)

Personnel Monitoring

Personnel monitoring requires oral health care professionals to wear a radiation monitoring device or **dosimeter** (Figures 6-16 and 6-17) such as a **film badge, TLD, OSL monitor,** or **DIS monitor** (Table 6-2). For a fee, radiation monitoring companies provide the measuring devices and services to the oral health care team. After use, the devices are returned to the company or the information recorded by the device is transmitted to the company via the Internet. The company evaluates the information captured by the device and provides the dental practice with a report regarding exposure. This report compares the operator's exposure reading with the maximum allowable level, and the monitoring company updates the subscriber's records to keep the wearer in full compliance with all federal and state safety regulations. The reports from a radiation monitoring service provide a reliable permanent record of accumulated doses of occupational radiation exposure. The types of personnel monitoring devices currently on the market are listed in Table 6-2.

The likelihood of dental radiation exposing an oral health care professional who is following ALARA is so small that only a few states consider dental radiation monitoring mandatory. Even so, more and more oral health care professionals are deciding to secure monitoring devices and services for themselves and their employees, even when not mandated by law. As a risk management tool, monitoring radiation exposure—or more likely, documenting the lack of exposure—helps to determine whether the operator is maintaining radiation safety protocols; aids in providing the radiographer with peace of mind; and assists with risk management by providing a health record of exposure, or more likely, the lack of exposure, for personnel.

Although **personnel monitoring devices** play a valuable role, it should be noted that they are limited in their ability to be precise at estimating very low levels of exposure. Advancing technology in this area continue to improve the ability of

TABLE 6-2	Types of Personnel Monitoring Devices		
TYPE	HOW IT WORKS	ADVANTAGES	LIMITATIONS
Film badge	Radiosensitive film in a plastic/metal holder lined with filters of different materials varying in thickness. Exposure is determined by "reading" the processed film electronically.	Film itself provides a permanent record of exposures Reliable technology	Film must be changed and returned to the monitoring company monthly
TLD (thermo-luminescent dosimeter)	Contains crystals, usually lithium fluoride, that absorb radiation. Crystals are heated after being exposed, and the energy emitted, in the form of visible light, is proportional to the amount of radiation absorbed.	Extremely accurate One-piece construction	Badge must be returned to the monitoring company every 3 months
OSL monitor (optically stimulated luminescence)	Absorbs radiation similar to TLD, but crystals release energy during optical stimulation instead of heat.	Allows multiple read-outs for reanalysis New technology	Badge can only be used once
DIS monitor (direct ion storage)	Uses a miniature ion chamber to absorb radiation. Exposure is determined through digital processing.	Instant real-time unlim-ited readouts New technology	Requires on-site reader or computer connec-tion to the Internet

dosimeters to estimate low-dose exposures. Monitors that have been approved by the National Voluntary Laboratory Accreditation Program (NVLAP) can be expected to be accurate. It should be noted that personnel monitoring devices do not "protect" the wearer from radiation.

Organizations Responsible for Recommending/Setting Exposure Limits

As early as 1902, studies were undertaken to determine the effect of radiation exposure on the body and to consider setting limits on radiation exposure. The International Commission on Radiological Protection (ICRP) was formed in 1928, and in 1929 the National Council on Radiation Protection and Measurements (NCRP) was created in the United States. The ICRP and the NCRP do not actually set the laws governing the use of ionizing radiation, but their suggestions and recommendations are so highly regarded that most all regulatory bodies use recommendations from these organizations to formulate legislation controlling the use of radiation. The American Dental Association (ADA) and its various committees and affiliated organizations, such as the American Academy of Oral and Maxillofacial Radiology (AAOMR), work closely with all organizations to ensure that oral health care patients receive state-of-the-art treatment in radiation safety (Table 6-3).

Maximum Permissible Dose (MPD)

The United States Nuclear Regulatory Commission has developed radiation protection guidelines referred to as the **maximum permissible dose (MPD)** for the protection of radiation workers and the general public (Table 6-4). Maximum permissible dose is defined as the dose equivalent of ionizing radiation that, in the light of present knowledge, is not expected to cause detectable body damage to average persons at any time during their lifetime. These limits do not apply to medical or dental radiation used for diagnostic or therapeutic purposes. Over the

years, the acceptable limits have been constantly revised downward; they are now about 700 times smaller than those originally proposed in 1902, mainly because many aspects of tissue damage from radiation are still not clearly understood.

Maximum limits are set higher for workers than for the public, but the suggested limits of the maximum permissible accumulated dose for both groups are purposely set far lower than it is believed the human body can safely accept.

- **Radiation workers.** The maximum permissible dose (MPD) for oral health care professionals is the same as for other **radiation workers.** According to these guidelines, the whole-body dose may not exceed 50 mSv (5 rem) per year. There is no established weekly limit, but state public health personnel usually use a weekly dose of 1.0 mSv (0.1 rem) when inspecting dental offices.

    The 50 mSv (5 rem) yearly limit for radiation workers has two very important exceptions. It does not apply to persons under 18 years or to any female members of the oral health care team who are known to be pregnant. Persons under 18 years are classified as part of the general public and can accumulate only 5 mSv (0.5 rem) per year. In the case of pregnant women, it is recommended that exposure to the fetus be limited to 5 mSv (0.5 rem), not to be received at a rate greater than 0.5 mSv (0.05 rem) per month.

- **General public.** The general public is permitted 5 mSv (0.5 rem) per year, or one-tenth the dose permitted radiation workers. It should be noted that the MPD has been established for incidental or accidental exposures and does not include doses from medical and dental diagnostic or therapeutic radiation. Necessary medical and dental diagnostic or therapeutic radiation is not counted in the permissible dose limits. If a patient needs radiographic services, then that patient needs the radiographic services. An oral health care team member who requires medical, dental diagnostic, or therapeutic radiation would become the "patient," and then the general public MPD would apply.

TABLE 6-3 Radiation Protection Organizations	
ORGANIZATION	WEB SITE
International Commission on Radiological Units and Measurements (ICRU)	www.icru.org
International Commission on Radiological Protection (ICRP)	www.icrp.org
National Council on Radiation Protection and Measurements (NCRP)	www.ncrp.com
U.S. Nuclear Regulatory Commission (NRC)	www.nrc.gov
U.S. Environmental Protection Agency (EPA)	www.epa.gov
U.S. Food and Drug Administration (FDA)	www.fda.gov
U.S. Occupational Safety and Health Administration (OSHA)	www.osha.gov
American Academy of Oral and Maxillofacial Radiology (AAOMR)	www.aaomr.org
American Dental Association (ADA)	www.ada.org

TABLE 6-4   U.S. Nuclear Regulatory Commission Occupational Dose Limits

TISSUE	ANNUAL DOSE LIMIT
Whole body	50 mSv (5 rem)
Any organ	500 mSv (50 rem)
Skin	500 mSv (50 rem)
Extremity	500 mSv (50 rem)
Lens of eye	150 mSv (15 rem)

U.S. Nuclear Regulatory Commission. (2007, December 4). Standards for protection against radiation, Title 10, Part 20, of the *Code of Federal Regulations*. Retrieved April 11, 2010, from http://www.nrc.gov/reading-rm/doc-collections/cfr/part020/part020-1201.html

Guidelines for Maintaining Safe Radiation Levels

Radiation Safety Legislation

The Tenth Amendment gives the states the constitutional authority to regulate health. Because many federal agencies are involved in the development and use of atomic energy, the federal government has preempted the control of radiation. Certain provisions of the Constitution and Public Law 86-373 have enabled the states to assume this preempted power and pass laws that spell out radiation safety measures to protect the patient, the operator, or anyone (the general public) near the source of radiation. In fact, even counties and cities have passed ordinances to protect their citizens from radiation hazards. Most states and a few localities require periodic inspection or monitoring of the equipment and its surroundings.

The entry of the federal government into the regulation of x-ray machines began in 1968 with the enactment of the Radiation Control for Health and Safety Act, which standardized the performance of x-ray equipment. Subsequently, the Consumer-Patient Radiation Health and Safety Act of 1981 was passed, requiring the various states to develop minimum standards for operators of dental x-ray equipment. Several states responded to this by enacting educational requirements for the certification of individuals who place and expose dental radiographs.

Because the laws concerning radiation control vary from state to state, individuals working with x-rays must be familiar with the regulations governing the use of ionizing radiation in their locale. Regardless of laws, failure to observe safety protocol cannot be justified ethically.

REVIEW—Chapter summary

Oral health care professionals have an ethical responsibility to adopt the ALARA concept—as low as reasonably achievable—which implies that any dose that can be reduced without major difficulty, great expense, or inconvenience should be reduced or eliminated.

The most important step in keeping the patient's exposure to a minimum is the use of evidence-based selection criteria to assess patients for radiographic need.

The technical ability of the radiographer will aid in preventing unnecessary radiation exposure to the patient. Technical ability includes communication, working knowledge of quality radiographs, and education. Technique standards, including the choice of paralleling or bisecting technique, and the selection of exposure factors also aid in preventing unnecessary radiation exposure. Equipment standards that play important roles in reducing patient radiation dose include filtration, collimation, and PID length.

Filtration is the absorption of long wavelength, less penetrating x-rays from the x-ray beam by passage through a sheet of material called a filter. The half-value layer (HVL) of an x-ray beam is the thickness (measured in millimeters) of aluminum that will reduce the intensity of the beam by one-half. Present safety standards require an equivalent of 1.5 mm aluminum filtration for dental x-ray machines operating in ranges below 70 kVp and a minimum of 2.5 mm aluminum for machines operating at or above 70 kVp. Total filtration is the sum of inherent and added filtration.

Collimation is the control of the size and shape of the useful beam. Federal regulations require that round opening collimators restrict the x-ray beam to 2.75 in. (7 cm) at the patient end of the PID. Rectangular collimation reduces patient radiation dose by 70 percent over round collimation. Collimation reduces scattered radiation that contributes to poor contrast of radiographic images.

The position indicating device (PID) is an extension of the tube housing and is used to direct the primary x-ray beam. The length of the PID helps to establish the desired target–surface distance; the longer the PID, the less radiation dose to the patient. PIDs have either a round or rectangular shape and are available in lengths of 8 in. (20.5 cm), 12 in. (30 cm), and 16 in. (41 cm).

Fast film requires less radiation for exposure. Film speed groups D, E, or F are currently available for use in dental radiography. Film speed F reduces patient radiation exposure by 20 percent over film speed E. Film speed E reduces patient radiation exposure by 50 percent over film speed D. The use of digital image receptors can further reduce the radiation dose to the patient.

The use of image receptor holders eliminates using the patient's fingers to stabilize the receptor intraorally, avoiding unnecessary radiation exposure to the patient's fingers.

A lead or lead-equivalent thyroid collar with apron should be placed on all patients during intraoral x-ray exposures. The thyroid collar is most important in protecting children and pregnant women and women of child-bearing age.

Optimum film processing using time-temperature techniques in an adequately equipped darkroom will help avoid retakes that lead to an increase in patient radiation exposure.

To reduce the chance of operator exposure, time spent near the source of radiation should be reduced; structural shielding employed; or the operator should be in a position at least 6 feet away from the source of radiation at a 45 degree angle to the exiting primary beam.

Area and personnel radiation monitoring can be used to measure radiation exposures. The International Commission on Radiological Protection (ICRP) and the National Council on

Radiation Protection and Measurements (NCRP) recommend dose limits. Federal, state, and local agencies set regulations governing exposure. The American Dental Association and the American Academy of Oral and Maxillofacial Radiology work closely with all agencies responsible for radiation safety.

The maximum permissible dose (MPD) is 50 mSv (5 rem) per year for radiation workers and 5 mSv (0.5 rem) for the general public, radiation workers who are pregnant, and children under 18 years of age.

RECALL—Study questions

1. Who has an ethical responsibility to adopt ALARA?
   a. The dental assistant
   b. The dental hygienist
   c. The dentist
   d. All of the above

2. Based on the selection criteria guidelines, what is the radiographic recommendation for bitewing radiographs on an adult recall patient with no clinical caries and no high-risk factors for caries?
   a. Every 6–12 months
   b. Every 12–18 months
   c. Every 18–24 months
   d. Every 24–36 months

3. Communication, working knowledge of a quality radiographic image, and education all aid in protecting the patient against unnecessary radiation exposure by
   a. using lower exposure factors.
   b. reducing the risk of retake radiographs.
   c. collimating and filtering the primary beam.
   d. creating a longer target–surface distance.

4. What is the minimum total filtration that is required by an x-ray machine that can operate in ranges above 70 kVp?
   a. 1.5 mm of aluminum equivalent
   b. 1.5 mm of lead equivalent
   c. 2.5 mm of aluminum equivalent
   d. 2.5 mm of lead equivalent

5. What is the federally mandated size of the diameter of the primary beam at the end of the PID (at the skin of the patient's face)?
   a. 1.75 in. (4.5 cm)
   b. 2.75 in. (7 cm)
   c. 3.75 in. (10 cm)
   d. 4.75 in. (12 cm)

6. Radiation protection from secondary radiation may be increased by the use of an aluminum filter and a lead collimator *because* the filter regulates the size of the tissue area that is exposed and the collimator prevents low-energy radiation from reaching the tissue.
   a. Both statement and reason are correct.
   b. Both statement and reason are NOT correct.
   c. The statement is correct, but the reason is NOT correct.
   d. The statement is NOT correct, but the reason is correct.

7. Which of the following exposes the patient to less radiation?
   a. 8 in. (20.5 cm) round PID
   b. 12 in. (30 cm) round PID
   c. 16 in. (41 cm) round PID
   d. 16 in. (41 cm) rectangular PID

8. Which of the following contributes the most to reducing patient radiation exposure?
   a. D speed film
   b. E speed film
   c. F speed film

9. During dental x-ray exposure, the lead/lead-equivalent thyroid collar with apron should be placed on
   a. children.
   b. females.
   c. males.
   d. all patients.

10. Each of the following aids in reducing patient radiation exposure EXCEPT one. Which one is the EXCEPTION?
    a. Slow-speed film
    b. Careful film handling
    c. Darkroom protocol
    d. Image receptor holders

11. If a protective barrier is not present, what is the recommended minimum distance that the operator should stand from the source of the radiation?
    a. 3 ft (0.91 m)
    b. 6 ft (1.83 m)
    c. 9 ft (2.74m)
    d. 12 ft (3.66m)

12. Film badges, TLDs, and OSL and DIS monitors are used to
    a. protect the operator from unnecessary radiation exposure.
    b. reduce the radiation exposure received by the patient.
    c. monitor radiation exposure the dental radiographer may incur.
    d. record an on-site survey of the radiation output of the x-ray unit.

13. The annual maximum permissible whole-body dose for oral health care personnel is
    a. 0.5 mSv.
    b. 5.0 mSv.
    c. 50 mSv.
    d. 500 mSv.

14. The annual maximum permissible whole-body dose for the general public is
    a. 0.5 mSv.
    b. 5.0 mSv.
    c. 50 mSv.
    d. 500 mSv.

15. List three radiation protection organizations.

a. _____

b. _____

c. _____

REFLECT—Case study

Use the selection criteria guidelines to make a preliminary recommendation and/or to explain to the patient why the dentist has prescribed or has not prescribed radiographs. Consider the following three cases:

1. A 17-year-old patient presents with a healthy oral assessment. No active caries were clinically detected. No periodontal pockets were noted. His record indicates that his last radiographs were bitewings taken 6 months ago. Based on the evidence-based selection criteria guidelines, what would be the most likely recommendation for radiographs for this patient?

2. A 25-year-old female recall patient presents for her 6-month check-up. Although her homecare is good, Class II (multisurface) restorations are present on several molars and premolars. Her last radiographs were bitewings taken 3 years ago. Based on the evidence-based selection criteria guidelines, what would be the most likely recommendation for radiographs for this patient?

3. A 45-year-old male patient, new to your practice, presents with a moderate periodontal condition and evidence of generalized dental disease. He reveals that he has not had professional oral care in several years, but is here today to begin to "take care of his teeth." Based on the evidence-based selection criteria guidelines, what would be the most likely recommendation for radiographs for this patient?

RELATE—Laboratory application

Using Box 6-1, Summary of Protection Methods for the Patient, and Box 6-2, Summary of Methods to Protect the Radiographer, as a guide, perform an inventory of your facility. Make a list of all the radiation protection methods used at your facility. Compare and contrast these with the safety protocols you learned in this chapter.

Begin with the first patient radiation protection method listed in Box 6-1, evidence-based prescribing. Investigate how the dentist at your facility determines who will need radiographs. What guidelines do the dental hygienist and the dental assistant use to help them in explaining the need for necessary radiographs to the patient? Does your facility use guidelines similar to the evidence-based guidelines you learned about in this chapter? Describe them. Compare and contrast the methods your facility uses to determine radiographic need to the guidelines you learned about in this chapter. Is your facility meeting or exceeeding this safety method for reducing patient radiation dose? If not, what is the rationale for not meeting this standard?

Proceed to the next item on the list in Box 6-1, Communication. Observe the communication between the oral health care professionals at your facility prior to, during, and following patient x-ray exposure. What are some examples of dialogue that contributed to aiding in the protection of patients from unnecessary radiation exposure? Was there any communication that you think could have been added? Again, compare and contrast the communication standards the professionals at your facility use to decrease the likelihood of unnecessary radiation exposure using the guidelines you learned about in this chapter. Is your facility meeting or exceeding this safety method for reducing patient radiation dose? If not, what is the rationale for not meeting this standard?

Proceed through the list of items in Box 6-1 and Box 6-2. Use observation and interviewing techniques to thoroughly investigate how each of these items is applied at your facility. Based on what you learned in this chapter, determine whether your facility is adequately applying all possible methods of reducing radiation exposure to patients and radiographers.

REFERENCES

American Dental Association Council on Scientific Affairs. (2001). An update on radiographic practices: Information and recommendations. *Journal of the American Dental Association, 132,* 234–238.

American Dental Association Council on Scientific Affairs. (2006). The use of dental radiographs: Update and recommendations. *Journal of the American Dental Association, 137,* 1304–1312.

Carestream Health, Inc. (2007). *Kodak Dental Systems: Radiation safety in dental radiography.* Pub. N-414. Rochester, NY: Author.

Health Canada. (2008). *Environmental and work place health. Technology comparison.* HC Pub.: 4429. :Author.

International Commission on Radiological Protection. (1991). *1990 recommendations of ICRP.* Publication 60. Stockholm: Annuals of the ICRP, 21, 1–3.

Kuroyanagi, K., Yoshihiko, H., Hisao, F., & Tadashi, S. (1998). Distribution of scattered radiation during intraoral radiography with the patient in supine position. *Oral Surgery, Oral Medicine, Oral Pathology, 85*(6), 736-741.

National Council on Radiation Protection and Measurements. (1991). *Implementation of the principle of as low as reasonably achievable (ALARA) for medical and dental personnel.* NCRP Report No. 107. Washington, DC: NCRP.

National Council on Radiation Protection and Measurements. (2003). *Radiation protection in dentistry.* NCRP Report No. 145. Washington, DC: NCRP.

Public Health Service, Food and Drug Administration, American Dental Association Council on Dental Benefit Program, Council on Dental Practice, Council on Scientific Affairs. (2004). *The selection of patients for dental radiographic examinations.* Washington, DC: U.S. Dept. of Health and Human Services.

Thomson, E. M. (2006). Radiation safety update. *Contemporary Oral Hygiene, 6*(3), 10–18.

CHAPTER

7

PART III • DENTAL X-RAY IMAGE RECEPTORS AND FILM PROCESSING TECHNIQUES

Dental X-ray Film

OBJECTIVES

Following successful completion of this chapter, you should be able to:

1. Define the key words.
2. List and describe the four parts of an intraoral film.
3. Describe latent image formation.
4. List and describe the four parts of an intraoral film packet.
5. Differentiate between the tube side and the back side of an intraoral film packet.
6. Identify the intraoral film speeds currently available for dental radiographs.
7. Match the intraoral film size with customary usage.
8. Match the type of intraoral projection with radiographic need.
9. Explain the difference between intraoral and extraoral film.
10. List typical extraoral film sizes.
11. Compare and contrast duplicating film with radiographic film.
12. List the seven conditions that fog stored film.

KEY WORDS

Antihalation coating
Bitewing radiograph
Duplicating film
Emulsion
Extraoral film
Film packet
Film speed
Gelatin
Halide
Identification dot

Intensifying screen
Intraoral film
Latent image
Occlusal radiograph
Pedodontic film
Periapical radiograph
Screen film
Silver halide crystals
Solarized emulsion
Tube side

Introduction

Technological advances in digital imaging may one day render film-based radiography obsolete. Until that day, film remains a reliable method for acquiring diagnostic images to assess oral health and plan treatment for oral disease. Because radiation's interaction with film is what allows for the use of x-rays in preventive oral health care, the dental assistant and dental hygienist should possess a working knowledge of how radiographic film records an image. Additionally, determining how film can best be used to provide the greatest amount of diagnostic information while exposing the patient to the least amount of radiation possible is key to radiation safety. The purpose of this chapter is to explain film composition, introduce film category types, and discuss film protection and storage to aid the dental assistant and dental hygienist in making appropriate decisions regarding film use and handling.

Composition of Dental X-ray Film

The film used in dental radiography is photographic film that has been especially adapted in size, emulsion, speed, and packaging for dental uses. Figure 7-1 illustrates the composition of dental x-ray film.

Film Base

The purpose of the film base is to provide support for the fragile emulsion and to provide strength for handling. Films used in dental radiography have a thin, flexible, clear, or blue-tinted polyester base. The blue tint enhances contrast and image quality. The base is covered with a photographic emulsion on both sides.

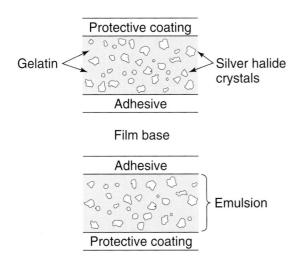

FIGURE 7-1 Schematic cross-section drawing of dental x-ray film. The rigid but flexible film base is coated on both sides with an emulsion consisting of silver halide (bromide and iodide) crystals embedded in gelatin. Each emulsion layer is attached to the base by a thin layer of adhesive. The emulsion layers are covered by a supercoating of gelatin to protect the emulsion from scratching and handling.

Adhesive

Each emulsion layer is attached to the base by a thin layer of adhesive.

Emulsion

The **emulsion** is composed of **gelatin** in which crystals of silver **halide** salts are suspended. The function of the gelatin is to keep the silver halide crystals evenly suspended over the base. The gelatin will not dissolve in cold water, but swells, exposing the silver halide crystals to the chemicals in the developing solution. The gelatin shrinks as it dries, leaving a smooth surface that becomes the radiograph.

The **silver halide crystals** are compounds of a halogen (either bromine or iodine) with another element. In radiography, as well as in photography, that element is silver. Dental film emulsion is about 90 to 99 percent silver bromide and 1 to 10 percent silver iodide. Silver halide crystals are sensitive to radiation. It is the silver halide crystals that, when exposed to x-rays, retain the latent image.

Protective Layer

The supercoating of gelatin to protect the emulsion from scratching and rough handling that covers the emulsion layers is called the protective layer.

Latent Image Formation

During radiation exposure x-rays strike and ionize some, but not all, of the silver halide crystals, resulting in the formation of a **latent** (invisible) **image.** Not all the radiation penetrating the patient's tissue will reach the film emulsion. For example, metal restorations such as amalgam or crowns will absorb the x-ray energy and stop the radiation from reaching the film. It should be noted that varying amounts of radiation will reach the film. The varying thicknesses of the objects in the path of the beam will allow more or less radiation to pass through and reach the film emulsion. For example, enamel and bone will absorb, or stop, more x-rays from reaching the film than the less dense structures such as the dentin or pulp chambers of the teeth. When radiation does reach the emulsion, the silver halide crystals are ionized, or separated into silver and bromide and iodide ions that store this energy as a latent image. These energy centers store the invisible image pattern until the processing procedure produces a visual image (see Chapter 8).

During the developing stage of the processing procedure, the exposed silver halide crystals—which have stored a latent image—are changed into black specks of silver, resulting in the black or radiolucent areas observed on a dental radiograph. The amount of black silver specks varies depending on the structures radiographed and whether or not those structures allowed the x-rays to pass through and reach the film emulsion. The less dense or thin structures permit the passage of x-rays; thick, dense structures will not. These dense structures will appear clear/white or radiopaque on the radiograph as a result of the fixer step during film processing (see Chapter 8).

Types of Dental X-ray Film

Depending on where the film is to be used—inside or outside the mouth—the film is classified as intraoral or extraoral.

Intraoral Films

Intraoral films are designed for use inside the oral cavity. The use of an intraoral film outside the oral cavity is contraindicated because of the increased dose of radiation needed to produce an acceptable radiographic density.

FILM PACKET   The film manufacturer cuts the films to the sizes required in dentistry. Small films suitable for intraoral (inside the mouth) radiography are made into what is called a **film packet.** The terms *film packet* and *film* are often used interchangeably. Figure 7-2 shows the front or **tube side** and the back side of an intraoral film packet.

All intraoral film packets are assembled similarly. The film is first surrounded by black, light-protective paper. Next, a thin sheet of lead foil to shield the film from backscatter radiation is placed on the side of the film that will be away from the radiation source. An outer wrapping of moisture-resistant paper or plastic completes the assembly (Figures 7-3 and 7-4).

The film packet consists of:

1. Film
2. Black paper wrapping
3. Lead foil
4. Moisture-resistant outer wrapping

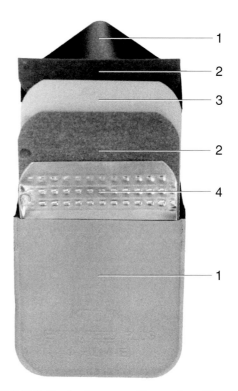

FIGURE 7-3 **Back of an open film packet. (1)** Moisture-resistant outer wrap. (**2**) Black paper. (**3**) Film. (**4**) Lead foil backing.

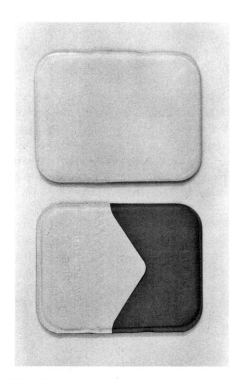

FIGURE 7-2 **Intraoral film packets** showing the front or tube side (white, unprinted side of the film packet) *(top)* and the back side (color-coded side) of the film packet *(bottom).*

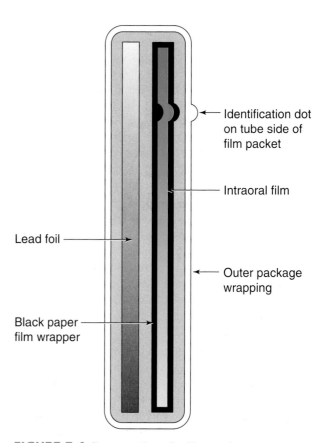

FIGURE 7-4 **Cross-section of a film packet.**

- **Film.** Film packets contain one or two films. When a packet containing two radiographic films is exposed, a duplicate radiograph results at no additional radiation exposure to the patient. One radiograph must be kept as part of the patient record. The copy can serve as a duplicate radiograph. Duplicate radiographs may be sent to a specialist for consultation regarding treatment, to another professional as a referral, to a third-party payer or insurance company as evidence for needed treatment, to document legal evidence, or given to the patient who is moving to another location and will seek treatment at another oral health care facility.

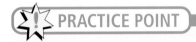

PRACTICE POINT

The patient has a right to access their dental records, including radiographs. The use of double film packets produces two original radiographs, allowing the practice to keep one as part of the patient's permanent record and provides a ready copy to give to the patient when requested.

A small raised **identification dot** is located in one corner of the film. The raised dot is used to determine film orientation and is used to distinguish between radiographs of the patient's right and left sides (see Chapter 21).

- **Black paper wrapping** surrounds the film inside the packet to protect it from light.
- **Lead foil.** A sheet of lead foil is located in the back of the film packet, behind the film. The purpose of the lead foil backing is to absorb scattered radiation. Scattered x-rays strike the film emulsion from the back side of the film (the side away from the tube), fogging or reducing the clarity of the image. The lead foil is embossed with a pattern that becomes visible on the developed radiograph in the event that the packet is accidentally positioned backward during the exposure.
- **Moisture-resistant outer wrapping** consisting of paper or soft vinyl plastic holds the packet contents and protects the film from light and moisture. This wrapping is either smooth or slightly pebbly to prevent slippage. Each film packet has two sides, a front side or tube side that faces the tube (radiation source) and a back side that faces away from the source of radiation (Figure 7-2).
  - **Tube side.** The tube side is usually solid white. A small embossed dot is evident near one of the film packet corners. The embossed dot will be used later to aid in identifying the image as either the patient's right or left side; however, it is important to know which corner it is located on during the film placement step.

In intraoral radiography, the tube side of the film faces the source of radiation. When placing the film intraorally, the tube side will face the lingual surfaces of the teeth of interest.

TABLE 7-1	Kodak Film Packet Color Codes	
	ONE-FILM PACKET	TWO-FILM PACKET
Ultra-speed (D)	Green	Gray
Insight (F)	Lavender	Tan

- **Back side.** The back side containing the tab for opening the film packet is white or may be color coded (Table 7-1). To aid in determining which is the front and the back side of the film packet, the following information is usually printed on the back side:
  - Manufacturer's name
  - Film speed
  - Number of films in the packet (one or two)
  - Circle or mark indicating the location of the identifying dot
  - The statement "Opposite side toward tube"

PRACTICE POINT

During intraoral film packet placement, the embossed dot should be positioned away from the area of interest. Usually, when taking periapical radiographs, the area of interest is the apices of the teeth; therefore, the embossed dot should be positioned toward the occlusal. To assist with positioning the embossed dot out of the way, intraoral film manufacturers have packaged film so that the embossed dot can be observed on the outer moisture-resistant wrapping.

FILM PACKAGING   Intraoral film packets are packaged in cardboard boxes or plastic trays. Depending on the size, intraoral films are packaged 25, 50, 130, or 150 to a box, the most popular being the 130- or 150-film packages. A layer of protective foil surrounds the films inside the container to protect against damage while being stored.

FILM EMULSION SPEEDS (SENSITIVITY)   Speed refers to the amount of radiation required to produce a radiograph of acceptable density. The faster the **film speed,** the less radiation required to produce a radiograph of acceptable density. Factors that determine film speed are

- **Size of silver halide crystals.** The larger the crystals, the faster the film speed.
- **Thickness of emulsion.** Emulsion is coated on both sides of the film base to increase film speed. The thicker the emulsion, the faster the film speed.
- **Special radiosensitive dyes.** Manufacturers add special dyes that help to increase the film speed.

Although the thickness of the emulsion and the addition of radiosensitive dyes aid in increasing film speed (film sensitivity), the most important factor in increasing film speed is the size of the silver halide crystals in the emulsion. The larger the crystals, the faster the film speed, resulting in less radiation exposure to produce an acceptable image. However, image sharpness is more distinct when the crystals are small. The larger crystals used in high-speed (fast) film result in a certain amount of graininess that reduces the sharpness of the radiographic image. It has been determined that this slight loss of image sharpness does not interfere with diagnosis and is tolerated because of the reduction in patient radiation exposure.

SPEED GROUPS Trademark names like *Ultra*-speed or *Insight* are names assigned by the manufacturer and do not indicate the actual film speed. The American National Standards Institute (ANSI) groups film speed using letters of the alphabet: speed group A for the slowest through F for the fastest. At the present time, F-speed is the fastest film available, and film speeds slower than D are no longer used. In addition to labeling the film packages, film speed is printed on the back side of each individual film packet.

Currently only D-speed, E-speed, and F-speed films are available. Some manufacturers have stopped producing E-speed film. Both the American Dental Association and the American Association of Oral and Maxillofacial Radiology recommend using the fastest speed film currently available to aid in reducing unnecessary radiation to patients. Although F-speed film requires less radiation to produce an acceptable image, some practitioners have not stopped using the slower D-speed film. Faster-speed films contain a larger crystal size that may contribute to a slight decrease in image resolution. Some practitioners who are accustomed to viewing D-speed images resist the change. However, it should be noted that changes in the visual acuity of today's films have improved the image of the faster-speed films. Additionally, it should be noted that studies of film speed comparisons have failed to indicate that faster-speed films are less diagnostic. The use of high-speed film has made it possible to reduce patient exposure to radiation to a fraction of the time formerly deemed necessary.

FILM SIZE There are five sizes of intraoral film: #0, #1, #2, #3, and #4. The larger the number, the larger the size of the film (Figure 7-5).

- **Size No. 0.** The #0 film is especially designed for small children and is often called pedo (from the Greek word *paidos,* child) or **pedodontic film.**

- **Size No. 1.** The #1 film may also be used for children. In adults, the use of the narrow #1 film is normally limited to exposing radiographs of the anterior teeth. Although it images only two or three teeth, this film is ideal for areas where the oral cavity is narrow.

- **Size No. 2.** The wider #2 film is generally referred to as the standard film, or PA for periapical film. This film size is used in probably 75 percent of all intraoral radiography. The #2 film is commonly used on both larger children, especially those with a mixed dentition, and adults.

- **Size No. 3.** The extra-long #3 film is called a long bitewing film. These films usually come with a preattached bite tab.

- **Size No. 4.** The #4 film is the largest of the intraoral films. Size #4 films are generally referred to as occlusal films.

TYPES OF PROJECTIONS These five film sizes are used to expose three types of intraoral film projections: bitewing, periapical, and occlusal.

- **Bitewing radiographs** (Figure 7-6) image the coronal portions of both the maxillary (upper) and mandibular (lower) teeth and crestal bone on the same film. Bitewing radiographs are used to examine the surfaces of the crowns of the teeth that touch each other and are particularly valuable in determining the extent of proximal caries. Bitewing radiographs image a portion of the alveolar bone crests, and vertical bitewing radiographs (see Chapter 16) provide added information regarding the supporting periodontia. Both vertical and horizontal bitewing radiographs may be exposed using film sizes #0, #1, or #2. Film size #3 is especially designed to expose horizontal bitewing radiographs. Bitewing film sizes, especially the size #3 film packet, may be purchased with an attached flap or tab on which the patient must bite to hold the film packet in place between the occlusal surfaces of the maxillary and mandibular teeth.

- **Periapical radiographs** (Figure 7-7) (from the Greek word *peri,* for around and the Latin word *apex* for the root tip) are used to record a detailed examination of the entire tooth, from crown to root tip or apex. Periapical radiographs image the supporting structures of the teeth such as the periodontal ligament space and the surrounding bone. Periapical radiographs may be exposed using film sizes #0, #1, or #2.

- **Occlusal radiographs** (see Figure 17-1) image a larger area than periapical radiographs. These projections are ideal for recording a large area of the maxilla, mandible, and floor of the mouth. They can reveal gross pathological lesions, root fragments, bone and tooth fractures, and impacted or supernumerary teeth and many other conditions. Occlusal radiographs can be used to survey an edentulous (without teeth) mouth. The size #4 film packet is especially designed as an occlusal film. Film size #2 may also be used with the occlusal radiographic technique, especially for young children who may not be able to tolerate the film packet placement necessary for periapical radiographs.

Extraoral Films

Extraoral films are designed for use outside the mouth. These large films are classified as screen film. **Screen film** (indirect-exposure film) is exposed primarily by a fluorescent type of light given off by special emulsion-coated **intensifying screens** that are positioned between the film and the x-ray source. The intensity of the fluorescent light emitted by the intensifying screens permits a significant reduction in the amount of radiation required to produce an image. The image produced on an extraoral film results from exposure to this fluorescent light, instead of directly from the x-rays.

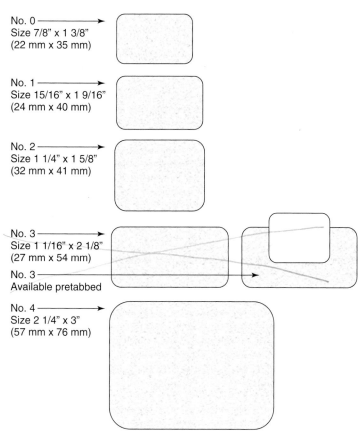

No. 0
Size 7/8" x 1 3/8"
(22 mm x 35 mm)

No. 1
Size 15/16" x 1 9/16"
(24 mm x 40 mm)

No. 2
Size 1 1/4" x 1 5/8"
(32 mm x 41 mm)

No. 3
Size 1 1/16" x 2 1/8"
(27 mm x 54 mm)

No. 3
Available pretabbed

No. 4
Size 2 1/4" x 3"
(57 mm x 76 mm)

FIGURE 7-5 Intraoral film sizes.

PACKAGING   Larger extraoral films are generally packaged 25, 50, or 100 to a box (Figure 7-8). The films are sometimes sandwiched between two pieces of protective paper, and the entire group is wrapped in protective foil. Because these films are designed for extraoral use with a cassette, discussed in detail in Chapter 29, they require neither individual lead backing nor moisture-resistant wrappings.

FILM SIZE   Extraoral films vary in size. Different sizes can accommodate imaging the oral cavity and various regions of the head and neck. The most common sizes are

- 5 × 7 in. (13 × 18 cm), used mainly for lateral views of the jaw or the temporomandibular joint (TMJ)
- 8 × 10 in. (20 × 26 cm), used for cephalometric profiles and posteroanterior views of the skull
- 5 or 6 in. × 12 in. (13 or 15 cm × 30 cm), used for panoramic radiographs of the entire dentition

Duplicating Film

When a duplicate radiograph, a copy identical to an original, is needed, oral health care practices often use two- or double-film

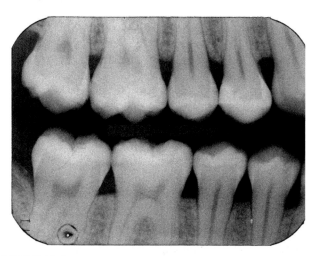

FIGURE 7-6 Bitewing radiograph.

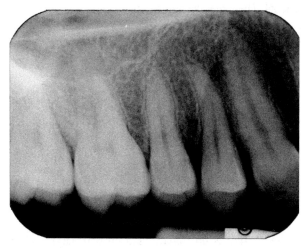

FIGURE 7-7 Periapical radiograph.

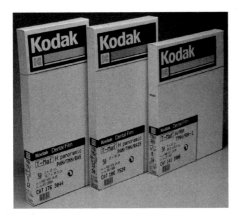

FIGURE 7-8 Extraoral film packages.
5 × 12-in. (13 × 30 cm), 6 × 12-in (15 × 30 cm), and
8 × 10 in. (20 × 26 cm) size extraoral film packages. (Used with permission of Eastman Kodak Company.)

intraoral packets. However, if an additional copy is needed or a two-film packet was not used when the original radiograph was exposed, a duplicating machine with special duplicating film can be used.

Duplicating film is different than x-ray film and is exposed by the action of infrared and ultraviolet light rather than by x-rays. Only one side of the duplicating film is coated with emulsion. The emulsion side appears dull and lighter under safe light conditions in the darkroom where it is used. The nonemulsion side is shiny and appears darker under safe light conditions. To make a copy of a radiograph, the emulsion side of the film is placed against the original radiograph with the nonemulsion side up (see Chapter 28). When the duplicating film is exposed to ultraviolet light from the duplicating machine, the **solarized emulsion** records the copy. Solarized emulsion is different than x-ray film emulsion in that the image produced in response to light exposure gets darker with less light exposure and lighter with more light exposure. The nonemulsion side contains an **antihalation coating.** The dye in the antihalation coating absorbs the ultraviolet light coming through the film to prevent back-scattered light from reexposing the film and creating an unsharp image.

Duplicating film, boxed in quantities of 50, 100, or 150 sheets, is available in periapical sizes and in 5 or 6 × 12 in. (13 or 15 × 30 cm) and 8 × 10 in. (20 × 26 cm) sheets.

Film Storage and Protection

All radiographic film is extremely sensitive to radiation, light, heat, humidity, chemical fumes, and physical pressure. Additionally, film is sensitive to aging, having a shelf life determined by the manufacturer. Precautions for safely storing and protecting films from these conditions must be followed. Film fogging is the darkening of the finished radiograph caused by one or more of these factors.

Radiation

Stray radiation, not intended for primary exposure, can fog film. Film should be stored in its original packaging in an area shielded

from radiation. Individual film packets should also be kept in a shielded area. This is especially important while in the process of exposing several radiographs at one time, as is the case when exposing a set of bitewings or full mouth series on a patient. Once a film has been exposed to radiation, the crystals within the emulsion increase in their sensitivity. The exposed film should be placed in a shielded area while the next film is exposed. All exposed films should be kept safe from radiation until processing.

Light

Care should be taken when handling intraoral film packets so as not to tear the outer light-tight wrap. Extraoral cassettes must be closed tightly to prevent light leaks. Safe lighting in the darkroom must be periodically examined to ensure safe light conditions (see Chapter 19).

Heat and Humidity

To prevent fogging, film should be stored in a cool, dry place. Ideally, all unexposed film should be stored at 50°F to 70°F (10°C–21°C) and 30 to 50 percent relative humidity.

Chemical Fumes

Film should be stored away from the possibility of contamination by chemical fumes. Film should not be stored in the darkroom near processing chemicals.

Physical Pressure

Physical pressure and bending can fog film. When storing, boxes of film must not be stacked so high as to increase the pressure on the packets. Heavy objects should not be placed or stored on top of film.

Shelf Life

Dental x-ray film has a limited shelf life. The expiration date is printed on the film packaging (Figure 7-9). All intraoral film should be stored so that the expiration date can be readily seen and the appropriate films used first. Expired film compromises the diagnostic quality of the image and should not be used.

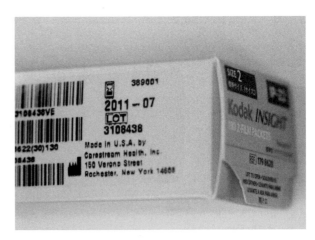

FIGURE 7-9 Film package showing expiration date.

REVIEW—Chapter summary

X-ray film serves as a radiographic image receptor. The film used in dental radiography is photographic film that has been especially adapted in size, emulsion, film speed, and packaging for dental uses. All x-ray film has a polyester base that is coated with a gelatin emulsion containing silver halide (bromide and iodide) crystals.

During radiation exposure, the x-rays strike and ionize some of the silver halide crystals, forming a latent image. The image does not become visible until the film is processed.

An intraoral film packet consists of film, white-light tight black paper wrapping, lead foil, and a moisture-resistant outer wrapping. Intraoral film packets have a white, unprinted front or tube side. The lead foil and the tab for opening the film packet are on the back side.

Film speed (sensitivity) refers to the amount of radiation required to produce a radiograph of acceptable density. Film speed groups range from A (for the slowest) through F (for the fastest). Currently only D-, E-, and F-speed films are available for dental radiographs.

The five intraoral film sizes are #0, #1, #2, #3, and #4. The three types of intraoral radiographic projections are bitewing, for imaging proximal tooth surfaces and alveolar bone crests; periapical, for examining the entire tooth and supporting structures; and occlusal, for surveying larger areas of the maxilla and the mandible.

Larger extraoral films designed for use outside the mouth are classified as screen films because fluorescent light from intensifying screens is used to help the x-rays produce the image. Extraoral films are used for lateral jaw exposures and cephalometric and panoramic radiographs.

Duplicating film is used in conjunction with a duplicating machine that emits light to make copies of radiographs. Duplicating film differs from radiographic film in that the solarized emulsion gets darker with less light exposure and lighter with more light exposure.

X-ray film is sensitive to radiation, light, heat, humidity, chemical fumes, physical pressure, and aging. Care must be exercised in storing and in handling the film before, during, and after exposure.

RECALL—Study questions

1. Which of these provides support for the fragile film emulsion?
   a. Base
   b. Adhesive
   c. Silver halide crystals
   d. Protective coating

2. Which of these is light and x-ray sensitive?
   a. Lead foil
   b. Adhesive
   c. Gelatin
   d. Silver halide crystals

3. During x-ray exposure, crystals within the film emulsion become energized with a(n)
   a. visible image.
   b. slow image.
   c. latent image.
   d. intensified image.

4. What is the function of the lead foil in the film packet?
   a. Moisture protection
   b. Absorb backscatter radiation
   c. Give rigidity to the packet
   d. Protect against fluorescence

5. Each of the following can be found on the back side of an intraoral film packet EXCEPT one. Which one is the EXCEPTION?
   a. Film speed
   b. Film size
   c. Embossed dot location
   d. Number of films in packet

6. Which of these films has the greatest sensitivity to radiation?
   a. D-speed
   b. E-speed
   c. F-speed

7. A size #4 intraoral film packet would most likely be used to expose a(n)
   a. bitewing radiograph.
   b. periapical radigraph.
   c. occlusal radigraph.
   d. pedodontic radiograph.

8. Which of these projections will the dentist most likely prescribe for evaluation of a specific tooth and its surrounding structures?
   a. Bitewing radiograph
   b. Periapical radigraph
   c. Occlusal radiograph
   d. Panoramic radiograph

9. Intensifying screens will
   a. reduce exposure time.
   b. decrease processing time.
   c. increase x-ray intensity.
   d. increase image detail.

10. Which of the following is considered to be a screen film?
    a. Occlusal
    b. Periapical
    c. Bitewing
    d. Panoramic

11. Which type of film is used to copy a radiograph?
    a. Duplicating film
    b. Screen film
    c. Nonscreen film
    d. X-ray film

12. X-ray films should be stored
    a. away from heat and humidity.
    b. near the source of radiation.
    c. in the darkroom.
    d. stacked in columns.

REFLECT—Case study

Utilize what you learned in this chapter about the sizes and types of projections to make a preliminary recommendation and/or to explain to the patient why the dentist has prescribed: (1) the type of projection; (2) the size of the film; and/or (3) the number of films to use for each of the following three cases.

1. An adult patient with suspected carious lesions on the proximal surfaces of posterior teeth. Additionally, this patient is considered to have a periodontal condition for which he is under maintenance treatment.
   a. The recommended type of projection will most likely be:
   b. The size of the film(s) will most likely be:
   c. The number of films to be exposed will most likely be:
2. An adult patient with a toothache in the area of the maxillary right molar.
   a. The recommended type of projection will most likely be:
   b. The size of film(s) will most likely be:
   c. The number of films to be exposed will most likely be:
3. An 8-year-old patient who, while skateboarding, seems to have suffered a traumatic injury to the anterior teeth.
   a. The recommended type of projection will most likely be:
   b. The size of film(s) will most likely be:
   c. The number of films to be exposed will most likely be:

RELATE—Laboratory applicaton

Obtain one each of a size #0, size #1, size #2, size #3, and size #4 intraoral film packet. Beginning with the size #0 film packet, consider the following. Repeat with each of the film sizes. Write out your observations.

1. What is the film speed? How did you get the answer to this question?
2. What information is written on the outside of the film packet? Where is this information written: on the front or back of the film packet?
3. How many films do you expect to find inside this packet? How did you get the answer to this question?
4. Where is the embossed dot located? How did you find it? What is this used for?
5. What type of projection (bitewing, periapical, or occlusal) could be taken with this film size? Explain your answer.
6. What about this film packet's size makes it ideal; less than ideal; or not suited for the adult patient? A child patient?
7. For what area(s) of the oral cavity will this film packet be best suited? Not suited?
8. Now open the film packet. List the four parts of the packet and explain the purpose of each.
9. Next, hold the film up horizontally (parallel to the floor) at eye level and observe it from the edge. Can you see the film base with the emulsion coating on the top and the bottom?
10. Next, observe the metal foil. What is the reason for the embossed imprint?
11. When you opened the film packet, did you utilize the black paper's tab? The tab plays an important role in opening a contaminated film packet aseptically. This is discussed in detail in Chapter 10.

REFERENCE

Carestream Health, Inc. (2007). *Kodak Dental Systems: Exposure and processing for dental film radiography.* Pub. N-414. Rochester, NY.

Dental X-ray Film Processing

OBJECTIVES

Following successful completion of this chapter, you should be able to:

1. Define the key words.
2. Explain how a latent image becomes a visible image.
3. List in sequence the steps in processing dental films.
4. List the four chemicals in the developer solution, and explain the function of each ingredient.
5. List the four chemicals in the fixer solution, and explain the function of each ingredient.
6. Discuss location, size, and lighting as considerations for setting up a darkroom.
7. Discuss the factors that affect safelighting.
8. Identify equipment needed for manual film processing
9. Demonstrate the steps of manual film processing.
10. Describe the role of rapid (chairside) processing.
11. Identify equipment needed for automatic film processing.
12. Demonstrate the steps of automatic film processing.
13. Compare manual and automatic processing methods stating advantages and disadvantages of each.
14. Explain the role chemical replenishment and solution changes play in maintaining optimal processing chemistry.

KEY WORDS

Acetic acid	Film feed slot
Acidifier	Film hanger
Activator	Film recovery slot
Automatic processor	Fixer
Darkroom	Fixing agent
Daylight loader	Hardening agent
Developer	Hydroquinone
Developing agent	Latent image
Elon	LED (light-emitting diode)

Introduction

Film **processing** is a series of steps that converts the invisible latent image on the dental x-ray film into a visible permanent image called a radiograph. The diagnostic quality of the visible image depends on strictly adhering to these processing steps. Film processing may be accomplished either manually or automatically. The purpose of this chapter is to explain the fundamentals of film processing and identify the roles processing solutions play in producing a visible image. Because most processing is accomplished in a **darkroom** equipped with special lights, darkroom design and equipment will be described.

Overview of Film Processing

Processing transforms the **latent** (hidden) **image,** which is produced when the x-ray photons are absorbed by the **silver halide crystals** in the emulsion, into a visible, stable image by means of chemicals. The basic steps of processing dental x-ray film are:

1. Developing
2. Rinsing (automatic processors often omit this step)
3. Fixing
4. Washing
5. Drying

Developing

The initial step in the processing sequence is the development of the film. The role of the **developer** solution is to reduce the exposed silver halide crystals within the film emulsion to black metallic silver. The unexposed silver halide crystals (in those areas of the film opposite metallic or dense structures that absorb and prevent the passage of x-rays) are unaffected at this time.

Rinsing

The purpose of the rinsing step is to remove as much of the alkaline developer as possible before placing the film in the fixer solution. Rinsing preserves the acidity of the fixer and prolongs its useful life.

Fixing

After brief rinsing, the film is immersed in the **fixer** solution. The role of the fixer is to remove the unexposed and/or undeveloped silver halide crystals from the film emulsion.

Washing

After the film is completely fixed, it is washed in running water to remove any remaining traces of the chemicals.

Drying

The final step is drying the film for storage as a part of the patient's permanent record. Films may be air-dried at room temperature or they may be dried in a heated cabinet especially made for this purpose.

The processed films are now called radiographs. The images on the radiograph are made up of microscopic grains of black metallic silver. The amount of silver deposited will vary with the thickness of the tissues penetrated. As discussed in Chapter 4, tissues that are not very dense, such as the pulp chamber of the tooth, allow more radiation to reach the film emulsion, resulting in black (**radiolucent**) areas on the film, whereas dense structures such as metal restorations will block the passage of x-rays, resulting in white (**radiopaque**) areas on the film. Basically, the developer is responsible for creating the film's radiolucent appearance, and the fixer is responsible for creating the film's radiopaque appearance.

Film Processing Solutions

Dental x-ray film processing requires the use of developer and fixer. These chemicals may be obtained in three forms (Figure 8-1):

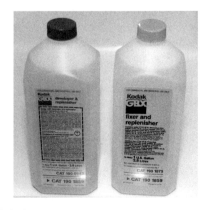

FIGURE 8-1 Processing chemicals. Liquid concentrate of developer and fixer. When mixed with distilled water, each bottle yields 1 gal (3.8 L) of solution.

TABLE 8-1   Composition of Developer

INGREDIENT	CHEMICAL	ACTION
Developing agents (reducing agents)	Hydroquinone	Reduces (converts) exposed silver halide crystals to black metallic silver. Slowly builds up black tones and contrast.
	Elon	Reduces (converts) exposed silver halide crystals to black metallic silver. Quickly builds up gray tones.
Preservative	Sodium sulfite	Prevents rapid oxidation of the developing agents.
Activator	Sodium carbonate	Activates developing agents by providing required alkalinity.
Restrainer	Potassium bromide	Restrains the developing agents from developing the unexposed silver halide crystals, which produce film fog.

- Powder
- Liquid concentrate
- Ready-to-use solutions

The powdered and liquid concentrate forms must be mixed with water prior to using. Chemical manufacturers usually recommend the use of distilled water when mixing chemistry to avoid potential problems with other chemicals that are sometimes present in tap water.

Developer

The main purpose of the developer is to convert the exposed silver halide crystals into metallic silver grains.

There are four chemicals in the developer (Table 8-1):

1. Developing agents (also called reducing agents)
2. Preservative
3. Activator (also called alkalizer)
4. Restrainer

The **developing agent** reduces the exposed silver halide crystals to metallic silver but has no effect on the unexposed crystals at recommended time–temperatures. This is called **selective reduction,** meaning that only the nonmetallic elements, the halides, are removed, and the exposed silver remains (Figure 8-2).

Developer contains two chemicals, **hydroquinone** and **elon.** The hydroquinone works slowly but steadily to build up density and contrast in the image. The elon works fast to bring out the gray shades (contrast) of the image. Both chemicals are affected by extreme temperatures. The higher the temperature, the less time required to develop the film; therefore, regulating the temperature of the developer is critical.

The **preservative, sodium sulfite,** protects the developing agents by slowing down the rapid oxidation rate of the developer.

The **activator,** usually **sodium carbonate,** provides the necessary alkaline medium required by the developing agents. It also softens and swells the gelatin, allowing more of the exposed silver halide crystals to come into contact with the developing agents.

The **restrainer, potassium bromide,** restrains the developing agents from developing the unexposed silver halide crystals and therefore inhibits the tendency of the solution to fog the film.

Fixer

The fixer plays three roles: (1) stops further film development—thereby establishing the image permanently on the film; (2) removes (dissolves) the unexposed/undeveloped silver halide crystals (those that were not exposed to x-rays); and (3) hardens (fixes) the emulsion.

There are four chemicals in the fixer (Table 8-2):

1. Fixing agent (also called a clearing agent)
2. Preservative
3. Hardening agent
4. Acidifier

The **fixing** (clearing) **agent,** ammonium thiosulfate or **sodium thiosulfate,** also known as "hypo" or hyposulfate of sodium, removes all unexposed and any remaining undeveloped silver halide crystals from the emulsion.

The preservative, sodium sulfite (the same chemical as used in the developer), slows the rate of oxidation and prevents the deterioration of the hypo and the precipitation of sulfur.

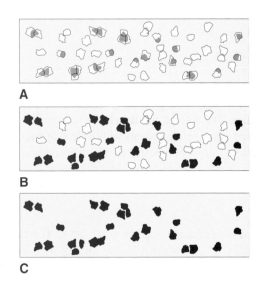

FIGURE 8-2 Cross section of dental x-ray film emulsion. (**A**) X-rays strike silver halide crystals, forming latent image sites (shown in gray). (**B**) After development, crystals struck by x-rays (latent image sites) reduced to black metallic silver. (**C**) Fixer removes unexposed, undeveloped crystals, leaving the black metallic silver.

TABLE 8-2	Composition of Fixer	
INGREDIENT	CHEMICAL	ACTION
Fixing agent (clearing agent)	Ammonium thiosulfate or sodium thiosulfate	Removes the unexposed and any remaining undeveloped silver halide crystals.
Preservative	Sodium sulfite	Slows the rate of oxidation and prevents deterioration of the fixing agent.
Hardening agent	Potassium alum	Shrinks and hardens the gelatin emulsion.
Acidifier	Acetic acid	Stops further development by neutralizing the alkali of the developer.

The **hardening agent, potassium alum,** shrinks and hardens the gelatin emulsion. This hardening continues until the film is dry, thus protecting it from abrasion.

The **acidifier, acetic acid,** provides the acid medium to stop further development by neutralizing the alkali of the developer.

Hardening Agents

Special hardening agents are sometimes added to the developer used in automatic processors to facilitate the transportation of the films through the roller systems.

Replenisher

Replenisher is a superconcentrated solution of developer or fixer. Replenisher is added to the developer or fixer in the processing tanks to compensate for the loss of volume and strength of the solutions due to oxidation and other causes. Processing solutions lose their potency over time and with use. Adding replenisher helps to maintain solution strength.

Darkroom

The purpose of the **darkroom** is to provide an area where x-ray films can be safely handled and processed. A well-equipped room with adequate safelighting aids in producing high-quality radiographic images. Films can be processed outside the darkroom with chairside manual processing mini-darkrooms (Figure 8-3) or with a **daylight loader**–equipped automatic processor (Figure 8-4). A darkroom remains the standard in most film-based practices, especially because safelight conditions are required to handle larger tasks such as extraoral film cassette loading and processing. The darkroom should be located near the area where radiographs will be exposed for convenient access and should be large enough to meet the requirements of the practice. The darkroom should be equipped with correct lighting, be well ventilated, and have adequate storage space for radiographic supplies.

The ability to store radiographic supplies such as extraoral film cassettes, duplicating film, and processing chemicals and cleaning supplies in the darkroom will add to the convenience of maintaining the ideal darkroom. Although storing unused film in the darkroom may seem convenient, it is not recommended. In addition to being sensitive to radiation and white light exposure, unexposed film is sensitive to heat, humidity and chemical fumes, all of which may be increased in the darkroom.

Lighting

X-ray film is sensitive to white light. Any white light in the darkroom can blacken the film or cause film fog. Therefore, the darkroom must be **light-tight.** A light-tight room is one that is completely dark and excludes all light. Felt strips may have to be installed around the door(s) to the darkroom or any other area such as around water pipes where a light leak is discovered. Although darkroom walls are sometimes painted black, this is not necessary if the room is completely sealed to white light. The following forms of illumination are desirable in the well-equipped darkroom.

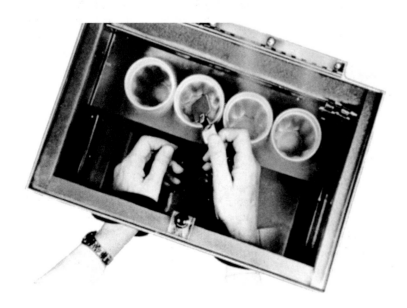

FIGURE 8-3 Chair-side mini-darkroom box with view-through plastic filtered top. First cup is filled with developer, second cup with rinse water, third cup with fixer, and fourth cup with wash water. A heater with a thermostat keeps the solutions at optimum temperature for rapid processing. (Courtesy of Dentsply Rinn.)

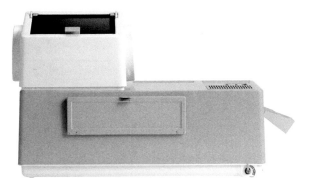

FIGURE 8-4 **Automatic processor with daylight loader attachment for use outside the darkroom.** (Courtesy of Air Techniques, Inc.)

1. **White ceiling light.** An overhead white ceiling light that provides adequate illumination for the size of the room will allow the clinician to perform equipment maintenance and other tasks requiring visibility.
2. **Safelight.** Safelighting is achieved through the use of a filtered white lightbulb or a special **LED (light-emitting diode)** bulb (Figure 8-5) that provide enough light in the darkroom to allow the clinician to perform activities without exposing or fogging the film. Traditional **safelights** consist of a 7 1/2 or 15 watt white incandescent light bulb with a **safelight filter** placed over it (Figure 8-6). The safelight filter removes the short wavelengths in the blue-green region of the visible light spectrum. The longer wavelength red-orange light is allowed to pass through the filter to illuminate the darkroom. A variety of filters are available. Orange or yellow filters allow for safe handling of D-speed film, but E- and F-speed film and most extraoral films require a red filter. The type of safelight required for film processing can usually be found written on the film package. LED (light-emitting diode) safelights emit pure red light and are safe for all film speeds and types.

   The term "safe" light is relative. Film emulsion can be damaged by prolonged exposure even to filtered safelight. Film handling should be limited to 2 1/2 minutes under safelight conditions or fogging (film darkening) may occur. The distance between the lamp and the film is critical. The rule is 2 1/4 watts per ft (0.3 m) and a 4-ft (1.2 m) minimum

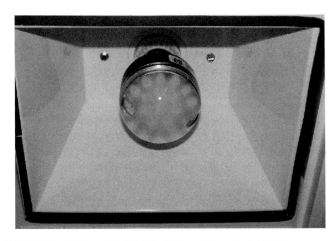

FIGURE 8-5 **Safelight.** LED (light-emitting diode) bulb.

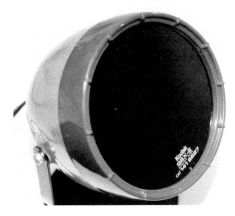

FIGURE 8-6 **Safelight.** A commercially available bracket-type lamp with safelight filter shielding the short wavelength, blue-green region of the visible light spectrum given off by the bulb. The light given off by this filter would appear dark red.

distance from the source of light and the counter space where the film will be handled. A summary of the factors to be considered for safelighting are listed in Box 8-1.

3. **Viewbox.** A **viewbox** or illuminator is a light source (generally a lamp behind an opaque glass) used for viewing radiographs. A darkroom equipped with a wall-mounted or countertop viewbox or illuminator will allow the clinician the opportunity for a quick reading, viewing the radiograph without leaving the darkroom. A viewbox emits considerable white light, and care must be taken not to turn it on when film packets are unwrapped. Additionally, if films are undergoing the developing process in a manual processor, the manual processor tank cover must remain on during the use of a view box.
4. **In-use Light.** The darkroom door should be locked when processing films to prevent someone from entering and inadvertently allowing white light into the darkroom. Some darkrooms are equipped with a warning light outside the darkroom, which indicates that it is not safe to open the door.

Maintenance

Cleanliness and orderliness are essential for the production of quality radiographs and the safety and health of the clinician using the area. Infection control protocol for opening film packets (see Chapter 10) must be strictly adhered to, and chemicals and other radiographic wastes must be properly handled and disposed (see Chapter 20). Because safelight conditions reduce visibility,

---

BOX 8-1   Safelight Considerations

- LED safelight that emits pure red light.
- 7 1/2 or 15 watt white incandescent bulb with filter.
- Darker red filters provide safer conditions for both intra and extraoral film handling than amber or yellow colored filters.
- Scratched or cracked filters allow white light to escape.
- 4-ft (1.2-m) minimum distance between lamp and counter surface where film is to be handled.
- Films should not be subjected to safelight exposure over 2 1/2 minutes.

the clinician must be skilled in the procedures to be performed. Needed materials should be within easy reach, and the person doing the processing should be familiar with where each item is located. The workspace counter must be free of substances that can contaminate films such as water, chemicals, and dust.

A utility sink large enough to accommodate cleaning the processing equipment should be available in the darkroom. A wastebasket should be placed in the darkroom for the disposal of general waste items. Lead foil is separated from other film wrappings and placed in an appropriate container for safe disposal, and the remainder of the film packet placed in a biohazard container for disposal (see Chapter 20).

Manual Film Processing

Manual processing is a method used to process films by hand in a series of steps. Although no longer in widespread use, advantages of manual film processing are that it is reliable and not subject to equipment malfunction. The clinician has more control over the processing procedure, including the ability to adjust the time–temperature and the ability to read the radiographs prior to the end of the processing procedure (wet reading). Clinicians often make use of the manual processing procedure to "rapid" or "hot" process working films discussed at the end of this section. The biggest disadvantage of manual processing is the time required to produce a finished radiograph.

Equipment

Manual processing requires the use of:

- Processing tank
- Thermometer
- Timer
- Stirring paddles
- Film hangers, drying racks, and drip pans

   1. **Processing tank.** The **processing tank** has two insert tanks placed inside the master tank (Figure 8-7). The insert tanks hold the developer and fixer solutions. Usually, the left insert tank holds the developer solution, and the right insert tank contains the fixer solution. However, these tanks should be labeled to prevent confusion as to which tank contains which chemical. The master tank holds water between the insert tanks for rinsing and washing the films.

Most tanks are made of stainless steel, which does not react with processing chemicals. Insert tanks are large enough to accept an 8 × 10 in. (20 × 26 cm) extraoral film. The capacity of an insert tank is 1 gallon (3.8 L).

The insert tanks are removable to facilitate cleaning. The master tank is connected to the water intake and to the drain. When in use, fresh water circulates constantly. An overflow pipe keeps the level of the water constant when the tank is full. Some tanks are equipped with a temperature control device, a water-mixing valve that mixes the hot and cold water in the pipes to any desired temperature. A close-fitting lightproof cover completes the tank assembly.

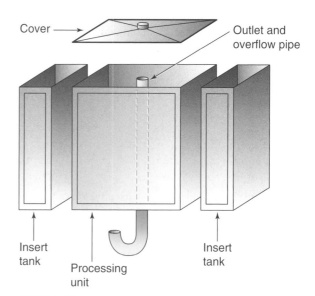

FIGURE 8-7 **Processing tank with removable inserts.** The central compartment holds the rinse/wash water. Usually, the insert on the left is filled with the developer solution, and the insert on the right is filled with the fixer solution.

   2. **Thermometer.** A thermometer is necessary to determine the temperature of the developing solution for time–temperature manual processing (Figure 8-8).
   3. **Timer.** An accurate interval timer is necessary for time–temperature manual processing. The timer is used to indicate how long the film is placed in the developing and fixing solutions and in the rinse and wash water baths. The timer should have an audible alarm to alert the radiographer to remove the films from each of the solutions. Timers with a digital readout should emit red light only so as not to fog the film.
   4. **Stirring paddles.** Two stirring paddles must be available for mixing the chemicals used for manual processing. To avoid contamination, the developer and the fixer each need their own stirring paddle. The paddles should be made of stainless steel or other material that will not corrode in the processing chemicals.

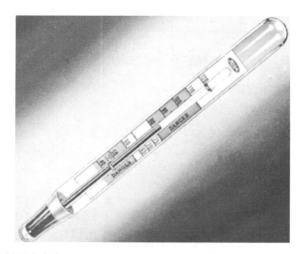

FIGURE 8-8 **Floating thermometer** used to record the temperature of the developer when manual processing.

5. **Film hangers, drying racks, and drip pans.** A **film hanger** is a stainless steel frame to which the films can be attached. A film hanger allows the radiographer to transport the films to and from each of the processing solutions (Figure 8-9). Various film hanger sizes are available that accommodate from 1 to 20 films. Film hangers have an identification tag near the curved handle on which the patient's name can be written. When manual processing was the norm, films would be dried with a commercial film dryer. Film dryers are not as readily available today. Instead, drying racks (towel racks) can be mounted for hanging film hangers to air dry. Drip pans are placed underneath the drying racks to catch water from wet films.

Preparation

The key to manually processing dental radiographs is adequate preparation.

1. **Solution levels must be checked** to be sure the developer and fixer will cover the top clips of the film hanger. The tanks are full when the solution levels are about one inch from the top. Add fresh solution if necessary.

2. **Developer and fixer must be stirred** thoroughly to prevent the heavier chemicals from settling to the bottom and to equalize the temperature of the solution throughout the tanks.

3. **The temperature of the developing solution must be determined** using a thermometer after stirring (Figure 8-8). The ideal manual processing temperature is 68°F (20°C)

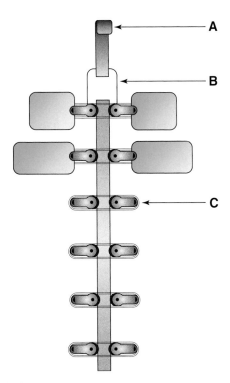

FIGURE 8-9 Intraoral film hanger with 12 clips. (**A**) Curved portion at the top allows the radiographer to rest the hanger on the rim of the tank insert for the duration of the time required. (**B**) White plastic identification tag on which the patient's name can be written in pencil and later erased. (**C**) Clamps with three-point positive grip hold the film securely in place. (Courtesy of Dentsply Rinn.)

with a development time of five minutes. Lower temperatures make the chemical reaction sluggish, and higher temperatures increase film fog. Temperature variations from the ideal may be acceptable as long as the developing time is correspondingly adjusted. The radiographer should consult a **time–temperature** development chart similar to the one in Table 8-3 to adjust developing time appropriately.

4. **The film hanger should be selected and examined.** The clips need to be in proper working order. Loose clips may cause films to fall off in the tank during the process. Extraoral film hangers have channels into which the film fits and is secured by a hinged retaining channel over the open end of the hanger. Film hangers should be labeled with the patient's name or otherwise identified.

Procedure (Procedure Box 8-1)

The manual film processing sequence consists of these five steps:

1. **Develop.** The film hanger with the attached films should be immersed into the developer tank first. Gently agitating the hanger up and down a few times—taking care not to splash—will keep air bubbles from clinging to the film. Air bubbles prevent the developer from contacting all areas of the film. Safelight conditions must be maintained throughout the development step unless the light-tight cover is in place on the processing tank.

2. **Rinse.** The purpose of the rinsing step is to remove as much of the alkaline developer as possible before placing the film into the fixer. When the timed developing step is complete, under safelight conditions, the film hanger should be lifted above the developing insert tank and allowed to drain a few seconds to minimize the amount of developer that will be removed from the tank. After gently agitating the film hanger in the rinse water, it should be held above the rinse water to drain for a few seconds to prevent diluting the fixer solution with excess water.

3. **Fix.** The film hanger with the attached films should be immersed into the fixer insert tank next, gently agitating the hanger to keep air bubbles from clinging to the film. Safelight conditions must be maintained for the first two or three minutes of the recommended fixing time. If the radiograph is needed immediately for a quick reading of the image, the film may be read under white light conditions after two or three minutes of fixing. This is called a

TABLE 8-3	Time–Temperature Chart	
TEMPERATURE		**DEVELOPMENT TIME (MIN)**
60°F (15.5°C)		9
65°F (18.3°C)		7
68°F (20°C)	optimum	5
70°F (21.1°C)		4.5
75°F (23.9°C)		4
80°F (26.7°C)		3

PROCEDURE 8-1
Manual film processing

1. Maintain infection control (see Chapter 10).
2. Select a film hanger and label with patient information.
3. Open the light-tight cover of the manual processing tank.
4. Stir the developer and fixer solutions to ensure even concentration throughout the tank. Use a different stirring paddle for each, developer and fixer, to prevent contamination of solutions.
5. Check the developer temperature.
6. Refer to the time–temperature recommendations of the solution manufacturer and set timer. (Optimal time–temperature for manually processed radiographs is 68°F for five minutes.)
7. Lock the darkroom door, turn off the white light, and turn on the safelight.
8. Open the film packets (see Procedure Box 10–5) and place films on hanger.
9. Immerse the films into the developer solution and agitate film hanger for five seconds to release trapped air bubbles.
10. Set the timer. (Time is dependent on temperature of the developer solution.)
11. Close the light-tight cover while the film is developing.
12. When the developing time is complete, under safelight conditions, open the light-tight cover and remove film hanger with films attached from developer solution.
13. Pause a few seconds over the developer tank to allow the excess solution to drain from the films.
14. Immerse the film hanger into the water rinse and agitate for 30 seconds.
15. Pause a few seconds over the water tank to allow the excess water to drain from the films.
16. Immerse the film hanger into the fixer solution and agitate for five seconds to release trapped air bubbles.
17. Activate the timer for double the time in the developer or 10 minutes.
18. Close the light-tight cover for the first two to three minutes of fixation. (It is safe to view the films under white light after two or three minutes of fixation for a wet reading, following which the films must be returned to the fixer solution for completion of the fixation time for archival quality.)
19. Remove the film hanger from the fixer solution when the time is up.
20. Pause a few seconds over the fixer tank to allow the excess solution to drain from the films.
21. Immerse the films into the water wash for 20 minutes.
22. Remove the film hanger from the water wash when the time is up.
23. Place the film hanger in a commercially made film dryer or hang to air dry when the wash is complete.
24. Mount and label the dried films.

wet reading. The film can be rinsed in water for a short interval and viewed at a viewbox. The film must be returned to the fixer as soon as possible to complete fixation and permit further shrinking of the emulsion. If this is not done, some of the unexposed silver halide grains may be left on the film, giving it a fogged and discolored appearance after it dries. Also, the emulsion may not completely harden.

The recommended fixing time is double the development time, or 10 minutes. The fixing time is not as critical as the developing time, so films may remain in the fixer slightly longer. When the fixing time is too short, the result can be slow drying, poor hardening of the emulsion, a possible partial loss of detail, and darkening over time. When the fixing time is excessively long, the image will lighten.

4. **Wash.** Washing the film removes all remaining chemicals. When the fixing step is complete, the film hanger should be lifted above the fixer insert tank and allowed to drain a few seconds to minimize the amount of fixer that will be removed from the tank. The films should be placed in the circulating water for 20 minutes. Leaving the films in the water slightly longer than 20 minutes is permissible, but leaving a film in water more than a few hours will begin to dissolve the emulsion, and the emulsion may peel away from the film base. The processing tank cover should remain in place during the washing step; however, it is not necessary to maintain safelight conditions during this step.

5. **Drying.** Following the wash step, the film hanger should be lifted above the water tank and allowed to drain. Excess

water may be removed by gently shaking the film hanger over the water tank. Films may be dried in a commercial heated drying cabinet if available or suspended from a rack until dry.

Following the Procedure

The steps taken to secure the darkroom are equally important to the preparation steps.

1. Once the white lights are turned on and visibility improves, the radiographer should check to see that none of the films have loosened from the clips and dropped on the floor or the bottom of the tank.

2. The work area should be cleaned as needed. Any moisture caused by dripping or accidental splashing of the water or chemical solutions must be wiped up.

3. After dry, films should be removed from the hangers and placed in properly identified protective envelopes or on film mounts with identifying data (see Chapter 21).

4. Identification markings should be removed or erased from the hangers. The hangers should be cleaned and dried as needed.

5. At the end of the workday, turn off the water to the tank, drain the water compartment, and turn off all lights in the darkroom. Leave the cover in place over the developer and fixer tanks to prevent oxidation and to contain chemical fumes.

Rapid (Chairside) Film Processing

Manual processing can be used to produce a **working radiograph** without a darkroom in about 30 seconds. **Rapid** or **chair-side processing** with the use of special, faster-acting chemicals and a compact light-tight box that acts as a miniature darkroom (Figure 8-3) can be valuable in endodontic, oral surgery practices and at remote sites, such as community outreach oral health projects where a darkroom is not available. A significant amount of time can be saved, for example, when it is necessary to expose a series of single films to check the progress in opening and cleaning out a root canal during endodontic treatment. However, rapid processing has definite limitations and is not intended to replace conventional processing.

Films processed in this manner are seldom suitable for filing with the patient's permanent record. Short developing and fixing times, combined with minimal washing, result in a substandard radiograph. Rapid processing chemistry does not produce archival (permanent) results, and the films will eventually discolor. In the event that the film is to be retained with the permanent record, it should be refixed for 4 minutes and washed for 20 minutes at normal conventional darkroom temperatures and conditions. Although rapid processing fulfills the dentist's need to receive information quickly, it is at the expense of image quality and longevity.

Equipment

Rapid processing requires the use of a **light-tight** countertop box that has two light-tight openings, or baffles, through which the radiographer's hands can be passed into the working compartment when the lid is closed. A transparent plastic top functions to filter out unsafe light while permitting the operator to see into the box to unwrap the film packet and manually proceed through the processing steps. Four cups are set up inside the box containing developer, rinse water, fixer, and wash water. Developing and fixing solutions made especially for rapid processing can be heated to 85°F (29.4°C) by a calibrated heater in the unit. Chemicals used for chairside processing are used for processing a limited number of films and then discarded appropriately (see Chapter 20). A small film hanger with a single clip is used to manually transfer the film from solution to solution.

Procedure

The steps for processing films using the rapid processing method are identical to the steps used for manual processing (Procedure Box 8-1). The film is placed in the developer first, then rinsed and placed in the fixer, then washed and dried. The development time ranges from 5 to 15 seconds; the fix time is approximately 30 seconds.

Following the Procedure

1. Turn off the heater.

2. Empty, rinse, and dry each of the cups. Dispose of the used fixer appropriately (see Chapter 20).

3. Clean and disinfect the inside of the chairside darkroom. Wipe off the transparent plastic top as needed.

4. Continue fixing and complete the washing and drying steps to convert a working film to a permanent image.

Automatic Film Processing

Automatic processing is more commonly employed to process dental x-ray film. Because of its ability to produce a large volume of radiographs in less time (usually five minutes from developer to dried finished radiograph), it is often preferred over manual processing. Another advantage of an **automatic processor** is the machine's ability to regulate automatically the temperature of the processing solutions and the time of the development process. Automatic processing has several disadvantages, however, including initial unit expense, possible equipment malfunction, increased maintenance required for optimal output, and more rapid chemical depletion than with manual processing chemistry.

Equipment

Automatic processing equipment varies in size and complexity (Figures 8-4 and 8-10). Some processors have a limited capacity and process only intraoral or certain sizes of extraoral films; others can handle any dental film regardless of size. Most are intended for use in the darkroom under safelight conditions. Automatic processors equipped with daylight loaders have a light-tight baffle for inserting the hands while unwrapping the film and can be used under normal white light conditions with a filter that acts as a safelight over the film entry slots (Figure 8-4).

Most automatic processors consist of three tanks or compartments, one each for the developer, fixer, and water, and a drying chamber (Figure 8-11). All automatic processors require water. Some machines are connected to existing plumbing, whereas others have a self-contained water supply. A heating unit warms the

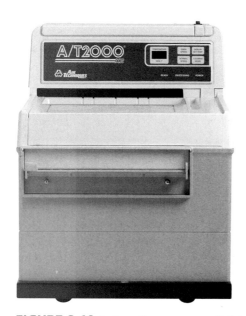
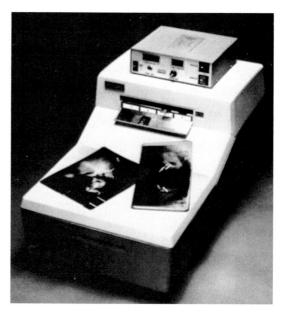

FIGURE 8-10 **Automatic processors.** (Left image: Courtesy of Air Techniques, Inc.)

processing chemicals to the required temperature so there may be a warming-up period before the unit is operational.

The automatic film processing sequence usually consists of only four steps: developing, fixing, washing, and drying. The use of a **roller transport system** helps "squeeze" excess solution from the film surface, allowing the automatic processor to omit the rinsing step between developing and fixing.

Unwrapped film is fed into the **film feed slot** on the outside of the processor. The roller transport system moves the film through the developer, fixer, water, and drying compartments. Motor-driven gears or belts propel the roller transport system. The film emerges from the processor through an opening on the outside of the processor called the **film recovery slot.** Most machines process a film in approximately five minutes. Some automatic processors have a two-minute setting for producing working radiographs for a quick reading.

Preparation

To prepare the automatic processor:

1. **The water supply to the automatic processor should be turned on.** If the processor uses a self-contained water supply, the water bottles should be checked and filled as needed.

2. **The chemicals should be replenished or changed** as necessary. Ensure that the tanks are filled to the levels indicated by the manufacturer.

3. **The automatic processor should be turned on** and allowed to warm up according to the manufacturer's recommendations.

4. **A special cleaning film** designed to remove debris from the unit rollers should be run at the beginning of the day or if the machine has been idle several hours.

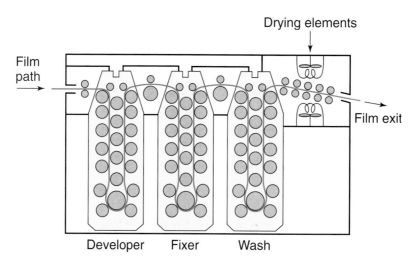

FIGURE 8-11 **Schematic illustration of automatic film processor.**
Film is transported by roller assemblies through each of the processing steps.

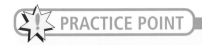

In addition to being less effective, a breakdown in the integrity of the processing chemicals will occur if chemicals are not replenished or changed at the recommended intervals. This breakdown causes the solutions to become slick. Slick solutions cause the films to slide or slip through the roller transport system of the automatic processor, making it difficult for the rollers to advance the film and resulting in films that get stuck inside the machine.

Procedure (Procedure Box 8-2)

Unless the automatic processor is equipped with daylight loader baffles, the processing procedure should begin under safelight conditions. An unwrapped film is placed into the designated feed slot on the processor. Once the film is completely inside the automatic processing unit, safelighting is no longer necessary.

When processing multiple films, each should be placed into alternating feed slots, one at a time, to prevent the films from overlapping and getting stuck in the machine. Five to ten seconds should elapse between the insertion of each film. Inserting the films too rapidly after each other will also result in overlapping films.

When more than one operator uses the processor, or when processing more than one patient's films, a method of labeling the feed slots for film identification is necessary. Depending on the processor model, the films will exit the processor in about five minutes, dried and ready for mounting.

Following the Procedure

1. Once the white lights are turned on and visibility improves, the radiographer should check to see that all the films have exited the processor.

2. Unless equipped with an automatic shutoff, the unit should be turned off or placed in stand-by mode to conserve water that would continue to run after the films have finished processing.

3. The work area should be cleaned as needed. Any moisture caused by dripping or accidental splashing of chemical solutions during replenishment must be wiped up.

4. At the end of the workday, the main power and water supply to the unit should be turned off. Leave the cover in place over the developer and fixer tanks to prevent oxidation and to contain chemical fumes. Turn off all lights in the darkroom.

Processing Chemical Maintenance

Both manual and automatic processing methods require chemical maintenance and solution replenishing and changing. Protective eyewear, mask, utility gloves, and a plastic or rubber apron should be worn when cleaning the processing tanks or changing the solutions.

Processing chemistry becomes weakened or lost in several ways. A small amount of developer and fixer is lost when chemicals adhere to the film surfaces during transfer from solution to solution. During manual processing stirring paddles, the thermometer, and film hangers all contribute to the loss of solution. Additionally, transfer of films between solutions will slowly contaminate the chemicals and weaken them.

PROCEDURE 8-2
Automatic film processing

1. Maintain infection control (see Chapter 10).

2. Turn on water supply.

3. Check for replenishment of chemicals.

4. Turn on the automatic processor.

5. Set the appropriate time/temperature as indicated by the manufacturer.

6. If it is the beginning of the day, or after several hours of inactivity, run a specially manufactured cleaning film through the processor and discard.

7. Lock the darkroom door, turn off the white light, and turn on the safelight.

8. Open the film packets (see Procedure Box 10-5) and place films into the automatic processor feed slot.

9. Allow the rollers to take the film before releasing.

10. Wait 10 seconds before placing an additional film into the same slot to avoid overlapping films.

11. Retrieve the processed films when the cycle is complete, usually about five minutes.

12. Mount and label the dried radiographs.

Weakened chemistry also occurs through **oxidation,** the union of a substance—in this case, the developer and fixer—with the oxygen in the air. The developer is especially subject to oxidation in the presence of air and loses its effectiveness very quickly. Whenever possible, the processing tank covers should remain in place to slow oxidation and evaporation. The cover should be removed only when adding solutions to the proper level; when checking the temperature of the developer, and when inserting, removing, or changing the film hangers from one compartment or insert to another (manual processing). Care must be taken not to rotate the processor cover when it is removed. Causing only a few drops of condensed developer to fall into the fixer or vice versa will contaminate and weaken the solutions. All chemistry must be changed periodically to avoid diminishing quality. The useful life of the solutions depends on:

- The original quality or concentration of the solution
- The original freshness of the solution used
- The number of films that are processed
- Contamination, oxidation, and evaporation of the chemicals

Many chemical manufacturers recommend that processing solutions be changed at least every four weeks under "normal" use. Because normal use may be defined differently among different practices, refer to the manufacturer recommendations to determine reasonable intervals to change solutions. One way to maintain solution strength in between changes is through replenishment.

Replenishment consists of removing a small amount of developer and fixer and replacing with fresh chemistry or chemical replenisher specifically made for this purpose. For every 30 intraoral films processed, it is recommended that 6 to 8 ounces of developer and fixer be removed and discarded. (See Chapter 20 for safe and environmentally sound protocols for discarding radiographic wastes.) Fresh chemicals should be added to raise the solution levels in the tanks to the full level.

Some processors automatically replenish the solutions; others depend on the operator to keep them at the correct level.

Automatic processors require strict adherence to manufacturers' instructions for chemical replenishment and changes and for cleaning the unit to maintain optimal performance. Few pieces of equipment in the oral health care practice require such diligence and regular care.

Depending on the workload, automatic processors require daily, weekly, or monthly cleaning. A specially made cleaning film may be run through the processor to remove any dirt and residual gelatin from the rollers daily or more often if the processor sits idle for several hours (Figure 8-12). However, complete cleaning and maintenance of the roller transports and solution-holding tanks is also required. If the rollers are not kept clean, the radiographs emerge streaked, stained, or worse, with scratched emulsion. Most manufacturers recommend that the roller assembly be removed and cleaned weekly, in warm, running water and special cleansers. It is important to follow the manufacturer's instructions concerning care and maintenance.

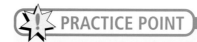

PRACTICE POINT

It is important to note that the processing chemicals used in automatic processors differ from those used in manual procedures. Solutions for use in automatic processors are supersaturated, and the developer contains more hardening agents. The chemical solutions in automatic processors are heated to temperatures much higher than those used in manual processing—as high as 125°F (52°C) in some units. Advanced film technology has produced film emulsions that can withstand these temperatures for the short times required in automated processing without excessive softening or melting.

REVIEW—Chapter summary

Film processing is a series of steps that converts the invisible latent image on the dental x-ray film into a visible permanent image called a radiograph. The sequence of processing steps is developing, rinsing, fixing, washing, and drying. Developing reduces the exposed silver halide crystals within the film emulsion to black metallic silver. Rinsing removes the alkaline developer before the film enters the fixer solution. Fixing removes the unexposed and/or undeveloped silver halide crystals from the film emulsion. Washing removes any remaining traces of the chemicals. Drying preserves the film for storage as a part of the patient's permanent record.

Two processing chemicals are used—an alkaline developer and a slightly acidic fixer. The four ingredients that make up the developer are developing agents (hydroquinone and elon), a preservative (sodium sulfite), an activator (sodium carbonate), and a restrainer (potassium bromide). The purpose of the developing solution is to reduce the exposed silver halide crystals to

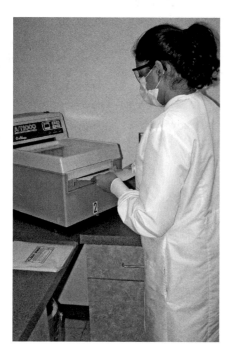

FIGURE 8-12 Cleaning sheet or specially prepared film run through the processor to remove any residual debris from the rollers.

black metallic silver. The four ingredients that make up the fixer are a fixing agent (sodium thiosulfate), a preservative (sodium sulfite), a hardening agent (potassium alum), and an acidifier (acetic acid). The purpose of the fixing solution is to remove the undeveloped silver halide crystals and harden the emulsion.

A darkroom must shut out all white light. With the exception of automatic processors equipped with daylight loaders and chairside rapid processing miniature darkroom boxes, all processing must be done in the darkroom under safelight conditions. Safelighting is achieved with a red LED (light-emitting diode) or a white incandescent lightbulb with a filter that eliminates short wavelength, blue-green colored light. Unwrapped film should not be exposed to safelight longer than about 2½ minutes.

Advantages of manual film processing include reliability, no equipment to malfunction, control over the time and temperature, and the ability to produce a wet reading. The biggest disadvantage of manual processing is the long time required to produce a finished radiograph. Manual processing requires a processing tank, thermometer, timer, stirring paddles, film hangers, and drying racks. The ideal time–temperature for manual processing is 68°F (20°C) for five minutes. Colder developer solution requires a longer developing time; warmer developer solution requires a shorter developing time.

A chairside miniature darkroom is utilized to produce working radiographs by the rapid processing method. Films are manually processed with special developer and fixer, which produce a radiographic image in less than 1 minute. Rapid processing chemistry does not produce archival results, and the films will eventually discolor. The advantage of rapid processing is that it fulfills the need to receive rapid information. However, image quality will be diminished.

The biggest advantage of automatic film processing is the short time required to produce a finished radiograph. Automatic processors equipped with daylight loader attachments can be used to process film without a darkroom. Disadvantages include initial unit expense, possible equipment malfunction, increased maintenance required for optimal output, and rapid chemical depletion. Automatic processors use a roller transport assembly to advance the films automatically from solution to solution, producing a finished radiograph in five minutes.

Step-by-step procedures for manual, rapid, and automatic processing are presented in this chapter.

Oxidation over time and chemical contamination through normal use prompt solution changes and regularly scheduled equipment maintenance and cleaning. The useful life of the solutions is determined by the original quality or concentration of the solution, the freshness of the solution, the number of films that are processed, and the contamination of the chemicals. Replenishment helps prolong the life of the processing solutions.

RECALL—Study questions

1. Which term best describes the process by which the latent image becomes visible?
   a. Reticulation
   b. Reduction
   c. Activation
   d. Preservation

2. Which of these is the correct processing sequence?
   a. Rinse, fix, wash, develop, dry
   b. Fix, rinse, develop, wash, dry
   c. Develop, rinse, fix, wash, dry
   d. Rinse, develop, wash, fix, dry

3. The basic constituents of the developer solution are
   a. reducing agent, activator, preservative, restrainer.
   b. reducing agent, acidifier, preservative, restrainer.
   c. clearing agent, activator, preservative, restrainer.
   d. clearing agent, preservative, hardener, acidifier.

4. During which step of the processing procedure are the exposed silver halide crystals reduced to metallic silver?
   a. Developing
   b. Fixing
   c. Rinsing
   d. Washing

5. Which ingredient removes the unexposed/undeveloped silver halide crystals from the film emulsion?
   a. Acetic acid
   b. Potassium bromide
   c. Sodium thiosulfate
   d. Hydroquinone

6. Which ingredient causes the emulsion to soften and swell?
   a. Acidifier
   b. Preservative
   c. Restrainer
   d. Activator

7. Which ingredient hardens the emulsion?
   a. Elon
   b. Potassium alum
   c. Sodium carbonate
   d. Sodium sulfite

8. Chemically, the developer used in an automatic processor contains more _____ than developer used for manual processing.
   a. activator
   b. acid
   c. preservative
   d. hardener

9. Each of the following should be considered when setting up an ideal darkroom EXCEPT one. Which one is the EXCEPTION?
   a. Black walls
   b. Location
   c. Lighting
   d. Size

10. Which of the following colors of safelight filters is safe for processing all film speeds?
    a. Yellow
    b. Green
    c. Red
    d. Blue

11. What is the minimum safe distance to position the safelight above the work area in the darkroom?

    a. 2 ft (0.6 m)
    b. 4 ft (1.2 m)
    c. 6 ft (1.8 m)
    d. 8 ft (2.4 m)

12. What is the appearance of the radiographic image if a film is exposed to a safelight too long?

    a. Oxidized
    b. Fogged
    c. Fixed
    d. Attenuated

13. Which of these is considered a disadvantage of manual processing over automatic processing?

    a. Darkroom required
    b. Processing time is long
    c. Chemicals must be replenished
    d. Temperature must be regulated

14. A thermometer is used for manual processing to determine the temperature of the

    a. developer solution.
    b. water.
    c. fixer solution.
    d. Both a and c

15. Each of the following is necessary and required for manual processing EXCEPT one. Which one is the EXCEPTION?

    a. Thermometer
    b. Timer
    c. Film dryer
    d. Film hanger

16. What is the ideal temperature for processing film manually?

    a. 60°F (15.5°C)
    b. 68°F (20°C)
    c. 75°F (23.9°C)
    d. 83°F (28.3°C)

17. A film may be safely exposed to white light for a wet reading after two or three minutes of

    a. developing.
    b. rinsing.
    c. fixing.
    d. washing.

18. Each of the following is true regarding rapid film processing EXCEPT one. Which one is the EXCEPTION?

    a. Uses a miniature darkroom placed on the counter in the operatory
    b. Produces archival (permanent) quality radiographs
    c. May use developer that is super heated to high temperatures
    d. Produces a radiographic image in about 1 or 2 minutes

19. Each of the following is an advantage of automatic processing over manual processing EXCEPT one. Which one is the EXCEPTION?

    a. Less maintenance
    b. Decreased processing time
    c. Increased capacity for processing
    d. Self-regulation of time and temperature

20. Replenisher is added to the developing solution to compensate for

    a. oxidation.
    b. loss of volume.
    c. loss of solution strength.
    d. All of the above

21. Which processing method requires the most maintenance and the strictest adherence to regular replenishment and cleaning?

    a. Manual
    b. Rapid
    c. Automatic

REFLECT—Case study

You work for a temporary agency that provides staffing for oral health care practices in your area. Today your employer has sent you to a practice organized and set up for a left-handed practitioner. Your first patient requires a bitewing series of radiographs. You expose the films and proceed to the darkroom for processing. Unknown to you, this practice has set up the manual processing tanks with the developing solution tank on the right and the fixer tank on the left. You are used to working with processing tanks set up with the developing solution on the left and the fixer on the right, and you proceed to process your films in this manner. What effect will this have on the resultant radiographs? Why will they look this way? Explain why the processing solutions will produce this result. What can you do to avoid this mistake in the future? What can this practice do to prevent this mistake from happening again?

RELATE—Laboratory application

For a comprehensive laboratory practice exercise on this topic, see Thomson, E. M. (2012). *Exercises in oral radiography techniques: A laboratory manual* (3rd ed.). Upper Saddle River, NJ: Pearson. Chapter 1, "Introduction to Radiation Safety and Dental Radiographic Equipment"

REFERENCE

Carestream Health, Inc. (2007). *Kodak Dental Systems: Exposure and processing for dental film radiography.* Pub. N-414. Rochester, NY.

Digital Radiography

OBJECTIVES

Following successful completion of this chapter, you should be able to:

1. Define the key words.
2. Explain the fundamental concept of digital radiography.
3. Differentiate between direct and indirect digital imaging.
4. List the equipment used in digital imaging.
5. List and describe three types of digital image receptors.
6. Discuss digital radiography's effect on radiation exposure.
7. List and describe five software features used to enhance digital image interpretation.
8. Identify advantages and limitations of digital radiography.

KEY WORDS

Analog

Artificial intelligence

Charge-coupled device (CCD)

Complementary metal oxide semiconductor (CMOS)

Digital image

Digital Imaging and Communications in Medicine (DICOM)

Digital radiograph

Digital subtraction

Digitize

Direct digital imaging

Gray scale

Gray value

Indirect digital imaging

Line pair

Noise

Photostimuable phosphor (PSP)

Pixel

Sensor

Solid state

Spatial resolution

Storage phosphor

x-coordinate

y-coordinate

Introduction

Digital radiographs, or filmless imaging, is rapidly becoming an integral part of the paperless oral health care practice (Figure 9-1). The introduction of a computer approach to x-rays with almost instant images has the potential to improve the quality of oral health care while reducing radiation exposure for the patient. Although the fundamentals of film-based radiography are necessary, it is important that the dental assistant and dental hygienist have an understanding of the basic concepts of digital radiography and be prepared to utilize digital technology.

The purpose of this chapter is to present the fundamental concepts of digital radiography, to introduce the types of digital imaging currently available, and to discuss the advantages and limitations of digital radiography.

Fundamental Concepts

The term *radiography* is derived from the words *radiation* and *photography,* meaning that a radiograph is a photographic image created using radiation. Digital imaging systems used in dentistry replace film with a **solid state** (no moving parts) image receptor called a **sensor** (Figure 9-2) or a polyester plate covered with phosphor crystals called a **photostimuable phosphor (PSP)** plate (Figure 9-3). Images made within a computer using these image receptors no longer need the photographic process. The term *imaging* has come to replace the term *radiography* when referring to these images. In radiography, we "take a radiograph," whereas in digital imaging we "acquire an image." Table 9-1 lists several terms pertaining to digital imaging that you should be familiar with.

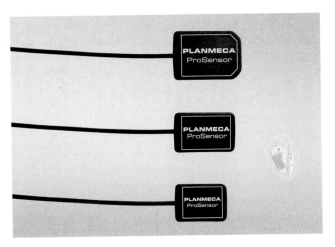

FIGURE 9-2 Solid-state digital sensors in sizes comparable to film. (Courtesy of Planmeca.)

The difference between a digital image and a film-based radiograph is that a **digital image** has no physical form. Digital images exist only as bits of information in a computer file that tell the computer how to construct an image on a monitor or other viewing device (Figure 9-4). Digital radiography systems are not limited to intraoral images. Panoramic and other extraoral radiographic digital imaging systems are also available.

Uses

Digital radiography is used for the same reasons one would use film-based radiography, including to:

- Detect, confirm, and classify oral diseases and lesions
- Detect and evaluate trauma

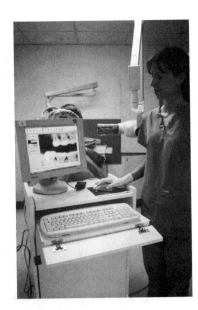

FIGURE 9-1 Digital intraoral radiographic system. The radiographic image is displayed on the computer monitor within seconds of exposure.

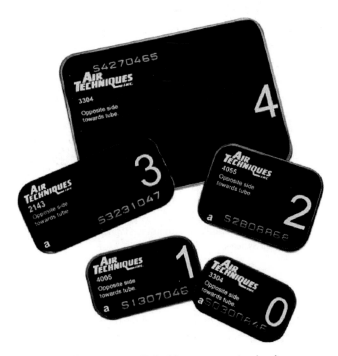

FIGURE 9-3 PSP plate digital image receptor in sizes comparable to film. (Courtesy of Air Techniques, Inc.)

TABLE 9-1 Terminology

TERM	DEFINITION
Analog	Relating to a mechanism in which data is represented by continuously variable physical quantities.
Artificial intelligence	Ability of a computer to perform decision making similar to a human being.
CCD and CMOS	CCD = charge-coupled device. CMOS = complementary metal oxide semiconductor. Solid-state detectors used in electronic devices such as digital cameras (CCD) and memory chips of a CPU (central processing unit; CMOS). In direct digital radiography, a CCD or CMOS (which one is used will depend on the manufacturer) sensor image receptor converts x-rays to an electronic signal that is then reconstructed by the computer and displayed on a monitor.
Digital subtraction	A process of digitally merging two images to show changes that occur over time or as the result of treatment intervention. The like images "cancel" each other out, clearly imaging the differences.
Digitize	To convert analog data, such as a film-based image, into a digital form that can be processed by a computer.
Electronic noise	An electrical disturbance that clutters the digital image.
Gray value	The number that corresponds to the amount of radiation received by a pixel. or cell
Gray scale	Refers to the number of shades of gray visible in an image.
lp/mm	Line pairs per millimeter. A term used to refer to the spatial resolution or sharpness of the image.
Pixel	Short for *picture element* (*pix,* plural of *pic*ture and *el,* short for *el*ement). Discrete units of information that together constitute an image.
PSP plate	PSP = photostimuable phosphor. Indirect digital image receptor composed of a polyester plate covered with storage phosphor crystals that "store" x-ray energy as a latent image. A laser scanning device releases the stored energy and sends it to a computer that reconstructs the image to display on a computer monitor.
Spatial resolution	The discernable separation of closely adjacent image details.
x- and y-coordinates	Values assigned to dimensions of a pixel that tell the computer where the pixel is located.

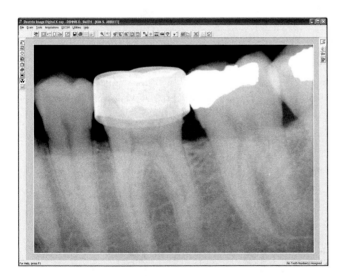

FIGURE 9-4 An example of a digital radiographic image. (Courtesy of Dentrix Dental Systems)

- Evaluate growth and development
- Provide information during dental procedures such as root canal therapy and surgery

The techniques and methods learned for exposing intra- and extraoral radiographs are the same whether using traditional film or a digital image receptor. The significant difference between film-based radiography and digital imaging is that the film is replaced with a digital image receptor.

Methods of Acquiring a Digital Image

It is sometimes desirable to convert film-based radiographs to digital images, for example, when updating to a paperless practice or to send an image electronically to another practice. Radiographs taken with film can be **digitized** by scanning or by digitally photographing the existing radiograph. A device called a transparency adapter can be mounted in the lid of a paper document scanner that will allow the scanner to scan film-based radiographs (Figure 9-5). Or existing radiographs can be placed on a viewbox and photographed with a digital camera. Although digitizing film-based radiographs with these methods can play a valuable role, the quality of the scanned or photographed images will most likely be inferior to an original digital image because the resultant image is essentially a copy. It should be noted that some practitioners call the process of digitizing film-based radiographs indirect digital imaging. In this text we will refer to images obtained via a photostimuable phosphor (PSP) plate indirect imaging. This will be explained in the next section.

True digital images are obtained via either **direct digital imaging** and **indirect digital imaging.**

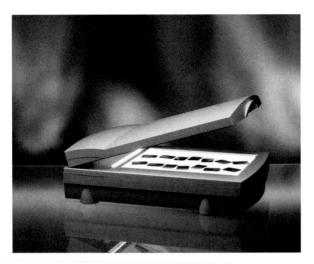

FIGURE 9-5 Digitizing film-based radiographs is accomplished by scanning into the computer. (Courtesy of DEXIS, LLC.)

Direct Digital Imaging

A solid state **sensor,** containing an electronic chip based on either **charge-coupled device (CCD)** technology or **complementary metal oxide semiconductor (CMOS)** technology, replaces conventional film as the image receptor. Both CCD and CMOS technologies work equally well at converting x-rays into an electronic signal that is sent to the computer. The difference between the two is in the architecture of the electronic chip. The use of CCD or CMOS technology depends on the manufacturer of the digital imaging system.

CCD and CMOS sensors are made up of a grid of x-ray or light sensitive cells (Figure 9-6). Each cell represents one **pixel** in the final image. A pixel serves as a small box or "well" into which the electrons produced by the x-ray exposure are deposited. A pixel is the digital equivalent of a silver halide crystal used in film-based radiography. As opposed to film emulsion that contains a random arrangement of silver halide crystals, pixels are arranged in a structured order in rows and columns. Each pixel has an *x*-coordinate, a *y*-coordinate, and a gray value. The **x- and y-coordinates** are numbers that represent where the pixel is located (what row and column) in the grid. When x-rays strike the sensor, the pixels are excited in such a way that an electronic charge is produced on the surface of the sensor. The number that represents the **gray value** increases or decreases in proportion to the number of x-rays striking each pixel. The sensor then transmits the *x*- and *y*-coordinates and the gray value, through a wire or wirelessly via radio frequency to a circuit board inside the computer. The computer software processes the *x*- and *y*-coordinates and a gray value number to reconstruct an image to display on the monitor.

Indirect Digital Imaging

Photostimuable phosphor (PSP) plate sensor technology, also called a storage phosphor system, replaces conventional film as the image receptor, but uses very different technology than CCD and CMOS systems. PSP sensors very closely parallel film in the way they look and in the way the radiographic image is captured as **analog** data and then processed (Figure 9-7). PSP technology uses polyester plates coated with something called a **storage phosphor** (europium activated barium fluorohalide). When exposed to x-rays this storage phosphor "stores" the x-ray energy as a latent image similar to the way silver halide crystals within film emulsion store a latent image. After exposure the PSP plate is placed into a laser scanning device (Figure 9-8). As the laser beam passes over the PSP plate, energy in proportion to the amount of x-ray energy absorbed is released. The released energy, in the form of light, is converted to an electrical signal that is then converted into digital values. The computer uses these digital values to reconstruct an image on the computer monitor. The laser scanner processing step makes PSP technology seem similar to film-based radiography

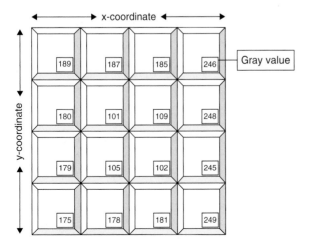

FIGURE 9-6 Diagram of sensor grid. Each square represents a pixel. Pixels store a number from 0 to 255, representing pure black at 0 to pure white at 255 that the computer will re-construct into an image.

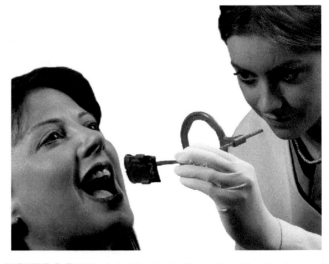

FIGURE 9-7 PSP plate. The similar dimensions allow for the use of a film holder to place the PSP plate. (Courtesy of Gendex Dental Systems.)

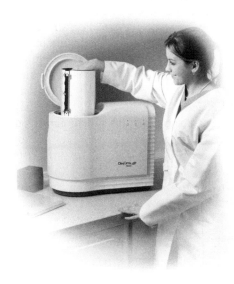

FIGURE 9-8 **PSP scanner.** Operator placing the exposed PSP sensor plates in to the laser scanning device. (Courtesy of Gendex Dental Systems.)

in that the image receptor is exposed and then "developed" later. Because of this additional laser scanning step, this method of acquiring a digital image is referred to as indirect digital imaging. After processing with the laser scanner, PSP plates must be erased by exposing them to bright light before using again.

Equipment

Both direct and indirect digital radiography use a dental x-ray machine, an image receptor capable of capturing digital information, a computer, and specialized software (Procedure Box 9-1).

PROCEDURE 9-1
Procedure for obtaining digital images

Equipment preparation*

1. Turn on the computer. Using the keyboard or mouse, activate the computer exam window and select the type of exam from the task bar (i.e., bitewings, periapicals, full mouth series).

2. Using the keyboard, type the patient identification information (i.e., name) and date of exam.

3. Wipe the sensor with an intermediate-level disinfectant approved by the sensor manufacturer. Place an FDA-cleared plastic sheath over the sensor (Figures 9-9 and 9-10).

4. Place the sensor into the appropriate biteblock and attach to the holding device (Figures 9-7 and 9-11).

5. Turn on the x-ray machine and adjust exposure settings. Refer to the manufacturer's recommendations for reducing film exposure settings by up to one-half those used for F-speed film-based exposures.

*Follow the manufacturer's instructions for your digital system. Only general guidelines concerning patient preparation and sensor placement are included here.

(Continued)

PROCEDURE 9-1
Procedure for obtaining digital images (continued)

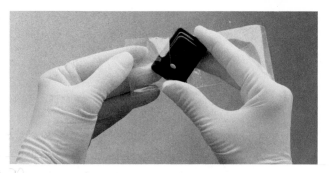

FIGURE 9-9 **Wireless sensor** being covered with a disposable plastic barrier for placement intraorally. (Courtesy of Schick Technologies, Inc.)

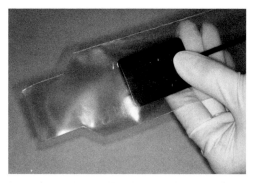

FIGURE 9-10 **Infection control.** Wired digital sensor being covered with a disposable plastic barrier for placement intraorally.

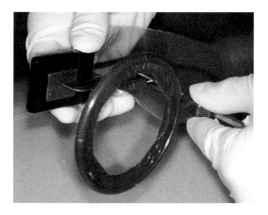

FIGURE 9-11 **Wired digital sensor** being placed into the image receptor holder.

Patient preparation

1. Request that the patient remove objects from the mouth that can interfere with the procedure and remove eyeglasses.

2. Adjust chair to a comfortable working level.

3. Adjust headrest to position patient's head so that the occlusal plane is parallel to the floor and the midsagittal plane (midline) is perpendicular to the floor.

4. Place the lead/lead equivalent apron and thyroid collar on the patient.

5. Perform a cursory inspection of the oral cavity and note possible obstructions (tori, shallow palatal vault, malaligned teeth) that may require an alteration of technique or placement of the sensor. Note the patient's occlusion to assist with aligning the sensor with the maxillary or mandibular teeth.

Exposure

1. Place the sensor intraorally into position (Figure 9-12).

2. Utilize the paralleling technique to position the sensor parallel to the long axes of the teeth of interest. Align the tube head and PID to direct the central rays of the x-ray beam perpendicular to the sensor. Direct the central rays to the middle (center) of the sensor to avoid conecut error (Figure 9-13).

PROCEDURE 9-1

Procedure for obtaining digital images (continued)

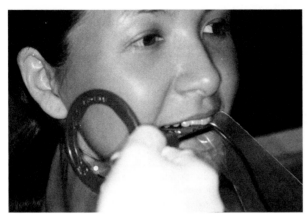

FIGURE 9-12 Sensor being placed intraorally.

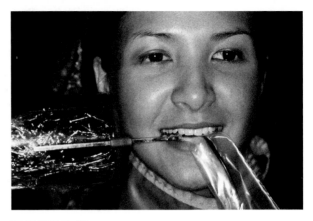

FIGURE 9-13 PID aligned with sensor held in place by holder.

3. Using the keyboard or mouse, activate the sensor for exposure.
4. Depress the exposure button to expose the sensor.

CCD (Charge-Coupled Device) or CMOS (Complementary Metal Oxide Semiconductor)

5. Wait for the image to appear on the computer monitor and evaluate technique. If a technique error has occurred that compromises diagnostic quality and requires a retake, do the following:

   a. Do not remove the sensor from the patient's oral cavity.

   b. Request that the patient remain still, in position.

   c. Observe the error and decide the corrective action. For example, if a conecut error has resulted in the posterior section of the image being blank, the appropriate corrective action would be to move the PID toward the posterior to align the central rays of the x-ray beam to the center of the sensor.

   d. Realign the PID to correct. To correct sensor placement errors, request that the patient open the mouth slightly, allowing you to perform the corrective action and then occlude on the biteblock holding the sensor in this new position.

   e. Using the keyboard or mouse, activate the retake window and make the exposure. Repeat step 5 to produce a diagnostic quality image.

PSP (Photostimuable Phosphor) plate

5. Remove the sensor (plate) from the patient's oral cavity.

6. Remove the sensor from the holding device.

7. Remove the plastic barrier and clean and disinfect sensor according to manufacturer's instructions.

8. Place the plate in light-tight box until ready for scanning (Figure 9-14) or place directly into the laser scanner and activate (Figure 9-8).

9. Observe the image on the monitor and evaluate technique. If a technique error has occurred that compromises diagnostic quality, retake the exposure. You may choose to use another prepared sensor or perform the following steps:

   a. Erase the used sensor plate according to manufacturer's instructions.

   b. Repeat the Equipment Preparation, Patient Preparation, and Exposure steps.

10. If the image is satisfactory, remove the sensor from the scanner and erase the used sensor plate according to the manufacturer's instructions. If additional images are required, repeat the Equipment Preparation, Patient Preparation, and Exposure steps or use additional sensors.

11. Repeat steps 1 through 10 until all exposures are acquired.

(Continued)

PROCEDURE 9-1
Procedure for obtaining digital images (continued)

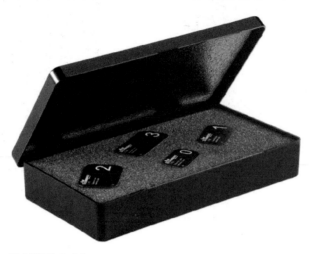

FIGURE 9-14 **Box to keep exposed PSP plates shielded from bright light until scanned.** (Courtesy of Air Techniques.)

6. If the image is satisfactory, remove the sensor from the patient's oral cavity. If additional images are required, reposition the sensor for the next exposure. (It may not be necessary to completely remove the sensor from the patient's oral cavity. Depending on the cooperation of the patient, the sensor may be positioned for the next image without completely removing the sensor from the oral cavity.)

7. Repeat steps 1 through 6 until all exposures are acquired.

Following exposure

1. Remove the sensor from the holding device.

2. Remove the plastic barrier and clean and disinfect according to manufacturer's instructions.

3. Save the patient's exam in the archived files. Back up the file on the computer or supplemental storage system. If required, print out a hard copy of the images.

X-ray Machine

Most digital x-ray systems can be used with existing dental x-ray machines that have electronic timers capable of producing very short exposure times (Figure 9-15). Older x-ray machines using impulse timers may need to be updated with electronic timers for use with digital systems. An x-ray machine adapted for digital radiography can still be used for conventional film-based radiography. Dental x-ray machines that are capable of producing low kilovoltage (60 kV), have low millamperage (5 mA), and have a direct current (DC) circuit are ideally suited to digital radiography.

Image Receptors

Both intra- and extraoral digital radiography use either a solid state sensor (CCD or CMOS) or a photostimuable phosphor (PSP) plate instead of film. CCD or CMOS intraoral sensors may be wired, connected to the computer by a fiber optic cable that records the generated signal or wireless. The cable may vary in length, with popular lengths from 3 to 9 ft (1 to 3 m). The shorter the cable, the more limited the range of motion. Intraoral dental x-ray machines are available with a conveniently attached wired sensor (Figure 9-16). Wireless sensors use a radio frequency to communicate with the computer and

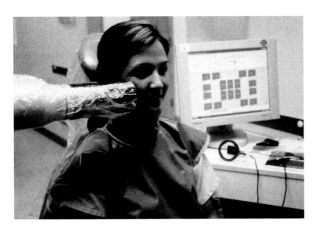

FIGURE 9-15 Digital radiography system. An existing dental x-ray unit being used with a digital imaging system.

are not connected by a cable (Figure 9-17). Eliminating the wire from the sensor has potential benefits such as increased mobility to position the sensor intraorally and increased patient comfort from not having to occlude carefully to avoid the wire. However, wireless sensors are usually thicker than wired sensors, and the technology used to communicate with the computer without being physically attached via a wire is sensitive to other signals or noise in the area, such as from other electronic devices being used in the vicinity. Digital images are usually displayed on a computer monitor within

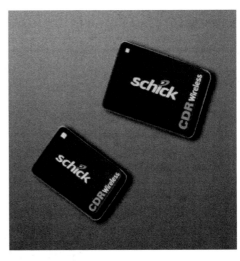

FIGURE 9-17 Wireless digital sensor in sizes similar to film. (Courtesy of Schick Technologies, Inc.)

0.5 to 120 seconds after the sensor is exposed. The sensor design is unique to the manufacturer. Sensors are available with contoured edges and angled wire attachments (Figure 9-18), and others have been reduced to just over 3 mm in width (thickness), all characteristics designed to enhance patient comfort during sensor placement intraorally.

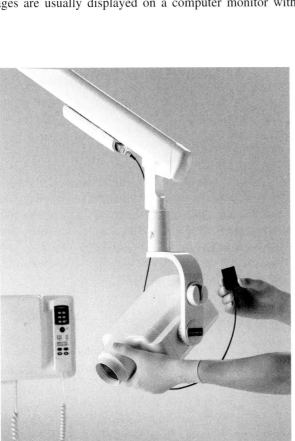

FIGURE 9-16 Digital radiography system with conveniently attached sensor. (Courtesy of Planmeca.)

PRACTICE POINT

The ability to view a digital image immediately allows for quick assessment of diagnostic quality and accurate correction of technique errors. For example, if a technique error results in overlapping or conecut images, the operator can make the necessary adjustments to the sensor placement or tube head alignment without removing the sensor from the patient's mouth, greatly increasing the likelihood that the corrective action will produce a quality image.

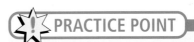

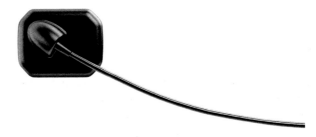

FIGURE 9-18 Digital wired sensor. Note the contoured edges and the angled attachment of the wire designed to facilitate placement intraorally. (Courtesy of DEXIS, LLC.)

Intraoral PSP plates very closely resemble intraoral film packets, and extraoral PSP plates are placed into a cassette (without intensifying screens) in the same manner as extraoral film (see Chapter 30). Intraoral PSP plates are thin and slightly flexible. (Figure 9-7) Care should be taken to not bend the plate, or damage will occur. There is no wire connection directly to the computer. Each plate is exposed and then kept protected from bright light until ready for the scanning step (Figure 9-14). Each plate is then arranged in a special mount and inserted into the laser scanner that is attached to the computer (Figure 9-8). The scanner uses a laser beam to convert the digital signal contained as a latent image in the plate to a visible image on a computer monitor. The scanning time can take between 10 seconds to produce an image for a single periapical radiograph and 5 minutes to produce a high-resolution panoramic image. PSP plates must be erased by exposing to bright light before they can be reused.

Both CCD and CMOS sensors and PSP plates are available in the sizes that approximate the different sizes of an intraoral film packet and extraoral film sizes, but PSP plates have a greater variety of sizes available, including a size suitable for exposing occlusal radiograph (Figure 9-3; see Chapter 17).

Computer

Digital radiography requires a computer to capture and a monitor to view the image (Figure 9-19). The computer digitizes, processes, and stores information received from the sensor. The type and size of computer required depends on the digital imaging software to be used. The computer must have a large enough memory to store the images and be equipped to support visual image displays on a monitor. Flat panel monitors have largely replaced large cathode ray tube (CRT) monitors (Figure 9-20). However, older CRT monitors, with tested technology, continue to provide high-quality image viewing (Figure 9-21). Technology has recently made available hand-held image viewers that store images, similar to a portable hard drive. The images can then be transferred wirelessly to a nearby computer via radio waves for permanent storage. When choosing a monitor with newer technology such as liquid crystal display (LCD) or plasma displays, careful

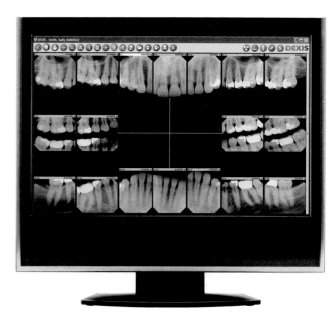

FIGURE 9-20 Flat panel computer monitor. (Courtesy of DEXIS, LLC.)

attention should be given to match the digital imaging system with the monitor recommended by the manufacturer.

The computer may be connected to the Internet to allow for electronic transfer of the images to insurance companies or when referring to other health care specialists. Connecting a printer to the computer will allow the operator to print out a photo- or plain-paper copy for the patient record if desired.

Software

Manufacturers of digital radiographic systems provide software programs that when loaded onto the computer will allow the operator to manipulate the images. Digital systems offer a variety of features to aid in viewing and interpreting the images. Some of the features offered by manufacturers of digital software include the following:

- **Side-by-side displays of images.** Allows the operator to view and compare multiple images on the monitor at one time. This feature is helpful when comparing current images with images taken previously (Figure 9-20).

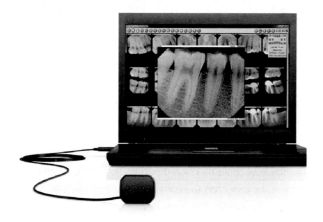

FIGURE 9-19 Digital imaging system for use with a laptop computer. (Courtesy of DEXIS, LLC.)

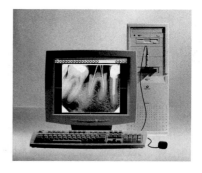

FIGURE 9-21 Computer with CRT monitor continue to provide high quality image viewing. (Courtesy of DEXIS, LLC.)

- **Magnification.** Allows specific images to be magnified. This feature is helpful when evaluating subtle changes not easily detected by the unaided human eye.

- **Density and contrast** Changes can be made to image density and contrast without retaking the radiograph. For example, when an image appears too light, this software tool allows the operator to increase the image darkness.

- **Measurement tools.** Linear and angular measurements can be obtained with a software "ruler" or measuring feature. Measurement tools are useful in measuring the length of root canals in endodontic therapy and for estimating periodontal bone levels.

- **Charting.** Software programs allow the operator to place interpretive notes directly on the radiographic images (Figures 9-22 and 9-23). An arrow or circle may be drawn directly on an area of interest, in much the same manner as an entry would be made on the patient's paper record or chart.

- **Digital subtraction.** This feature allows for comparison of digitally stored images to detect changes over time or prior to and after treatment interventions. **Digital subtraction** merges two radiographic images of the same area, taken at different times. Merged together electronically, those portions of the images that are alike (i.e., did not change over time) will cancel each other out as they are subtracted from each other. The portions of the images where change occurred will stand out conspicuously. Digital subtraction eliminates distracting background information that is similar in both images and highlights the changes (differences). Digital subtraction is an effective method of measuring periodontal changes such as bone loss or regeneration, assessment of implants, and healing of periapical pathosis.

In the past, for digital subtraction to be effective, the technique used to acquire the two images had to be closely standardized. The positions of the sensor, the patient, and the tube head all had to be the same for both images. This was accomplished with fabrication of a custom biteblock

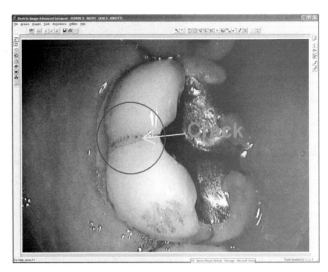

FIGURE 9-23 **Charting software** allows the radiographer to place notes directly on the image. (Courtesy of Dentrix Dental Systems.)

so that the patient could bite down in the same place with each radiograph. Technological advances in software that match gray values between subsequent images have made digital subtraction easier to achieve.

- **Artificial intelligence.** Software technology continues to find ways to improve the diagnostic yields from digital imaging. Predictions have been made that **artificial intelligence,** programming a computer to make decisions regarding the diagnosis of the images acquired, will one day be used to assist the practitioner with reading and interpreting digital images. Possible uses for artificial intelligence would be to develop computer software to analyze bone around a dental implant to determine if osseointegration (anchoring in bone) has occurred or to analyze bone densities of the jaws to screen for osteoporosis with a dental radiograph. Although certainly very beneficial ideas, these uses of artificial intelligence are still being studied.

PRACTICE POINT

A future possible use of artificial intelligence. Because the computer can record more data than the human eye can detect, in the future software features might be constructed that alert the practitioner to subtle dental disease that may go undetected. For example, the computer could be directed to color all healthy enamel, with a certain level of density, yellow. Any enamel density that falls below a certain established healthy level could be colored purple. Therefore, when interpreting the image on the computer monitor, the practitioner could easily identify the caries indicated by the purple areas.

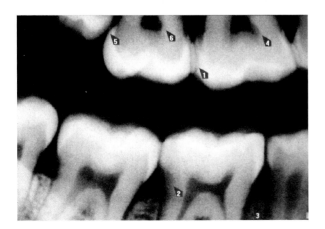

FIGURE 9-22 **Charting software** allows the radiographer to place notes directly on the image.

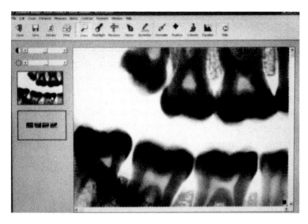

FIGURE 9-24 Reversing the gray scale. Digital software can change the image's radiopacities to radiolucencies and vice versa.

- **Other features.** Other features of specialized software promoted by manufacturers include reversing the gray scale, embossing (Figures 9-24 and 9-25), and colorization, where different densities can be assigned a different color value on the monitor. Some practitioners find these features helpful aids to interpreting images, whereas others view them as visual gimmicks because these features currently do not have the power to take the place of the dental practitioner. Interpreting digital images with or without these features requires practice. A practitioner must spend time developing the skills required for interpreting digital images. Currently software cannot match the ability of a skilled practitioner at interpreting dental disease and deviations from the normal.

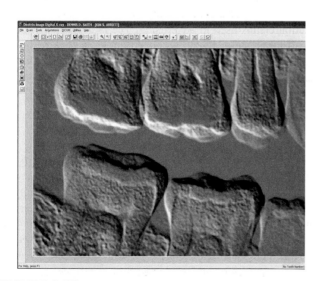

FIGURE 9-25 Embossing. An example of a digital software feature that can be used to manipulate the image to enhance interpretation. (Courtesy of Dentrix Dental Systems.)

Characteristics of a Digital Image

The term *digital image* is used to distinguish it from an analog image. An **analog** image can be compared to a painting that has a continuous smooth blend from one color to another. A digital image is like a mosaic, made up of many small pieces put together to make a whole. The digital image is composed of structurally ordered areas called **pixels.** Pixels, short for "picture elements," are tiny dots that make up a digital image. Each pixel is a single dot in a digital image. The more pixels in an image, the higher the resolution and the sharper the image. Studies continue to compare different digital imaging systems and find that all systems currently on the market produce acceptable images in terms of spatial resolution and gray scale when compared to intraoral film.

Spatial Resolution

The number and size of pixels determines the **spatial resolution** of an image. When the number of pixels is low, the image appears to have jagged edges and is difficult to see (Figure 9-26). Spatial resolution is measured in terms of line pairs. A **line pair** refers to the greatest number of paired lines visible in 1 millimeter (mm) of an image. For example, a resolution of 10 line pairs/mm would mean that when 10 ruled lines are squeezed into 1 mm of an image, the individual lines can still be distinguished from each other. The greater the spatial resolution in an image, the sharper it looks.

Gray Scale

Gray scale refers to the number of shades of gray visible in an image. The gray scale of a radiographic image is probably the most important characteristic of a radiographic image. Detection and diagnosis of oral conditions depend on the gray scale to provide the appropriate image contrast. The practitioner most often relies on the radiograph's contrast, its radiolucency and radiopacity, to determine the presence or absence of disease. The ability to record subtle changes in the gray areas of images improves diagnosis. Digital radiographic systems claim the ability to produce up to 65,500 gray levels. However, computer monitors can display only 256 gray levels. A number stored for each pixel determines the number of shades of gray

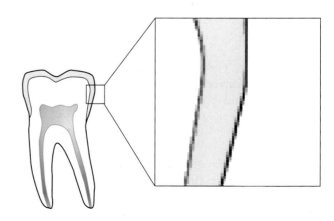

FIGURE 9-26 Example of pixel size effect on the image.

visible (Figure 9-6). Each pixel has a number from 0 to 255, representing pure black at 0 to pure white at 255 for a total of 256 gray levels in an image.

The human eye can distinguish only about 32 shades of gray unaided. However, this does not necessarily mean that the large range of gray scale captured by digital imaging systems is wasted. When aided by the computer software features, which can be used to enhance the gray levels, it may be possible to detect changes that might be overlooked in film-based images.

The goal of digital imaging systems is to produce high-quality diagnostic images. It is the combination of pixels, spatial resolution, and gray scale that determines the quality of the final image. Manufacturers are continuing to improve the capability of digital equipment and software to aid in the early detection of oral diseases.

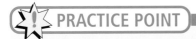

PRACTICE POINT

The ability to increase or decrease digital image density will not compensate for a severely under- or overexposed image. For example, if the exposure setting is too low, the resultant image will be too light. Often a light image will not reveal such subtle changes as an early or incipient carious lesion. If the original image does not detect the radiolucency of the caries because it was underexposed (too light), then merely darkening the image with the digital software density control tool will not "put" the caries into the picture. If it was not detected to begin with, the software will not reveal it.

Radiation Exposure

The advantages of digital imaging over film-based radiography are significant (Table 9-2). One of these advantages that is often a major benefit touted by digital imaging system manufacturers is the reduction in radiation exposure to the patient. However, with fast-speed intraoral film and the fast-speed extraoral film and screen combinations (see Chapter 29) used today, the actual radiation reduction may be 0 to 50%. Claims for up to 80% radiation reduction are most often accurate when the digital exposure is compared to slower D-speed film.

Solid-state CCD and CMOS digital imaging sensors are more efficient at capturing x-rays than conventional dental x-ray film and would most likely produce a bigger reduction in exposure. For example, if a 12-impulse (0.2-second) exposure time is required for a radiograph taken with F-speed intraoral film, the exposure time for this same image acquired utilizing CCD or CMOS technology could possibly be reduced to 6 impulses (0.1 second). However, the operator should evaluate the actual result in practice and adjust the exposure time as necessary to produce a diagnostically acceptable image. This large of a reduction in radiation dose

may not be realized in practice with PSP plate technology, as a low radiation exposure produces an increase in **noise,** an electrical disturbance that clutters the image, at very low exposure times. The practitioner will often increase the exposure time to eliminate the noise. Additionally, PSP technology has the unique ability to produce an acceptable image at longer exposure times. Overexposed PSP plates will not alert the radiographer that too much radiation is being used to produce the image. What this means in practice is that the radiographer may be setting the exposure time higher than needed.

There may be no radiation reduction realized when comparing extraoral CCD, CMOS, or PSP technology to extraoral film-screen combinations. In fact, some extraoral systems using PSP technology actually require an increase in radiation exposure over film-screen radiographs.

Another important consideration when discussing radiation exposure is that studies have indicated a higher retake rate and more exposures taken with direct digital imaging when compared with film-based radiographs. Increased exposures lead to increased patient radiation doses. Possible explanations for this higher incidence of exposure with direct digital imaging include:

- The ease with which retakes can be immediately taken without removing the sensor from the patient's mouth.
- The real and the perceived radiation dose reduction expected by digital imaging makes retakes seem easily justifiable.
- The recording dimensions of the sensors are smaller than a film requiring multiple exposures of the same region.
- The size and rigidity of the sensor and the wire and plastic infection-control barrier protruding from the oral cavity make placement difficult, which leads to increased chance of errors.

Although a reduction in radiation dose is an advantage of digital imaging technologies, the International Commission on Radiological Protection has recently indicated interest in investigating how some digital imaging systems arrive at radiation reduction claims used in advertising. The radiographer should critically evaluate a digital system to determine the radiation dose reduction and be aware of the pitfalls that negate the beneficial reductions in radiation exposures.

Digital Imaging and Communications in Medicine (DICOM)

When digital imaging began to replace film-based radiography, the medical community, where digital imaging is more widely utilized, adopted the **Digital Imaging and Communications in Medicine (DICOM)** standard to allow different digital systems to interface with each other. Exporting and importing digital images can require complex steps and considerable computer knowledge. Without standards, system compatibility will be an issue when digital images are transferred electronically between systems. The American Dental Association Informatics Task Group has recommended that the DICOM standard be used for dental imaging systems as

TABLE 9-2 Advantages and Limitations of Digital Radiography

ADVANTAGES	LIMITATIONS
• Less radiation exposure • Almost instantaneous viewing of the image • Elimination of the photographic process and darkroom • No generation of hazardous wastes such as used fixer and lead foils and elimination of cost of disposal • Elimination of darkroom processing errors • Dark/light images may be improved with software to avoid reexposing the patient • Images can be manipulated to enhance interpretation • Improved grayscale resolution enhances contrast discrimination • Software features such as charting and measuring tools assist with interpretation and diagnosis • Remote electronic consultation and sending of images • Effective patient viewing that enhances discussion of treatment plan and oral hygiene education (Figure 9-28) • Long-term costs may be less when compared to costs associated with purchasing film and processing chemicals	• The ease of retakes may result in excess radiation exposure • Bulky, thicker sensor size (CCD and CMOS) and attached wire may elicit patient complaints of discomfort or excite a gag reflex • Plastic barrier sheaths placed over the sensor to maintain infection control add additional bulk. • Infection control requires careful adherence to manufacturer's recommendations to avoid damage to the sensor. Infection control must be maintained for computer keyboard and/or mouse (Figure 9-27) • Smaller overall sensor dimensions limits recording area. Additional exposures may be required to image an area entirely. • Initial investment costs to convert from film-based radiography • Special image receptor holders may need to be purchased • Technology concerns, when to make the change from film-based imaging, and what type of digital system to buy can be a difficult decision • Concern with reliability of digital imaging. Computer crashes, system malfunction, and computer viruses are real risks. • Concern regarding a possible temporary inability to access the images in the computer's memory due to a computer glitch or power failure that can delay patient treatment • Archival storage (to keep patient records for the time required or recommended by law) and backup storage (to protect files from computer malfunction) need to be considered. Media used to store the images will have to be updated continually to be accessible over time. • Learning curve required to read digital images on a computer monitor • Viewing digital images will be restricted to the area where the computer and monitor are located. (Although technology is now producing portable viewers.) • Although environmentally friendly in the short term, disposal of broken, obsolete digital equipment is a concern.

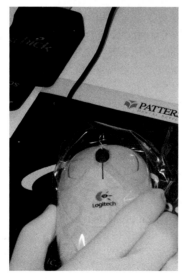

FIGURE 9-27 Infection control. A disposable plastic barrier protects the computer mouse.

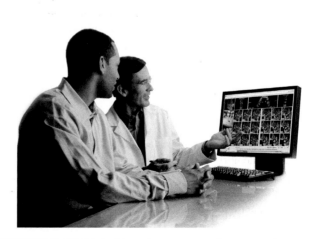

FIGURE 9-28 Digital imaging system enhances patient consult. (Courtesy of Gendex Dental Systems.)

well. As manufacturers of digital imaging equipment adopt the DICOM standard, the ease with which information can be shared will improve. Currently manufacturers of dental digital imaging systems are being encouraged to produce systems that are compatible with each other.

Studies indicate that although the adoption of digital imaging by oral health care practices is increasing, it has not replaced film-based radiography. Oral health care will most likely continue to implement digital imaging into patient care as improvements and standardizations of the technology continue. The oral health care practice of the near future will most likely see a decreased use of film-based radiography.

REVIEW—Chapter summary

Digital radiography is a method of capturing a radiographic image and displaying it on a computer screen. A solid-state sensor or phosphor plate replaces film. Digital images have no physical form, but exist as bits of information in a computer file. Film-based radiographs may be digitized by scanning or photographing to convert these analog images to digital files.

Direct digital imaging replaces film with a solid-state sensor, containing an electronic chip based on either charge-coupled device (CCD) technology or complementary metal oxide semiconductor (CMOS) technology. Grids made up of pixels arranged in columns and rows make up the sensor. When x-rays strike the sensor an electronic signal is produced and transmitted to a computer. The computer uses the *x*- and *y*-coordinates and the gray value for each pixel to reconstruct the image for viewing on a monitor. Indirect digital imaging replaces film with a photostimuable phosphor (PSP) plate covered with a storage phosphor that captures the analog image similar to the action of film. PSP sensor "stores" x-ray energy until read later in a laser scanner.

Digital imaging requires the use of a conventional dental x-ray unit, CCD or CMOS sensor or PSP plate, computer, and special software. Ideal x-ray machines have an electronic timer, low kVp, low mA, and direct current (DC). CCD and CMOS sensors may be wired or wireless, with contoured edges, and with angled wire attachments. PSP plates are not attached to the computer with a wire. After exposure to x-rays PSP plates must be kept away from bright light until scanned. PSP plates are placed into a laser scanner that converts the digital signal to an image on a computer monitor. PSP plates must be erased by exposing to bright light before reusing.

All digital imaging systems require the use of a computer with enough memory to run the special software and to store the images generated. Consideration should be given to choosing a monitor that provides ease of reading and interpreting the images. A printer attached to the computer will allow the operator to print hard copies of the radiographic images if desired.

Special software is required to run the digital radiographic systems. Digital software packages allow the radiographer to manipulate the image. Common features include the ability to view multiple radiographic images on one screen, magnification, measuring, and charting tools. Digital subtraction is a software process where two images are merged electronically, canceling out like portions of the image and revealing changes. Artificial intelligence may one day assist practitioners with determining the presence of diseases.

The digital image is composed of pixels, short for picture elements. Each pixel is a single dot in the digital image. The number and size of pixels determines the spatial resolution and the sharpness of the image. Spatial resolution is measured as line pairs. A line pair refers to the number of paired lines visible in 1 mm of an image. The greater the spatial resolution, the sharper the image appears. Pixels also determine the gray scale of the image. Each pixel has a number from 0 to 255, representing pure black at 0 to pure white at 255. The higher the gray scale, the more likely the image is to record subtle changes in the patient's condition.

A major advantage of digital radiography is radiation dose reduction, between 0 and 50% over film-based radiography. Other advantages include almost instant images, elimination of the darkroom and chemicals and hazardous wastes, potential for improved interpretation through image manipulation, ability to transmit the images electronically, and effective patient education. Limitations include too easily making retakes that might lead to excess radiation exposure and the need for digital system manufacturers to adhere to DICOM (digital imaging and communications in medicine) to allow transfer of images between different systems. Other limitations include increased sensor width and decreased recording area, initial costs to convert to digital imaging, infection control protocols, issues with the technology including memory storage, computer crashes, and interrupted access to the data. There is a learning curve to gain proficiency with interpretation.

RECALL—Study questions

For questions 1 to 5, match each term with its definition.

  a. analog
  b. gray scale
  c. line pair
  d. pixel
  e. spatial resolution

  _D_ 1. Discrete units of information that together constitute an image.

  _E_ 2. The discernable separation of closely adjacent image details.

  _C_ 3. Refers to the number of paired lines visible in 1 mm of an image.

  _A_ 4. Relating to a mechanism in which data is represented by continuously variable physical quantities.

  _B_ 5. Refers to the total number of shades of gray visible in an image.

6. A digital radiographic image exists as bits of information in a computer file.

   The computer converts this information into an image that appears on the computer monitor.

   a. The first statement is true. The second statement is false.

   b. The first statement is false. The second statement is true.

   c. Both statements are true.

   d. Both statements are false.

7. Digital radiography can be used for which of the following?

   a. To detect caries

   b. To monitor an endodontic procedure

   c. To detect dental disease

   d. All of the above

8. Digital radiography systems can be used for which of the following?

   a. Bitewing images

   b. Periapical images

   c. Panoramic images

   d. All of the above

9. When a transparency scanner or digital camera is used to convert an existing film-based radiograph to a digital file, the process is called

   a. digital radiography.

   b. digital subtraction.

   c. direct digital imaging.

   d. digitization.

10. Each of the following is a digital image receptor EXCEPT one. Which one is the EXCEPTION?

    a. CCD

    b. CMOS

    c. XCP

    d. PSP

11. Which of the following stores the x-ray energy until later stimulation by a laser beam reads the electric signal and converts it into a digital image?

    a. CCD

    b. CMOS

    c. XCP

    d. PSP

12. Each of the following is necessary for digital radiography EXCEPT one. Which one is the EXCEPTION?

    a. X-ray machine

    b. Solid-state sensor or phosphor coated plate

    c. Computer and monitor

    d. Special software

    e. Darkroom

13. To maintain infection control, most manufacturers recommend that the sensor used in digital radiography be

    a. packaged for steam sterilization and autoclaved.

    b. disposed of after use, with biohazard wastes.

    c. decontaminated with soap and water and disinfected with a high-level disinfectant.

    d. wiped with an intermediate-level disinfectant and covered with a plastic barrier.

    e. sanitized and immersed in a chemical sterilant.

14. List five features offered by digital software that can be used to enhance the radiographic image.

    a. _____

    b. _____

    c. _____

    d. _____

    e. _____

15. The smaller the number of pixels in the image the sharper the spatial resolution.

    Each pixel stores a number representing a different shade of gray.

    a. The first statement is true. The second statement is false.

    b. The first statement is false. The second statement is true.

    c. Both statements are true.

    d. Both statements are false.

16. Digital radiography requires less radiation exposure to produce an image than film-based radiography because the

    a. chemical processing steps are eliminated.

    b. radiation used for digital imaging is different than radiation used for film-based imaging.

    c. image receptor (CCD or CMOS) is more sensitive to x-rays than film.

    d. computer can control the amount of radiation output better than the radiographer.

17. Each of the following is true regarding digital radiography in comparison to film-based radiography EXCEPT one. Which one is the EXCEPTION?

    a. Provides a more legal document.

    b. Less time is required to obtain a diagnostic image.

    c. Eliminates film and chemical wastes.

    d. Patient radiation is reduced 0 to 50 percent.

    e. Software features enhance interpretation.

18. Each of the following is a disadvantage of digital radiography when compared to film-based radiography EXCEPT one. Which one is the EXCEPTION?

    a. Initial cost of setting up the system

    b. Being able to magnify the image for diagnosis

    c. Risk of computer crashes and lost files

    d. Learning curve required to transfer interpretation skills

    e. Management of infection control

REFLECT—Case study

The oral health care practice where you are employed is considering purchasing a digital radiography system. Using the Internet, search for companies that manufacture and sell dental digital imaging products. From your research, choose two companies and compare their two products. Prepare an analysis to help your practice decide what digital radiography system will be the best choice. Contact the company for literature or additional information as needed to answer the following questions about each of the products.

    a. What are the names of the companies that manufacture the products you chose to compare?

    b. What are the names of the digital radiography systems they manufacture/sell?

    c. Do these digital systems have special computer requirements, or can they be used with the computer currently in use at your practice?

    d. What type of sensor does each offer? How are they alike? How are they different?

    e. What size sensors are available?

    f. Are special sensor holding devices required for positioning the sensor intraorally? Where can these be purchased?

    g. What are the infection control guidelines for the sensor? Does the company make custom-sized plastic barriers that fit the sensor?

    h. Does software come with the purchase of the digital radiography system? What features are included that will allow the operator to enhance the image for interpretation?

    i. Are the companies adhering to DICOM standards?

    j. Does the company offer training for your oral health care team to learn to operate the system? Is there training in digital radiographic interpretation? Is there a fee for service and/or maintenance to the system after purchase?

    k. Does the company offer articles or reviews of their products by outside agencies that support their marketing claims?

    l. Based on what you learned in this chapter, prepare a list of advantages and limitations of each of these products.

    m. Based on your research, which product would you recommend your practice purchase, and why?

RELATE—Laboratory application

For a comprehensive laboratory practice exercise on this topic, see Thomson, E. M. (2012). *Exercises in oral radiography techniques: A laboratory manual* (3rd ed.). Upper Saddle River, NJ: Pearson Education. Chapter 3, "Introduction to digital imaging."

REFERENCES

American Dental Association Council on Scientific Affairs. (2006). The use of dental radiographs: Update and recommendations. *J Am Dent Assn, 137,* 1304–1312.

American Dental Association Standards Committee on Dental Informatics. (2005). *Implementation requirements for DICOM in dentistry.* Technical report no. 1023-2005. Chicago: Author.

Farman, A. G., & Farman, T. T. (2005). A comparison of 18 different x-ray detectors currently used in dentistry. *Oral Surgery, Oral Medicine, Oral Pathology, 99,* 485–489.

Francisco, E. F., Horlak, D., & Azevedo, S. (2010). The balance between safety and efficacy: Understanding the technology available that will produce high quality radiographs while reducing patient risk to ionizing radiation. *Dimensions of Dental Hygiene, 8,* 26–30.

Horner, K., Drage, N., & Brettle, D. (2008). *21st century imaging.* London: Quintessence Publishing.

Palenik, C. J. (2004). Infection control for dental radiography. *Dentistry Today, 23,* 52–55.

Van der Stelt, P. F. (2005). Filmless imaging: The uses of digital radiography in dental practice. *Journal of the American Dental Association, 136,* 1379–1387.

Van der Stelt, P. F. (2008). Better imaging: The advantages of digital radiography. *Journal of the American Dental Association, 139,* 7S–13S

White, S. C., & Pharoah, M. J. (2008). *Oral radiology: Principles and interpretation* (6th ed.). St. Louis: Elsevier.

Williamson, G. F. (2005). Digital radiography in dentistry. *Journal of Practical Hygiene,* 13–14.

CHAPTER

10 Infection Control

CHAPTER OUTLINE

OBJECTIVES

Following successful completion of this chapter, you should be able to:

1. Define the key words.
2. State the purpose of infection control.
3. Describe the possible routes of disease transmission.
4. Identify conditions for the chain of infection and methods of breaking the chain.
5. Identify agencies responsible for recommending and regulating infection control guidelines.
6. List the personal protective equipment recommended for the dental radiographer.
7. Explain disinfection and sterilization.
8. Differentiate between semicritical and noncritical objects used during radiographic procedures.
9. Demonstrate competency in following infection control protocol prior to radiographic procedures.
10. Demonstrate competency in following infection control protocol during radiographic procedures.
11. Demonstrate competency in following infection control protocol after radiographic procedures.
12. Demonstrate competency in following infection control protocol for handling and processing intraoral image receptors.
13. Demonstrate competency in following the infection control protocol when using an automatic processor with a daylight loader attachment.

KEY WORDS

Acquired immunodeficiency syndrome (AIDS)

Antiseptic

Asepsis

Barrier envelope

Contamination

Cross-contamination

Disinfect

Hepatitis B

Human immunodeficiency virus (HIV)

Immunization

Infection control

Intraoral dental film

Microbial aerosol

Pathogen

Personal protective equipment (PPE)

Protective barrier

Sepsis

Spatter

Standard precautions

Sterilize

Universal precautions

Introduction

The purpose of **infection control** procedures used in oral health care is to prevent the transmission of disease among patients and between patients and oral health care practitioners. Maintaining infection control throughout the radiographic procedure can be challenging. The radiographer must possess a thorough understanding of the recommended infection control protocols that should be followed before, during, and after radiographic exposures. The specific steps of these protocols require practice to achieve competency in skilled handling of contaminated radiographic equipment and supplies.

The purpose of this chapter is to identify infection control terminology (Table 10-1), present the need for infection control during radiographic procedures, and describe step-by-step infection control procedures used in dental radiology.

Purpose of Infection Control

Infectious diseases may be transmitted from patient to oral health care personnel, from oral health care personnel to patient, and from patient to patient. The primary purpose of infection control is to prevent the transmission of infectious diseases. Human beings have always lived with the possibility of infection occurring through invasion of the body by pathogens such as bacteria or viruses. A **pathogen** is a microorganism capable of causing disease. Because of the special risk these diseases carry, of particular concern to the oral health care professionals are **acquired immunodeficiency syndrome (AIDS),** the **human immunodeficiency**

virus **(HIV),** viral hepatitis, including the highly infectious **hepatitis B** virus (HBV), tuberculosis (TB), and herpesvirus diseases.

Routes of infection transmission are

* Direct contact with pathogens in open lesions, blood, saliva, or respiratory secretions.
* Direct contact with airborne contaminants present in aerosols of oral and respiratory fluids.
* Indirect contact with contaminated objects or instruments.

Chain of Infection

For infection to occur, four conditions must be present (Figure 10-1).

1. A susceptible (i.e., not immune) host
2. A disease-causing microorganism (pathogen)
3. Sufficient numbers of the pathogen to initiate infection
4. An appropriate route (portal of entry) for the pathogen to enter the host

The purpose of infection control is to alter one of these four conditions to prevent the transmission of disease.

Breaking the Chain of Infection

The chain of infection can be broken by:

1. **Immunization** of the susceptible host. The Centers for Disease Control and Prevention (CDC) recommends that dental personnel working with blood or blood-contaminated substances be vaccinated for hepatitis B virus (HBV).

TABLE 10-1 Terminology

TERM	DEFINITION
Antiseptic	Agent used on living tissues to destroy or stop the growth of bacteria
Asepsis	Absence of septic matter or freedom from infection (*a* means without; *sepsis* means infection)
Contamination	Soiling by contact or mixing
Cross-contamination	To contaminate from one place or person to another place or person
Disinfect	The use of a chemical or physical procedure to reduce the disease-producing microorganisms to an acceptable level on inanimate objects
Immunization	The process of making someone immune to a disease
Infection control	The prevention and reduction of disease-causing (pathogenic) microorganisms
Microbial aerosol	Suspension of microorganisms that may be capable of causing disease produced during normal breathing and speaking
Pathogen	A microorganism that can cause disease (*pathos* means disease)
Protective barrier	Any material that prevents the transmission of infective microorganisms
Sepsis	Infection, or the presence of septic matter
Spatter	A heavier concentration of microbial aerosols, such as visible particles from a cough or sneeze
Standard precautions	A practice of care to protect persons from pathogens spread via blood or any other body fluid, excretion, or secretion (except sweat)
Sterilize	The total destruction of spores and disease-producing microorganisms, accomplished by autoclaving or dry heat processes
Universal precautions	Concept of infection control where the focus was on blood-borne pathogens. The all-inclusive "standard precautions" has replaced this concept

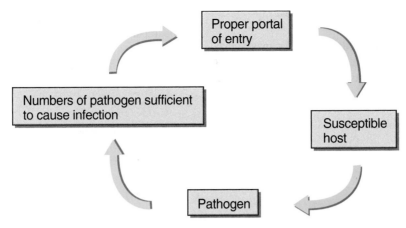

FIGURE 10-1 Chain of infection.

Additionally, all oral health care workers should be vaccinated against influenza, measles, mumps, rubella, and tetanus.

2. **Removing the pathogen.** Use sterilization techniques and/or protective barriers.

3. **Reducing the sufficient numbers of pathogens.** Use disinfection and sterilization techniques and/or protective barriers.

4. **Blocking the portal of entry.** Use personal protective equipment (PPE) barriers such as protective clothes, masks, eyewear, and gloves.

Guidelines for Infection Control

In the past, there may have been a tendency to use a double standard in that certain infection control precautions were used only if the patient was known to be infectious. It is a fact that some patients are reluctant to admit their infectious condition. Taking a thorough medical history and performing an oral examination will not always identify potential infected patients. Failure to use a single standard for all patients put everyone at risk. Therefore, the use of **standard precautions,** where all body fluids (except sweat) of all patients, whether known to be infected or not, are assumed to be infected requires that the necessary infection control procedures must be applied to all patients.

The following government agencies are responsible for developing, recommending, and/or regulating infection control guidelines:

- **Centers for Disease Control and Prevention (CDC)** Although it does not enforce regulations, the CDC is a major influence in the development and recommendation of guidelines for preventing disease and controlling infection.
- **Occupational Safety and Health Administration (OHSA)** Enforces regulations that protect the radiographer from infection in the oral health care workplace.
- **U.S. Food and Drug Administration (FDA)** Regulates oral health care products to ensure safe use. Although we associate the FDA with drug testing, the products tested by this agency include protective plastic barriers for use with digital intraoral image receptors.
- **U.S. Environmental Protection Agency (EPA)** The EPA is most often associated with its efforts to promote a clean environment, but its regulation of waste products, chemicals, and disinfectants influence radiographic infection control practices.

Each oral health care practice should have a written infection control policy that incorporates practical procedures that are compatible with recommendations and regulations stated by these agencies and are in accordance with state and local regulations. The dentist (or designated personnel) has the authority and the responsibility to see that the infection control policy is correctly carried out. The CDC's infection control guidelines that directly relate to dental radiology are listed in Box 10-1.

BOX 10-1   The Centers for Disease Control and Prevention (CDC) Recommended Infection-Control Practices for Oral Radiography

- Wear patient treatment gloves when exposing radiographs and handling contaminated image receptors.
- Use protective eyewear, mask, and gown as appropriate if spattering of blood or other body fluids is likely.
- Use heat-tolerant or disposable image receptor holding devices whenever possible (at a minimum, disinfect semicritical heat-sensitive devices such as digital radiographic sensors, according to the manufacturer's instructions).
- Clean and heat-sterilize image receptor holding devices between patients.
- Transport and handle exposed image receptors in an aseptic manner to prevent contamination of processing equipment.
- Use FDA-cleared protective barriers on digital radiographic image receptors.

Personal Protective Equipment (PPE)

Personal protective equipment or **PPE** (clothing, masks, eyewear, and gloves) worn by dental personnel acts as a **protective barrier** (Figure 10-2). PPE prevents the transmission of infective microorganisms between oral health care practitioners and patients.

Protective Clothing

Protective clothing, such as scrubs, gowns, and uniforms, provides protection from exposure to body fluids. Protective clothing should be changed daily, or more frequently if soiled or wet. Protective clothing should be removed before leaving the treatment facility. Protective clothing should be laundered separately with bleach to prevent contamination of other items. Ideally, protective clothing should be laundered by a commercial biohazard laundry service that can safely remove the items from the practice for laundering.

Masks

Although radiographic procedures are much less likely than other dental procedures to produce spatter, protection from microbial aerosols may be achieved through the use of a mask. Masks should be changed when soiled or wet and between patients.

Protective Eyewear

Although radiographic procedures are much less likely than other types of dental procedures to subject the radiographer to physical eye accidents, the use of protective eyewear will protect against microbial aerosols and spatter. Types of protective eyewear include glasses with side shields, goggles, and full-face shields. Protective eyewear must be washed with appropriate cleaning agents following treatment and as needed.

Gloves

Gloves must be worn at all times throughout the radiographic procedure. A variety of gloves is available for specialized uses. Sterile gloves are used for surgical procedures; medical examination (nonsterile) gloves are used for most dental procedures, including radiographic procedures; plastic overgloves have temporary applications such as protecting or containing patient treatment gloves; and utility gloves are appropriate for cleaning and disinfection. Medical examination gloves are made of latex or vinyl material. Powdered gloves should be avoided, as the powder residue can cause radiographic artifacts (see Chapter 18.) Gloves should never be washed with soap or disinfected for reuse. Soap may damage gloves in a way that would allow the flow of liquid through undetected holes. Punctured, torn, or cut gloves should be changed immediately. Gloves should always be changed and discarded between patients.

All unprotected surfaces not directly associated with the procedure such as doorknobs to access the darkroom, unexposed film packets or unprotected digital sensors, or patient records should not be touched with contaminated gloves.

Handwashing

Protective clothing, mask, and eyewear should all be in place to prepare for handwashing prior to putting on medical examination gloves. Hands should be cleaned thoroughly before and after treating each patient (before gloving and after removing gloves; see Procedure Box 10-1). Potentially infectious pathogens can grow rapidly inside a warm, moist glove.

When hands are visibly dirty, they must be washed with an antimicrobial soap and water. If hands are not visibly soiled, an alcohol-containing preparation designed for reducing the number of viable microorganisms on the hands may be used. All jewelry, including a watch and rings, should be removed prior to handwashing. Long fingernails, false fingernails, and nail polish should be avoided, as these may harbor pathogens and have the potential to puncture treatment gloves. Handwashing is most effective when nails are cut short and well manicured. Hands must be dried thoroughly before putting on treatment gloves.

Disinfection and Sterilization of Radiographic Instruments and Equipment

Prior to and following radiographic procedures, the treatment area and the equipment must be cleaned and disinfected. Cleaning instruments and equipment to prepare for sterilization and prior to disinfecting provides for effective infection control. Cleaning, disinfection, and sterilization break the chain of infection to prevent the transmission of infective microorganisms.

Disinfection

Disinfection is the use of a chemical or physical procedure to reduce the disease-producing microorganisms (pathogens) to an acceptable level on inanimate objects. Spores are not necessarily destroyed. Disinfecting agents are too toxic for use on living tissue, so are only used on clinical surfaces and on some instruments that cannot be heat sterilized.

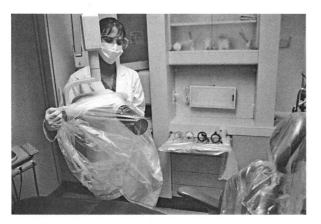

FIGURE 10-2 Radiographer preparing x-ray equipment.
Wearing PPE (barrier gown, protective eyewear, mask, gloves) to place barriers to cover the x-ray tube head and PID. In the background, note that image receptor holders have been assembled and placed on a plastic barrier on the countertop.

PROCEDURE 10-1
Procedure for handwashing for radiographic procedures

1. Put on protective gown, eyewear, and mask.
2. Remove rings, wristwatch,* and other jewelry.
3. Wet hands with cool/tepid water and apply liquid antimicrobial soap.
4. Vigorously lather for 15 seconds; interlace fingers and thumbs, and move hands back and forth; work lather under nails.
5. Rinse well, allowing water to run from fingertips.
6. Dry each hand thoroughly with a separate paper towel.
7. Unless equipped with a foot pedal, turn off the water by placing a clean paper towel between clean, dry hand and the faucet.

*Wristwatch may be replaced after handwashing as long as it will remain protected under the gown or covered with the glove during the procedure.

EPA-registered disinfectants are classified as:

- **High-level disinfectant.** Chemical germicides inactivate spores and can be used to disinfect heat-sensitive semicritical dental instruments.
- **Intermediate-level disinfectant.** Chemical germicides labeled as both hospital-grade disinfectants and tuberculocidals. Examples are iodophors, phenolics, and chlorine-containing compounds. These do not destroy spores.
- **Low-level disinfectant.** Chemical germicides labeled as hospital-grade disinfectants. Cannot destroy spores, tubercle bacilli, or nonlipid viruses.

Because of their corrosive and toxic properties, the CDC discourages the use of disinfectants. Additionally, disinfectants have the potential to affect electrical connections, so directly spraying or saturating the x-ray control panel, dials, or exposure button may damage the x-ray machine. Therefore, protective barriers should be used whenever practical. Plastic wrap or barriers are commonly used to cover those surfaces most likely to be contaminated during the radiographic procedure such as the PID and tube head, control panel, exposure switch, and counter surfaces (Figures 10-2 and 10-3). Surfaces not covered must be cleaned and disinfected after the radiographic procedures are completed.

Sterilization

Sterilization is the total destruction of spores and disease-producing microorganisms. Sterilization is usually accomplished by autoclaving or dry heat processes. Ideally, all equipment and instruments should be sterilized. Acceptable methods of sterilization in the oral health care facility include

- Steam under pressure (steam autoclave)
- Dry heat
- Heat/chemical vapor (chemical autoclave)
- EPA-registered high-level disinfectant

Classification of Objects Used in Radiographic Procedures

Radiographic instruments and clinical contact surfaces are classified according to their risk of transmitting infection and to the need to sterilize between uses (Table 10-2). All surfaces that will be used for or contacted during the procedure must be cleaned and disinfected or sterilized according to the object's classification as critical, semicritical, or noncritical.

- Critical instruments are those used to penetrate soft tissue or bone. Examples are needles, forceps, and scalers. Critical objects must be discarded or sterilized after each use. No critical instruments or equipment are used in radiographic procedures.
- Semicritical instruments are those that contact oral mucosa without penetrating soft tissue or bone, such as intraoral dental mirrors. Radiographic image receptor holding

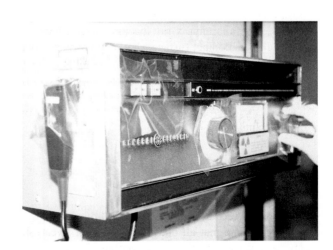

FIGURE 10-3 Plastic barrier wrap covering x-ray control panel.

TABLE 10-2 Risk of Transmitting Disease Classification of Objects Used in Radiographic Procedures

CATEGORY	RADIOGRAPHIC EQUIPMENT	STERILIZE OR DISINFECT OR DISCARD
Critical	None	N/A
Semicritical	Image receptor holders	Sterilize or use disposable devices
	Digital sensor/phosphor plate*	
	Panoramic biteblocks	
Noncritical/clinical contact surface	X-ray tube head, PID, support arms	Clean and disinfect with an appropriate level EPA-registered disinfectant
	Exposure controls**	
	Lead/lead-equivalent apron and thyroid collar	
	Countertop in operatory and darkroom	
	Extraoral radiographic machine parts such as chin/forehead rest, side head positioner guides; cephalostat	

*Some phosphor plates can be gas sterilized, but most digital radiographic sensor manufacturers recommend against sterilizing these fragile devices. Instead, wipe with an appropriate level EPA-registered disinfectant before covering with an FDA-cleared barrier and wipe again following barrier removal after the procedure. Consult manufacturer's recommendations.

**Liquid disinfectants may damage the electrical components of the dental x-ray control panel. Therefore, most dental x-ray equipment manufacturers recommend covering the control panel exposure dials and exposure button with an FDA-cleared barrier. Consult manufacturer's recommendations.

devices and the bite block of the panoramic x-ray machine (see Chapter 30) fall into this category. Semicritical instruments must be sterilized after use or discarded. Although most image receptor holders can be sterilized or are disposable, some devices on the market may be heat sensitive. Although heat-sensitive semicritical instruments may be sterilized under certain conditions with EPA-registered chemicals classified as high-level disinfectant, using instruments that can be heat-sterilized or that are disposable is recommended.

• Noncritical instruments and clinical contact surfaces are those devices and surfaces of the treatment area that may contact intact skin or may become contaminated by microbial aerosols or spatter, but do not come into contact with the mucous membranes. Examples include the lead apron, the PID (position indicating device), and the chin rest and head positioner guides of extraoral radiographic equipment such as the panoramic x-ray machine. (See Chapter 30.) Other clinical contact surfaces that may become contaminated during the procedure include the x-ray machine tube head, the exposure button, and the countertop. Noncritical instruments and clinical contact surfaces can be disinfected using EPA-registered intermediate- or low-level disinfectants. use ↑ level

Infection Control Protocol for the Radiographic Procedure

Using standard precautions, infection control procedures for radiography assume that all body fluids (except sweat) of all patients have the potential to be infectious. Infection control procedures for exposing radiographs can be divided into three categories: prior to, during, and after exposure.

Infection Control Prior to the Radiographic Procedure (Procedure Box 10-2)

PREPARE THE TREATMENT AREA All treatment area surfaces likely to come in contact with the patient either directly or indirectly must be sterilized, or cleaned and disinfected, and/or covered with a protective barrier. All supplies, image receptors, and holding devices should be obtained and placed for easy access during the procedure.

Intraoral dental film inside its original packaging is not sterile, but rather is considered "industrially clean," which means that it is not expected to be contaminated with pathogens. To avoid contamination prior to use, intraoral film packets should be dispensed just prior to use in disposable containers such as a paper cup or small envelope. The film packets must be handled carefully to prevent cross-contamination. Because they are heat-sensitive, film packets cannot be sterilized, and the liquid saturation required for disinfecting is not recommended.

Another method used to prevent the transmission of microorganisms by the film packet is to use **barrier envelopes.** Barrier envelopes are commercially available for film sizes #0, #1, and #2. Film packets placed and sealed in these plastic envelopes (Figure 10-4) are protected from contact with fluids in the oral cavity during exposure. Film packets already sealed in barrier plastic envelopes by the manufacturer are also available commercially. Following removal from the patient's oral cavity, the barrier envelope is opened (Figure 10-5) and discarded appropriately. The film packet that was sealed in the barrier envelope may now be handled with clean hands (or new gloves) to complete the processing procedure.

DIGITAL IMAGE RECEPTORS Phosphor plates used to obtain radiographic images digitally (see Chapter 9) must also be sealed in plastic barrier envelops prior to use intraorally

PROCEDURE 10-2
Infection control prior to the radiographic procedure

1. Follow handwashing described in Procedure Box 10-1 or apply an antiseptic hand rub following the manufacturer's directions for use.*

2. Put on utility gloves.

3. Clean and disinfect with appropriate disinfectant all surfaces that will come in contact either directly or indirectly with the patient. See the following list:

    a. PID

    b. X-ray tube head

    c. Tube head support arms and handles

    d. Exposure button**

    e. Control panel dials (impulse timer, kVp, and MA controls)**

    f. Treatment chair, including headrest, back support, arm rests, body and back of the chair

    g. Bracket table or countertop or other clinical contact surfaces that will be used during the procedure

    h. Digital sensor or phosphor plates

    i. Lead/lead equivalent apron/thyroid collar

4. Wash, dry, and remove utility gloves. Disinfect.

5. Wash hands with an antimicrobial soap or apply an antiseptic hand rub.*

6. Put on clean overgloves.

7. Obtain plastic barriers and cover all surfaces that will come in contact either directly or indirectly with the patient. See the following list:

    a. PID

    b. X-ray tube head (Figure 10-2)

    c. Tube head support arms and handles

    d. Exposure button

    e. Control panel dials (impulse timer, kVp, and MA controls; Figure 10-3)

    f. Treatment chair including headrest, back support, arm rests, body and back of the chair

    g. Bracket table or countertop or other clinical contact surface that will be used during the procedure

    h. Computer keyboard and mouse (digital imaging)

    i. Digital sensor or phosphor plates

    j. Lead/lead equivalent apron/thyroid collar (optional)

    k. Film packets (optional; Figure 10-4)

    l. Digital sensors or phosphor plates

8. Obtain radiographic supplies. See the following list:

    a. Image receptors (film packets/digital sensors/phosphor plates)

    b. Sterile or disposable image receptor holding devices

    c. Film mount (for film-based radiography)

    d. Disposable paper/plastic cup

    e. Paper towels

    f. Miscellaneous supplies (i.e., cotton rolls, extra disposable image receptor holding devices)

9. Place the film mount under the plastic barrier on the counter work space.

PROCEDURE 10-2
Infection control prior to the radiographic procedure (continued)

10. Place the film packets on the plastic barrier placed over the film mount.

11. Saturate a folded paper towel with disinfectant and place next to the film mount on top of the plastic barrier.

12. Prepare antimicrobial mouth rinse for patient use prior to procedure.***

*When hands are visibly dirty, they must be washed with an antimicrobial soap and water. If hands are not visibly soiled, an alcohol-containing preparation designed for reducing the number of viable microorganisms on the hands may be used. Refer to manufacturer's recommendations for use.

**Exposure switches and control panel dials may be damaged by the use of a disinfectant solution. Manufacturer's recommendations should be consulted. Saturating a paper towel with disinfectant and then carefully wiping the switches may be an option. Infection control may also be achieved by protecting with a plastic barrier (Figure 10-3). (Foot pedal exposure switches do not require disinfection.)

***Scientific evidence does not indicate that preprocedural mouth rinsing prevents the spread of infections. However, antimicrobial mouth rinses (e.g., chlorhexidine gluconate, essential oils, or povidone-iodine) can reduce the number of microorganisms the patient might release in the form of aerosols or spatter.

(Figure 10-6). The same careful handling recommended for film packets should be followed to avoid cross-contamination. Solid-state digital sensors cannot withstand sterilization procedures, so they must be wiped with disinfectant and covered with a plastic barrier prior to placing intraorally (Figure 10-7).

There are many sizes and styles of plastic barriers for phosphor plates and plastic sheaths for digital sensors designed to protect these image receptors from contamination (see Figures 9-9 and 9-10). However, these barriers are subject to tearing and are not always totally protective. The use of an FDA-cleared disposable plastic barrier will help decrease the risk of a breach in asepsis. Additionally, wiping the sensor or phosphor plate with an appropriate level disinfectant prior to and after placement of the plastic barrier is usually recommended (Figure 10-7). Although the manufacturer's instructions for maintaining infection control should

be consulted to prevent damage to the sensor or phosphor plate, options for substitutes for harsh chemical disinfection and sterilants are not usually offered. Infection control techniques for digital radiography have not yet been perfected and remain a problem to be solved through rigorous testing as this technology evolves.

A laser scanning device (for use with phosphor plates) and a computer keyboard and/or mouse (for use with solid state sensors) must be operated to produce images and activate the exposure sequence, so these should also be covered with a plastic barrier that is changed between patients (see Figure 9-28). As digital technology advances, infection control protocols are expected to advance as well. In fact, medical grade computer monitors that have glass fronts that are easy to clean and can be disinfected are becoming increasingly available for mounting in a dental operatory in close proximity to patient treatment.

damp, not dripping

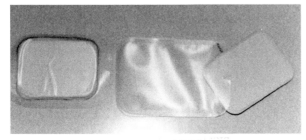

FIGURE 10-4 Barrier envelope. (*left*) Film available from manufacturer sealed in barrier packet ready for use. (*right*) Barrier envelopes may be purchased separately.

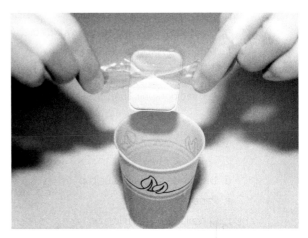

FIGURE 10-5 Opening the barrier envelope. A steady pull is used, allowing the film packet to drop into a clean cup.

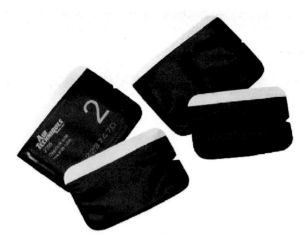

FIGURE 10-6 Barrier envelopes for phosphor plates. (Courtesy of Air Techniques, Inc.)

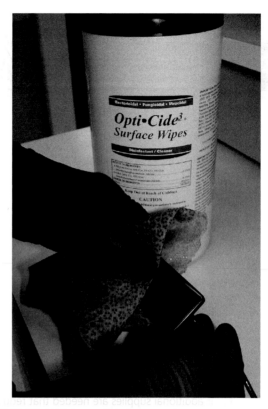

FIGURE 10-7 Using a disinfectant wipe to prepare a digital sensor prior to placing plastic barrier.

Protocol During the Radiographic Procedure (Procedure Box 10-3)

PATIENT PREPARATION   The patient is seated after the treatment area is prepared and supplies are readied. The patient may be asked to rinse with an antimicrobial mouth rinse to reduce oral microorganisms that contribute to infectious aerosols. The patient is draped with the lead/lead-equivalent apron and thyroid collar. Care must be taken when making adjustments to the treatment chair and headrest so as not to compromise the infection control process. Covering the treatment chair controls with a plastic barrier will aid in the infection control process.

Any object that may interfere with the procedure, such as patient's eyeglasses, dentures, etc., should be removed by the patient and placed in an area so they do not become contaminated and do not contaminate other objects.

DURING EXPOSURES   Once the procedure has begun, care must be taken to touch only covered surfaces. The best way to minimize contamination is to touch as few surfaces as possible. If drawers or cabinets must be opened to retrieve additional supplies, or the radiographer must leave the treatment area during the procedure, the patient treatment gloves should be removed and the hands washed. New treatment gloves must be used when restarting the procedure. Overgloves may also be used, if treatment must be interrupted. The patient treatment gloves may be rinsed briefly with water only (do not use soap, as it will compromise the integrity of the protection), dried, and covered with plastic overgloves. To restart the exposure procedure, the overgloves are removed.

FILM PACKETS AND PHOSPHOR PLATES   Immediately after removing the image receptor from the oral cavity it should be swiped across a disinfectant-soaked paper towel that was prepared during setup to remove excess saliva (Figure 10-8). The film should next be dropped into a paper cup without touching the outside edges of the cup. The cup will serve as the transport method of getting the contaminated film packets safely into the darkroom. Phosphor plates should be dropped into the containment light-tight box for transport to the laser scanner (see Figure 9-14).

If using a film packet covered with a plastic barrier, the infection control protocol is the same as that used for phosphor plates. Hold the image receptor over the cup designated for containment (film packets) or the containment light-tight box (phosphor plates) and tear open the plastic barrier (Figure 10-5), allowing the sealed image receptor to drop into the containment receptacle untouched by gloved hands. Once all the image receptors are exposed and opened in this manner, the containment cup of film packets can be transported to the darkroom for processing, and the containment box of phosphor plates can be transported to the location of the laser scanner.

DIGITAL IMAGE RECEPTORS   The plastic barrier placed prior to use will remain in place until the completion of all exposures. Excess saliva should be removed with a paper towel. When the procedure is complete, the plastic barrier should be carefully removed to avoid tearing and contaminating the sensor (Figure 10-9).

IMAGE RECEPTOR HOLDERS   The image receptor holding devices should be transferred from a barrier-protected surface to the patient's oral cavity and then back to the same covered surface. Never place contaminated instruments on an uncovered surface.

PROCEDURE 10-3
Infection control during the radiographic procedure

1. Follow handwashing described in Procedure Box 10-1 or apply an antiseptic hand rub following the manufacturer's directions for use.
2. Put on patient treatment gloves.
3. Place overgloves over patient treatment gloves.
4. Place the lead/lead equivalent apron and thyroid collar on the patient.
5. Remove overgloves and place on the counter.
6. Assemble the image receptor into the appropriate holding device, place intraorally, and position the x-ray tube head and PID.
7. Depress the exposure button, and remove the image receptor and holding device from the patient's oral cavity.
8. Remove the image receptor from the holding device.
9. Film or phosphor plate: swipe the image receptor across the disinfectant-soaked paper towel and drop into the containment cup/box.*

   Digital sensor: remove excess saliva with paper towel.
10. Proceed to place and expose all radiographs in this manner.
11. If additional supplies are needed that requires the operator to contact noncovered surfaces or the procedure must otherwise be interrupted:

    a. Rinse treatment gloves with plain water (no soap) and dry.**
    b. Place overgloves over treatment gloves.
    c. To restart the procedure, remove overgloves.

*Phosphor plates and film packets sealed in plastic barrier envelopes should be opened immediately using aseptic technique.

**If the procedure must be interrupted, the treatment gloves may be removed and discarded and the hands washed. Prior to restarting the procedure, the hands should be washed again and new treatment gloves put on.

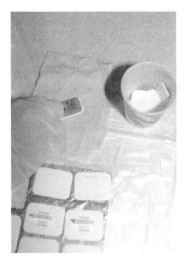

FIGURE 10-8 Remove saliva. Radiographer is swiping the film packet across a disinfectant-soaked paper towel prior to dropping the film into the containment cup.

Protocol After the Radiographic Procedure (Procedure Box 10-4)

Once the radiographic procedure is complete, patient gloves should be removed and discarded, and hands washed with an antimicrobial soap or an alcohol-based hand rub. The lead/lead equivalent apron with thyroid collar can now be removed from the patient and the cup containing the exposed films, carried to the darkroom for processing or phosphor plates to the laser scanner.

Once the patient is dismissed, the radiographer should place utility gloves on for cleaning and disinfecting the treatment area. With utility gloves on, the image receptor holders are cleaned and prepared for sterilization according to the manufacturer's recommendations. Usually these holders can be washed with soap and water or ultrasonic cleaned in detergent and dried and packaged in an autoclave bag for sterilization. All disposable holders and other disposable supplies, such as cotton rolls, should be discarded. Dispose of all contaminated items according to local and state regulations. Plastic barriers, including those covering the digital sensor, should be carefully removed, making sure not to touch the surfaces underneath. The digital sensor should be wiped with a

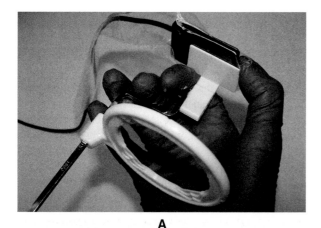

A

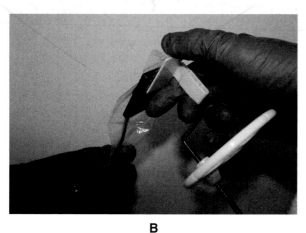

B

FIGURE 10-9 Removing the plastic barrier from a digital sensor. Removal of sticky-backed biteblocks is easier if the image receptor holder remains in place attached to the barrier. **(A)** Grasping the holder in the palm of one hand, press on the sensor with the thumb. **(B)** As the sensor begins to move, guide it out of the plastic sheath with the other hand.

PROCEDURE 10-4
Infection control after the radiographic procedure

1. Rinse, remove, and discard patient treatment gloves and wash hands. Follow handwashing described in Procedure Box 10-1 or apply an antiseptic hand rub following the manufacturer's directions for use.
2. Remove lead/lead equivalent apron with thyroid collar and dismiss patient.
3. Put on utility gloves.
4. Prepare and package image receptor holders for sterilization.*
5. Sterilize image receptor holders according to manufacturer's recommendations.
6. Discard all disposable contaminated items (i.e., disposable image receptor holders, paper towels, cotton rolls).
7. Remove and discard all plastic barriers.
8. Clean and disinfect any uncovered surface.
9. Wipe digital sensor/phosphor plates with disinfectant.
10. Clean and disinfect lead/lead equivalent apron and thyroid collar.
11. Wash, dry and remove utility gloves. Disinfect.
12. Wash hands with antimicrobial soap. Follow handwashing described in Procedure Box 10-1 or apply an antiseptic hand rub following the manufacturer's directions for use.

*Refer to manufacturer's recommendations for cleaning with soap and water or ultrasonic detergents.

disinfectant. All areas not covered should be cleaned and disinfected, including the lead/lead equivalent apron and thyroid collar. When cleanup is complete, utility gloves should be washed with soap and water, removed, and disinfected. The radiographer should wash hands again after removing utility gloves.

Infection Control Protocol for Radiographic Processing

Film-handling procedures for processing will depend on whether or not barrier envelopes are used to protect the film packets.

Film Handling Without the Use of Barrier Envelopes (Procedure Box 10-5)

The use of commercial plastic film barrier envelopes protects the film packet while in the oral cavity. Once the film packet is aseptically removed from the barrier envelope, it is safe to handle with clean, dry hands or clean treatment gloves. Although readily available, the use of protective plastic envelopes for intraoral films is not universal. For this reason, it is important that the dental radiographer be skilled at handling film packets without barrier envelopes.

Once the film packets have been transported to the darkroom, the operator must put on treatment gloves and proceed to open the

---

PROCEDURE 10-5
Infection control for processing radiographic films without barrier envelopes

1. Transport the contaminated film packets to the darkroom in the paper/plastic cup used for containment.
2. Place one paper towel on the counter work space, and place the cup with contaminated films on this paper towel.
3. Place a second paper towel on the counter work space adjacent to the first paper towel and designate it as the uncontaminated area.
4. Secure darkroom door.
5. Turn off white overhead light and turn on safelight.
6. Put on clean patient treatment gloves.
7. Open each film packet (Figure 10-10).

    a. Peel back the outer plastic/paper wrap using the tab on the back of the packet.

    b. Grasp the black paper with film sandwiched in between, and pull straight out.

    c. Hold the black paper–film assembly over the designated uncontaminated paper towel and pull out slowly.

    d. Allow the film to drop out onto the paper towel. Do not touch the film with contaminated patient treatment gloves.

8. Drop the contaminated film packet outer plastic/paper wrap, black paper, and lead foil onto the contaminated paper towel.
9. Repeat steps 7 and 8 until all film packets have been opened.
10. Remove and discard patient treatment gloves and wash and dry hands.
11. With clean, dry hands, grasp by the edges and place films into the automatic processor feeder slots or load onto manual processing film racks for processing.
12. When the films are safely in the automatic processor, or the manual processing cover is securely closed, turn on the overhead white light.
13. Put on utility gloves.
14. Separate lead foil from film packets and discard into lead recycling waste.
15. Gather the contaminated paper towel with all waste and discard appropriately.
16. Clean and disinfect the counter work space and any other area that may have been touched during the procedure.
17. Wash, dry, and remove utility gloves. Disinfect.
18. Wash and dry hands.*

*If hands are not visibly soiled, an alcohol-containing preparation designed for reducing the number of viable microorganisms on the hands may be used. Refer to manufacturer's recommendations for use.

packets aseptically (Figure 10-10). Skill in this procedure will help avoid dropping and potentially losing films in the darkroom's dim lighting. In addition, the radiographer should be able to open all film packets, especially when processing a full mouth series, in two minutes or less to avoid prolonged exposure of the film to safelight. Prolonged exposure to light, even if it is called safelight, increases the risk of film fog (see Chapter 8.) After the last film is placed into the automatic processor or into the manual processing tank and the cover is closed, the darkroom must be cleaned and disinfected. Discard all materials appropriately, including the film packets, lead foil (see Chapter 20), and any materials used as protective barriers. Clean and disinfect darkroom counter surfaces and/or any other areas touched by gloved hands.

Film Handling with the Use of Barrier Envelopes and Phosphor Plates

Although protected while in the oral cavity, film packets and phosphor plates that were secured in barrier envelopes must still be handled carefully. Once these image receptors have been removed from the plastic barrier envelopes, they may be handled with clean, dry hands, or with new treatment gloves. To avoid damage, handle these image receptors by the edges. The use of powdered gloves should be avoided because powder residue will leave artifacts on the radiograph (see Chapter 18).

Infection Control for Processors with a Daylight Loader

Daylight loader attachments on automatic processors have light-tight flaps or sleeves that allow the radiographer's hands to slide through to access the intake slots on the front of the processor. A processor equipped with daylight loader attachment does not require a darkroom. Daylight loader attachments require special infection control considerations (Procedure Box 10-6). With strict adherence to proper infection control protocol, the use of daylight loaders should not compromise infection control. The radiographer should be discouraged from shortcutting these procedures, which would pose a health threat not only for the operator, but also for others who use the device.

The key to infection control using the daylight loader is to open the light-filter cover when placing and removing items (Figure 10-11). Never attempt to push items through the light-tight baffles. After removing the light-filter cover from the daylight loader, the cup containing the contaminated film packets, an additional, uncontaminated cup, and unused treatment gloves should be placed inside the unit on top of a plastic or paper towel barrier. With the light-filter cover closed, clean, dry hands can be slid through the light-tight baffles to

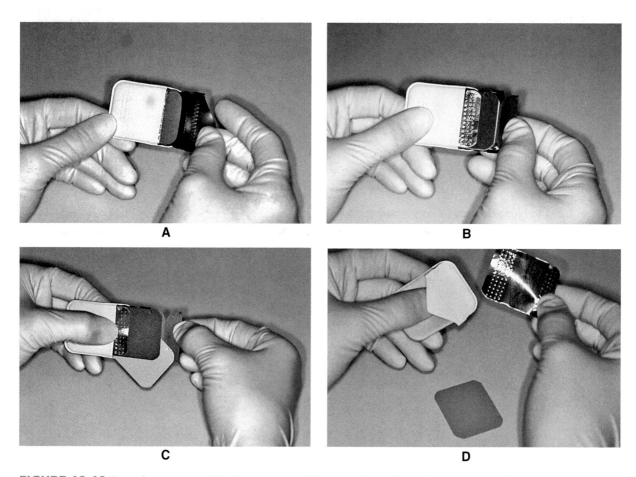

A

B

C

D

FIGURE 10-10 **Steps for removing film from packet without touching film with contaminated gloves.** (**A**) Open the film packet by lifting the plastic tab. (**B**) Locate the folded tab of black paper and grasp with finger and thumb. (**C**) Gently pull on the black paper tab, sliding the film out of the packet. (**D**) Allow the film to drop out onto the plastic or paper towel barrier placed on the counter. Separate the lead foil from the rest of the packet and dispose of all materials appropriately.

PROCEDURE 10-6
Infection control for an automatic processor with a daylight loader attachment

1. Transport the contaminated film packets to the automatic processor equipped with the daylight loader attachment.

2. Obtain a clean pair of patient treatment gloves.

3. Open the light-filter cover and line the floor of the daylight loader compartment with a clean paper towel or plastic barrier. Designate one side as the contaminated side and the other side as uncontaminated.

4. Place the cup with the film packets on the contaminated side and a clean pair of patient treatment gloves on the uncontaminated side inside the daylight loader.

5. Close the light-filter cover.

6. Slide clean, dry hands through the light-tight baffles.

7. Once inside, put on the pair of clean patient treatment gloves.

8. Open each film packet (Figure 10-10).

   a. Peel back the outer plastic/paper wrap using the tab on the back of the packet.

   b. Grasp the black paper with film sandwiched in between and pull straight out.

   c. Allow the film to drop onto the paper towel or plastic barrier on the uncontaminated side of the floor of the compartment. Do not touch the film with contaminated client gloves.

9. Drop the contaminated film packet onto the paper towel on the contaminated side of the floor of the compartment.

10. Repeat steps 8 and 9 until all film packets have been opened.

11. Remove patient treatment gloves and place on the contaminated side of the paper towel on the floor of the compartment.

12. With clean, dry hands, grasp by the edges and place films into the automatic processor feeder slots for processing.

13. When the films are safely in the automatic processor, remove ungloved hands through the light-tight baffles.

14. Wash and dry hands.*

15. Put on utility gloves.

16. Open the light-filter cover and separate the lead foil from the film packets, and dispose of appropriately. Remove the cup, contaminated film packet outer plastic/paper wrap, and paper towels or plastic barrier and discard appropriately.

17. Clean and disinfect the inside of the compartment.

18. Wash, dry and remove utility gloves. Disinfect.

19. Wash and dry hands.*

*If hands are not visibly soiled, an alcohol-containing preparation designed for reducing the number of viable microorganisms on the hands may be used. Refer to manufacturer's recommendations for use.

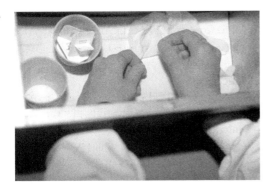

FIGURE 10-11 Daylight loader with cover opened. The operator placed clean, dry hands through the baffles. Note that gloves will be put on once the hands are inside the unit.

access the unit. With hands inside, the radiographer will place the treatment gloves on, open the film packets, separate the lead foil, and contain all contaminated items. Once all the film packets have been opened, the gloves are removed and placed with the contaminated items, and the films can be loaded in the automatic processor with clean, dry hands. The ungloved hands are removed through the light-tight baffles, and the light-filter cover is opened to remove the discarded items and clean and disinfect the inside of the unit wearing utility gloves. The key to infection control using the daylight loader is never to slide anything through the light-tight baffles except clean, dry hands.

Although film packets with and without plastic barrier envelopes can be processed in an automatic processor with a daylight loader attachment, because of the complexity of the infection protocol for its use, using film packets with barriers is recommended.

REVIEW—Chapter summary

The purpose of infection control is to prevent the transmission of disease between patients and operators and between patients. Standard precautions treat every patient as if known to be infectious. The chain of infection involves a susceptible host, pathogens in sufficient numbers to initiate infection, and an appropriate route for the pathogen to enter the host. The oral health care practice should have a written infection control policy. The Centers for Disease Control and Prevention (CDC), the Occupational Safety and Health Administration (OHSA), the U.S. Food and Drug Administration (FDA), and the U.S. Environmental Protection Agency (EPA) each play a role in developing, recommending, and/or enforcing guidelines for infection control.

Personal protective equipment (PPE) includes protective clothing, masks, eyewear, and gloves that act as barriers to prevent the transmission of infective microorganisms. Hands should be washed thoroughly before and after treating each patient.

Disinfection and sterilization breaks the chain of infection to prevent the transmission of infective microorganisms. Radiographic equipment and instruments may be classified as semicritical or noncritical and clinical contact surfaces, and they should be sterilized or disinfected accordingly. Specific step-by-step infection control procedures must be performed prior to, during, and after the radiographic procedure.

Recommended step-by-step procedures for handling image receptors with and without barrier envelopes is presented. Darkroom infection control protocol must be mastered to prevent lost or fogged radiographs. Strict infection control protocol must be followed when using an automatic processor with a daylight loader.

RECALL—Study questions

1. The purpose of infection control is to prevent the transmission of disease between
   a. patients.
   b. patient and operator.
   c. operator and patient.
   d. All of the above

2. Each of the following will break the chain of infection EXCEPT one. Which one is the EXCEPTION?
   a. Use of a digital sensor
   b. Use of personal protective equipment
   c. Sterilizaton of radiographic equipment
   d. Immunization of oral health care practitioners

3. An approach to infection control that states that the body fluids (except sweat) of all patients should be treated as if infected is
   a. universal precautions.
   b. standard precautions.
   c. protective barriers.
   d. cross-contaminations.

4. Which of these agencies develops and provides recommendations for adoption of infection control guidelines, but does not act as an enforcer of these guidelines?
   a. Centers for Disease Control and Prevention (CDC)
   b. Occupational Safety and Health Administration (OHSA)
   c. U.S. Food and Drug Administration (FDA)
   d. U.S. Environmental Protection Agency (EPA)

5. List four items of PPE (personal protective equipment) recommended for the dental radiographer:
   a. Gloves
   b. Masks
   c. eyewear
   d. Jacket / clothing

6. The use of a chemical or physical procedure to reduce the disease-producing microorganisms to an acceptable level on inanimate objects is the definition of
   a. asepsis.
   b. antiseptic.
   c. disinfection.
   d. sterilizaton.

7. Radiographic image receptor holders are classified as
   a. critical instruments.
   b. semicritical instruments.
   c. noncritical instruments.
   d. clinical contact surfaces.

8. The lead/lead equivalent apron and thyroid collar is classified as a
   a. critical object.
   b. semicritical object.
   c. noncritical object.
   d. cross-contaminated object.

9. Spraying disinfectant directly on which of these should be avoided?
   a. Digital sensor
   b. Lead/lead equivalent apron and thyroid collar
   c. X-ray machine exposure switch
   d. Bracket table or countertop

10. Each of the following may be protected with a plastic barrier to maintain infection control during the radiographic procedure EXCEPT one. Which one is the EXCEPTION?
   a. Image receptor
   b. Image receptor holder
   c. Exposure button
   d. PID and tube head

11. Which of the following is correct infection control for digital image receptors such as phosphor plates and solid state sensors?
   a. Protect with a plastic barrier prior to use. Sterilize following use.
   b. Protect with a plastic barrier prior to use. Disinfect following use.
   c. Disinfect prior to use. Protect with a plastic barrier prior to use. Sterilize following use.
   d. Disinfect prior to use. Protect with a plastic barrier prior to use. Disinfect following use.

12. Which of the following can be heat-sterilized following use?
   a. Digital sensor
   b. Phosphor plate
   c. Film packet
   d. Image receptor holder

13. What should be done with the image receptor immediately after removing it from the patient's mouth?
   a. Remove and reapply a clean plastic barrier.
   b. Remove excess saliva with a dry or disinfectant-soaked paper towel.
   c. Drop it into a containment cup or box without touching the sides.
   d. Rinse briefly with plain water, do not use soap.

14. Following the radiographic procedure, the patient treatment area should be cleaned and disinfected using
   a. clean, dry hands.
   b. patient treatment gloves.
   c. plastic overgloves.
   d. utility gloves.

15. Which of the following is the correct order for maintaining infection control after the radiographic procedure?
   a. Remove patient treatment gloves, remove lead/lead equivalent apron, put on utility gloves, clean and disinfect
   b. Remove lead/lead equivalent apron, remove patient treatment gloves, put on utility gloves, clean and disinfect
   c. Remove lead/lead equivalent apron, clean and disinfect, remove patient treatment gloves, put on utility gloves
   d. Put on utility gloves, remove lead/lead equivalent apron, clean and disinfect, remove patient treatment gloves

16. Which of the following is aseptically correct after using the tab to open an exposed, contaminated film packet without a plastic barrier?
   a. Grasp the film holding by the edges between the index finger and thumb.
   b. Remove the lead foil first to get it out of the way to allow for easier removal of the film.
   c. Pull the black paper tab to allow the film to drop out onto a paper towel.
   d. Continue peeling back the outer plastic/paper wrap until all contents of the packet are readily accessible.

17. Which of the following is recommended for use with an automatic processor with a daylight loader attachment?
   a. Digital sensors that used plastic barrier sheaths
   b. Phosphor plates that used plastic barrier envelopes
   c. Film packets that used plastic barrier envelopes
   d. Film packets that did not use plastic barrier envelopes

REFLECT—Case study

While exposing a full mouth series of radiographs on your patient, you accidentally drop the image receptor holding device on the floor. Because you still have additional exposures to complete, you need the use of this device. Explain in detail what infection control protocol you would follow to deal with this dilemma.

RELATE—Laboratory application

For a comprehensive laboratory practice exercise on this topic, see Thomson, E. M. (2012). *Exercises in oral radiography techniques: A laboratory manual* (3rd ed.). Upper Saddle River, NJ: Pearson Education. Chapter 8, "Infection control and student partner practice."

REFERENCES

American Dental Association Council on Scientific Affairs. (2006). The use of dental radiographs: Update and recommendations. *Journal of the American Dental Association, 137*(9), 1304–1312.

Darby, M. L., & Walsh, M. M. (2010). *Dental hygiene theory and practice* (3rd ed.). St. Louis: Saunders Elsevier.

Dietz-Bourguignon E., & Badavinac R. (2002). *Safety standards and infection control for dental hygienists.* Albany, NY: Delmar, Thomson Learning.

Hokett, S. D., Honey, J. R., Ruiz, F., Baisden, M. K., & Hoen, M. M. (2000). Assessing the effectiveness of direct digital radiography barrier sheaths and finger cots. *Journal of the American Dental Association, 131,* 463–467.

Huber, M. A., Holton, R. H., & Terezhalmy, G. T. (2005). Cost analysis of hand hygiene using antimicrobial soap and water versus an alcohol-based hand rub. *Oral Surgery, Oral Medicine, Oral Pathology, 99,* 4.

Kalathingal, S. M., Moore, S., Kwon, S., Schuster, G. S., Shrout, M. K., & Plummer, K. (2009). An evaluation of microbiologic contamination on phosphor plates in a dental school. *Oral Surgery, Oral Medicine, Oral Pathology, 107,* 279–282.

Kalathingal, S. M., Youngpeter, A., Minton, J., Shrout, M. K., Dickinson, D., Plummer, K., & Looney, S. (2010). An evaluation of microbiologic contamination on a phosphor plate system: Is weekly gas sterilization enough? *Oral Surgery, Oral Medicine, Oral Pathology, 109,* 457–462.

Kohn, W. G., Harte, J. A., Malvitz, D. M., Collins, A. S., Cleveland, J. L., & Eklund, K. J. (2004). Guidelines for infection control in dental health care settings—2003. *Journal of the American Dental Association, 135,* 33–47.

Negron, W., Mauriello, S. M., Peterson, C. A., & Arnold, R. (2005). Cross-contamination of the PSP sensor in a preclinical setting. *Journal of Dental Hygiene, 79*(3), 1–10.

Organization for Safety, Asepsis and Prevention. (2004, January). *Infection Control in Practice, 3*(1), entire issue. Retrieved from http://www.osap.org

Organization for Safety, Asepsis Prevention. (2004). OSAP check-up: 2003 CDC guidelines. Is your infection control program up to date? *Infection Control in Practice. Dentistry's Newsletter for Infection Control and Safety, 3*(1), 1–11.

Palenik, C. J. (2004). Infection control for dental radiography. *AADMRT Newsletter* Retrieved from www.aadmrt.com/currents/palenik_fall_04_print.htm

U.S. Dept. of Health and Human Services for Disease Control and Prevention, Centers for Disease Control and Prevention. (2003, December 19). Guidelines for infection control in dental health-care settings. *MMWR, 52*(RR17), 1–61.

U.S. Dept. of Health and Human Services for Disease Control and Prevention, Centers for Disease Control and Prevention. (2002, October 25). Guidelines for hand hygiene in health care settings: Recommendations of the Healthcare Infection Control Practices Advisory Committee and the HICPAC/SHEA/APIC/IDSA Hand Hygiene Task Force. *MMWR, 51*(RR16), 1–44.

Wilkins, E. M. (2009). *Clinical practice of the dental hygienist* (10th ed.). Philadelphia: Lippincott Williams & Wilkins.

Legal and Ethical Responsibilities

OBJECTIVES

Following successful completion of this chapter, you should be able to:

1. Define the key words.
2. Discuss the federal and state regulations concerning the use of dental x-ray equipment.
3. Describe licensure requirements for exposing dental radiographs.
4. Identify specific risk management strategies for radiography.
5. Recognize negative remarks about radiographic equipment that should be avoided.
6. List the five aspects of informed consent.
7. List the radiographic items that must be documented in the patient's record.
8. Explain what should be said to patients who refuse radiographs.
9. Identify the role professional ethics play in guiding the radiographer's behavior.

KEY WORDS

American Dental Assistants Association (ADAA)

American Dental Association (ADA)

American Dental Hygienists' Association (ADHA)

Code of Ethics

Confidentiality

Consumer-Patient Radiation Health and Safety Act

Direct supervision

Disclosure

Ethics

Federal Performance Act of 1974

Health Insurance Portability and Accountability Act (HIPAA)

Informed consent

Liable

Malpractice

Negligence

Risk management

Self-determination

Statute of limitations

Introduction

Legal and ethical issues directly relate to radiation safety. The dental radiographer must understand and respect the law governing the use of ionizing radiation. Additionally, the radiographer should be aware of the dental profession's codes of ethics that guide decisions regarding the use of ionizing radiation. The purpose of this chapter is to discuss regulations that apply to dental radiography and to present the ethical use of dental radiographs.

Regulations and Licensure

To perform radiographic services for patients safely and legally, the dental radiographer should be aware of the laws and regulations pertaining to dental radiology. This is especially important because laws vary from state to state and often change to meet the changing needs of society.

Equipment Regulations

Both federal and state regulations control the manufacture and use of x-ray equipment. The **Federal Performance Act of 1974** requires that all x-ray equipment manufactured or sold in the United States meet federal performance standards. These standards include safety requirements for filtration, collimation, and other x-ray machine characteristics.

In addition to federal regulations, city, county, and state laws affect the use of dental x-ray equipment. State laws require registration and inspection of x-ray machines. Inspections are conducted every 2 to 4 years, and usually fees are collected for this service. Because laws and regulations vary for each state and are subject to change, the dental radiographer should contact the state's bureau of radiological health for specific information.

Licensure Requirements

Additionally, there are laws that establish guidelines regarding who can place and expose radiographs. In 1981, then updated in 1991, the federal **Consumer-Patient Radiation Health and Safety Act** was passed and signed into law to protect patients from unnecessary radiation. This act established minimum standards for state certification and licensure of personnel who administer radiation in medical and dental radiographic procedures. The intent of the act was to minimize unnecessary exposure to potentially hazardous radiation.

Adoption of the act's standards was made discretionary with each state. As a result, not all states have voluntarily established licensure laws for personnel who place and expose dental radiographs. Nevertheless, most state laws require that operators of x-ray equipment be trained and certified or licensed to take dental radiographs. Many states consider dental hygienists and dental assistants who have passed the National Board Dental Hygiene Examine (NBDHE) and the Dental Assisting National Board Examination (DANB), respectively, and hold a license to practice in the state as a Registered Dental Hygienist or Certified Dental Assistant, respectively, to meet this requirement. However, some states require dental hygienists and dental assistants to take an additional examination or to fulfill continuing education requirements annually to be certified specifically in radiation safety or radiographic technique competency.

State laws regulating personnel who expose dental radiographs vary considerably for on-the-job trained dental assistants. Whereas many states have a mandatory state examination or a continuing education requirement, some states allow these uncertified dental assistants with proper training to take radiographs under the direct supervision of a dentist without certification. **Direct supervision** means the dentist is present in the office when the radiographs are taken. Each state's Dental Commission controls the scope of practice for assistants and hygienists. Because laws and regulations vary for each state and are subject to change, the dental radiographer should contact the state's Dental Commission directly to learn about legal requirements for placing and exposing dental radiographs in that state. A complete list of state Dental Commisions can be viewed on the American Dental Association's Web site (www.ada.org) (Box 11-1).

Legal Aspects

To aid in ensuring that one is practicing within the scope of the law, the dental radiographer should be familiar with all laws and regulations pertaining to dental radiography.

Risk Management

The most important legal aspect of dental radiology is **risk management.** Risk management can be defined as the policies and procedures to be followed by the radiographer to reduce the chances that a patient will file legal action against the dentist and oral health care team. Malpractice actions have increased in number and amount of awards in recent years. All members of the oral health care team must participate to make an effective

---

BOX 11-1 Web Sites for Professional Organizations

American Dental Assistant Association (ADAA)	www.dentalassistant.org
American Dental Hygienists' Association (ADHA)	www.adha.org
American Dental Association (ADA)	www.ada.org
Hispanic Dental Association (HDA)	www.hdassoc.org
National Dental Association (NDA)	www.ndaonline.org
National Dental Assistants Association (NDAA)	Link from www.ndaonline.org
National Dental Hygienists Association (NDHA)	www.ndhaonline.org

risk management program. Following standard procedures and performing procedures correctly will help reach the goal of providing quality care and minimizing risk. (See Box 11-2 for a radiography mini-audit for avoiding risk.)

Specific risk management procedures that can be a good defense when performed correctly or a liability if performed poorly include attempting to obtain a duplicate copy of a new patient's radiographs before reexposing the patient to ionizing radiation; using the best equipment currently available, including fast-speed film, leaded aprons and thyroid collars, film-holding devices, and collimination; and establishing a written quality assurance system for the darkroom to include daily, weekly, and monthly evaluation. Providing all radiographers with a radiation monitoring badge, whether required by law or not, is also a good risk management tool (Figure 11-1). Monitoring radiation exposure, or more precisely the lack of exposure, will provide the practice with documentation of safe work habits.

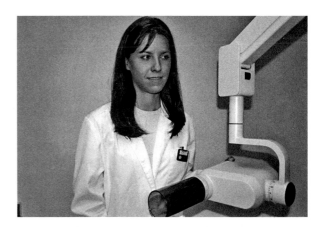

FIGURE 11-1 **Radiographer wearing a radiation monitoring badge.**

Patient Relations

Patient relations refers to the relationship between the patient and the dental radiographer. It is important to make the patient feel comfortable by establishing a relaxing and confident chairside manner (see Chapter 12). Always explain to the patient what and how procedures are to be performed. Answer all questions the patient may have concerning the procedures. Good patient relations reduces the risk of possible legal action.

Avoid negative remarks about procedures, equipment, and the dental staff. Statements like, "The films got stuck in the processor again" or "This tube head always drifts" should never be made to the patient or in front of the patient. These statements imply that you have chosen to use known defective equipment on a patient. This is not the same as saying, "The films got stuck in the processor. They must be retaken. However, we will not process the new films until a thorough investigation is made to correct the problem with the processor." or "This tube head is drifting. Because this is a problem, we cannot use it to take your x-rays until it is repaired. Let's move to another room for your procedure." If equipment is not working properly, it should be repaired or serviced.

Informed Consent

Informed consent is the consent the patient gives for treatment after being informed of the nature and purpose of all treatment procedures.

All patients have the legal right to make choices about the health care they receive. This is called **self-determination.** Self-determination includes the right to refuse treatment. To make

---

BOX 11-2 Radiography Safety Audit for Risk Management

- Are all radiographers legally licensed, or certified, or properly trained to work with the x-ray equipment?
- Are radiographers' licenses, registrations, certificates, and continuing education achievements posted for public view?
- Are equipment inspection certificates posted near or on the x-ray equipment as may be required by law?
- Are accident prevention signs in place as needed (i.e., to watch head when pulling x-ray tube head away from the wall)?
- Are signs posted regarding the use of ionizing radiation as may be required by law?
- Does the radiographer wear personal protective equipment (PPE) during the procedure?
- Are all radiographers required to wear a radiation dosimeter?
- Are radiation safety rules posted near the x-ray units?
- Are exposure settings for types of projections and patients posted near the control panel?
- Is a signed informed consent from the patient secured prior to radiography procedure?
- Are adequate records kept on patient exposures (consent, assessment of need, number and type of exposures, retakes, name of radiographer who took the radiographs)?
- Are patient radiographs kept confidential? How?
- Will patient radiographs be interpreted thoroughly and findings documented and communicated to the patient following the appointment?
- Is x-ray equipment up to date on all required inspections?
- Is documentation on quality control tests performed on all darkroom equipment kept?
- Does the radiographer wear impervious gloves and gowns and safety goggles when handling processing chemistry?
- Is an emergency eye wash station near where processing chemistry is handled?
- Do all radiographers or handlers of chemicals know the location of the hazardous chemicals lists and material safety data sheets? (See chapter 20)
- Is emergency spill equipment available?

a decision regarding informed consent, the patient must be informed of the following:

- The purpose of taking radiographs
- The benefits the radiographs will supply
- The possible risks of radiation exposure
- The possible risks of refusing the radiographs
- The person who will perform the procedure

It is the responsibility of the dentist to explain the nature and purpose of all treatment procedures. When taking radiographs, the risks and benefits must be explained in lay terms. The informing process is called **disclosure.** The patient should be given the opportunity to ask questions prior to radiography. Answer all questions completely in terms the patient understands. State laws vary concerning informed consent. Be sure to become familiar with your state laws.

Liability

Liable means to be legally obligated to make good any loss or damage that may occur. Many states have laws that require dentists to supervise the performance of dental radiographers. Both dentists and dental radiographers are liable for procedures performed by the dental radiographer. Therefore, it is important to understand that even though radiographers work under the supervision of the dentist, they are legally liable for their own actions. In malpractice cases, both the supervising dentist and the dental radiographer may be sued for the actions of the radiographer.

Patient Records

A record of all aspects of dental care must be kept for every patient. Dental radiographs are considered a part of the patient's record and are therefore legal documents.

DOCUMENTATION   The exposure of dental radiographs should be documented in the patient's record. Entries in the patient's record should be made by the dentist or under the dentist's supervision. The following items must be documented in the patient's record.

- The patient's informed consent
- The number and type of radiographs, including retakes

- The date the radiographs are taken and the name of the radiographer who took them
- The reason for taking the radiographs
- The interpretive and diagnostic results

CONFIDENTIALITY   State laws have always governed **confidentiality** to protect the patient's privacy. On April 14, 2003, the federal government signed into law privacy standards to protect patients' medical records and other health information, including radiographs. Developed by the Department of Health and Human Services (DHHS) as part of the **Health Insurance Portability and Accountability Act** of 1996 **(HIPAA),** this federal law is designed to provide patients with control over how their personal health information is used and disclosed. Radiographs are confidential and should never be shown or discussed with anyone outside the oral health care practice without first obtaining a current, signed release from the patient. A patient will usually be asked to sign a notice that indicates how their radiographs may be used and their privacy rights under this law.

OWNERSHIP   The courts have ruled that radiographs are the property of the dentist. The patient pays for the dentist's ability to interpret the radiographs and to arrive at a diagnosis. However, patients may have reasonable access to their radiographs. They may request a copy of their radiographs if they decide to change dentists or request a consultation with a dental specialist (Procedure Box 11-1). The original radiographs, however, belong to the dentist. Because of statute of limitation laws, it is recommended that all records (including radiographs) be retained indefinitely.

RETENTION   Dental radiographs must be retained for seven years after the patient ceases to be a patient. Legal action that can be brought against the dentist depend on the malpractice and limitation statues that vary from state to state. For adult patients, the statute of limitations generally begins to run at the time of the injury, or when the injury should have reasonably been discovered. For children, the statute of limitations does not begin until the child reaches the age of majority (18 to 21 years old, depending on the state). If you work for a governmental entity, the statute of limitations may be affected by certain notice statutes, which

PROCEDURE 11-1
Procedure for releasing a copy of the patient's radiographs

1. Patient requests copy of radiographs in writing.
2. Keep the letter requesting radiographs in the patient's record.
3. Duplicate the original radiographs or print out a paper copy of digital images.
4. Send the duplicate radiographs or paper copy of digital images by the U.S. Postal Service's Certified Mail™.
5. Keep the postal receipt in the patient's record.

may greatly reduce the time in which a suit may be brought. Because the time period is so indefinite, it is recommended that radiographs be retained forever.

INSURANCE CLAIMS Insurance companies have the right to request pretreatment radiographs to evaluate the dental treatment plan for services that they will be paying for. Again, only duplicate radiographs should be sent. The oral health care practice should keep the originals. It may be acceptable to send digital images electronically. The number of insurance companies that except digital images electronically is increasing.

Malpractice Issues

Malpractice results when one is negligent. Negligence occurs when the dental diagnosis or treatment is below the standard of care provided by dentists in a similar locality and under similar conditions.

NEGLIGENCE **Negligence** is defined as the failure to use a reasonable amount of care when failure results in injury or damage to another. Negligence may result from the care (or lack of care) of either the dentist or the dental radiographer.

Statute of Limitations is the time period during which a patient may bring a malpractice action against a dentist or radiographer. State laws govern this time period, which begins when the patient discovers, or should have discovered, an injury due to negligent dental treatment.

Sometimes negligence is not discovered until years later, when a patient changes dentists and discovers an injury has occurred. In such cases, the statute of limitations begins years after the negligent dental treatment occurred. An example would be where appropriate radiographs were not taken on a patient with periodontal disease. Years later, the patient is examined by another dentist and is informed of the irreversible periodontal condition that might have been prevented if detected earlier.

Besides the statute of limitations, many states have separate malpractice laws that may limit damages or, in the case of governmental entities, may provide limited or complete immunity from suit, under certain circumstances. Because the laws vary greatly from state to state, it is desirable to consult a lawyer experienced in this area to provide training and answer questions for the entire oral health care practice team as part of the risk management program.

PATIENTS WHO REFUSE RADIOGRAPHS Occasionally, for a variety of reasons, patients express opposition to the dentist's proposal that x-rays be taken. Often these patients believe that such radiographs are unnecessary or that they will add to the cost of treatment, or the patient may be fearful that dental x-ray exposure will be hazardous to their health. When this happens, the dentist and radiographer must carefully explain in clear terms why the radiographs are needed to supplement the diagnosis, prognosis, or treatment plan and therefore benefit the patient.

Frequently a patient may offer to sign a paper to assume the responsibility for not taking radiographs. The patient must be informed in a diplomatic manner that legally, such documents do not release the dentist from liability and are not valid because the patient cannot legally consent to negligent care. If the patient still refuses the radiographs, the dentist must carefully decide whether treatment can be provided. Usually, in such cases, the dentist cannot treat the patient.

Ethics

In addition to the law, the ethics of a profession also guide the behavior of the health care practitioner. **Ethics** is defined as a sense of moral obligation regarding right and wrong behavior. Professional ethics define a standard by which all members of the profession are obligated to conform. These professional rules of conduct are called a profession's **Code of Ethics.** See Box 11-1 for a list of Web sites where you can locate the Code of Ethics for the **American Dental Association (ADA)**, **American Dental Hygienists' Association (ADHA)**, and **American Dental Assistants Association (ADAA)**. A professional Code of Ethics helps to define the rules of conduct for its members.

Goals

Managing risk, knowing the law, and applying ethics, the dental radiographer should strive for practice that is safe, is professional, and places the patient's well-being first. One achieves this by setting goals. Such goals are closely related, and all are equally important. Goals of the dental radiographer include the following:

- **Achieve perfection with each radiograph.** This is accomplished by careful attention to details. Each step in the process, whether in image receptor placement, exposure technique, or processing and identification, is significant.
- **Perform confidently and with authority.** Patients are more likely to cooperate with someone who demonstrates self-confidence. Communicate with patients in a respectful manner.
- **Take pride in services rendered and professional advancement.** Obtain certification in radiation safety, whether or not required by law. Improve skills and update techniques by attending continuing education lectures and workshops, participating in professional association meetings, and reading professional journals and books.
- **Keep radiation exposure as low as possible.** Take the time to use protective devices that minimize radiation to the patient and follow strict protocols to protect yourself during exposures. Maintain an environment that minimizes the risk of harm.
- **Avoid retakes.** Be familiar with common errors to avoid. Do not retake any exposure when you are not sure of the corrective action. If the patient cannot tolerate placement of the image receptor or cannot cooperate with the procedure, stop and get assistance, or try an acceptable alternative procedure.
- **Develop integrity, dedication, and competence** that promotes ethical behavior and high standards of care. Provide patients with information to assist them in making informed decisions regarding their consent to radiographic procedures. Serve all patients without discrimination.

REVIEW—Chapter summary

The dental radiographer should be aware of the laws and regulations pertaining to dental radiography. Both federal and state regulations control the manufacture and use of x-ray equipment.

State laws require that operators of x-ray equipment be trained and certified or licensed to take dental radiographs. Some states may require the registered dental hygienist and the certified dental assistant to take an additional examination or a continuing education course to be certified to take radiographs. Other states allow an on-the-job-trained dental assistant with proper training to place and expose radiographs under the direct supervision of the dentist.

Risk management strategies and good patient relations reduce the risk of possible legal actions. Informed consent allows the patient to make decisions regarding the procedure. Disclosure informs the patient about the radiographic procedure and answers all questions the patient may have concerning the procedures. Both the dentist and the dental radiographer are liable for procedures performed by the dental radiographer.

The patient's records, including the radiographs, are confidential. The courts have ruled that radiographs are the property of the dentist; the patient pays only for the diagnosis. However, patients may have access to their radiographs via copies.

When an individual ceases to be a patient, the radiographs should be retained for at least seven years. Risk management and the statutes of limitation suggest that radiographs be retained indefinitely.

The patient who refuses radiographs may not legally consent to negligent care. The professional's code of ethics guides the behavior of the radiographer. Goals for the dental radiographer are presented.

RECALL—Study questions

1. Registration and inspection of x-ray machines is regulated by the
   a. federal government.
   b. state government.
   c. local government.
   d. Any of the above

2. The laws allowing individuals to place and expose dental radiographs vary from state to state.
   a. True
   b. False

3. Which of the following is a risk management strategy?
   a. The use of fast-speed film, film-holding devices, and collimation
   b. Monitoring the dental radiographer with radiation dosimeters
   c. Obtaining a copy of a new patient's radiographs from a previous dentist
   d. All of the above

4. Which of these comments should be avoided when talking to the patient?
   a. "We have switched to a fast-speed film."
   b. "This exposure button sticks sometimes."
   c. "You must stay still during the exposure."
   d. "I'm certified to take your radiographs."

5. List five aspects of informed consent.
   a. _____
   b. _____
   c. _____
   d. _____
   e. _____

6. Every patient has the legal right to make choices about the oral health care they receive. This is called
   a. disclosure.
   b. informed consent.
   c. self-determination.
   d. liability.

7. List five items regarding the radiographic procedure that should be documented in the patient's record.
   a. _____
   b. _____
   c. _____
   d. _____
   e. _____

8. Legally dental radiographs should be retained for an individual who ceases to be a patient for
   a. three years.
   b. five years.
   c. seven years.
   d. nine years.

9. Both the dentist and the dental radiographer are liable for procedures performed by the dental radiographer.
   a. True
   b. False

10. Failure to use a reasonable amount of care that results in injury is termed
    a. risk.
    b. liability.
    c. confidentiality.
    d. negligence.

11. The courts have ruled that radiographs are the property of the
    a. patient.
    b. dentist.
    c. dental radiographer.
    d. state.

12. When patients express opposition to having dental radiographs taken, the radiographer should
    a. ask the patient to sign a document to release the dentist of liability.
    b. consult the professional code of ethics about what to do next.
    c. postpone the procedure and ask the patient to return at a later date.
    d. explain why the radiographs are needed and what the benefits will be.

13. A professional code of ethics
    a. makes the laws that govern the use of dental radiographs.
    b. establishes the time frame for taking dental radiographs.
    c. helps to define the rules of conduct for its members.
    d. protects the dental radiographer in cases of legal action.

14. Each of the following is a goal of the radiographer EXCEPT one. Which one is the EXCEPTION?
    a. Increasing the demand for dental x-ray services
    b. Reducing the radiation dose used during an exposure
    c. Professional improvement and advancement
    d. Presenting confidence to gain patient acceptance

REFLECT—Case study

Consider the following scenario.

You have been working in a practice for over a year and have developed a friendship with another dental assistant. You often socialize together outside work, and your children play together. One evening during dinner, your dental assistant friend tells you that even though she has been exposing dental radiographs on patients since she was hired by the practice over two years ago, she does not have the state-required radiation safety certification. She tells you that the dentist never asked to see her certificate during the job interview. She wasn't planning to "break the law" but the first day on the job, the dentist explained to a patient that she would be taking the full mouth series, and "not to worry, because she was a competent clinician." Your friend explains to you that it would have been embarrassing to tell the dentist at that point that she was not certified, so she exposed the radiographs. After that, she thought about taking a course to prepare for the state examination, but didn't want to get "caught" taking the exam after she had already been placing and exposing radiographs all this time. She hopes you will keep her confidence because you are friends.

Reflect on this scenario and answer the following questions.

1. How has your friend broken the law?
2. How has this behavior endangered the patient? Your friend? Your employer?
3. Describe the legal and/or ethical situation she faces.
4. Describe the legal and/or ethical dilemma you face.
5. How could your employer have prevented this situation?
6. What aspects of the Dental Assisting or Dental Hygiene Code of Ethics apply to this situation?
7. Take the role of your friend; what would you have done if you were she?

RELATE—Laboratory practice

Using the computer, visit the Web sites for the board of radiological health or the board of dentistry in all 50 states and the District of Columbia. Compile a listing of states with certification requirements for dental radiographers and answer the following questions.

1. How many states require all radiographers to be certified for performing radiographic procedures?
2. What states accept a registered dental hygienist's or certified dental assistant's credentials as certification for performing radiographic procedures?
3. Do any states require additional tests or continuing education classes for a dental assistant or dental hygienist to maintain radiographic certification?
4. Why do you think some states do not require certification for those individuals who place and expose dental radiographs?
5. What are the advantages to the oral health care practice to hire only certified radiographers?
6. How should the public be educated on these laws governing the certification of individuals to place and expose dental radiographs?

REFERENCES

Bundy, A. L. (1988). *Radiology and the law.* Rockville, MD: Aspen.

Darby, M. L., & Walsh, M. M. (2010). *Dental hygiene theory and practice* (3rd ed.). St. Louis, MO: Elsevier.

Davison, J. A. (2000). *Legal and ethical considerations for dental hygienists and assistants.* St. Louis, MO: Mosby Elsevier.

U.S. Dept. of Health and Human Services. (n.d.). *Fact sheet: Protecting the privacy of patients' health information.* Retrieved from www.hhs.gov/news/facts/privacy.html

CHAPTER

12

Patient Relations and Education

OBJECTIVES

Following successful completion of this chapter, you should be able to:

1. Define key words.
2. Value the need for patient cooperation in producing quality radiographs.
3. List the aspects of patient relations that help to gain confidence and cooperation.
4. Explain how appearance and first impression affect patient relations.
5. Identify five areas where the radiographer's positive attitude will foster patient confidence.
6. State examples of interpersonal skills that are used to communicate effectively.
7. Explain the relationship between verbal and nonverbal communication.
8. Give an example of a negative-sounding word that should be avoided when explaining the radiographic procedure.
9. Explain the communication method show-tell-do and give three examples of when this method would be effective.
10. State the two reasons patient education in radiography is valuable.
11. Respond to a patient's concern regarding unnecessary exposure to x-rays.
12. Describe two methods by which the patient can be educated to appreciate the value of dental radiographs.

KEY WORDS

Appearance

Attitude

Chairside manner

Communication

Empathy

Frequently asked questions (FAQs)

Interpersonal skills

Nonverbal communication

Patient education

Patient relations

Show-tell-do

Verbal communication

Introduction

Effective communication is essential to producing quality radiographic images. The radiographic procedure requires that the patient understand and cooperate with the process. The radiographer must be able to communicate specific directions for success of the procedure. Precise patient positioning, the sometimes difficult placement of an image sensor in the oral cavity, and the potentially harmful nature of ionizing radiation make clear communication and good interpersonal skills especially important. The purpose of this chapter is to discuss how interpersonal skills affect the radiographic process, present guidelines for effective communication, and investigate the role the dental assistant and the dental hygienist play in educating the patient regarding the need for dental radiographs.

Patient Relations

Patient relations refers to the relationship between the patient and the oral health care professional. Appearance, attitude, interpersonal skills, and communication help gain patient confidence and cooperation, the outcome of which will be the production of quality radiographs.

Appearance

The patient's first impression of the dental radiographer is important. The first impression is often made based on the radiographer's **appearance.** The dental radiographer should always maintain a professional appearance. The careful attention given to personal hygiene and grooming such as trimmed nails, clean hands, and fresh breath convey an understanding of the importance of maintaining all aspects of infection control. A clean, neat appearance builds confidence in patients.

Attitude

Attitude is defined as the position assumed by the body in connection with a feeling or mood. Attitude will play a significant role in gaining the patient's trust in the radiographer's ability. The attitude of the radiographer toward the procedure will be conveyed to the patient. If the radiographer feels that the procedure is uncomfortable or unnecessary, these feelings will be conveyed to the patient. The radiographer should not impose his/her own feelings onto the patient. Although the radiographer may have had a less than ideal experience with a certain procedure, this does not necessarily mean that the patient will experience the same discomfort. For example, the radiographer may have experienced a gag reflex when posterior periapicals were taken on him/her. If this radiographer approaches the patient with the attitude that posterior periapicals will excite a gag reflex, the outcome is likely to be just that. A fresh, positive attitude with each new patient will more likely produce a cooperative patient. This is especially true if the patient perceives the radiographer as possessing a nonjudgmental attitude.

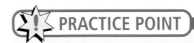

Always greet the patient by name. Address the patient using their proper title (Miss, Mrs., Ms., Mr., Dr., etc.) and last name. If you are uncertain of the correct pronunciation of the patient's name, ask the patient to pronounce it for you. Always introduce yourself to the patient, using both your name and title. For example: "Good morning, Ms. Washington. My name is Maria Melendez. I'm the dental assistant who will be taking your radiographs today. Please follow me to the x-ray room, and we will get started."

The radiographer's attitude toward his/her own technical ability will also be conveyed to the patient. Because a demonstration of technical skill will build patient confidence, the radiographer should feel that his/her training and education provided adequate preparation for this role. Having confidence in oneself fosters confidence in others.

Additionally, the unique close working relationship of the oral health care team requires that everyone work well together. Attitudes toward an employer and coworkers also play a role in determining the degree of successful patient management. Patients can sense the professional's attitude by the way he/she walks, talks, and behaves. For example, the patient will easily sense a disgruntled dental assistant who had to interrupt what he/she was doing to take radiographs for a dental hygienist who was running behind in the schedule. Maintaining a pleasant, positive attitude will help generate the same from patients.

Interpersonal Skills

Interpersonal skills are used to communicate with others successfully. Respectfulness, courtesy, empathy, and patient, honest, and tactful communication are examples of interpersonal skills. When explaining the need for radiographs, consider how the patient will feel. If the patient has concerns regarding the need for x-ray exposure, respect their views. Statements such as, "Don't worry" and "Everything will be okay," may convey an attitude of apathy, or imply that the patient's apprehensions don't matter. If placement of an intraoral imaging receptor during the radiographic procedure is uncomfortable, show empathy. **Empathy** is defined as the ability to share in another's emotions or feelings. Be courteous and polite at all times even in difficult situations. However, if discomfort must be tolerated to produce the necessary radiograph, empathetic, yet direct and tactful communication can help bring about the desired result.

An important aspect of interpersonal skills is the radiographer's chairside manner. **Chairside manner** refers to the conduct of the radiographer while working at the patient's chairside. The radiographer should strive to always make the patient feel comfortable. Working in a confident manner will help put the patient at ease. Comments that indicate a lack of control, such as "Oops!" must be avoided. An important consideration during the radiographic procedure is to praise the patient for any assistance they provide. Positive reinforcement and feedback that the procedure is going well will help foster even more cooperation. For example, letting a patient know that you appreciated their ability to hold the image receptor in place long enough to make the exposure will help to motivate the patient to continue working together with you to complete the procedure. Likewise, showing frustration with a patient who is having difficulty managing the the procedure will most likely only increase the patient's anxiety.

PRACTICE POINT

If it is necessary to place the image receptor into a particularly sensitive area, encourage the patient to cooperate and praise him/her for the willingness to tolerate the difficult placement. Show empathy, but let the patient know that the placement is correct and if he/she can tolerate the discomfort for the short time required for exposure, the result will be a diagnostic quality radiograph. Avoid asking, "Does that feel okay?" The patient will perceive this to mean that discomfort equals incorrect positioning and will feel obligated to inform you of any and all feelings associated with the procedure. The patient will now be acutely aware of the feeling of the image receptor in the mouth and continue to inform you regarding the "feeling" of each subsequent placement, possibly making the procedure more difficult. Saying, "Are you doing okay so far?" is a better way to let the patient know you are aware of their efforts to cooperate.

Communication

Communication is defined as the process by which information is exchanged between two or more persons. This may be accomplished verbally (with words) or nonverbally (without words). Effective communication is communication that works (Box 12-1).

HONESTY Verbal and nonverbal communication are essential to building patient confidence. Patient questions must be answered honestly. It is very important that the radiographic procedure be explained honestly, including any possible discomfort anticipated, to gain cooperation and assistance. Honesty develops trust. When a patient trusts the dental radiographer, the patient is more likely to cooperate with the radiographic procedure.

BOX 12-1   Guidelines for Effective Communication

- Introduce yourself and show interest.
- Face the patient and make eye contact.
- Lean forward to demonstrate listening.
- Be honest to build trust.
- Show courtesy and respectfulness.
- Maintain a positive attitude.
- Demonstrate empathy when appropriate.
- Use clear commands.
- Make nonverbal communication in agreement with verbal communication.

Verbal Communication

Effective use of words in **verbal communication** begins with facing the patient directly and maintaining eye contact. Because a face mask is recommended PPE (personal protective equipment; see Chapter 10) during radiographic procedures, it is very important that the verbal requests and commands used to communicate specific directions during the radiographic procedures be understood by the patient. Once the image receptor is in place, the operator needs to give explicit directions to complete the procedure quickly. For example, once the receptor holding device is placed in the mouth, the patient must be requested to bite firmly and to hold completely still while the operator leaves the area to make the exposure. The process will be hindered and prolonged if the patient does not understand the requests or the operator must repeat the commands.

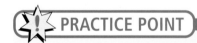

PRACTICE POINT

Always give a command, and not a question, to request that the patient hold still during the exposure. For example, asking the patient, "Can you hold still, please?" will most likely cause the patient to attempt to move to answer you, defeating the purpose of your request. The command, "Hold still, please" is less likely to prompt the patient to move.

The radiographer's choice of words and sentence structure are also important. Words used should be at a level the patient can understand. For example, young children may better understand, "These are pictures of the teeth made with a special dental camera" (Box 12-2). An adult would appreciate hearing a more professional sounding, "Here's a radiograph showing your periodontal condition." However, too many highly technical words may confuse the patient and result in misunderstandings. Words that imply negative images such as "zap," "shot," and "irradiate" are better avoided.

BOX 12-2 Guidelines for Communicating with Children

- Use guidelines for effective communication.
- Use age-level appropriate language.
- Do not talk down or use baby talk.
- Avoid threatening-sounding words.
- Expain the procedure simply and clearly.
- Use show-tell-do.
- Tell the truth whenever possible.

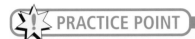

PRACTICE POINT

Sentence structure is important for the short, precise directions needed for radiographic procedures. For example, requesting that the patient bite down on the image receptor holder by saying, "Close slowly please" may prompt the patient to close before the operator says the word *slowly*. Rearranging the words to say, "Slowly close please," may be more likely to produce the desired result.

BOX 12-3 Guidelines for Communicating with the Elderly

- Use guidelines for effective communication.
- Address by the person's title unless they instruct you otherwise.
- Avoid condescending salutations such as "Honey" and "Dear."
- Be aware of generational differences.
- Be aware of sensory or cognitive impairments such as hearing loss, effects of stroke.
- Encourage the use of eyeglasses and hearing aids during the procedure and especially when showing radiographs during patient education.

BOX 12-4 Guidelines for Communicating with People of Different Cultures

- Use guidelines for effective communication.
- Learn about the cultures in your community.
- Be accepting and nonjudgmental.
- Be aware that gestures may be interpreted differently.
- Be aware that touch and personal space are sometimes considered differently by different cultures.
- Speak slowly and avoid the use of slang or uncommon terms.
- Verify that the listener has understood what you said.

Nonverbal Communication

Nonverbal communication includes gestures, facial expressions, body movement, and listening. A nod of the head indicates yes or agreement, and a shake of the head indicates no or disagreement. We usually use a combination of verbal and nonverbal communication. Nonverbal communication is very believable. When verbal and nonverbal communications are not in synch, it is often the nonverbal communication that conveys the strongest message. For example, if you tell the patient that you don't mind that they have to stop and take a break in between each radiograph placement, but you roll your eyes or tap your foot while waiting for them to feel ready to begin again, the patient will probably not believe you because your actions speak louder than your words. Facial expressions strongly convey the attitude of the radiographer. A smile by the radiographer will likely relax the patient and reduce apprehension.

It is just as important that the radiographer practice good listening skills. Careful attention to listening results in fewer misunderstandings. Eye contact and attentive body posturing communicates warmth and caring to the patient. Additionally, the radiographer should observe the patient's nonverbal communication. There is most likely something wrong with a patient who is clutching the arms of the treatment chair with tears in her eyes, even if she has not verbally communicated with you.

The use of **show-tell-do** as a method of combined verbal and nonverbal communication is useful in dental radiography, especially when barriers to communication exist such as in the case of a language or cultural difference, a sensory impairment, or a cognitive impairment (Boxes 12-3 and 12-4). Showing the patient the image receptor and holder and demonstrating PID placement prior to beginning to procedure can help alleviate apprehension.

Patient Education

Educating patients about the importance of dental radiographs in comprehensive oral health care depends on the radiographer's ability to communicate (Figures 12-1 and 12-2). This communication ability is based on the radiographer's knowledge, education, and training in the area of dental radiology. It is surprising how many patients do not comprehend the

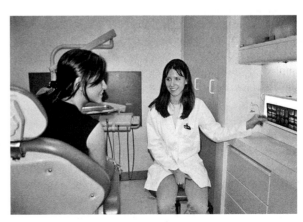

FIGURE 12-1 Patient education The dental radiographer educates the patient on the value of radiographs.

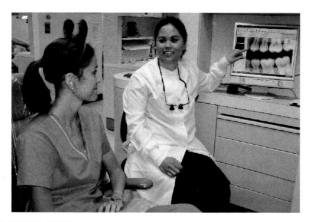

FIGURE 12-2 Incorporating digital radiographic images in patient education.

enormous value of a radiographic examination of their teeth and the supporting oral structures.

Value of Patient Education

The value of **patient education** is twofold. First is the understanding that dental radiographs disclose pathology (disease) that might otherwise go undetected and become an increasing threat to the patient's health if not treated in a timely manner. Second is that the educated patient is more inclined to understand and accept dental treatment plans and embrace suggestions for oral health promotion and disease prevention. Such patient acceptance helps develop a spirit of confidence and mutual trust in the oral health care practice.

Necessity for Patient Education

Most people have heard negative reports regarding the effects of overexposure to radiation. The dental patient, when faced with a treatment plan recommending radiographs, will rightfully question the necessity of being exposed to x-radiation. It is the responsibility of the entire dental team to provide the patient with clear, concise, and satisfactory answers regarding any questions or concerns he/she may have. Acceptance of the dental treatment plan is more likely not only when a satisfactory explanation of need is presented, but also when the patient is given an explanation of the ethical safeguards the practice has adopted to reduce the risk of harm.

Identifying with the patient's concerns is the first step to open communication. The radiographer can verbally agree with the patient that excess radiation exposure is a concern and that the practice has adopted a strict radiation safety program. Patient acceptance and confidence increase when he/she is made aware of the many safety protocols the practice has put into place.

To begin the conversation, the patient should be told about the evidence-based selection criteria guidelines developed by an expert panel of health care professionals and updated in 2004 by the American Dental Association that aid the dentist in deciding when, what type, and how many radiographs should be taken (see Chapter 6). These evidence-based guidelines are the single biggest factor in eliminating unnecessary radiographs.

Further, the patient should be informed that all standard safety protocols as suggested by federal agencies, such as the National Council on Radiation Protection and Measurements, and the state and local laws governing inspections, calibrations, and the use of radiological equipment are being adhered to. Many people may not realize that x-ray equipment is strictly regulated by law.

In some locations, laws also regulate who can operate the dental x-ray machine. Where applicable, individuals who place and expose radiographs must be educated and trained and pass an examination prior to being certified to place and expose dental radiographs. If the state issues a license or a certificate of compliance to show that a radiation safety examination has been passed, that can be offered in evidence. Many radiographers display their certificates near the x-ray machine. Patient confidence in the radiographer increases when he/she knows that the professional has been educated or trained and has passed a certification exam in the safety protocols governing the use of x-radiation.

The patient should be assured that everyone in the office who works with the dental x-ray machine, regardless of state-mandated certification, is trained in its use and the safety aspects of radiation. Continuing education courses in radiology taken by the radiographer also boost patient confidence and elevate the practice as one that values competency.

Finally, the patient and radiographer may have a discussion about equipment specially designed to reduce radiation exposure, such as collimated position indicating devices (PIDs), thyroid collars and protective lead aprons, fast-speed film, and modern equipment that is better constructed to prevent unnecessary radiation. The patient may not be aware of the reasoning behind the use of these devices. Many patients assume the lead apron is only for pregnant females and may be unaware that utilizing a holder to position the image receptor prevents them from having to hold the film in their mouth and unnecessarily expose their fingers.

Methods of Patient Education

The patient can be educated on the value of radiographs through verbal discussion, printed literature, or a combination of the two. Backing up your verbal explanation with a printed brochure is very effective at getting the message across. Literature may be obtained from professional organizations, commercial dental product companies, or off the Web. However, care should be taken to use reliable sources of literature. The radiographer should be aware of misleading sources of information, especially those readily available to patients on the Web. The radiographer should be prepared to help the patient separate correct information from incorrect or misleading information.

ORAL PRESENTATION An effective method of educating the patient is to give an oral presentation using a series of radiographs showing typical dental conditions, both normal and abnormal. Placed in convenient mounts, the radiographs are shown to the patient on a lighted view box or a computer

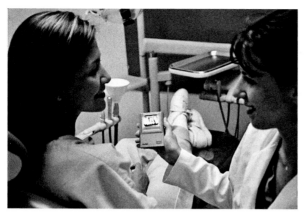

FIGURE 12-3 Handheld viewer-enlarger is a helpful adjunct to patient education.

monitor (Figures 12-1 and 12-2). The handheld viewer shown in Figure 12-3 is well suited for an up-close chairside view of film-based radiographs. Patients are generally able to identify the areas that are pointed out to them on the radiographs better if the images are magnified and the brightness of the light is controlled. A sample set of radiographs will allow the radiographer to explain the value of the use of radiographs in the patient's oral care plan. When viewing the patient's own radiographs, the radiographer should remember that all members of the oral health care team can interpret radiographs, but it is the dentist's responsibility to make the final interpretation and diagnosis. The difference between interpretation and diagnosis is discussed in Chapter 21.

PRINTED LITERATURE An effective education method is to place printed literature in the reception area or to give it to patients before their appointment. Giving pamphlets to the patient opens the door for two-way communication on the advisability and necessity of regular radiographic examinations. All too often the patient is simply told that the doctor requires radiographs and will not treat the patient unless they are taken, or else the explanation is limited to a few short and often unsatisfactory answers.

Literature may be obtained from one's professional association (American Dental Association, American Dental Hygienists' Association, American Dental Assistants Association) or can be custom produced to meet the needs of the practice (Table 12-1).

Frequently Asked Questions

Here are some examples of **frequently asked questions (FAQs)** and answers reprinted from the American Dental Association brochure Dental X-ray Examinations: Your Dentist's Advice and Web site (www.ada.org/public/topics/xrays_Faq.asp) and from the Academy of General Dentistry's Web site (http://www.knowyour teeth.com/infobites/abc/article/?abc=w&iid=342&aid=1373).

QUESTION: What are the benefits of dental x-rays?

ANSWER: Many diseases of the teeth and surrounding tissues cannot be seen through a visual examination alone. An x-ray examination may reveal

- Small areas of decay between the teeth
- Infections in the bone
- Abscesses or cysts
- Developmental abnormalities
- Some types of tumors

Finding and treating oral health problems at an early stage can save time, money, and unnecessary discomfort. Radiographs can detect damage to oral structures not visible during a regular exam. If you have a hidden tumor, radiographs may even help save your life.

QUESTION: How often should x-rays be taken?

ANSWER: How often radiographs (dental x-rays) should be taken depends on the patient's individual health needs. It is important to recognize that just as each patient is different from the next, so should the scheduling of x-ray exams be individualized for each patient. The dentist will review your history, examine your mouth, and then decide whether you need radiographs and what type. If you are a new patient, the dentist may recommend radiographs to determine the present status of the hidden areas of your mouth and to help analyze changes that may occur later.

The schedule for needing radiographs at recall visits varies according to your age, risk for disease, and signs and symptoms. Updated radiographs may be needed to detect new cavities, to determine the status of gum disease, or for evaluation of growth and development. Children may need x-rays more often than adults. This is because their teeth and jaws are still developing and because their teeth are more likely to be affected by tooth decay than those of adults.

TABLE 12-1 Web Site Resources for Patient Education Materials	
SOURCE	URL
American Dental Association	http://www.ada.org/2760.aspx?currentTab=2
Academy of General Dentistry	http://www.knowyourteeth.com/infobites/abc/article/?abc=X&iid=342&aid=1373
U.S. National Library of Medicine	www.nlm.nih.gov/medlineplus/ency/article/003801.htm
Colgate	http://www.colgate.com/app/Colgate/US/OC/Information/OralHealthBasics/ CheckupsDentProc/XRays/XRaysandIntraoralPictures.cvsp
WebMD Health	http://www.webmd.com/oral-health/guide/dental-x-rays-when-get-them

QUESTION: Can I refuse dental x-rays and still be treated?

ANSWER: No. Treatment without necessary radiographs is considered negligent care. Even if you signed a paper stating that you refused radiographs and released the dentist from all liability, you would be consenting to negligent care. You cannot, legally, consent to negligent care. (Negligent care is discussed in Chapter 11.)

QUESTION: What kind of radiographs does my dentist usually recommend?

ANSWER: Typically, most dental patients have periapical or bitewing radiographs taken. These require a film or digital sensor be placed into the mouth, and the patient must stabilize it by biting down on the holder. Bitewing radiographs can be used to determine the presence of decay in between teeth, whereas periapical radiographs show root structure, bone levels, cysts, and abscesses.

QUESTION: My dentist has prescribed a panoramic radiograph. What is that?

ANSWER: Just as a panoramic photograph allows you to see a broad view, a panoramic radiograph allows your dentist to see the entire structure of your mouth in a single image. All teeth of both the maxilla and the mandible plus the surrounding tissues and supporting bone are imaged.

QUESTION: Why do I need both types of radiographs?

ANSWER: A periapical or bitewing radiograph shows only a few teeth on one image. The panoramic radiograph is a comprehensive view of all of the teeth plus the surrounding supporting structures. Both may be needed because although the panoramic radiograph images more tissues, the periapical or bitewing radiographs provide a more detailed image, making it easier to see decay or cavities between your teeth and early or subtle changes in the periodontal tissues. Radiographs are not prescribed indiscriminately. Your dentist has a need for the different information that each radiograph can provide to formulate a diagnosis.

QUESTION: How is x-ray exposure measured?

ANSWER: Special units are used to measure x-rays. When human tissue or other materials are exposed to x-rays, some of the energy is absorbed and some passes through without effect. The amount of energy absorbed by the tissue is the dose. The dose is often measured in sieverts (Sv). In modern diagnostic dental x-ray procedures, the exposures are usually so small that they are expressed in "milli" units—that is, units that are equal to one-thousandth of a Sv, or mSv.

QUESTION: What effects can x-rays have on the body?

ANSWER: Scientists have known for some time that exposure to very large amounts of x-radiation is harmful. Changes can occur in the reproductive system, altering the genetic material that determines the health of future generations. Large amounts of radiation can cause changes in the tissues of the body, including the possibility of cancer.

On the other hand, diagnostic procedures involve very low doses. With modern techniques and equipment, the amount of radiation received in a dental exam is minuscule. Also only a small part of the body is exposed (approximately the region corresponding to the size of the image receptor). Therefore, the risk of harmful effects from dental x-ray exams is extremely small.

QUESTION: How do dental x-rays compare to other sources of radiation?

ANSWER: We are exposed to radiation every day from various sources, including outer space, minerals in the soil, and appliances in our homes (like smoke detectors and television screens). Here is a sample of a comparison of radiation doses from different sources:

Source	Estimated Exposure (mSv*)
Dental radiographs	
Bitewings (4 films)	0.038
Full mouth series (about 19 films)	0.150
Medical radiographs	
Lower GI series	4.060
Upper GI series	2.440
Chest	0.080
Average radiation from outer space in Denver, CO (per year)	0.510
Average radiation in the United States from natural sources (per year)	5.500

*The term millisievert (mSv) is a unit of radiation measurement that allows for comparisons between different types of radiation.

Source: Frederiksen, N. L. (1995). X-rays: What is the risk? *Texas Dental Journal, 112*(2), 68–72.

QUESTION: Why do you use a lead apron?

ANSWER: Lead and other materials that simulate lead used in protective aprons and thyroid collars absorb potential scatter radiation and protect other parts of your body from unnecessary radiation.

QUESTION: Why does the radiographer leave the room when x-ray exposures are taken?

ANSWER: If the radiographer did not leave the room or stand behind a barrier, he/she would be exposed many times a day to radiation. Although the amount of radiation he/she would receive each time is quite small, over a long period of time they would receive a needless dose that provides no benefit to them.

QUESTION: If I am pregnant or think I may be pregnant, should dental x-ray exams be postponed?

ANSWER: A 2004 study published in the *Journal of the American Medical Association* (*JAMA, 291,* 16) suggests that dental radiography during pregnancy is associated with full-term, low-birth-weight pregnancies. It is currently unclear whether dental radiation affects the reproductive organs directly or whether exposure to the head and neck area affects the thyroid function and thereby indirectly affects pregnancy outcomes or whether factors unrelated to radiation are responsible for the low birth weight. Currently, the American Dental Association recommends that pregnant women postpone elective dental x-rays until after delivery and reinforces the importance of using lead/lead equivalent thyroid collars in addition to abdominal shielding (e.g., protective aprons). (Radiographs for the pregnant patient is discussed in Chapter 27.)

QUESTION: If I had radiation therapy for cancer of the head or neck, should I avoid dental x-rays?

ANSWER: No. The dose of radiation required for dental x-rays is extremely small compared to that used for radiation therapy. The effects of very high doses involved in therapeutic radiation may increase your susceptibility to diseases, such as tooth decay. This can occur as a result of a decrease in secretions of the salivary glands. It is especially important for you to have dental x-ray exams as needed, to detect problems at an early stage. (Radiographs for the cancer patient is discussed in Chapter 27.)

QUESTION: Can dental x-rays cause skin cancer?

ANSWER: There have been no recorded cases of patients developing cancer from modern diagnostic dental x-rays. In the early days, prior to radiation safety standards, dentists who repeatedly held the film in the patient's mouth during exposures developed cancer on their fingers.

QUESTION: What special precautions will you take to minimize the amount of radiation I receive?

ANSWER: There are several ways we minimize the amount of radiation that you receive. First and foremost, only necessary radiographs are taken. We use the fastest type of x-ray film currently available and use equipment that restricts the beam to the area that needs to be examined. A lead/lead equivalent apron and thyroid shield will be placed on you during the exposure, and the films will be developed according to the manufacturer's recommendations to produce a high-quality image.

QUESTION: Who owns my dental radiographs?

ANSWER: The dentist owns all your dental records, including the radiographs. You have the right of reasonable access to your dental records, but they remain the property of the dentist.

QUESTION: Should I have my previous radiographs sent to my new dentist?

ANSWER: Yes, if possible. These radiographs can reveal your previous disease activity and may assist in determining the need for a new x-ray exam. Although the dentist who treated you in the past is considered the owner of your records, including your x-rays, arrangements can usually be made to have x-rays duplicated and sent to your new dentist. You should contact your former dentist and request that this be done.

REVIEW—Chapter summary

Effective communication is the key to producing quality radiographs. The radiographer must be a skilled communicator.

Patient relations affect the confidence level of the patient and help the radiographer gain trust. The radiographer's appearance and attitude play a significant role in conveying professionalism.

The attitude of the radiographer toward the patient, the radiographic procedure and his/her own technical ability, coworkers, and employer will be conveyed to the patient. A positive, empathetic attitude will most likely generate a cooperative patient who will accept treatment recommendations and embrace oral health promotion and disease prevention. The radiographer should be cognizant of the roles interpersonal skills and chairside manner play in producing quality radiographs.

Honesty in verbal and nonverbal communication develops trust. Nonverbal communication is often stronger than verbal communication. Show-tell-do is an effective method of communication for all patients, especially when barriers to communication exist such as a language or cultural difference, a sensory impairment, or a cognitive impairment.

Patient education is valuable in securing acceptance of treatment and in addressing concerns about the safety of the radiographic procedures. The entire oral health care team must be able to provide the patient with complete explanations regarding the need for radiographs. The methods of patient education include oral presentations and the distribution of printed materials.

Examples of frequently asked questions and answers are provided.

RECALL—Study questions

1. The key to producing quality radiographic images is
   a. gaining patient trust and cooperation.
   b. presenting a confident, caring image.
   c. communicating effectively.
   d. All of the above

2. List four aspects of patient relations that help to gain confidence.
   a. _____
   b. _____
   c. _____
   d. _____

3. Dental radiographers with a positive attitude are more likely to produce high-quality radiographs.
   a. True
   b. False

4. When a patient trusts the radiographer, the patient is more likely to cooperate with the radiographic procedures.
   a. True
   b. False

5. The ability to share in the patient's emotions and feelings is called
   a. chairside manner.
   b. atitude.
   c. empathy.
   d. verbal communication.

6. Each of the following will enhance verbal communication EXCEPT one. Which one is the EXCEPTION?
   a. Face the patient.
   b. Make eye contact.
   c. Use clear commands.
   d. Use slang words.

7. Which of the following words should be avoided when discussing the radiographic procedure?
   a. Picture
   b. Zap
   c. X-ray
   d. Radiograph

8. The use of highly technical words may confuse the patient and result in miscommunication.
   a. True
   b. False

9. The method of show-tell-do is a beneficial way of communicating with
   a. someone who speaks a different language.
   b. children.
   c. hearing-impaired patients.
   d. All of the above

10. What is the value of patient education regarding dental radiographs?
    a. Radiographer is more likely to spend less time exposing radiographs.
    b. Radiographer is more likely to develop a positive attitude.
    c. Patient is more likely to accept the treatment plan.
    d. Patient is more likely to request radiographs at each appointment.

11. Patient education in radiography is necessary to
    a. increase the demand for oral health services.
    b. increase acceptance of oral health care recommendations.
    c. assure the patient that the radiographer is licensed.
    d. meet legally required mandates for it.

12. List four things you could tell the patient in response to his/her concerns regarding the necessity of dental x-rays and the reduction of excess radiation exposure.
    a. _____
    b. _____
    c. _____
    d. _____

REFLECT—Case study

A new patient to your practice has just been examined by the dentist, who has prescribed a set of vertical bitewings and a panoramic radiograph. You escort the patient to the x-ray room to prepare to expose the radiographs. At this time, the patient is having second thoughts about consenting to the radiographic surveys. She begins to question you about the procedure. Respond to the questions listed. Write out your answers. Together with a partner, role-play this scenario.

"Why do I need x-rays?"

"Why do I have to have bitewings and a panoramic x-ray?"

"How often should I have x-rays taken?"

"Are you going to take the x-rays, or will the dentist take them?"

"I'm a little nervous about having this done."

"How long will it take?"

"What will you do to protect me from excessive exposure?"

RELATE—Laboratory application

Produce your own brochure for the purpose of educating patients about the radiographic procedure. Give your brochure a title, for example, "Dental X-Rays for Your Health," or something similar. The narration should be simple and in language that is professional, yet not overly technical. You may direct your brochure to a target population. For example your brochure may be for children or for a particular culture (e.g., for Spanish speakers). Include pictures of radiographs illustrating conditions that can be identified easily. Search the Web for information and pictures to download (Table 12-1).

REFERENCES

American Dental Association. (2000). *The benefits of dental x-ray examinations*. Chicago: ADA.

American Dental Association. (2000). *Answers to common questions about dental x-rays*. Chicago: ADA.

Grubbs, P. A. (2003). *Essentials for today's nursing assistant*. Upper Saddle River, NJ: Prentice Hall.

Hujoel, P. P., Bollen, A. M., Noonan, C. J., & del Aguila, M. A. (2004). Antepartum dental radiography and infant low birth weight. *JAMA, 291*(16), 1987–1993.

Pulliam, J. L. (2006). *The nursing assistant: Acute, sub-acute and long-term care* (4th ed.). Upper Saddle River, NJ: Prentice Hall.

Thunthy, K. H. (1993). X-rays: Detailed answers to frequently asked questions. *Compendium of Continuing Education in Dentistry, 14*, 394–398.

PART V • INTRAORAL TECHNIQUES

Intraoral Radiographic Procedures

OBJECTIVES

Following successful completion of this chapter, you should be able to:

1. Define the key words.
2. Compare the three intraoral radiographic examinations.
3. Identify the two intraoral techniques.
4. List the five rules for shadow casting.
5. Determine conditions that effect the selection of image receptor size.
6. Select the type and number of image receptor required for a full mouth survey.
7. Explain horizontal and vertical angulation.
8. Explain point of entry.
9. List at least five contraindications for using the patient's finger to hold the image receptor during exposure.
10. Explain the basic design of image receptor positioners/holders.
11. Describe the proper patient seating position.
12. Demonstrate a systematic and orderly sequence of the exposure procedure.

KEY WORDS

Angulation
Bisecting technique
Biteblock
Bitewing radiograph
Conecut error
Film holder
Full mouth series (full mouth survey)
Horizontal angulation
Identification dot
Image receptor holder or positioner
Interproximal radiograph
Intraoral
Mean tangent

Midsaggital plane
Negative angulation
Occlusal plane
Occlusal radiograph
Paralleling technique
Periapical radiograph
Point of entry
Positive angulation
Rule of isometry
Shadow casting
Vertical angulation
Vertical bitewing radiograph

Introduction

Intraoral radiography consists of methods of exposing dental x-ray film, phosphor plates, or digital sensors within the oral cavity. Producing diagnostic quality dental radiographs depends on knowledge of and attention to:

- Positioning the patient in the chair
- Selecting a film, phosphor plate, or digital sensor of suitable size
- Determining how the image receptor is to be positioned and held in place
- Setting the radiation exposure variables
- Aiming the position indicating device (PID)

Each of these steps have specific applications for each of the three types of intraoral examinations and when utilizing the paralleling or the bisecting technique. The purpose of this chapter is to introduce the three types of intraoral examinations, explain the principles of producing intraoral images (shadow casting), and describe the fundamentals of image receptor holding devices to set the stage for Chapters 13, 14, and 15, where an in-depth explanation of the paralleling, bisecting, and bitewing techniques will follow.

Intraoral Procedures

Each of the three types of intraoral radiographic examinations has a specific imaging objective. *also technique*

1. **Bitewing examination.** Images the coronal portions of the teeth and the alveolar crests of bone of both the maxilla and mandible on a single radiograph (see Figure 7-6). The bitewing examination, sometimes referred to as an **interproximal radiograph,** is especially useful in detecting caries (dental decay) of the proximal surfaces where adjacent teeth contact each other in the arch. Bitewing radiographs are also used to examine crestal bone of patients with periodontal disease. The technique used to image **bitewing radiographs** is unique to the bitewing exam. However, because of the almost parallel relationship of the image receptor to the teeth, the bitewing technique could be considered to be a modification of the paralleling technique used for exposing periapical radiographs.

2. **Periapical examination.** The purpose of **periapical radiographs** is to image the apices of the teeth and the surrounding bone (see Figure 7-7). The word *periapical* is derived from the Greek word *peri* (meaning around) and the Latin word *apex*

(meaning highest point). Therefore, as the word suggests, the periapical radiograph images the entire tooth, including the root end and surrounding bone. The periapical radiograph may be used to examine a single tooth or condition or may be used in combination with other periapical and bitewing radiographs to image the entire dentition and supporting structures (full mouth series; Figure 13-1). Conditions prompting the exposure of a periapical radiograph include apical pathology (abscesses), fractures, large carious lesions (Figure 13-2), extensive periodontal involvement (Figure 13-3), examination of developmental anomalies such as missing teeth and abnormal eruption patterns, and any unexplained pain or bleeding. Periapical radiographs may be taken utilizing either the paralleling or the bisecting technique.

3. **Occlusal examination.** Images the entire maxillary or mandibular arch, or a portion thereof, on a single radiograph (see Figure 17-1). Occlusal radiographs are most often taken with a larger size #4 intraoral film, making this examination useful in imaging large areas of pathology that may not be adequately imaged on a smaller periapical radiograph. Conditions that may prompt the exposure of occlusal radiographs include cysts, fractures, impacted or supernumerary (extra) teeth, and in locating the buccal or lingual position of foreign objects (see Chapter 28). The technique used to image **occlusal radiographs** is unique to the occlusal exam. However, because of the image receptor placement required, the occlusal technique could be considered a modification of the bisecting technique.

Techniques   *PA's*

Two basic techniques are used in intraoral radiography: paralleling and bisecting. Either technique can be modified to meet special conditions and requirements. Although each technique will produce diagnostic quality radiographic images if the fundamental principles of the technique are followed, paralleling is the technique of choice because it is more likely to satisfy more of the shadow casting requirements.

The concept of the **bisecting technique** (also called the bisecting-angle or short-cone technique) originated in 1907 through the application of a geometric principle known as the **rule of isometry.** This theorem states that two triangles having equal angles and a common side are equal triangles (see Figure 15-1). The bisecting technique was the only method used for many years. However, because many radiographers

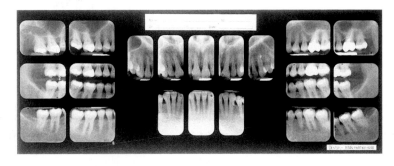

FIGURE 13-1 Full mouth series. The 20-film radiographic survey includes four bitewing radiographs and eight anterior and eight posterior periapical radiographs.

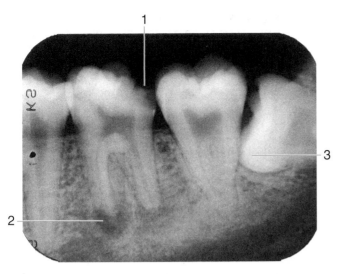

FIGURE 13-2 Periapical radiograph. Posterior periapical radiograph showing (**1**) extensive caries, (**2**) apical pathology, and (**3**) impacted third molar. Note the use of a size #2 film and the horizontal positioning of the long dimension of the film packet for imaging the posterior regions.

experienced difficulties and obtained unsatisfactory results, the search for a less-complicated technique that would produce better radiographs more consistently resulted in the development of the paralleling technique in 1920. The **paralleling technique** (also called right-angle, extension-cone, or long-cone technique) is considered to be the technique of choice because better-quality radiographs are produced with this technique. The specific steps of each of these two techniques are discussed in detail in Chapters 14 and 15.

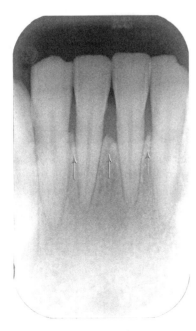

FIGURE 13-3 Periapical radiograph. Anterior periapical radiograph showing extensive periodontal involvement. Note the use of a size #1 film and the vertical positioning of the long dimension of the film packet for imaging the anterior regions.

Fundamentals of Shadow Casting

X-rays produce an image on a film, phosphor plate, or digital sensor in a similar manner as light casting a shadow of an object. When a hand is placed between a nearby light source such as an electric bulb and a flat object such as a tabletop, a shadow of the hand is seen on the tabletop. In dental radiography, x-rays cast a shadow of the teeth on to the image receptor.

The radiograph is essentially a shadow image. To produce an image that represents the teeth and supporting structures accurately, the x-ray beam must be directed at the structures and the image receptor at certain angles. The function of the image receptor is to record the shadow image. To produce the best image, it is important to understand the fundamentals of **shadow casting.** Shadow casting refers to five basic rules for casting a shadow image (see Chapter 4).

1. Use the smallest possible focal spot on the target (source of radiation).
2. The object (tooth) should be as far as practical from the target (source of radiation).
3. The object (tooth) and the image receptor (film, phosphor plate, or digital sensor) should be as close to each other as possible.
4. The object (tooth) and the image receptor (film, phosphor plate, or digital sensor) should be parallel to each other.
5. The radiation (central ray) must strike both the object (tooth) and the image receptor (film, phosphor plate, or digital sensor) at right angles (perpendicularly).

Neither the paralleling nor the bisecting technique completely meets all five requirements for accurate shadow casting in all regions of the oral cavity on all patient types. With the bisecting technique, it is often not possible to position the image receptor parallel to the object, preventing the radiation from striking the object and the image receptor at right angles. With the paralleling technique, the distance between the object and the image receptor is often greater than ideal in most regions of the oral cavity. However, the paralleling technique is more likely to meet most of these requirements, making the technique less likely to produce image distortion. For this reason, the paralleling technique is the recommended technique (Figures 13-4 and 13-5).

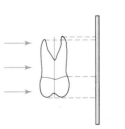

FIGURE 13-4 Principle of the paralleling technique. Positioning the recording plane parallel to the long axis of the tooth and directing the x-ray beam perpendicular to both the recording plane and the long axis of the tooth produces an image with less distortion. (Courtesy of Dentsply Rinn.)

Bisecting + Paralleling = PA's   Bitewing also technique

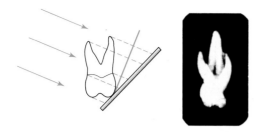

FIGURE 13-5 Principle of the bisecting technique. The x-ray beam is directed perpendicular to the imaginary line that bisects the angle formed by the recording plane and the long axis of the tooth. Because the tooth is a three–dimensional object, the part of the object farthest from the recording plane is projected in an incorrect relationship to the parts closest to the recording plane. (Courtesy of Dentsply Rinn.)

Although the paralleling technique produces superior diagnostic quality radiographs, not all patients present with conditions that allow for the use of the paralleling technique. When use of the paralleling technique is difficult, a reasonably acceptable quality radiograph may be produced using the bisecting technique. For this reason, the radiographer who is skilled in both paralleling and bisecting techniques will be better prepared to produce quality radiographs in most all situations.

The Radiographic Examination

Size, Number, and Placement of Image Receptors

The size #4 film or phosphor plate is used exclusively for occlusal radiographs of adult patients, and the size #3 film or phosphor plate is used exclusively for horizontal bitewing radiographs of adult patients. Bitewing and periapical radiographs of adults, adolescents, and children can be made with any of the three intraoral film, phosphor plates, or digital sensor sizes (#0, #1, #2) or any combination of these sizes. The size of the image receptor selected for use depends on:

- The age of the patient
- The size of the oral cavity
- The shape of the dental arches
- The presence or absence of unusual conditions or anatomical limitations
- The patient's ability to tolerate placement of the image receptor
- The image receptor positioner or holder and technique used

The bitewing survey may consist of two to eight radiographs. A complete set of seven or eight **vertical bitewing radiographs** may be exposed for the examination of a periodontally involved patient. This vertical bitewing set will include both posterior and anterior bitewings. When the patient does not require anterior bitewings, two or four posterior bitewing radiographs positioned either vertically or horizontally are usually taken (see Figure 15-5). When the periapical and bitewing examinations include a series of radiographs that image all the teeth, the term **full mouth series** or full mouth survey is used to describe the collection of radiographs (Figure 13-1).

The number and size of image receptors used for a full mouth series of bitewing and periapical radiographs varies among oral health care practices. A minimum of 4 bitewing and 14 periapical radiographs (Figure 13-6) make up a full mouth survey for most adult patients. The four bitewing radiographs are used to image the following regions:

- One radiograph each for the right and left premolar regions
- One radiograph each for the right and left molar regions

The 14 periapical radiographs are used to image the following regions:

- One radiograph each for the maxillary and mandibular incisor regions
- One radiograph each for the right and left maxillary and mandibular canine regions
- One radiograph each for the right and left maxillary and mandibular premolar regions
- One radiograph each for the right and left maxillary and mandibular molar regions

Although most oral health care practices will use eight size #2 image receptors for the exposure of the posterior periapicals on an adult patient, the number and size of image receptors used for the exposure of the anterior teeth varies. The general rule is to use the largest image receptor that can readily be positioned to minimize the number of exposures. However, more films or more exposures of a digital sensor may be required for unusual conditions or for narrow arches requiring a smaller size image receptor. A size #1 image receptor is often used instead of the size #2 image receptor for exposures of the anterior teeth. However, the narrow size #1 image receptor may require the use of additional exposures to completely record the region. Three examples of image receptor combinations for use in recording the images for anterior periapical radiographs using the narrow #1 size or the standard #2 size are:

- **Eight anterior exposures.** Five size #1 image receptors may be used for the exposure of the maxillary anterior teeth (Figure 13-7A). One image receptor is centered at the midline behind the central incisors, one image receptor each is centered behind the right and left lateral incisors, and one image receptor each is centered behind the right and left canines. Three size #1 image receptors are used for the exposure of the mandibular arch, where the teeth are smaller. One image receptor is centered behind the central and lateral incisors, and one image receptor each is centered behind the right and left canines.

- **Eight anterior exposure.** Four size #1 image receptors may be used for the exposure of the maxillary anterior teeth (Figure 13-7B). One image receptor each is centered behind the right and left central and lateral incisors, and one image receptor each is centered behind the right and left canines. Four size #1 image receptors are used for the exposure of the mandibular anterior teeth in much the same way as for the maxilla. One image receptor each is centered behind each of the right and left central and lateral incisors, and one image receptor each is centered behind the right and left canines.

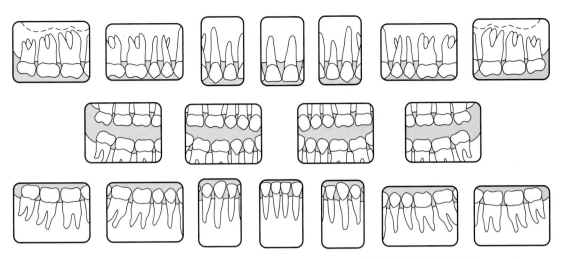

FIGURE 13-6 **Full mouth series.** Drawing of 18-image full mouth survey includes 14 periapical and 4 bitewing radiographs.

- **Six anterior exposures.** Three size #1 or three size #2 image receptors may be used for the exposure of the maxillary anterior teeth (Figure 13-7C). One image receptor is centered at the midline behind the central and lateral incisors, and one image receptor each is centered behind each of the right and left canines. The three size #1 or three size #2 image receptors used for the exposure of the mandibular arch are positioned in the same manner as

described earlier, where one image receptor is centered behind the central and lateral incisors and one image receptor each is centered behind the right and left canines. Although the use of size #2 image receptor for anterior periapical radiographs is acceptable, the narrower size #1 image receptor usually fits this area better. When using the size #2 film packet or phosphor plate in the anterior region, there is a tendency to bend the film packet or plate corners

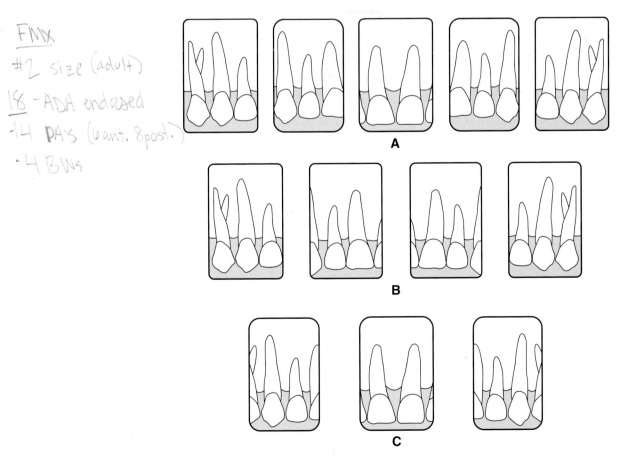

FIGURE 13-7 **Maxillary anterior image receptor placement.** (**A**) Five-image survey. (**B**) Four-image survey. (**C**) Three-image survey.

to make it fit more comfortably. Bending the image receptor will result in a distorted image and/or radiolucent or radiopaque creases. Some patients present with a narrow anterior region that may make positioning the size #2 digital sensor difficult. Some practices utilize one size #2 image receptor for the exposure of the maxillary central and lateral incisors, where the area is the widest, and use size #1 image receptors to expose the remaining five areas.

See Table 13-1 for a list of the various combinations of standard placements of the film packet, phosphor plate, or digital sensor for each of the periapical radiographs of a full mouth series.

Orientation of the Image Receptor

With few exceptions, for exposure of the anterior regions of the oral cavity the film packet, phosphor plate, or digital sensor is placed with the longer dimension vertical (described as vertical placement; Figure 13-3). For exposure of the posterior regions the image receptor should be placed with the longer dimension horizontal (described as horizontal placement; Figure 13-2). The white, unprinted side of the film packet (front side) must face the source of radiation. Depending on the manufacturer, the plain side of the phosphor plate, or side without the cord attachment of the digital sensor, should be placed to face the source of radiation.

When placing a film packet for periapical radiographs, it is important to make note of where the identification dot is located. The **identification dot,** embossed into the film by the manufacturer, will be utilized during interpretation of the radiograph to distinguish between the patient's right and left sides (see Chapter 21). There is a tendency for the embossed identification dot to distort images, so during film packet placement it is important to position the identification dot away from the area of interest. In the case of periapical radiographs, the identification dot should be positioned toward the incisal or occlusal edges, where it is least likely to interfere with diagnostic information.

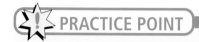

PRACTICE POINT

When using a film-holding device with a film slot, it is helpful to remember that "dot in the slot" will position the embossed identification dot away from the apices of the teeth where it could interfere with diagnosis. Dot in the slot will position the identification dot toward the incisal or occlusal edges for both maxillary and mandibular periapical radiographs.

Horizontal and Vertical Angulation Procedures

Angulation is defined as the procedure by which the tube head and PID are aligned to obtain the optimum angle at which the radiation is to be directed toward the image receptor. Angulation is changed by rotating the tube head horizontally and vertically. The x-ray machine is constructed with three swivel joints to support

TABLE 13-1 Standard Image Receptor Placements for Periapical Radiographs of a Full Mouth Series	
PERIAPICAL RADIOGRAPH	**IMAGE RECEPTOR PLACEMENT**
Maxillary central incisors (size #1 or size #2)	Center the image receptor to line up behind the central and lateral incisors; if using size #2, include the mesial halves of the canines.
Maxillary central and lateral incisors (size #1)	Center the image receptor to line up behind the central and lateral incisors; include the distal half of the central incisor on the opposite side and the mesial half of the canine.
Maxillary lateral incisor (size #1)	Center the image receptor to line up behind the lateral incisor; include the distal half of the central incisor and the mesial half of the canine.
Maxillary lateral incisor and canine (size #1)	Center the image receptor to line up behind the lateral incisor and canine; include the distal half of the central incisor and the mesial half of the premolar.
Maxillary canine (size #1 or size #2)	Center the image receptor to line up behind the canine; include the distal half of the lateral incisor and the mesial half of the first premolar.
Mandibular central incisors (size #1 or size #2)	Center the image receptor to line up behind the central and lateral incisors; if using a size #2 film, include the mesial halves of the canines.
Mandibular central and lateral incisors (size #1)	Center the image receptor to line up behind the central and lateral incisors; include the distal half of the central incisor on the opposite side and the mesial half of the canine.
Mandibular canine (size #1 or size #2)	Center the image receptor to line up behind the canine; include the distal half of the lateral incisor and the mesial half of the first premolar.
Maxillary and mandibular premolar (size #2)	Align the anterior edge of the image receptor to line up behind the distal half of the canine; include the entire first and second premolars and mesial half of the first molar.
Maxillary and mandibular molar (size #2)	Align the anterior edge of the image receptor to line up behind the distal half of the second premolar; include the entire first, second, and third molars.

the yoke and tube head. One of these, located at the top and center of the yoke where it attaches to the extension arm, permits horizontal movement of the tube head to control the anterior–posterior dimensions. The other two swivel joints are located at either side of the yoke. These permit the tube head to be rotated up or down in a vertical direction to control the longitudinal dimensions of the resulting image. Determining the correct direction of the central beam in the horizontal and vertical planes requires practice.

The correct horizontal and vertical angulations are critical to producing a quality radiograph.

Horizontal Angulation

Horizontal angulation is achieved by directing the central rays perpendicularly (at a right angle) toward the surface of the image receptor in a horizontal plane (Figure 13-8). To change direction, swivel the tube head from side to side. The central ray (PID) should be directed perpendicular to the curvature of the arch, through the contact points of the teeth. The horizontal angulation is established by directing the central rays perpendicularly through the **mean tangent** of the embrasures between the teeth of interest. Incorrect alignment in the horizontal plane caused by incorrect angulation toward the mesial or the distal results in overlapping of adjacent tooth structures shown on the radiograph. The steps to determining correct horizontal angulation are the same for both the bisecting and paralleling methods and for exposing bitewing radiographs.

Vertical Angulation

Vertical Angulation is achieved by directing the central rays perpendicularly (at a right angle) toward the surface of the image receptor in a vertical plane (Figure 13-9). Vertical angulation is customarily described in degrees. On most dental x-ray machines the vertical angles are scaled in intervals of 5 or 10 degrees on one or both sides of the yoke where the tube head is connected. The vertical angulation of the tube head and the PID begins at zero. In the zero position the PID is parallel to the plane of the floor. All deviations from zero in which the PID is tilted downward to direct the x-rays toward the floor are called

positive (plus) **angulations.** Those in which the PID is tipped upward to direct the x-rays toward the ceiling are called **negative** (minus) **angulations.** Positive (+) angulation, the positioning of the central ray (PID) downward toward the floor, is used for exposure of bitewing radiographs and generally used for the exposure of periapical radiographs of the maxillary arch. Negative (−) angulation, the positioning of the central ray (PID) upward toward the ceiling, is generally used for the exposure of periapical radiographs of the mandibular arch. Although the vertical angulation setting for the exposure of bitewing radiographs for the adult patient is +10 for all regions of the oral cavity, the precise vertical angulation setting for periapical radiographs is determined differently depending on the technique used (see Chapters 14 and 15).

Points of Entry

The image receptor must be centered within the beam of radiation to avoid **conecut error,** where a portion of the image is not recorded on the radiograph. The **point of entry** for the central ray should be in the middle for the image receptor. A film holder or image receptor postioner with an external aiming device will assist the radiographer with determining the point of entry. The portion of the holder, or biteblock, that extends from the oral cavity can be used to estimate the center of the image receptor when using a holder without an external indicator. The open end of the PID should be placed as close to the patient's skin as possible without touching. Failure to bring the end of the PID in close to the patient will result in an underexposed radiograph because as the beam of radiation spreads out, less radiation is available to strike the image receptor and produce a diagnostic quality image.

Film Holders and Image Receptor Postioners

Film holders and holders designed to position a phosphor plate or digital sensor are collectively called **image receptor holders** or **positioners.** These devices are used to hold the image receptor in place to expose intraoral radiographs. When the bisecting

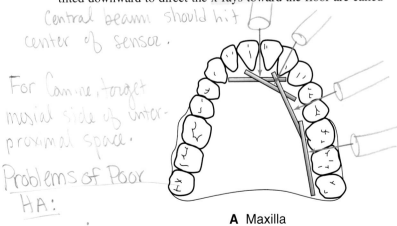
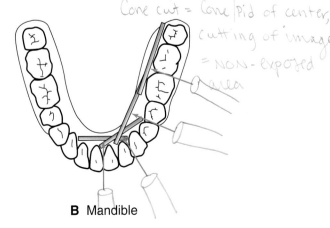

A Maxilla   **B** Mandible

FIGURE 13-8 Horizontal angulation. Horizontal angulation is determined by directing the x-ray beam directly through the interproximal spaces perpendicular to the mean tangent of the teeth. The image receptor must be positioned parallel to the teeth of interest so that the central ray will also strike the image receptor perpendicularly.

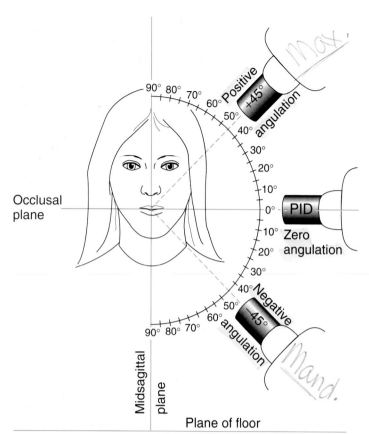

Handwritten note:
Problems of poor VA:
• forshortening - caused by too steep
• elongation - caused by too shallow

Handwritten labels on diagram: max., Mand.

FIGURE 13-9 Vertical angulation. Diagram showing patient sitting in the recommended position upright in dental chair with midsagittal plane perpendicular to and occlusal plane parallel with the floor. Zero angulation is achieved when the long axis of the PID is directed parallel with the floor. All angulations achieved with the PID pointed toward the floor are called positive, or plus (+) angulations. All angulations achieved with the PID is pointed toward the ceiling are called negative, or minus (−) angulations. Generally a positive angle is used for bitewing exposures and periapical exposures of the maxilla, and a negative angle is used for periapical exposures of the mandible.

technique was first introduced in 1907, film holders and image receptor positioners did not yet exist. Instead, the patient was directed to hold the film packet in the mouth using a finger or thumb. Asking the patient to hold the film packet in this manner has many disadvantages, and this practice is no longer acceptable (Box 13-1). Image receptor positioners and holders vary from simple disposable **biteblocks** that require no sterilization to complex devices that position the image receptor at the correct angles for directing the x-ray beam in relation to the teeth and image receptor (Figures 13-10 and 13-11.) Some commercially manufactured image receptor holders are designed specifically for use with the bisecting technique or specifically for use with the paralleling technique. Some holders may be slightly altered to accommodate both techniques (Figure 13-12). Other manufactures offer interchangeable biteblocks to accommodate either technique and placement of a film packet, phosphor plate, or digital sensor (Figure 13-13). It is important that the radiographer match the image receptor biteblock with the technique and type of receptor (film, phosphor plate, or sensor) for which it was designed, to achieve optimal results.

It is beneficial to have a variety of image receptor positioners available, because one type of holder may not be suitable for all patients, or even all areas of the same patient's mouth. Additionally, the operator may have to alternate between the paralleling and the bisecting technique to complete a full mouth series on a patient.

Preparations and Seating Positions

Unit Preparation

Prior to placing the image receptor intraorally, the x-ray unit should be turned on and the exposure settings selected. It is helpful to place the tube head and PID in the approximate position for the exposure to limit the time required for this step once the image receptor has been placed into the patient's oral cavity.

BOX 13-1 Contraindications for Using the Patient's Finger to Hold the Film Packet, Phosphor Plate, or Digital Sensor in Place

- Potential for bending the image receptor.
- Potential to move the image receptor from the correct position.
- Increased patient instruction and cooperation required.
- Potential patient objection to placing the fingers in the mouth.
- Radiation exposure to the patient's fingers.
- No external aiming device to assist with aligning the x-ray beam to the correct position.
- Potential to be viewed by the patient as unprofessional and unsanitary.

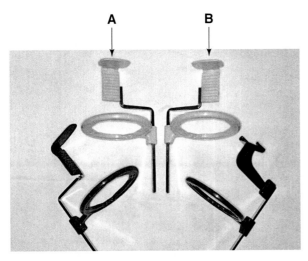

FIGURE 13-10 Rinn XCP™ **paralleling technique film holders.** Color-coded rings and biteblocks assist with assembly of multiple parts. Note the mirror-image assembly of these posterior periapical film holders. Assembly A is used for exposures on the maxillary right and the mandibular left, whereas assembly B is used for exposures on the maxillary left and on the mandibular right.

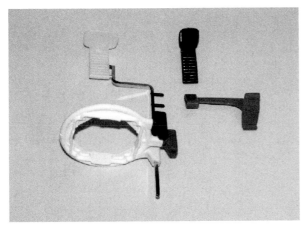

FIGURE 13-11 Rinn XCP ORA™ **(one ring and arm) positioning system.** Color-coded pins on the metal arm match the colored inserts on the plastic ring. When matched with the appropriate biteblocks, it can be configured for exposures in all regions of the oral cavity with either film or digital sensors.

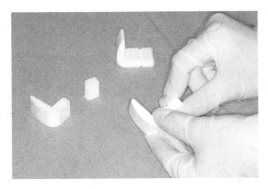

FIGURE 13-12 Stabe® **(Dentsply Rinn).** Bite extension required for use with the paralleling technique may be broken off for use with the bisecting technique.

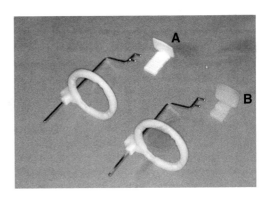

FIGURE 13-13 **Film holders.** The extension arm and aiming ring of the Rinn XCP® (Dentsply Rinn) instrument may be combined with a (**A**) biteblock suitable for the paralleling technique or a (**B**) biteblock suitable for the bisecting technique.

Patient Preparation

To help gain patient cooperation and confidence, it is important to explain the procedure. Include specific instructions regarding the need for patient cooperation and be honest about any difficulties anticipated (see Chapter 12). Perform a cursory oral inspection and ask the patient to remove any objects from the mouth that would interfere with the procedure, such as removable dentures or orthodontic appliances, chewing gum, and so on. Ask the patient to remove eyeglasses; if any metal or thick plastic parts of the eyeglasses remain in the path of the x-ray beam, they will be imaged onto the radiograph. Protect the patient with the lead or lead equivalent apron and thyroid collar barriers.

Patient Seating Position

If the image receptor holder has an external aiming device, the patient's head can be in any position. Without these special holders that indicate x-ray beam positions, patients must be seated upright with their head straight. This position is necessary for consistent results in determining the best horizontal

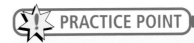

PRACTICE POINT

Seating the patient with the head against the headrest not only helps position the occlusal and midsaggital planes, but the patient is much less likely to move during the exposures when his/her head is firmly supported by the headrest. Additionally, Chapter 27 states that directing the patient's attention to the back of the head where it touches the headrest (the occipital protuberance) can serve as a distraction technique when needed (for example, when an exaggerated gag reflex presents).

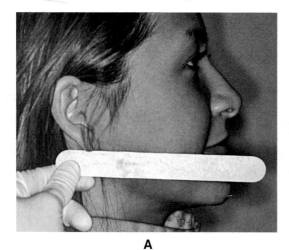
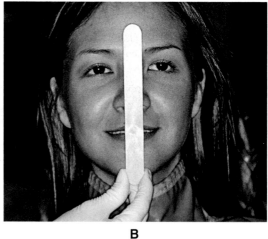

A **B**

FIGURE 13-14 Patient positioning. The patient is positioned with the head supported against the headrest with the (**A**) occlusal plane parallel to the floor and the (**B**) midsaggital plane perpendicular to the floor.

and vertical angulations of the x-ray beam and points of entry. Additionally, stabilizing the patient's head against the headrest is important to prevent movement during the exposure. Place the headrest against the occipital protuberance (the back, base of the skull) for greatest stability.

The recommended position is to seat the patient upright and adjust the headrest so that the **occlusal plane** for the arch being examined is parallel to the floor (Figure 13-14). The **midsagittal plane** that divides the patient's head into a right and left side should be positioned perpendicular to the floor (Figure 13-15). Although an experienced radiographer can

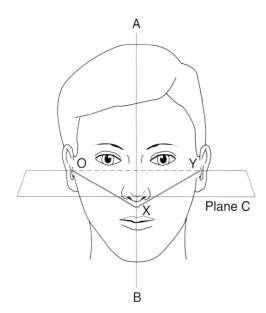

FIGURE 13-15 Head divided by midsagittal plane and occlusal plane. The midsagittal plane (**A–B**) must be perpendicular to the floor, and the occlusal plane (**C**) must be parallel with the floor unless an image receptor with an external aiming device is used. The lines **O–X** and **X–Y** are the lines of orientation for the maxillary teeth, also known as the ala–tragus line. The apices of the roots of the maxillary teeth are located close to this line.

expose radiographs with the patient either upright or supine, the use of predetermined head positions is recommended to standardize the procedure.

Sequence of Procedure

A definite sequence of positioning the image receptor should be followed to prevent omitting an area or exposing an area twice. Develop a set routine to prevent errors and save time.

Opinions differ as to which region should be exposed first when taking a full mouth series of periapical and bitewing radiographs. Some radiographers prefer to begin in the right maxillary molar region and continue in sequence to the left maxillary molar region, drop down to the left mandibular molar region, and finish in the right mandibular molar region.

Others begin with the anterior exposures, on the theory that the image receptor placement is more comfortable here and less likely to excite a gag reflex than when it is placed in the maxillary molar region, where the tissues may be more sensitive (see Chapter 27). If the first few placements produce no discomfort, the patient may become used to the feel of the image receptor and may more readily accept it as the procedure continues.

For an experienced radiographer who can place the image receptor skillfully and rapidly, it probably makes little difference which area is exposed first. However, the same order for placement of the image receptor should always be followed to make sure that all regions are exposed in an orderly and efficient manner. The following sequence of image receptor placements is suggested to help the student adopt a systematic routine:

- Maxillary anterior periapicals
- Mandibular anterior periapicals
- Maxillary posterior periapicals
- Mandibular posterior periapicals
- Anterior bitewings
- Posterior bitewings

Anterior image receptor placements are often more comfortable and allow the patient to become accustomed to the procedure. The bitewing examination (see Chapter 16) is last because the patient tolerates these fairly well, and the radiographic procedure can end pleasantly. In addition, it may be helpful for the radiographer not to have to break the sequence of exposing periapical radiographs by switching to a bitewing holder and changing techniques in the middle of the procedure. Procedure Box 13-1 summarizes the steps for exposing a full mouth series of radiographs.

PROCEDURE 13-1
Procedure for exposing a full mouth series of radiographs

1. Perform infection control procedures (see Procedure Box 10-2).

2. Prepare unit. Turn on and set exposure factors.

3. Seat patient and explain the procedure.

4. Request that the patient remove objects from the mouth that can interfere with the procedure and remove eyeglasses.

5. Adjust chair to a comfortable working level.

6. Adjust the headrest to position the patient's head so that the occlusal plane of the arch being imaged is parallel to the floor and the midsagittal plane (midline) is perpendicular to the floor.

7. Place the lead or lead-equivalent barrier apron and thyroid collar on the patient.

8. Perform a cursory inspection of the oral cavity and note possible obstructions (tori, shallow palatal vault, malaligned teeth) that may require an alteration of technique or number of exposures.

9. Place the image receptor into the positioner. When using film, place such that the embossed dot will be positioned toward the occlusal/incisal edge ("dot in the slot"). Position anterior image receptors vertically and posterior image receptors horizontally.

10. Insert the image receptor and positioner into the patient's oral cavity and center the receptor behind the teeth to be imaged. (See Table 14-5 for the exact placements for each of the maxillary and mandibular periapical radiographs and Table 16-3 for placements for each of the posterior and/or anterior bitewing radiographs in the procedure.) Visually locate the contact points of the teeth to be imaged and place the image receptor perpendicular to the embrasures.

11. Hold the image receptor holder against the occlusal/incisal surface of the maxillary/mandibular teeth while asking the patient to bite firmly onto the biteblock of the holder. (Use a sterilized cotton roll for stabilization if needed.)

12. Release the image receptor postioner when the patient has closed firmly, holding it in place.

13. Set the vertical angulation:

    a. For periapical radiographs: (See Table 14-5 for the recommended vertical angulation setting for the area being imaged.)

       1. Intersect the image receptor plane and the long axes of the teeth perpendicularly when utilizing the paralleling technique. If using an image receptor positioner with an external aiming device, align the open end of the PID with the indicator ring.

       2. Intersect the imaginary bisector of the receptor plane and the long axes of the teeth perpendicularly when utilizing the bisecting technique.

    b. For bitewing radiographs use +10 degrees.

14. Determine the correct horizontal angulation by directing the central ray of the x-ray beam perpendicular to the receptor in the horizontal plane through the contact point of the teeth of interest. (See Table 14-5 for the exact embrasure space through which to direct the central ray for each of the periapical radiographs and Table 16-3 for each of the bitewing radiographs in the procedure. Horizontal angulation is determined the same for both paralleling and bisecting techniques and for bitewing radiographs.) If using an image receptor positioner with an external aiming device, align the open end of the PID with the indicator ring.

(Continued)

PROCEDURE 13-1
Procedure for exposing a full mouth series of radiographs (continued)

15. Center the PID over the image receptor. If using an image receptor positioner with an external aiming device, align the open end of the PID with the indicator ring. (See Table 15-4 for point of entry recommendations when utilizing the bisecting technique.)

16. Make the exposure.

17. Remove the image receptor and positioner from the patient's oral cavity.

18. Repeat steps 9 through 17 until all radiographs in the series have been exposed.

19. Remove the lead or lead equivalent barrier apron and thyroid collar from the patient.

20. Perform infection control procedures following the exposures (see Procedure Box 10-4).

REVIEW—Chapter summary

The three types of intraoral radiographic procedures are the bitewing, periapical, and occlusal surveys. Each of these examinations differs in purpose, and a variety of image receptor sizes may be used to achieve the desired result.

Both the bisecting and the paralleling techniques are used to produce a shadow image of the tooth onto the radiograph. Although neither technique completely satisfies all the requirements for accurate shadow casting, the paralleling technique is more likely to produce superior results. Each technique has advantages and disadvantages. The skilled operator, within the limits of the equipment available, must select the technique that fits the situation.

The size and number of image receptors used for exposure of a full mouth radiographic survey depends on several factors. A bitewing series may consist of two to eight radiographs. A minimum of 14 periapical radiographs are required for a full mouth series of an adult patient—additional images may be needed if narrow size #1 image receptors are used in the anterior regions. Exposures include the central incisor, canine, premolar, and molar areas of the right and left maxilla and mandible. The image receptor should be positioned with the long dimension vertical in the anterior region and horizontal in the posterior region. The embossed identification dot present on radiographic film should be placed toward the incisal/occlusal edges of the teeth when positioning the film packet for periapical radiographs.

The horizontal angulation is determined by directing the central rays of the x-beam perpendicular to the plane of the image receptor through the mean tangent of the embrasures between the teeth of interest. Both paralleling and bisecting techniques and bitewing procedures determine horizontal angulation in the same manner.

With negative vertical angulation, the PID is pointing down toward the floor. With positive vertical angulation, the PID is pointing up toward the ceiling. The vertical angulation is determined by directing the central rays of the x-beam perpendicular to the plane of the image receptor and the long axes of the teeth when utilizing the paralleling technique. When utilizing the bisecting technique, the vertical angulation is determined by directing the central rays of the x-ray beam perpendicular to the imaginary bisector. The vertical angulation setting for exposing bitewings is +10.

The point of entry is used to center the image receptor within the beam of radiation.

Before image positioners were developed, the patient would hold the film packet in the oral cavity with the fingers or a thumb. With the variety of image receptor positioners currently on the market, this practice is unacceptable today. Film holders are designed for use with the paralleling or the bisecting technique or may be modified to use with both techniques.

Unless the image receptor holder has an external aiming device to indicate the correct angulation, care must be taken to seat the patient so that the occlusal plane is parallel with the floor and that the midsaggital plane is perpendicular to the floor.

An exposure sequence is recommended to avoid error and be efficient. Anterior image receptor placements may be more comfortable for some patients. Beginning the exposure sequence in the anterior may assist in gaining patient cooperation with the procedure.

RECALL—Study questions

1. Which of these is NOT an intraoral radiograph?
   a. Bitewing
   b. Occlusal
   c. Panoramic
   d. Periapical

2. Which radiograph is used most often to detect proximal surface dental decay?
   a. Bitewing
   b. Occlusal
   c. Panoramic
   d. Periapical

3. Which intraoral technique satisfies more shadow casting principles?
   a. Bisecting
   b. Paralleling

4. Which intraoral technique is based on the rule of isometry?
   a. Bisecting
   b. Paralleling

5. Each of the following is a shadow casting principle EXCEPT one. Which one is the EXCEPTION?
   a. Object and image receptor should be perpendicular to each other.
   b. Object and image receptor should be as close as possible to each other.
   c. Object should be as far as practical from the target (source of radiation).
   d. Radiation should strike the object and image receptor perpendicularly.

6. Which of these factors does NOT need to be considered when deciding which image receptor size to use when exposing a full mouth series?
   a. Age of the patient
   b. Shape of the dental arches
   c. Previous accumulated exposure
   d. Patient's ability to tolerate the image receptor

7. What is the minimum image receptor requirement for an adult full mouth series of periapical radiographs?
   a. 12
   b. 14
   c. 16
   d. 18

8. How many size #2 image receptors are required by most health care practices for the exposure of posterior radiographs of a full mouth series?
   a. 5
   b. 6
   c. 7
   d. 8

9. Lining the image receptor up behind the right and left central and lateral incisors to include the mesial half of the right and left canines describes the image receptor placement for which of the following periapical radiographs?
   a. Central incisors
   b. Canines
   c. Premolars
   d. Molars

10. Anterior periapical image receptors are placed _____ in the oral cavity. Posterior periapical image receptors are placed _____ in the oral cavity.
    a. vertically; horizontally
    b. horizontally; vertically
    c. vertically; vertically
    d. horizontally; horizontally

11. Where should the embossed identification dot be positioned when taking periapical radiographs?
    a. Toward the midline of the oral cavity
    b. Toward the incisal or occlusal edge of the tooth
    c. Toward the palate or floor of the mouth
    d. Toward the distal or back of the arch

12. The x-ray tube head must be swiveled from side to side to adjust the vertical angulation of the central ray.

    To avoid overlap error the central ray must be directed perpendicular to the curvature of the arch through the contact points of the teeth.
    a. Both statements are true.
    b. Both statements are false
    c. The first statement is true. The second statement is false.
    d. The first statement is false. The second statement is true.

13. At which of the following settings would the PID be pointing to the floor?
    a. −30
    b. 0
    c. +20

14. An incorrect point of entry will result in
    a. overlapping.
    b. foreshortening.
    c. cutting off the root apices.
    d. conecutting.

15. List five contraindications for using the patient's finger to hold a film packet in position during exposure.
    a. _____
    b. _____
    c. _____
    d. _____
    e. _____

16. An image receptor positioner/holder must be used with
    a. the paralleling technique.
    b. the bisecting technique.
    c. the bitewing technique.
    d. all of the above techniques.

17. Which of the following is the correct seating position for the patient during radiographic examinations when an image receptor without an external aiming device is used?
    a. Occlusal plane parallel and midsaggital plane perpendicular to the floor
    b. Occlusal plane perpendicular and midsaggital plane parallel to the floor
    c. Occlusal and midsaggital planes parallel to the floor
    d. Occlusal and midsaggital planes perpendicular to the floor

18. Which of the following is the best sequencing for exposing a full mouth series of periapical radiographs?

    a. Mandibular anteriors, maxillary anteriors, mandibular posteriors, maxillary posteriors

    b. Maxillary anteriors, mandibular anteriors, maxillary posteriors, mandibular posteriors

    c. Mandibular posteriors, maxillary posteriors, mandibular anteriors, maxillary anteriors

    d. Maxillary posteriors, mandibular posteriors, maxillary anteriors, mandibular anteriors

REFLECT—Case study

The dentist has prescribed a full mouth series of periapical and bitewing radiographs for a patient who represents with several areas of decay and a suspected abscess. This oral health care practice uses an 18-image full mouth series configuration. Consider the following and write out your answers:

1. Prepare a list of the specific periapical and bitewing radiographs you intend to expose. Include what size image receptor you will use and why, and which specific teeth must be imaged on each of the projections.

2. Which radiographic technique for exposing periapical radiographs will you choose for this exam? Why?

3. How will your patient be seated for the exposures? Why?

4. Will you be using the patient's finger or a holder to position the image receptor within the oral cavity? Explain your choice.

5. Describe how the image receptor will be positioned in relation to the teeth and how you will be directing the central ray of the x-ray beam for the specific technique you plan to use.

6. Summarize the steps you would take to locate the vertical and horizontal angulations.

7. Prepare a sequence of exposures and explain your choice.

RELATE—Laboratory application

Set up a teaching manikin or skull in the radiography operatory. Position the occlusal plane parallel to the floor and the mid-sagittal plane perpendicular to the floor. Obtain an image receptor and holder. Using Table 13-1 Standard Image Receptor Placements for Periapical Radiographs of a Full Mouth Series practice the standard image receptor placements for the periapical radiographs listed. Write out your answers to the following questions.

1. What size image receptors did you chose for each of the radiographs? List the considerations that prompted your decision.

2. Observe and describe the orientation of the image receptor in each position. Give a rationale for why the image receptor is positioned with the long dimension vertical or horizontal in different regions of the oral cavity.

3. If using intraoral film packets, where did you position the embossed dot? Why?

4. Explain the order you used to position each of the radiograph.

Next practice positioning the x-ray tube head in relation to each of the standard image receptor placements. Using the paralleling technique, determine the horizontal angulation by swiveling the tube head from side to side to direct the central rays of the x-ray beam perpendicular to the image receptor through the mean tangent of the embrasures between the teeth of interest. Determine the vertical angulation by moving the tube head up and down in the yoke to direct the central rays of the x-ray beam perpendicular to the image receptor.

5. List what teeth you used to determine where to horizontally direct the central rays of the x-ray beam for each of the standard image receptor placements. Why did you choose these teeth?

6. What error is most likely to occur if the horizontal angulation is not correctly aligned between the embrasures of the teeth of interest?

7. Observe the degrees of vertical angulation noted on the yoke of the x-ray tube head for each of the standard image receptor placements. Determine if using positive or negative angulation. Write down each of the settings.

8. Compare the vertical angulation settings you used for each of the standard image receptor placements with those noted in Table 15-2 Summary of Steps for Acquiring Periapical Radiographs–Bisecting Technique. Explain the difference between the vertical angulations you used for the paralleling technique with the vertical angulations recommended in Table 15-2 for use with the bisecting technique. What general statement can you make about the differences? Why?

REFERENCES

Eastman Kodak Company. (2002). *Successful intraoral radiography.* Rochester, NY: Author.

Rinn Corporation. (1983). *Intraoral radiography with Rinn XCP/BAI instruments.* Elgin, IL: Dentsply/Rinn Corporation.

White, S. C., & Pharoah, M. J. (2008). *Oral radiology: Principles and interpretation* (6th ed.). St. Louis: Elsevier.

The Periapical Examination—Paralleling Technique

OBJECTIVES

Following successful completion of this chapter, you should be able to:

1. Define the key words.
2. Discuss the principles of the paralleling technique.
3. List the advantages and disadvantages of the paralleling technique.
4. Identify and be able to assemble and position image receptor holders for use with the paralleling techniques.
5. Explain the importance of achieving accurate horizontal and vertical angulation in obtaining quality diagnostic radiographs using the paralleling technique.
6. Identify vertical angulation errors made when using the paralleling technique.
7. Demonstrate the image receptor positioning for maxillary and mandibular periapical exposures using the paralleling technique.

KEY WORDS

Biteblock
Embrasure
External aiming device

Film holder
Image receptor holder or positioner
Indicator ring

Introduction

Because of its ability to produce superior diagnostic quality radiographs, the paralleling technique should be the technique of choice when exposing periapical radiographs (Table 14-1). The purpose of this chapter is to present step-by-step procedures for exposing a full mouth series of periapical radiographs using the paralleling technique.

Fundamentals of Paralleling Technique

The basic principles of the paralleling technique meet the following two shadow casting principles:

- The image receptor (film packet, phosphor plate, or digital sensor) is placed parallel to the long axis of the object (tooth) being radiographed.

- The central ray of the x-ray beam is directed to intersect both the image receptor and the object (tooth) perpendicularly (Figure 14-1).

Oral structures, particularly the curvature of the palate and the outwardly inclined anterior teeth, make it difficult to place the image receptor parallel to the long axes of the teeth (Figure 14-2). The paralleling technique must achieve parallelism by placing the image receptor away from the crowns of the teeth. Parallelism is accomplished by using an **image receptor positioner** or **film holder** specifically designed to allow the patient to stabilize the image receptor in this position away from the crowns of the teeth. This position, however, does not meet the shadow cast principle that states that the image receptor (film, phosphor plate, or digital sensor) and the object (tooth) should be as close to each other as possible. To compensate for the increased object–image receptor distance needed to achieve parallelism, the target–image receptor distance should also be increased. The PID length contributes to the target–image receptor distance and satisfies the shadow cast principle that states that the object (tooth) should be as far as practical from the target

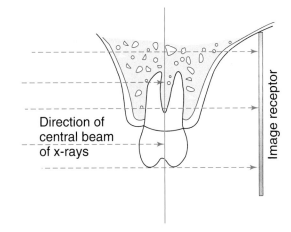

FIGURE 14-1 Paralleling technique. The x-ray beam is directed perpendicular to the recording plane of the image receptor, which has been positioned parallel to the long axis of the tooth.

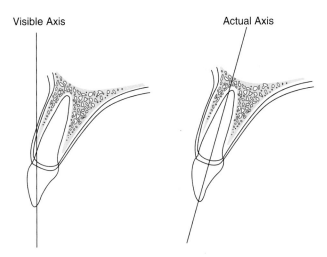

FIGURE 14-2 Visible and actual long axis of the tooth. The root portion of the tooth should be taken into consideration to accurately locate the long axis of the tooth.

TABLE 14-1	Advantages and Disadvantages of the Paralleling Technique
ADVANTAGES	**DISADVANTAGES**
• Produces images with minimal dimensional distortion. • Minimizes superimposition of adjacent structures. • Long axis of the tooth and recording plane of the image receptor can be visually located making it easier to direct the x-rays appropriately. • Many choices of image receptor holders on the market with external aiming devices specifically designed to make paralleling simple and easy to learn. • With appropriate image receptor holding devices, takes less time than trying to locate the position of an imaginary bisector. • When using a long PID (16 in./41 cm), patient radiation dose may be reduced.	• Parallel placement of the image receptor may be difficult to achieve on certain patients: children, adults with small mouths, low palatal vaults, or the presence of tori, patients with sensitive oral mucosa or an exaggerated gag reflex, edentulous regions. • These same conditions may increase patient discomfort when the image receptor impinges on oral tissues. • A short PID (8 in./20.5 cm) should not be used. The longer PID required may be more difficult to maneuver and stabilize for exposures.

Using 8 inch (20.5 cm) target-image receptor distance

Image receptor

Using 16 inch (41 cm) target-image receptor distance

Image receptor

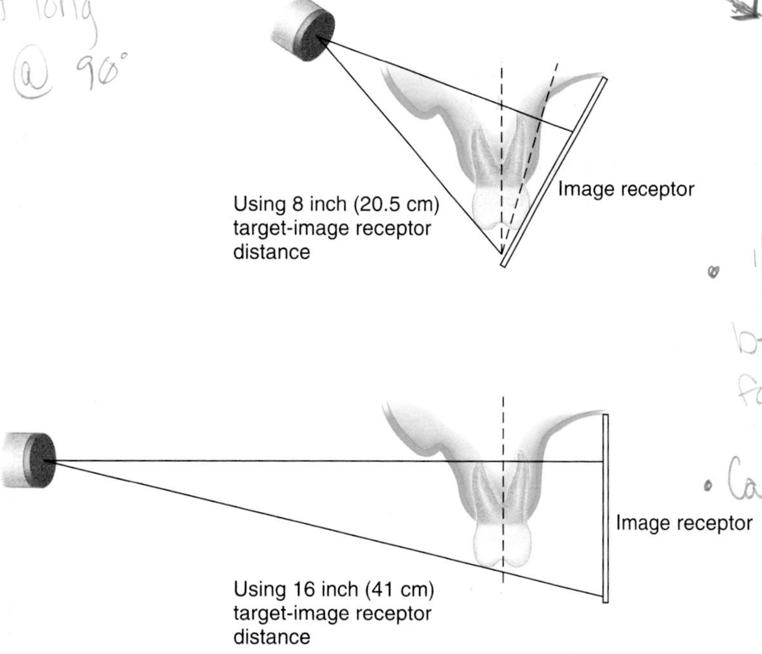

FIGURE 14-3 Comparison of the bisecting and paralleling methods.
With the bisecting technique, the image receptor is positioned adjacent to the tooth, making a target–image receptor distance of 8 in. (20.5 cm) acceptable. With the paralleling technique the image receptor is positioned near the center of the oral cavity, where it must be retained in a position parallel to the long axes of the teeth. This increased object–image receptor distance requires a longer (12 in./30 cm or 16 in./41 cm) target–image receptor distance to produce a quality radiograph.

(source of radiation). Ideally, the target–image receptor distance used with the paralleling technique is 16 in. (41 cm) or at least 12 in. (30 cm; Figure 14-3).

Holding the Periapical Image Receptor in Position

Image receptor holders designed for use with the paralleling technique usually have a long **biteblock** area for the purpose of achieving a parallel relationship between the recording plane of the image receptor and the long axes of the teeth and an L-shaped backing to help support the image receptor and keep it in position (Figure 14-4). Examples of paralleling positioners and holders are the XCP™ (which stands for Extension Cone Paralleling) for use with radiographic film (Figure 14-5) and the XCP-DS™ for use with digital sensors manufactured by Dentsply Rinn (www.rinncorp.com) and the RAPD® (which stands for Right Angle Positioning Device) manufactured by Flow Dental (www.flowdental.com; Figure 14-6). These instruments have an **external aiming device** to assist the radiographer in locating the correct angles and points of entry, making errors less likely. The external aiming device also eliminates the need to position the patient's head precisely.

It should be noted, however, that the extra size and weight of the external aiming device may make placement difficult or uncomfortable for some patients. If placement of the image

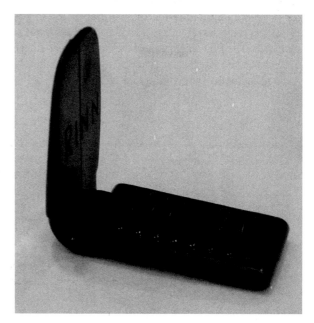

FIGURE 14-4 Paralleling image receptor holder. Anterior biteblock . The biting plane is at a right angle (90⁰) with the backing plate. The patient bites down far enough out on the bite extension to keep the image receptor and teeth parallel.

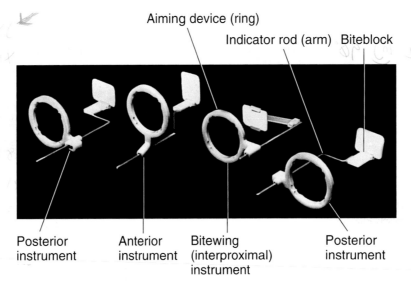

Aiming device (ring)

Indicator rod (arm) Biteblock

Posterior instrument | Anterior instrument | Bitewing (interproximal) instrument | Posterior instrument

FIGURE 14-5 **Rinn XCP™.** Note the external aiming device to assist with locating the correct angles and points of entry. The external aiming device eliminates the need to position the patient's head precisely. (Courtesy of Dentsply Rinn.)

receptor is compromised and therefore not positioned correctly, the aiming device will indicate directing the x-ray beam to the wrong place. Manufacturers have responded to the need to help reduce the size and weight of an external aiming device with products such as Dentsply Rinn's Uni-GripAR® (Figure 14-7) and Flip Ray™ (Figure 14-8). These holders with positioning arms and aiming rings are made of lightweight plastic for the purpose of improving patient comfort.

There are several image receptor positioners on the market that with slight modifications may be used with both the paralleling and the bisecting techniques. Examples include the Stabe® (Dentsply Rinn www.rinncorp.com) and the SUPA® (which stands for Single Use Positioning Aid), manufactured by Flow Dental (www.flowdental.com; Figure 14-9). These holders provide a long biteblock and L-shaped back support for use with the paralleling technique. However, the manufacturers have designed the holder with a scored groove that allows the radiographer to break off the bite extension and use the holder with the

bisecting technique as well (see Figure 13-12). The light, polystyrene single-part construction makes these holders comfortable and easy to place for most patients. However, because these positioners lack an external aiming ring, the radiographer must be skilled in estimating the correct angles and points of entry to utilize these devices. For this reason, it is important that the radiographer develop the skills necessary to evaluate image receptor placement for correctness, regardless of the holder used.

For illustration purposes, the Rinn XCP™ film holder with film packet is described and demonstrated here because its external aiming device attachment aids in directing the central ray at the teeth and image receptor perpendicularly. The Rinn XCP-ORA™ (Figure 14-10 and see Figure 13-11) may be used in the same manner while eliminating the need for multiple extension arms and rings. This holder allows the operator to insert the metal arm into color-coordinated openings in the aiming ring that match the biteblocks to accommodate placements for exposure of periapical and bitewing radiographs in all regions of

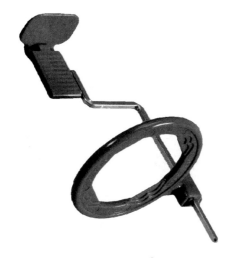

FIGURE 14-6 **Flow Dental's RAPD®.** (Courtesy of Flow Dental.)

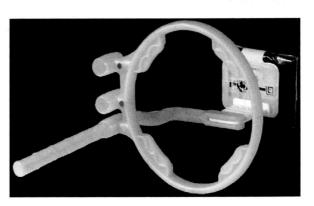

FIGURE 14-7 **Dentsply Rinn's Uni-GripAR®.** Note the wireless digital sensor image receptor. (Courtesy of Dentsply Rinn.)

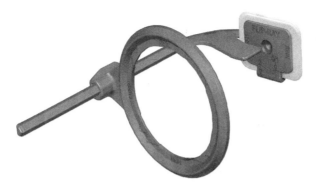

FIGURE 14-8 **Dentsply Rinn's Flip Ray™**. Note the film packet image receptor. (Courtesy of Dentsply Rinn.)

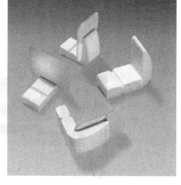

FIGURE 14-9 **Flow Dental's SUPA®**. Note the film packet image receptor. (Courtesy of Flow Dental.)

the oral cavity. Although the radiographer should refer to the manufacturer's instructions for use, important key points regarding image receptor holders with external aiming devices are:

- The patient must bite down on the biteblock as far away from the teeth as possible, utilizing the full extent of the biteblock. The exception to this rule is for the mandibular premolar and molar regions, where the image receptor can be close to the teeth and still remain parallel because of the nearly vertical position of the mandibular premolars and the slightly inward inclination of the mandibular molars (Figure 14-11).
- The patient must bite down on the biteblock firmly enough to hold the image recptor in place. A sterilized cotton roll may be placed on the opposite side of the biteblock to provide stabilization and add to patient comfort.
- The external **indicator ring** attachment must be slid all the way down the metal arm of the device to be as close to the

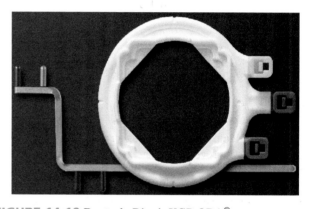

FIGURE 14-10 **Dentsply Rinn's XCP-ORA®**. (Courtesy of Dentsply Rinn.)

patient's skin as possible without touching the patient prior to the exposure.
- The open end of the PID is aligned to the indicator ring to achieve correct horizontal and vertical angulations and correct point of entry.

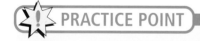

PRACTICE POINT

When using a sterile cotton roll to aid in stabilizing the image receptor, be sure that the cotton roll is placed on the opposite side from the teeth of interest. If the purpose of the radiograph is to image a maxillary tooth, the cotton roll should be placed under the biteblock so that the mandibular teeth contact the cotton roll when the patient occludes. If the purpose of the radiograph is to image a mandibular tooth, the cotton roll should be placed on top of the biteblock so that the maxillary teeth contact the cotton roll when the patient occludes. Placing the cotton roll on the biteblock on the same side as the teeth being imaged will prevent the patient from occluding all the way onto the biteblock and will result in cutting off the apices of the teeth on the image.

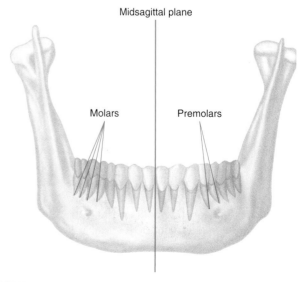

FIGURE 14-11 Long axes of the premolar and molar teeth.

Horizontal and Vertical Angulation Procedures

Horizontal Angulation

To rely on the image receptor holder's external aiming ring to accurately direct the central rays of the x-ray beam perpendicularly (at a right angle) toward the surface of the image receptor in a horizontal plane, the image receptor itself must be positioned parallel to the teeth of interest in the horizontal dimension. The image receptor must be positioned parallel to the interproximal space or **embrasure** of two predetermined teeth. The teeth selected depend on the region being radiographed. Table 14-2 lists the embrasure through which to align the image receptor and to direct the central ray for each projection. The central ray must be directed appropriately to avoid overlapping adjacent teeth on the resultant image.

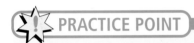

PRACTICE POINT

If the image receptor is correctly positioned parallel to the teeth of interest and the central ray is accurately directed through the appropriate embrasure and overlapping of other adjacent teeth on the image occurs, it is usually attributed to crowded or malaligned teeth. Crowded or malaligned teeth will most likely require additional exposures to achieve a clear view of all proximal surfaces (see Chapter 28).

Vertical Angulation

When utilizing the paralleling technique, the correct vertical angulation is achieved by directing the central rays of the x-ray beam perpendicular to the image receptor and perpendicular to the long axes of the teeth in the vertical plane. An image receptor holding device designed for use with the paralleling technique is used to position the image receptor parallel to the long axes of teeth so that directing the central rays perpendicular to the teeth will simultaneously direct the central rays perpendicular to the image receptor. To rely on a holder's external aiming ring to accurately direct the central ray perpendicularly (at a right angle) toward the surface of the image receptor in a vertical plane, the image receptor itself must be positioned parallel to the teeth of interest in the vertical dimension. Incorrect vertical angulation when utilizing the paralleling technique results in cutting off a portion of the area of interest from the image. When the vertical angulation is excessive (greater than perpendicular to the recording plane of the image receptor), the incisal or occlusal edges of the teeth will most likely be cut off, and when the vertical angulation is inadequate (less than perpendicular to the recording

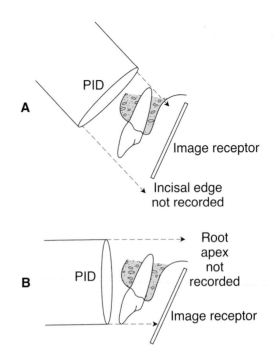

FIGURE 14-12 Vertical angulation error–paralleling technique. (A) Excessive vertical angulation results in incisal/occlusal edges being cut off the image. **(B)** Inadequate vertical angulation results in the apices being cut off the image.

plane of the image receptor), the root apices of the teeth will most likely be cut off (Figure 14-12).

Points of Entry

Point of Entry

The point of entry for directing the central ray at the image receptor when utilizing the paralleling technique for periapical radiographs may be located using the external aiming device of the image receptor positioner. Without an external indicator, care should be taken to center the image receptor within the beam of x-radiation. Use the portion of the holder, or biteblock, that extends from the oral cavity to estimate the center of the image receptor. Incorrect point of entry, or not centering the image receptor within the x-ray beam, will result in conecut error. (see Figure 18-7 and Figure 18-8)

The Periapical Examination: Paralleling Technique

Figures 14-13 through 14-20 illustrate the precise positions and the required angulations for each of the periapical radiographs in a basic 14-image full-mouth series utilizing the paralleling technique. See Table 14-2 for a summary of the four basic steps of the technique—placement, vertical angulation, horizontal angulation, and point of entry.

PERIAPICAL RADIOGRAPH	PLACEMENT	VERTICAL ANGULATION*	HORIZONTAL ANGULATION	POINT OF ENTRY
Maxillary incisors (image receptor size #1 or size #2) (Figure 14-13)	Center the image receptor to line up behind the central and lateral incisors; if using a size #2 image receptor, include the mesial halves of the canines. Align the image receptor parallel to the long axes of the incisors and parallel to the left and right central incisor embrasure.	Direct the central ray perpendicular to the plane of the image receptor and long axes of the incisors. PID will be pointing down.	Direct the central ray perpendicular to the image receptor through the left and right central incisor embrasure.	Center the image receptor within the x-ray beam by directing the central rays at the center of the image receptor.
Maxillary canine (image receptor #1 or size #2) (Figure 14-14)	Center the image receptor to line up behind the canine; include the distal half of the lateral incisor and the mesial half of the first premolar. Align the image receptor parallel to the long axes of the canines and parallel to the mesial and distal line angles of the canine.	Direct the central ray perpendicular to the plane of the image receptor and long axis of the canine. PID will be pointing down.	Direct the central ray perpendicular to the image receptor at the center of the canine.	Center the image receptor within the x-ray beam by directing the central rays at the center of the image receptor.
Maxillary premolar (image receptor #1 or size #2) (Figure 14-15) *always know where the mesial side of receptor is.*	Align the anterior edge of the image receptor to line up behind the distal half of the canine; include the first and second premolars and mesial half of the first molar. Align the image receptor parallel to the long axes of the premolars and parallel to the first and second premolar embrasure.	Direct the central ray perpendicular to the plane of the image receptor and long axes of the premolars. PID will be pointing down.	Direct the central ray perpendicular to the image receptor through the first and second premolar embrasure.	Center the image receptor within the x-ray beam by directing the central rays at the center of the image receptor.
Maxillary molar (image receptor size #2) (Figure 14-16)	Align the anterior edge of the image receptor to line up behind the distal half of the second premolar; include the first, second, and third molars. Align the image receptor parallel to the long axes of the molars and parallel to the first and second molar embrasure.	Direct the central ray perpendicular to the plane of the image receptor and long axes of the molars. PID will be pointing down.	Direct the central ray perpendicular to the image receptor through the first and second molar embrasure.	Center the image receptor within the x-ray beam by directing the central rays at the center of the image receptor.

(Continued)

TABLE 14-2 (Continued)

PERIAPICAL RADIOGRAPH	PLACEMENT	VERTICAL ANGULATION*	HORIZONTAL ANGULATION	POINT OF ENTRY
Mandibular incisors (image receptor size #1 or #2) (Figure 14-17)	Center the image receptor to line up behind the central and lateral incisors if using a size #2 image receptor; include the mesial halves of the canines. Align the image receptor parallel to the long axes of the incisors and parallel to the left and right central incisor embrasure.	Direct the central ray perpendicular to the plane of the image receptor and long axes of the incisors. PID will be pointing up.	Direct the central ray perpendicular to the image receptor through the left and right central incisor embrasure.	Center the image receptor within the x-ray beam by directing the central rays at the center of the image receptor.
Mandibular canine (image receptor size #1 or #2) (Figure 14-18)	Center the image receptor to line up behind the canine; include the distal half of the lateral incisor and the mesial half of the first premolar. Align the image receptor parallel to the long axes of the canines and parallel to the mesial and distal line angles of the canine.	Direct the central ray perpendicular to the plane of the image receptor and long axis of the canine. PID will be pointing up.	Direct the central ray perpendicular to the image receptor at the center of the canine.	Center the image receptor within the x-ray beam by directing the central rays at the center of the image receptor.
Mandibular premolar (image receptor size #2) (Figure 14-19)	Align the anterior edge of the image receptor to line up behind the distal half of the canine; include the first and second premolars and mesial half of the first molar. Align the image receptor parallel to the long axes of the premolars and parallel to the first and second premolar embrasure.	Direct the central ray perpendicular to the plane of the image receptor and long axes of the premolars. PID will be pointing up.	Direct the central ray perpendicular to the image receptor through the first and second premolar embrasure.	Center the image receptor within the x-ray beam by directing the central rays at the center of the image receptor.
Mandibular molar (image receptor size #2) (Figure 14-20)	Align the anterior edge of the image receptor to line up behind the distal half of the second premolar; include the first, second, and third molars. Align the image receptor parallel to the long axes of the molars and parallel to the first and second molar embrasure.	Direct the central ray perpendicular to the plane of the image receptor and long axes of the molars. PID will be pointing up.	Direct the central ray perpendicular to the image receptor through the first and second molar embrasure.	Center the image receptor within the x-ray beam by directing the central ray at the center of the image receptor.

*The patient must be seated in the correct position, with the occlusal plane of the arch being imaged parallel to the floor and the midsaggital plane perpendicular to the floor.

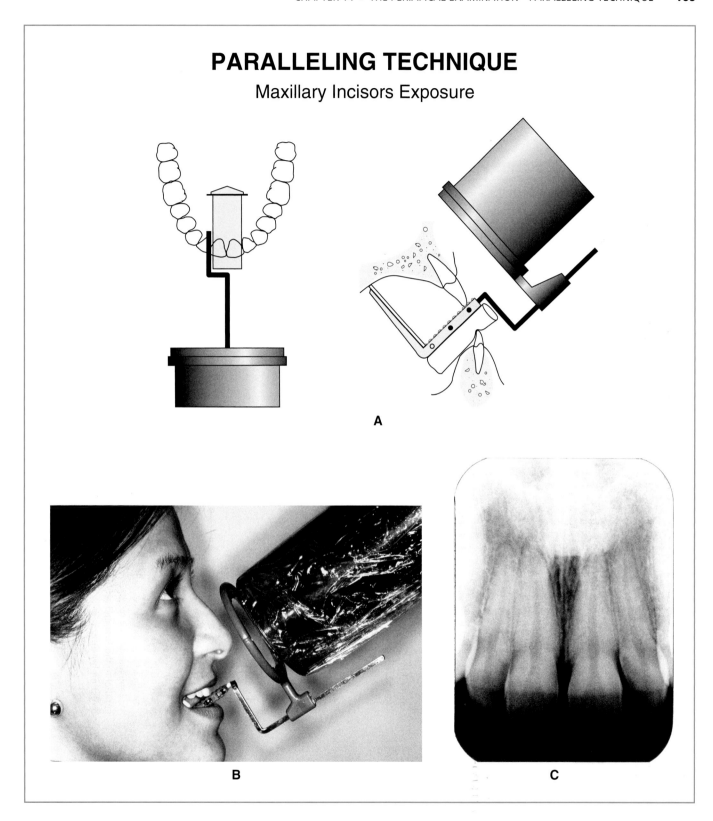

PARALLELING TECHNIQUE
Maxillary Incisors Exposure

A

B

C

FIGURE 14-13 Maxillary incisors exposure. (A) Diagrams show the relationship of the image receptor and holder, teeth, and PID. As in all anterior regions, the image receptor is positioned with the long dimension vertically. Image receptor is parallel to the teeth with the biteblock inserted to its full length to position the image receptor back toward the region of the first molars to achieve parallelism with the long axes of the incisors. A sterile cotton roll may be placed on the biteblock on the opposite side from the image receptor to help stabilize the placement. **(B)** Patient showing position of image receptor holder and 12 in. (30 cm) circular PID. **(C)** Maxillary incisors radiograph.

PARALLELING TECHNIQUE
Maxillary Canine Exposure

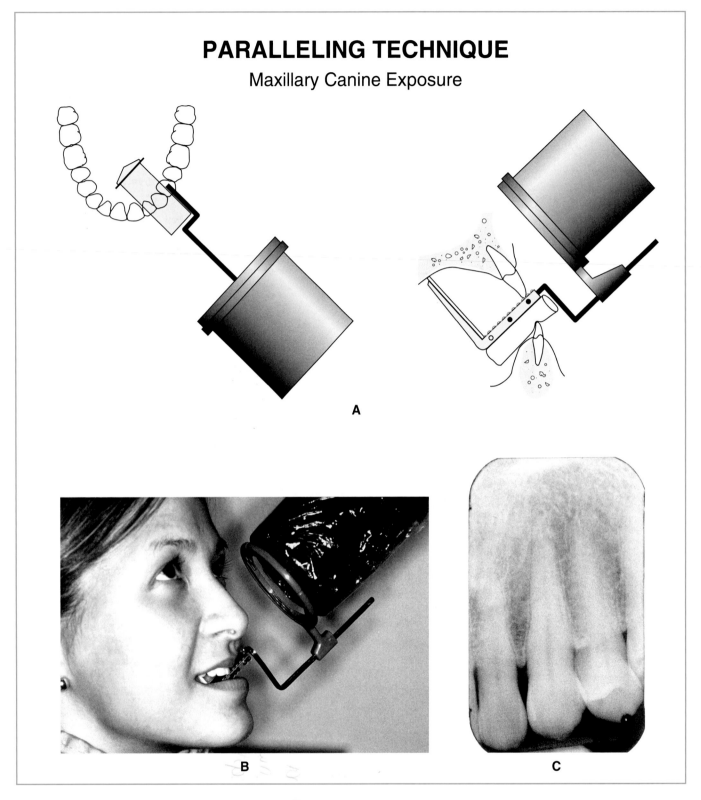

A

B

C

FIGURE 14-14 **Maxillary canine exposure.** (**A**) Diagrams show the relationship of the image receptor and holder, teeth, and PID. As in all anterior regions, the image receptor is positioned with the long dimension vertically. Image receptor is parallel to the teeth with the biteblock inserted to its full length to position the image receptor up into the midline of the palate to take advantage of the highest point and achieve parallelism with the long axis of the canine. A sterile cotton roll may be placed on the biteblock on the opposite side from the image receptor to help stabilize the placement (**B**) Patient showing position of image receptor holder and 12 in. (30 cm) circular PID. (**C**) Maxillary canine radiograph.

PARALLELING TECHNIQUE
Maxillary Premolar Exposure

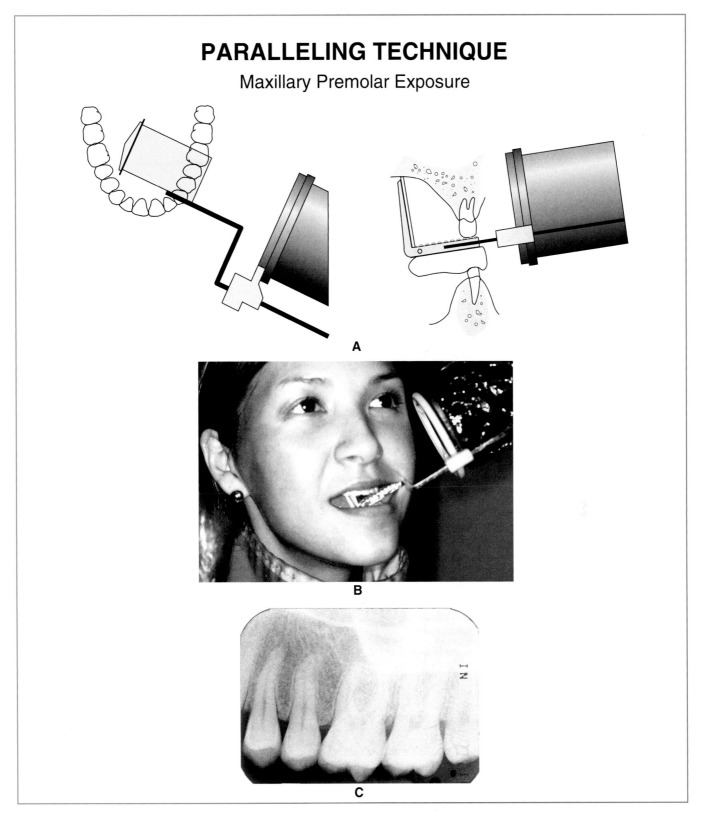

FIGURE 14-15 Maxillary premolar exposure. (A) Diagrams show the relationship of image receptor and holder, teeth, and PID. As in all posterior regions, the image receptor is positioned with the long dimension horizontally. Image receptor is parallel to the teeth with the biteblock inserted to its full length to position the image receptor up into the midline of the palate to take advantage of the highest point and achieve parallelism with the long axes of the premolars. A sterile cotton roll may be placed on the biteblock on the opposite side from the image receptor to help stabilize the placement. **(B)** Patient showing position of image receptor holder and 12 in. (30 cm) circular PID. **(C)** Maxillary premolar radiograph.

PARALLELING TECHNIQUE
Maxillary Molar Exposure

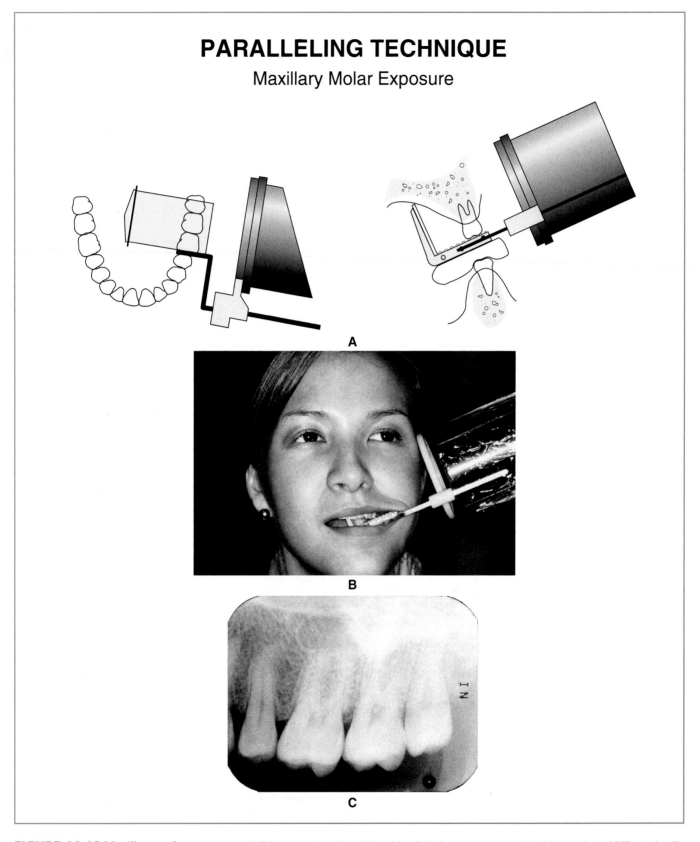

A

B

C

FIGURE 14-16 **Maxillary molar exposure.** (**A**) Diagrams show the relationship of the image receptor and holder, teeth, and PID. As in all posterior regions, the image receptor is positioned with the long dimension horizontally. Image receptor is parallel to the teeth with the biteblock inserted to its full length to position the image receptor up into the midline of the palate to take advantage of the highest point and achieve parallelism with the long axes of the molars. A sterile cotton roll may be placed on the biteblock on the opposite side from the image receptor to help stabilize the placement. (**B**) Patient showing position of image receptor holder and 12 in. (30 cm) circular PID. (**C**) Maxillary molar radiograph.

PARALLELING TECHNIQUE
Mandibular Incisors Exposure

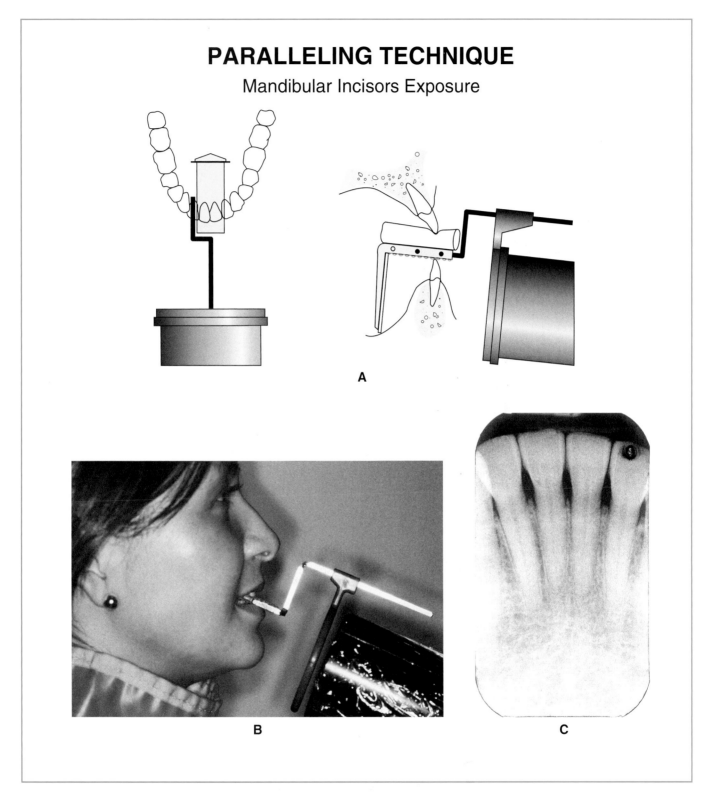

FIGURE 14-17 Mandibular incisors exposure. (A) Diagrams show the relationship of the image receptor and holder, teeth and PID. As in all anterior regions, the image receptor is positioned with the long dimension vertically. Image receptor is parallel to the teeth. A sterile cotton roll may be placed on the biteblock on the opposite side from the image receptor to help stabilize the placement. This will aid in forcing the biteblock down into position when the opposing teeth occlude. **(B)** Patient showing position of image receptor holder and 12 in. (30 cm) circular PID. **(C)** Mandibular incisors radiograph.

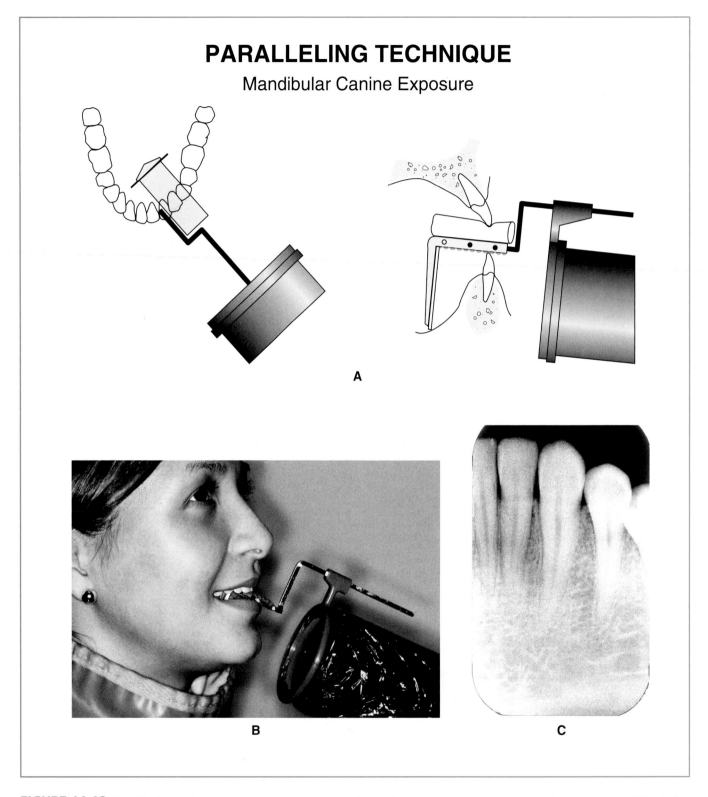

PARALLELING TECHNIQUE
Mandibular Canine Exposure

A

B

C

FIGURE 14-18 **Mandibular canine exposure.** (**A**) Diagrams show the relationship of the image receptor and holder, teeth, and PID. As in all anterior regions, the image receptor is positioned with the long dimension vertically. Image receptor is parallel to the teeth. A sterile cotton roll may be placed on the biteblock on the opposite side from the image receptor to help stabilize the placement. This will aid in forcing the biteblock down into position when the opposing teeth occlude. (**B**) Patient showing position of image receptor holder and 12 in. (30 cm) circular PID. (**C**) Mandibular canine radiograph.

PARALLELING TECHNIQUE
Mandibular Premolar Exposure

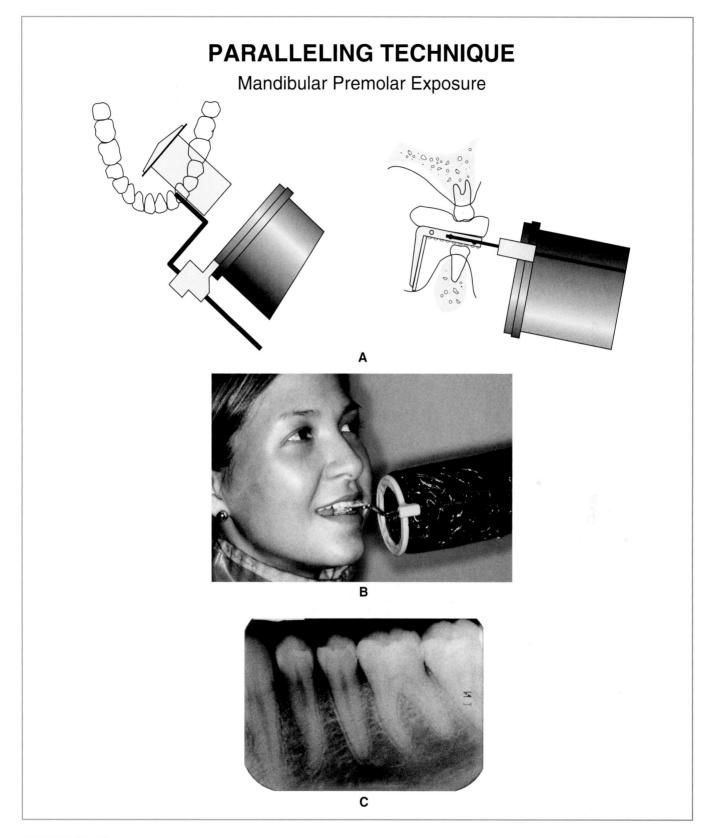

A

B

C

FIGURE 14-19 **Mandibular premolar exposure. (A)** Diagrams show the relationship of the image receptor and holder, teeth, and PID. As in all posterior regions, the image receptor is positioned with the long dimension horizontally. Image receptor is parallel to the teeth. A sterile cotton roll may be placed on the biteblock on the opposite side from the image receptor to help stabilize the placement. This will aid in forcing the biteblock down into position when the opposing teeth occlude. **(B)** Patient showing position of image receptor holder and 12 in. (30 cm) circular PID. **(C)** Mandibular premolar radiograph.

PARALLELING TECHNIQUE
Mandibular Molar Exposure

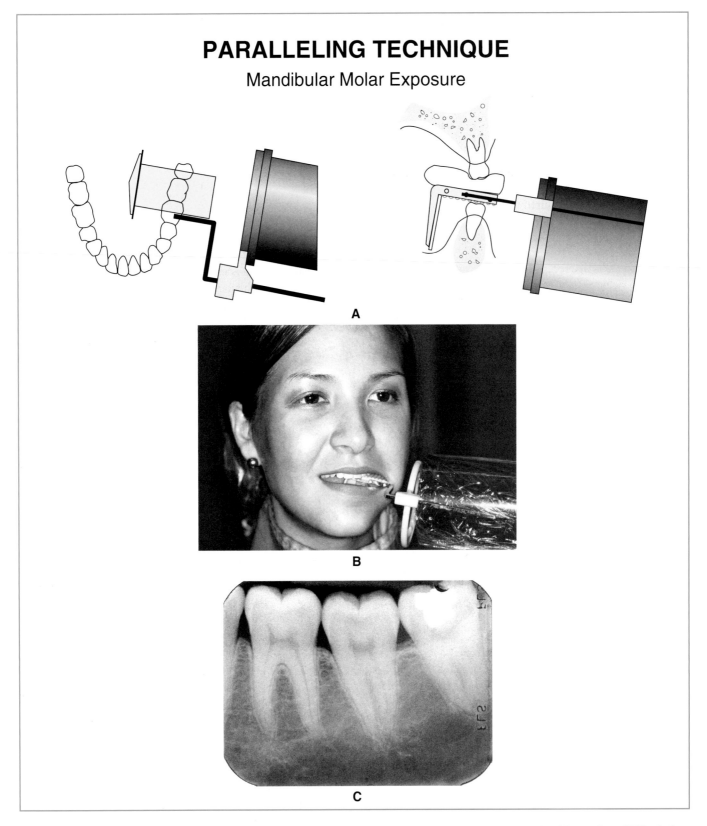

A

B

C

FIGURE 14-20 Mandibular molar exposure. (**A**) Diagrams show the relationship of the image receptor and holder, teeth, and PID. As in all posterior regions, the image receptor is positioned with the long dimension horizontally. Image receptor is parallel to the teeth. A sterile cotton roll may be placed on the biteblock on the opposite side from the image receptor to help stabilize the placement. This will aid in forcing the biteblock down into position when the opposing teeth occlude. (**B**) Patient showing position of image receptor holder and 12 in. (30 cm) circular PID. (**C**) Mandibular molar radiograph.

REVIEW—Chapter summary

The paralleling technique is the technique of choice when exposing periapical radiographs because of its ability to produce superior diagnostic-quality radiographs. The paralleling technique satisfies two key shadow casting principles—the image receptor is placed parallel to the long axes of the teeth, and the central ray of the x-ray beam is directed perpendicular to both the recording plane of the image receptor and the long axes of the teeth. A long PID (16 in/41 cm or 12 in/30 cm) compensates for the increased distance between the image receptor and the teeth required to achieve parallelism. A disadvantage of the paralleling technique is that a parallel object–image receptor relationship may be difficult to achieve on some patients.

Because the image receptor must be positioned farther from the teeth to achieve parallelism, a holding device with a long biteblock and L-shaped backing is required. Image receptor holders are designed for use with the paralleling or the bisecting technique or may be modified to use with both techniques. A holder with an external aiming device will assist in determining the correct horizontal and vertical angulations and with determining the precise point of entry. To rely on the holder's external aiming ring, the image receptor must be positioned parallel to the long axes of the teeth (in the vertical dimension) and parallel to the embrasure of two predetermined teeth (in the horizontal dimension).

If a holder without an external aiming device is used, the horizontal angulation is determined by directing the central ray of the x-beam perpendicular to the recording plane of the image receptor through the mean tangent of the embrasures between the teeth of interest, and the vertical angulation is determined by directing the central ray of the x-beam perpendicular to the long axes of the teeth and perpendicular to the recording plane of the image receptor. The point of entry is determined by using that portion of the biteblock that extends beyond the oral cavity to direct the central ray of the x-ray beam to the center of the image receptor.

The four basic steps to exposing a periapical radiograph are placement, vertical angulation, horizontal angulation, and point of entry. Step-by-step illustrated instructions for exposing a full mouth series of periapical radiographs utilizing the paralleling techniques are presented.

RECALL—Study questions

1. What shadow casting principle is NOT likely to be met when utilizing the paralleling technique?
   a. Radiation should strike the object (tooth) and image receptor perpendicularly.
   b. Object (tooth) should be as far as practical from the target (source of radiation).
   c. Object (tooth) and image receptor should be parallel to each other.
   d. Object (tooth) and image receptor should be as close as possible to each other.

2. To compensate for the increased object–image receptor distance needed to achieve parallelism, the target–image receptor distance should be
   a. increased.
   b. decreased.

3. Which of the following is NOT an advantage of the paralleling technique?
   a. Produces images with minimal dimensional distortion
   b. Minimizes superimposition of adjacent structures
   c. Satisfies more shadow casting principles
   d. Easy technique for children

4. The most important reason for using a holder when utilizing the paralleling technique is to stabilize the image receptor in a position
   a. at a right angle to the teeth.
   b. perpendicular to the teeth.
   c. parallel to the teeth.
   d. parallel to the bisector.

5. Film holders designed for use with the paralleling technique should have a
   a. short biteblock and L-shaped backing.
   b. long biteblock and L-shaped backing.
   c. short biteblock and no backing.
   d. long biteblock and no backing.

6. Which of the following is an example of a holder that can be used with both the paralleling and the bisecting techniques?
   a. SUPA®
   b. Uni-GripAR®
   c. XCP™
   d. Flip Ray™

7. Each of the following is a part of the assembled XCP® holder EXCEPT one. Which one is the EXCEPTION?
   a. Metal arm
   b. Indicator ring
   c. Long biteblock
   d. 105-degree angled backing

8. Lining the image receptor up behind the distal half of the canine to include the first and second premolars and mesial half of the first molar describes the placement for which of the following periapical radiographs?
   a. Central incisors
   b. Canine
   c. Premolar
   d. Molar

9. To determine the horizontal angulation for the maxillary molar periapical radiograph, the central rays of the x-ray beam should be directed at the image receptor perpendicularly through the embrasures of the
   a. first and second molars.
   b. second premolar and first molar.
   c. first and second premolars.
   d. canine and first premolar.

10. To determine the horizontal angulation for the mandibular premolar periapical radiograph, the central rays of the x-ray beam should be directed at the image receptor perpendicularly through the embrasures of the

    a. first and second molars.
    b. second premolar and first molar.
    c. first and second premolars.
    d. canine and first premolar.

11. Directing the central rays perpendicular to the plane of the image receptor and perpendicular to the long axes of the teeth describes which step of the paralleling technique?

    a. Placement
    b. Vertical angulation
    c. Horizontal angulation
    d. Point of entry

12. Cutting off the root apex portion of the image on a periapical radiograph results from

    a. excessive horizontal angulation.
    b. inadequate horizontal angulation.
    c. excessive vertical angulation.
    d. inadequate vertical angulation.

REFLECT—Case study

You have recently accepted a position in a general practice dental office. This week you discovered that the image receptor holding device for exposing a full mouth survey is the one pictured in Figure 14-9. You have always used the film-holding device pictured in Figures 14-13 through 14-20, and the new holder is unfamiliar to you. Based on what you have learned about image receptor holders designed for use with the paralleling technique, answer the following questions:

1. Which technique is the new holder designed to be used with? How can you tell?
2. How is the new holder similar to the one you have been using? Different?
3. Which holder would it be best to know how to use? Why?
4. What are the advantages/disadvantages of the new holder?
5. What are the advantages/disadvantages of the holder you have been using?
6. What is your recommendation for the practice? Should they continue to use this holder, or should they purchase the holder you are familiar with? Explain your answers.

RELATE—Laboratory application

For a comprehensive laboratory practice exercise on this topic, see Thomson, E. M. (2012). *Exercises in oral radiography techniques: A laboratory manual* (3rd ed.). Upper Saddle River, NJ: Pearson Education. Chapter 4, "Periapical radiographs—paralleling technique."

REFERENCES

Eastman Kodak Company. (2002). *Successful intraoral radiography.* Rochester, NY: Author.

Rinn Corporation. (1983). *Intraoral radiography with Rinn XCP/BAI instruments.* Elgin, IL: Dentsply/Rinn Corporation.

White, S. C., & Pharoah, M. J. (2008). *Oral radiology: Principles and interpretation* (6th ed.). St. Louis, MO: Elsevier.

The Periapical Examination—Bisecting Technique

OBJECTIVES

Following successful completion of this chapter, you should be able to:

1. Define the key words.
2. Discuss the principles of the bisecting technique.
3. List the advantages and disadvantages of the bisecting technique.
4. Identify and be able to assemble and position image receptor holders for use with the bisecting technique and distinguish these holders from those used with the paralleling technique.
5. Explain the importance of achieving accurate horizontal and vertical angulation in obtaining quality diagnostic radiographs using the bisecting technique.
6. List the recommended predetermined vertical angulation settings used with the bisecting technqiue.
7. Identify vertical angulation errors made when using the bisecting technique.
8. Locate facial landmarks used for determining the points of entry used with the bisecting technqiue.
9. Demonstrate image receptor positioning for maxillary and mandibular periapical exposures using the bisecting technique.

KEY WORDS

Ala
Bisector
Biteblock
Bite extension
Elongated image
Embrasure
Film holder

Foreshortened image
Horizontal angulation
Image receptor holder or positioner
Isometric triangle
Mean tangent
Symphysis
Vertical angulation

Introduction

Because it satisfies fewer shadow cast principles (see Chapter 13), the bisecting technique is less likely to produce superior diagnostic quality radiographs. However, some situations and conditions make the use of the paralleling technique difficult. When irregularities or obstructions of the oral tissues and the curvature of the palate prevent a parallel image receptor to long axes of the teeth placement, an acceptable diagnostic-quality radiograph may be obtained utilizing the bisecting technique (Table 15-1). The radiographer who possesses a working knowledge of both the paralleling and the bisecting techniques will be prepared to meet and overcome conditions that challenge the ability to produce diagnostic radiographs. Although the bisecting technique is not recommended because images produced contain inherent dimensional distortion, careful attention to the steps of the technique can produce acceptable results when needed. The purpose of this chapter is to present step-by-step procedures for exposing a full mouth series of periapical radiographs using the bisecting technique.

Fundamentals of Bisecting Technique

The bisecting principle is applied when the image receptor is not, or cannot, be placed parallel to the long axes of the teeth. This is often the case with children, with adults who have a shallow palatal vault or a large torus present, or when edentulous regions exist. If the image receptor is not positioned parallel to the long axes of teeth, it will not be possible to direct the central ray appropriately perpendicular to the long axes of the teeth simultaneously with perpendicular to the plane of the image receptor. To cast an accurate shadow representation of a tooth onto the image receptor, the angle formed by the long axis of the tooth and the plane of the image receptor must be bisected. One must first find the long axis of the tooth and then find the long axis of the image receptor as it is placed next to the tooth. After visualizing these two planes, one must imagine a line, called the **bisector,** which bisects the angle where the long axis of the tooth and the long axis of the image receptor plane meet. The central ray of the x-ray beam is directed perpendicular to this imaginary bisector (Figure 15-1).

Theoretically, two **isometric triangles** (triangles having equal measurements) are formed when the central ray is directed perpendicular to the bisector, and the image that results should

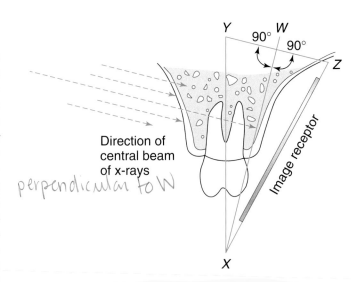

W = bisector

perpendicular to W

FIGURE 15-1 Rule of isometry applied to the bisecting technique. Line *XY* passes through the long axis of the tooth while the image receptor is positioned along line *XZ*. The central beam of radiation is directed perpendicularly through the apical area of the tooth toward the bisector *XW*. Because triangles *WXY* and *WXZ* are equal, the shadow image cast on the image receptor will be approximately equal to the length of the actual tooth, provided that the bisector line is correctly estimated.

be the same size as the tooth. In practice, this does not always happen (Figure 15-2 and see Figure 4-13). The diagnostic quality of the image is usually compromised, with some dimensional distortion that is inherent in the bisecting technique.

TARGET–IMAGE RECEPTOR DISTANCE Because the long axis of the tooth and the plane of the image receptor are not parallel, a shorter target–image receptor distance will limit magnification and distortion. The shorter 8-in. (20.5-cm) PID facilitates a shorter target–image receptor distance and is generally preferred for use with the bisecting technique. Whereas the paralleling technique is better matched with a longer target–image receptor distance, typically a 12-in. (30-cm) or ideally a 16-in. (41-cm) PID to compensate for the greater object–image receptor distance, the bisecting technique should be matched with a shorter target—image receptor distance, typically an 8-in. (20.5-cm) PID, to compensate for the lack of parallelism between the long axis of the tooth and the plane of the image receptor.

TABLE 15-1 Advantages and Disadvantages of the Bisecting Technique

ADVANTAGES	DISADVANTAGES
• Image receptor placement may be easier with certain patients: children, adults with small mouths, low palatal vaults, or the presence of tori, patients with sensitive oral mucosa or an exaggerated gag reflex, edentulous regions. • A short PID (8 in/20.5 cm) may be used. (Some operators find a short PID easier to maneuver.)	• Produces images with dimensional distortion. (Some elongation or foreshortening will occur even when the technique is performed correctly.) • Often superimposes adjacent structures. (The necessary vertical angle increase often causes a shadow of the zygomatic process of the maxilla to be superimposed over the molar roots in the maxillary regions.) • Estimating the location of the imaginary bisector may be difficult. • When using a short PID (8 in/20.5 cm), patient radiation dose may be increased.

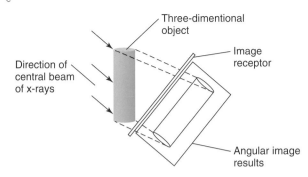

Three-dimentional object

Image receptor

Direction of central beam of x-rays

Angular image results

FIGURE 15-2 **Dimensional distortion** is inherent to the bisecting technique. When the image receptor is not positioned parallel to the object, the part of the object farthest from the image receptor is projected in an incorrect relationship to the parts closest to the image receptor. This occurs when a three-dimensional object, such as the tooth, is projected onto a two-dimensional surface, creating an angular relationship between the object and the image receptor. *Unequal magnification (80 or size) of an image in different areas*

PRACTICE POINT

To aid in estimating the imaginary bisector, utilize the two *visible* planes: the teeth and the image receptor. Looking at the teeth, locate the long axes. Then align the x-ray beam to intersect the long axes of the teeth perpendicularly. Study the PID and make a mental note of this angle. Next look at the image receptor. Note the plane of the image receptor as it is placed against the teeth. Then shift the PID so that the x-ray beam is aligned to intersect the plane of the image receptor perpendicularly. Note this angle while recalling the angle at which the x-ray beam intersected the long axes of the teeth. If you need to, repeat this process, shifting the PID to allow the x-ray beam to intersect the long axes of the teeth and then the image receptor plane perpendicularly until you can estimate a position halfway in between these two angles. This halfway point is the imaginary bisector.

OBJECT–IMAGE RECEPTOR DISTANCE It is important to note that when the image receptor is placed close to the teeth in both the anterior and the posterior regions of the maxilla and in the anterior region of the mandible, the bisecting technique must be utilized to compensate for the lack of parallelism between the image receptor and the long axes of the teeth. However, the mandibular posterior region, which includes the molars and premolars, is the exception to this generalization. If oral conditions present that allow for placement of the image receptor close to the teeth in these regions a parallel relationship may indeed result, and the paralleling technique may be used successfully (see Figure 14-11).

Holding the Periapical Image Receptor in Position

Image receptor holders or **positioners** designed for use with the bisecting technique will most likely have a short **biteblock.** Typically, a shorter biteblock or a holder that lacks the L-shaped support backing is considered an image receptor positioner better suited for use with the bisecting technique. The use of holders of this type allows the image receptor to be placed close to the lingual surface of the teeth and therefore not parallel to the long axes of the teeth. Examples of holders designed for use with the bisecting technique are the Snap-A-Ray® (manufactured by Dentsply Rinn www.rinncorp.com) and the Wing-A-Ray™ (manufactured by steri-shield www.steri-shield.com) both for use with radiographic film, phosphor plates, or digital sensors; Figure 15-3 and Figure 15-4).

As noted in Chapter 13, paralleling image receptor positioners are available that can be slightly modified for use with the bisecting technique. The **bite extension** of the Stabe® (Dentsply Rinn www.rinncorp.com) and the SUPA® (which stands for Single Use Positioning Aid) manufactured by Flow Dental (www.flowdental.com) that is needed for use with the

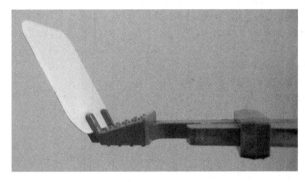

FIGURE 15-3 **Snap-A-Ray® image receptor holder.** The short biteblock and 105°; angled backing indicate that this holder be paired with the bisecting technique. Note the film packet image receptor.

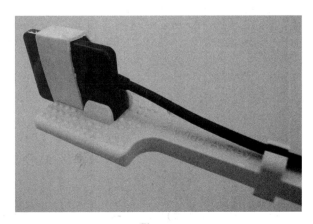

FIGURE 15-4 **Wing-A-Ray™ image receptor holder.** The short biteblock and lack of L-shaped backing indicate that this holder be paired with the bisecting technique. Note the digital sensor image receptor.

paralleling technique may be broken off for use with the bisecting technique (see Figure 13-12). Dentsply Rinn offers a bite-block with a raised platform and a 105-degree backing plate (Figure 15-5), called the BAI® (which stands for Bisecting Angle Instrument), for use with the positioning arm and aiming ring of the XCP® (which stands for Extension Cone Paralleling; see Figure 13-13). Replacing the 90-degree biteblock of the XCP® with the 105-degree biteblock of the BAI® converts this paralleling image receptor-holder into one that can be used with the bisecting technique.

Because of the variety of film, phosphor plate, and digital sensor holders available currently and that continue to come to market, it is important that the radiographer possess a working knowledge of the bisecting technique to better match the holder with the technique for optimal results.

For illustration purposes, the Rinn Stabe® **film holder** with film packet is described and demonstrated here. Its light-weight construction and small size allow for ease in placing the image receptor when the patient presents with conditions that make parallel image receptor placement difficult. Although the radiographer should refer to the manufacturer's instructions for use, important key points regarding this type of image receptor holder are:

- The patient should bite down on the biteblock as close to the teeth as necessary. This will most likely not position the image receptor parallel to the long axes of the teeth. The exception to this rule is for the mandibular premolar and molar regions, where the image receptor can be close to the teeth and still remain parallel because of the nearly vertical position of the mandibular premolars and the slightly inward inclination of the mandibular molars (see Figures 14-2 and 14-11).

- The patient must bite down on the biteblock firmly enough to hold the image receptor in place. A sterilized cotton roll may be placed on the opposite side of the biteblock to provide stabilization and add to patient comfort.

- Using the long axes of the teeth and the plane of the image receptor, the radiographer must determine the correct vertical angle and direct the central ray perpendicular to the imaginary bisector, adjusting the PID accordingly. If the patient is seated correctly with the midsaggital plane perpendicular to the floor and the occlusal plane parallel to the floor, predetermined vertical anglation settings may be used.

- Using the teeth contact points and the plane of the image receptor, the radiographer must determine the correct horizontal angle and direct the central ray perpendicular through the embrasures of the teeth of interest adjusting the PID accordingly.

- The radiographer must determine the correct point of entry and direct the central ray at the apices of the teeth of interest. If the patient is seated correctly with the midsaggital plane perpendicular to the floor and the occlusal plane parallel to the floor, predetermined anatomical landmarks may be used through which to direct the central ray of the x-ray beam.

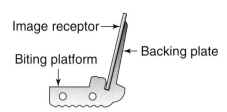

FIGURE 15-5 Bisecting technique image receptor holder. Anterior biteblock of BAI®. The backing plate is at a 105° angle with the short biteblock allowing for close placement of the image receptor to the teeth. (Courtesy of Dentsply Rinn.)

To limit magnification and distortion that results from lack of parallelism between the long axes of the teeth and the plane of the image receptor when using the bisecting technique, the target–image receptor distance is decreased to an 8-in. (30-cm) PID.

Horizontal and Vertical Angulation Procedures

Horizontal Angulation

The steps for determining correct horizontal angulation are the same for both the bisecting and paralleling techniques. First, the image receptor must be positioned parallel to the interproximal space, or **embrasure,** of two predetermined teeth. Then the **horizontal angulation** is achieved by directing the central ray of the x-ray beam perpendicular to the **mean tangent,** or curvature of the arch, through the contact points of these teeth (Table 15-2).

Vertical Angulation

With the bisecting technique the central ray of the x-ray beam can not be directed perpendicular to both the long axes of the teeth and the plane of the image receptor simultaneously. When utilizing the bisecting technique, the correct **vertical angulation** is achieved by directing the central ray of the x-ray beam perpendicular to the imaginary **bisector** between the long axes of the teeth and the plane of the image receptor. If the patient is seated with the head positioning correct, the occlusal plane parallel to the floor, and the midsaggital plane perpendicular to the floor, predetermined vertical settings may be utilized to position the PID at the correct vertical angulation (Table 15-2). It is important to check that the occlusal plane of the arch being imaged is parallel to the floor. Incorrect vertical angulation when utilizing the bisecting technique results in an image that appears elongated or foreshortened. When the vertical angulation is excessive (greater than perpendicular to the imaginary bisector) a **foreshortened image** will result, and when the vertical angulation is inadequate (less than perpendicular to the imaginary bisector), the result is an **elongated image** (Figure 15-6). Vertical angulation error is explained in Chapter 18.

TABLE 15-2   Summary of Steps for Acquiring Periapical Radiographs—Bisecting Technique

PERIAPICAL RADIOGRAPH	PLACEMENT	VERTICAL ANGULATION*	HORIZONTAL ANGULATION	POINT OF ENTRY*
Maxillary incisors (image receptor size #1 or size #2) (Figure 15-8)	Center the image receptor to line up behind the central and lateral incisors; if using a size #2 image receptor, include the mesial halves of the canines. Place the image receptor as close as possible to the lingual surfaces of the incisors, parallel to the left and right central incisor embrasure.	Direct the central ray toward the imaginary bisector between the long axes of the incisors and the plane of the image receptor in the vertical dimension at +40°.	Direct the central ray perpendicular to the image receptor through the left and right central incisor embrasure.	Center the image receptor within the x-ray beam by directing the central ray at a point near the tip of the nose. (Figure 14-7 maxillary point #1)
Maxillary canine (image receptor size #1 or size #2) (Figure 15-9)	Center the image receptor to line up behind the canine; include the distal half of the lateral incisor and the mesial half of the first premolar. Place the image receptor as close as possible to the lingual surface of the canine, parallel to the mesial and distal line angles of the canine.	Direct the central ray toward the imaginary bisector between the long axis of the canine and the plane of the image receptor in the vertical dimension at +45°.	Direct the central ray perpendicular to the image receptor at the center of the canine.	Center the image receptor within the x-ray beam by directing the central ray at the root of the canine, at the ala of the nose. (Figure 14-7 maxillary point #2)
Maxillary premolar (image receptor size #2) (Figure 15-10)	Align the anterior edge of the image receptor to line up behind the distal half of the canine; include the first and second premolars and mesial half of the first molar. Place the image receptor as close as possible to the lingual surfaces of the premolars, parallel to the first and second premolar embrasure.	Direct the central ray toward the imaginary bisector between the long axes of the premolars and the plane of the image receptor in the vertical dimension at +30°.	Direct the central ray perpendicular to the image receptor through the first and second premolar embrasure.	Center the image receptor within the x-ray beam by directing the central ray at a point on the ala–tragus line directly below the pupil of the eye. (Figure 14-7 maxillary point #3)
Maxillary molar (image receptor size #2) (Figure 15-11)	Align the anterior edge of the image receptor to line up behind the distal half of the second premolar; include the first, second, and third molars. Place the image receptor as close as possible to the lingual surfaces of the molars, parallel to the first and second molar embrasure.	Direct the central ray toward the imaginary bisector between the long axes of the molars and the plane of the image receptor in the vertical dimension at +20°.	Direct the central ray perpendicular to the image receptor through the first and second molar embrasure.	Center the image receptor within the x-ray beam by directing the center ray at a point on the ala–tragus line directly below the outer canthus of the eye. (Figure 14-7 maxillary point #4)

(Continued)

TABLE 15-2 (Continued)

PERIAPICAL RADIOGRAPH	PLACEMENT	VERTICAL ANGULATION*	HORIZONTAL ANGULATION	POINT OF ENTRY*
Mandibular incisors (image receptor size #1 or #2) (Figure 15-12)	Center the image receptor to line up behind the central and lateral incisors; if using a size #2 image receptor, include the mesial halves of the canines. Place the image receptor as close as possible to the lingual surfaces of the incisors, parallel to the left and right central incisor embrasure.	Direct the central ray toward the imaginary bisector between the long axes of the incisors and the plane of the image receptor in the vertical dimension at −15°.	Direct the central ray perpendicular to the image receptor through the left and right central incisor embrasure.	Center the image receptor within the x-ray beam by directing the central ray at a point in the middle of the chin (symphysis), 1 in. (2.5 cm) above the lower border of the mandible. (Figure 14-7 mandibular point #1)
Mandibular canine (image receptor size #1 or #2) (Figure 15-13)	Center the image receptor to line up behind the canine; include the distal half of the lateral incisor and the mesial half of the first premolar. Place the image receptor as close as possible to the lingual surfaces of the canine, parallel to the mesial and distal line angles of the canine.	Direct the central ray toward the imaginary bisector between the long axis of the canine and the plane of the image receptor in the vertical dimension at −20°.	Direct the central ray perpendicular to the image receptor at the center of the canine.	Center the image receptor within the x-ray beam by directing the central ray at the center of the root of the canine, 1 in. (2.5 cm) above the inferior border of the mandible. (Figure 14-7 mandibular point #2)
Mandibular premolar (image receptor size #2) (Figure 15-14)	Align the anterior edge of the image receptor to line up behind the distal half of the canine; include the first and second premolars and mesial half of the first molar. Place the image receptor as close as possible to the lingual surfaces of the premolars, parallel to the first and second premolar embrasure.	Direct the central ray toward the imaginary bisector between the long axes of the premolar and the plane of the image receptor in the vertical dimension at −10°.	Direct the central ray perpendicular to the image receptor through the first and second premolar embrasure.	Center the image receptor within the x-ray beam by directing the central ray at a point on the chin, 1 in. (2.5 cm) above the border of the mandible, directly inferior to the pupil of the eye. (Figure 14-7 mandibular point #3)
Mandibular molar (image receptor size #2) (Figure 15-15)	Align the anterior edge of the image receptor to line up behind the distal half of the second premolar; include the first, second, and third molars. Place the image receptor as close as possible to the lingual surfaces of the molars, parallel to the first and second molar embrasure.	Direct the central ray toward the imaginary bisector between the long axes of the molars and the plane of the image receptor in the vertical dimension at −5°.	Direct the central ray perpendicular to the image receptor through the first and second molar embrasure.	Center the image receptor within the x-ray beam by directing the central ray at a point on the center of the chin 1 in. (2.5 cm) above the lower border of the mandible, directly below the outer canthus of the eye. (Figure 14-7 mandibular point #4)

* The patient must be seated in the correct position, with the occlusal plane of the arch being imaged parallel to the floor and the midsaggital plane perpendicular to the floor.

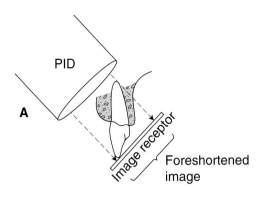

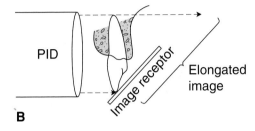

FIGURE 15-6 Vertical angulation error—bisecting technique. (**A**) Excessive vertical angulation results in a foreshortened image. (**B**) Inadequate vertical angulation results in an elongated image.

FIGURE 15-7 Points of entry. Facial landmarks can provide the radiographer with a reference for positioning the PID and directing the central ray of the x-ray beam. The patient must be seated upright with the midsagittal plane perpendicular to the floor and the occlusal plane parallel to the floor to use these landmarks accurately. Note the numbers that indicate the points of entry for each of the projections listed in Table 15-2.

Points of Entry

The image receptor must be centered within the beam of x-radiation to avoid conecut error. The central ray of the x-ray beam should be directed through the apices of the teeth of interest. When utilizing the bisecting technique, if the patient is seated with the correct head position, the point of entry may be estimated with the use of recommended landmarks (Table 15-2; Figure 15-7).

The Periapical Examination: Bisecting Technique

Figures 15-8 through 15-15 illustrate the precise image receptor positions and the required angulations for each of the periapical radiographs in a basic 14-film full mouth series utilizing the bisecting technique. See Table 15-2 for a summary of the four basic steps of the technique—placement, vertical angulation, horizontal angulation, and point of entry.

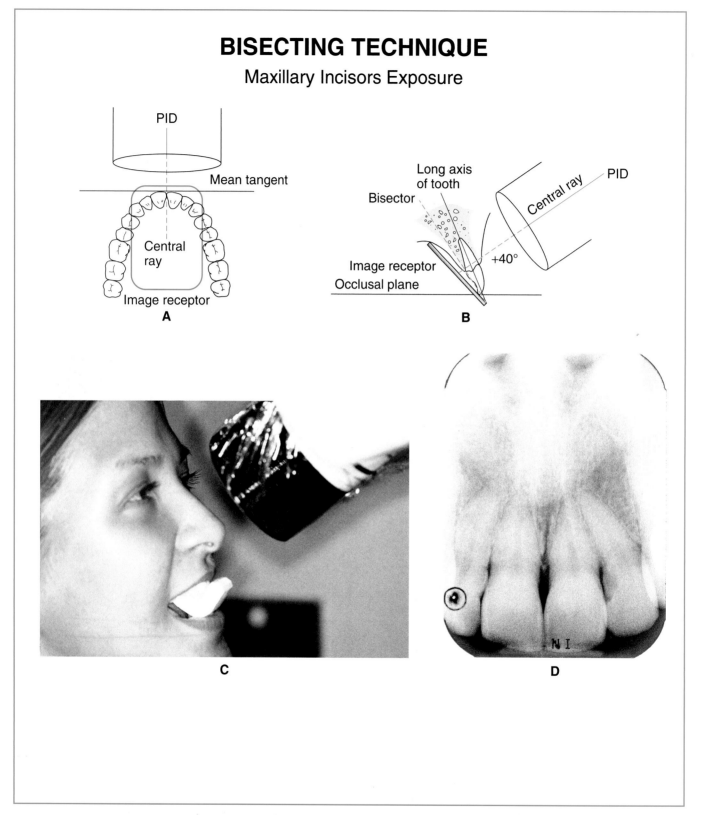

BISECTING TECHNIQUE
Maxillary Incisors Exposure

FIGURE 15-8 Maxillary incisors exposure. (A) Diagram shows horizontal angulation is directed through the central incisors embrasure and perpendicular to the mean tangent. **(B)** Vertical angulation is directed perpendicular to the bisector at approximately +40 degrees with the PID tilted downward. **(C)** Patient showing position of image receptor and holder, and 8-in. (20.5-cm) circular PID. **(D)** Maxillary incisors radiograph.

BISECTING TECHNIQUE
Maxillary Canine Exposure

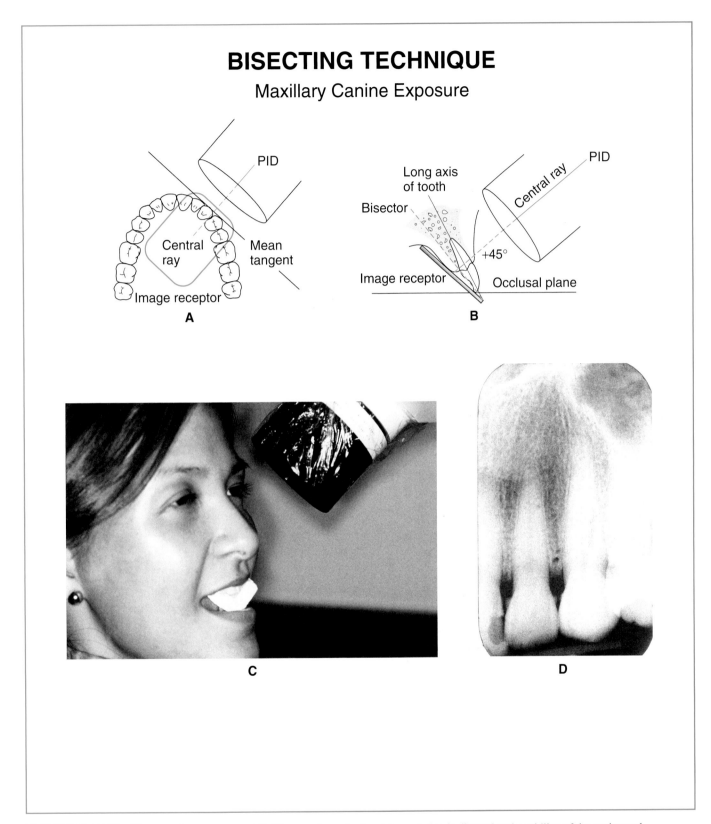

A

B

C

D

FIGURE 15-9 Maxillary canine exposure. (**A**) Diagram shows horizontal angulation is directed at the midline of the canine and perpendicular to the mean tangent. (**B**) Vertical angulation is directed perpendicular to the bisector at approximately +45 degrees with the PID tilted downward. (**C**) Patient showing position of image receptor and holder, and 8-in. (20.5-cm) circular PID. (**D**) Maxillary canine radiograph.

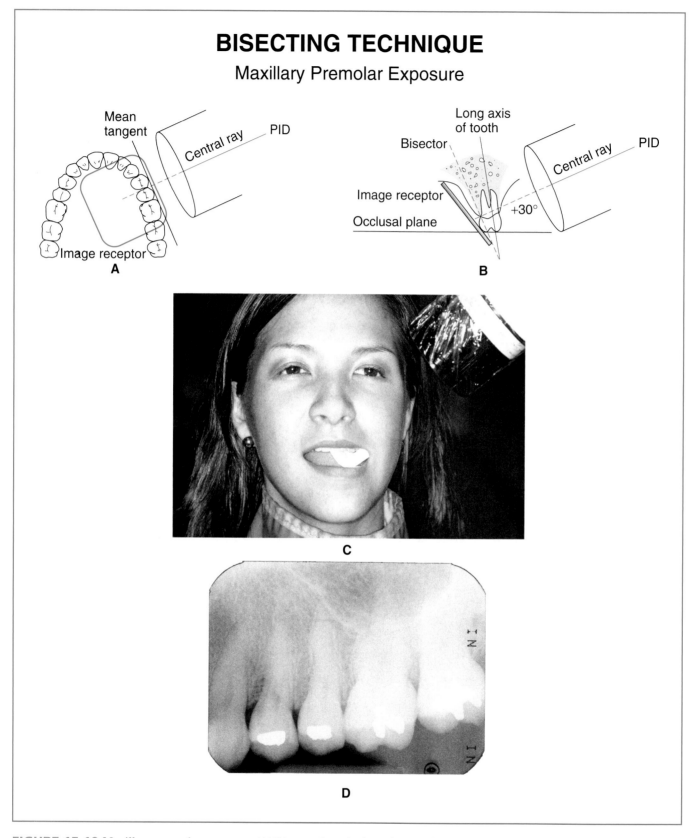

BISECTING TECHNIQUE
Maxillary Premolar Exposure

A
Mean tangent
Central ray
PID
Image receptor

B
Long axis of tooth
Bisector
Central ray
PID
Image receptor
Occlusal plane
+30°

C

D

FIGURE 15-10 Maxillary premolar exposure. (A) Diagram shows horizontal angulation is directed through the premolars embrasure and perpendicular to the mean tangent. **(B)** Vertical angulation is directed perpendicular to the bisector at approximately +30 degrees with the PID tilted downward. **(C)** Patient showing position of image receptor and holder, and 8-in. (20.5-cm) circular PID. **(D)** Maxillary premolar radiograph.

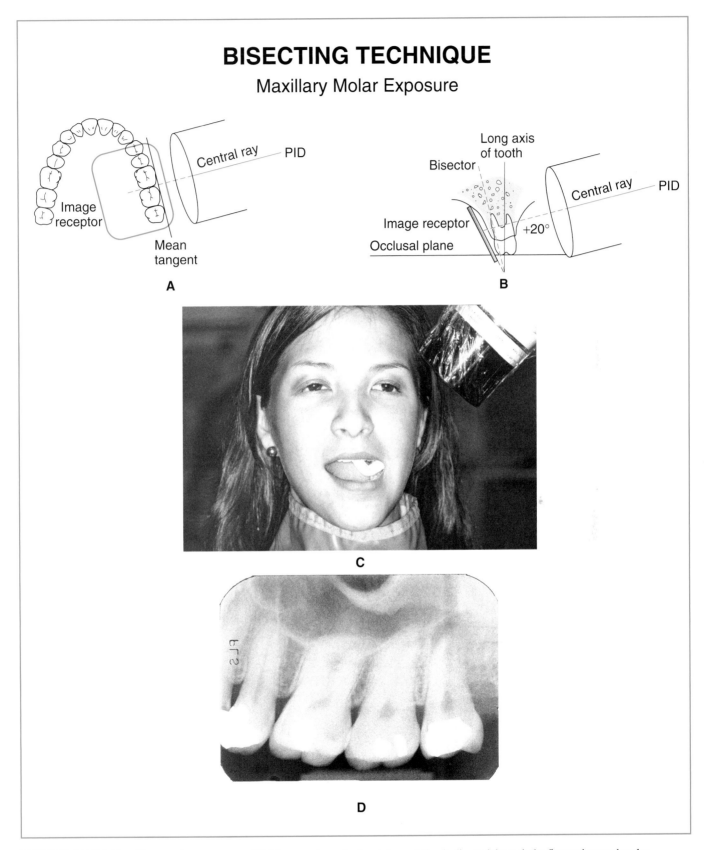

BISECTING TECHNIQUE
Maxillary Molar Exposure

A

B

C

D

FIGURE 15-11 **Maxillary molar exposure.** (**A**) Diagram shows horizontal angulation is directed through the first and second molar embrasure and perpendicular to the mean tangent. (**B**) Vertical angulation is directed perpendicular to the bisector at approximately +20 degrees with the PID tilted downward. (**C**) Patient showing position of image receptor and holder, and 8-in. (20.5-cm) circular PID. (**D**) Maxillary molar radiograph.

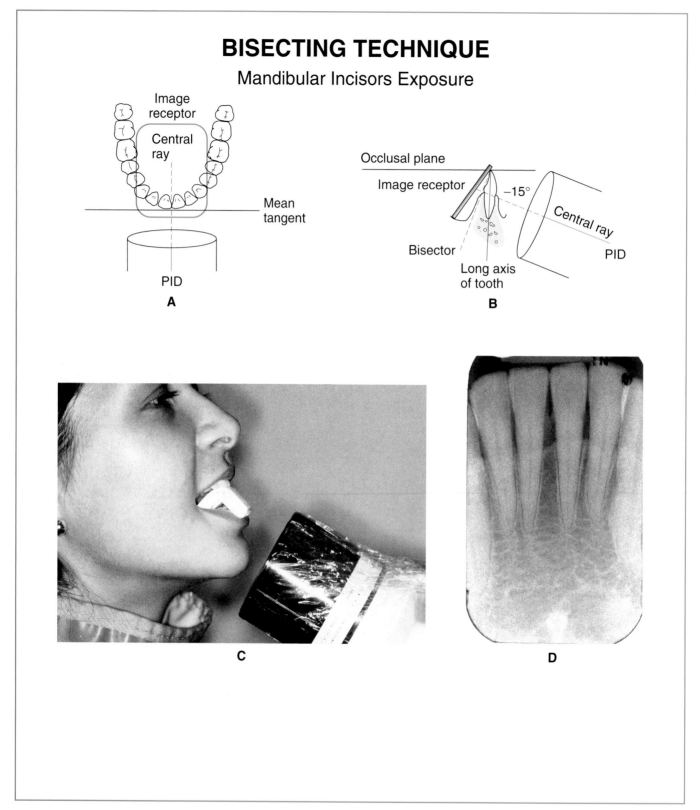

BISECTING TECHNIQUE
Mandibular Incisors Exposure

FIGURE 15-12 Mandibular incisors exposure. (**A**) Diagram shows horizontal angulation is directed through the central incisors embrasure and perpendicular to the mean tangent. (**B**) Vertical angulation is directed perpendicular to the bisector at approximately −15 degrees with the PID tilted upward. (**C**) Patient showing position of image receptor and holder, and 8-in. (20.5-cm) circular PID. (**D**) Mandibular incisors radiograph.

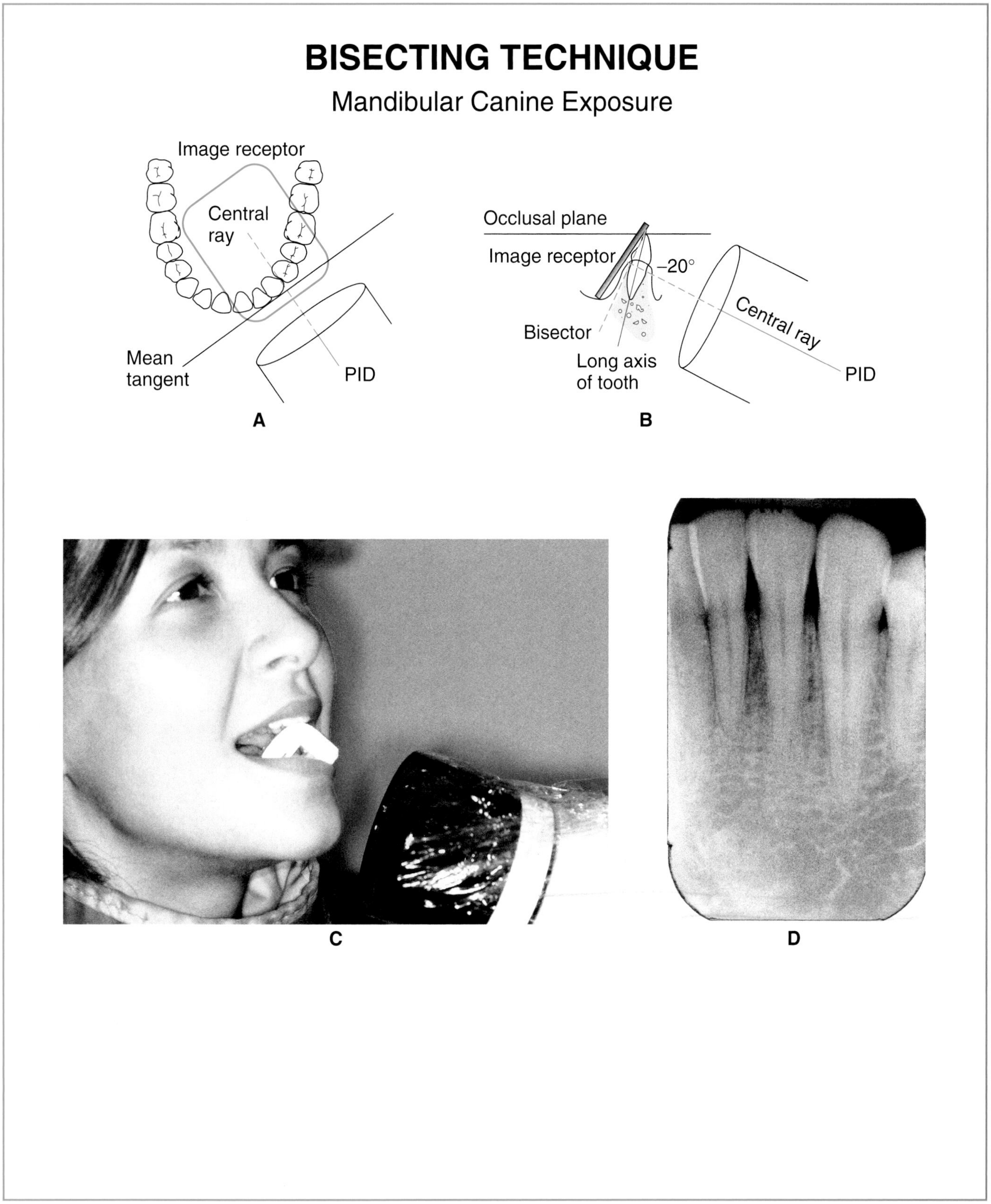

BISECTING TECHNIQUE
Mandibular Canine Exposure

A

B

C

D

FIGURE 15-13 **Mandibular canine exposure.** (**A**) Diagram shows horizontal angulation is directed at the midline of the canine and perpendicular to the mean tangent. (**B**) Vertical angulation is directed perpendicular to the bisector at approximately −20 degrees with the PID tilted upward. (**C**) Patient showing position of image receptor and holder, and 8-in. (20.5-cm) circular PID. (**D**) Mandibular canine radiograph.

BISECTING TECHNIQUE
Mandibular Premolar Exposure

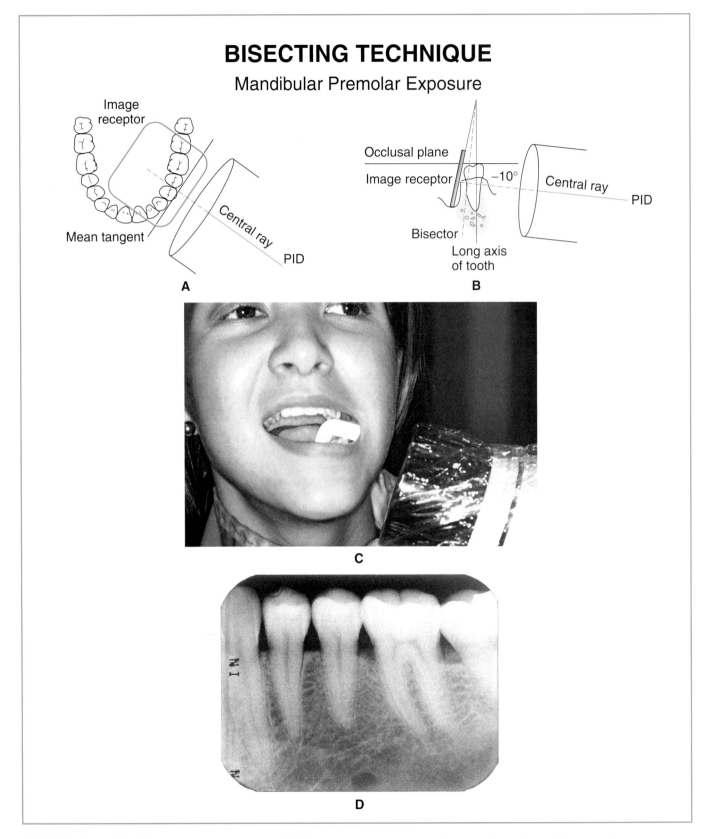

FIGURE 15-14 Mandibular premolar exposure. (**A**) Diagram shows horizontal angulation is directed through the premolar embrasure and perpendicular to the mean tangent. (**B**) Vertical angulation is directed perpendicular to the bisector at approximately −10 degrees with the PID tilted upward. (**C**) Patient showing position of image receptor and holder, and 8-in. (20.5-cm) circular PID. (**D**) Mandibular premolar radiograph.

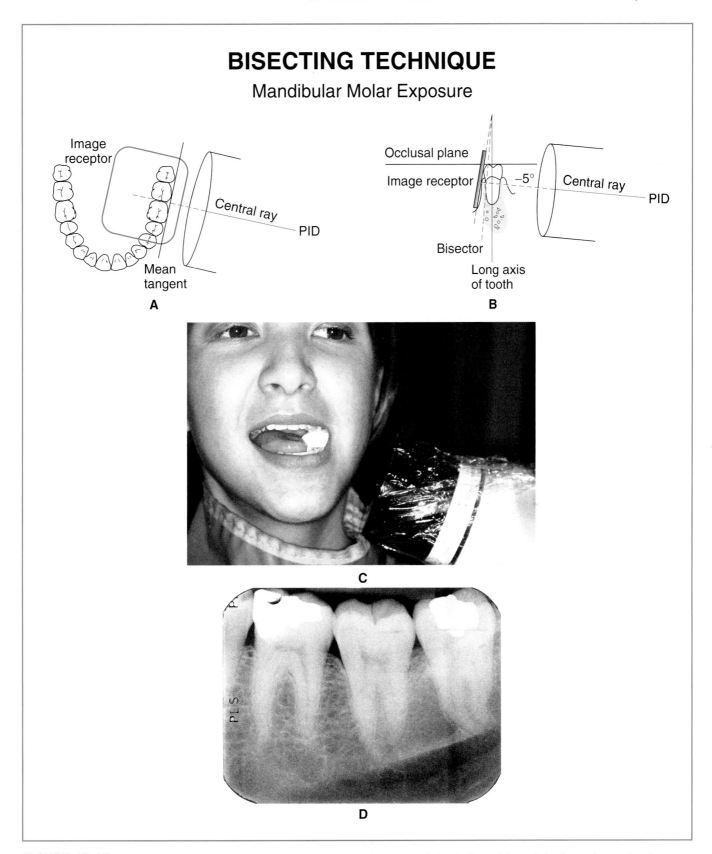

BISECTING TECHNIQUE
Mandibular Molar Exposure

A

B

C

D

FIGURE 15-15 Mandibular molar exposure. (A) Diagram shows horizontal angulation is directed through the first and second molar embrasure and perpendicular to the mean tangent. **(B)** Vertical angulation is directed perpendicular to the bisector at approximately −5 degrees with slight upward tilt of the PID. **(C)** Patient showing position of image receptor and holder, and 8-in. (20.5-cm) circular PID. **(D)** Mandibular molar radiograph.

REVIEW—Chapter summary

Meeting fewer shadow casting principles than the paralleling technique, the bisecting technique is less likely to produce superior diagnostic quality radiographs. The bisecting technique is based on the theory that two isometric triangles are formed when the central ray is directed perpendicular to the bisector. If irregularities or obstructions of the oral tissues prevent a parallel image receptor placement, the radiographer who is skilled in the bisecting technique can produce an acceptable diagnostic-quality radiograph when needed.

When the image receptor is positioned close to the tooth, parallelism is not likely. The exception to this occurs in the mandibular posterior region, where the molars and premolars are positioned near vertical in the arch. When parallelism cannot be established, to cast an accurate shadow representation of a tooth onto the image receptor, the angle formed by the long axis of the tooth and the plane of the image receptor must be bisected. The central ray of the x-ray beam is directed perpendicular to this imaginary bisector. A short target—image receptor distance (8-in/20.5-cm PID) will limit magnification that is inherent when parallelism is not established.

Image receptor holders designed for use with the bisecting technique generally have a short biteblock and lack the L-shaped back support. Holders are available that with modification can be used with either the bisecting or the paralleling technique.

The horizontal angulation is determined by directing the central ray of the x-beam perpendicular to the recording plane of the image receptor through the mean tangent of the embrasures between the teeth of interest. Both paralleling and bisecting techniques determine horizontal angulation in the same manner.

The vertical angulation is determined by directing the central ray of the x-beam perpendicular to the imaginary bisector. If the patient's head position is correct, predetermined vertical angle settings may be used.

The image receptor must be centered within the beam of radiation. If the patient's head position is correct, predetermined landmarks may be used to estimate the point of entry.

The four basic steps to exposing a periapical radiograph are placement, vertical angulation, horizontal angulation, and point of entry. Step-by-step illustrated instructions for exposing a full mouth series of periapical radiographs utilizing the bisecting technique are presented.

RECALL—Study questions

1. The bisecting technique satisfies more shadow casting rules than the paralleling technique.

    A better image results when the shadow casting rules are followed.
    a. The first statement is true. The second statement is false.
    b. The first statement is false. The second statement is true.
    c. Both statements are true.
    d. Both statements are false.

2. What shadow casting principle is most likely to be met when utilizing the bisecting technique?
    a. Object (tooth) and image receptor should be parallel to each other.
    b. Object (tooth) and image receptor should be as close as possible to each other.
    c. Object (tooth) should be as far as practical from the target (source of radiation).
    d. Radiation should strike the object (tooth) and image receptor perpendicularly.

3. What term describes the imaginary line between the long axis of the tooth and the plane of the image receptor?
    a. Tangent
    b. Median
    c. Midsagittal
    d. Bisector

4. When utilizing the bisecting technique, the image receptor is placed
    a. parallel to the tooth.
    b. as close as possible to the tooth.
    c. as close as possible to the bisector.
    d. parallel to the bisector.

5. When utilizing the bisecting technique, the central ray of the x-ray beam is directed
    a. perpendicular to the bisector.
    b. parallel to the bisector.
    c. perpendicular to the image receptor.
    d. parallel to the image receptor.

6. Which of these target–image receptor distances is recommended for use with the bisecting technique?
    a. 8 in. (20.5 cm)
    b. 12 in. (30 cm)
    c. 16 in. (41 cm)

7. Each of the following is a disadvantage of the bisecting technique EXCEPT one. Which one is the EXCEPTION?
    a. Produces images with dimensional distortion.
    b. Often superimposes adjacent structures.
    c. Estimating the location of the bisector may be difficult.
    d. May not be used with children or adults with small oral cavities.

8. Image receptor holders designed for use with the bisecting technique should have a
    a. short biteblock and L-shaped backing.
    b. long biteblock and L-shaped backing.
    c. short biteblock and 105° backing.
    d. long biteblock and 105° backing.

9. Which of the following is NOT an image receptor holder that can be used with the bisecting technique?
    a. Snap-A-Ray®
    b. SUPA®
    c. BAI®
    d. XCP®

10. Lining the image receptor up behind the distal half of the second premolar to include the first, second, and third molars describes the placement for which of the following periapical radiographs?

    a. Central incisors
    b. Canine
    c. Premolar
    d. Molar

11. To determine the horizontal angulation for the mandibular premolar periapical radiograph, the central rays of the x-ray beam should be directed at the image receptor perpendicularly through the embrasures of the

    a. canine and first premolar.
    b. first and second premolars.
    c. second premolar and first molar.
    d. first and second molars.

12. When utilizing the bisecting technique, the recommended vertical angle setting for the maxillary premolar periapical radiograph is

    a. +45 degrees
    b. +30 degrees
    c. −10 degrees
    d. −5 degrees

13. When utilizing the bisecting technique, the recommended vertical angle setting for the mandibular canine periapical radiograph is

    a. +40 degrees
    b. +20 degrees
    c. −15 degrees
    d. −20 degrees

14. With the bisecting technique, what is the effect on the radiographic image if the vertical angulation is significantly greater than necessary?

    a. Overlapping
    b. Conecutting
    c. Elongating
    d. Foreshortening

15. Elongation results from

    a. excessive horizontal angulation.
    b. inadequate horizontal angulation.
    c. excessive vertical angulation.
    d. inadequate vertical angulation.

16. Which of the following is the suggested point of entry for directing the central ray of the x-ray beam when exposing the maxillary incisors radiograph using the bisecting technique?

    a. The tip of the nose
    b. The ala of the nose
    c. A point on the ala-tragus line below the pupil of the eye
    d. A point on the ala-tragus line below the outer canthus of the eye

17. Which of the following points 1 in. (2.5 cm) above the lower border of the mandible is the suggested landmark for directing the central ray of the x-ray beam when exposing the mandibular premolar radiograph using the bisecting technique?

    a. The middle (symphysis) of the chin
    b. The center of the root of the canine
    c. Directly inferior to the pupil of the eye
    d. Directly inferior to the outer canthus of the eye

REFLECT—Case study

Compare the paralleling (Chapter 14) and the bisecting techniques. Include answers to the following questions in your discussion.

1. What are the major differences between the two techniques?
2. How are the two techniques similar?
3. What are the advantages/disadvantages of each of the two techniques?
4. When would use of the bisecting/paralleling technique be appropriate?
5. Describe the characteristics of the image receptor holder appropriate for use bisecting/paralleling technique.
6. How does each of the four steps for exposing periapical radiographs (placement, vertical and horizontal angulation, and point of entry) differ between the two techniques? How are they similar?
7. Which technique do you anticipate being easier/more difficult to master?
8. Would you recommend that radiographers learn one technique over the other? Why/why not?

RELATE—Laboratory application

For a comprehensive laboratory practice exercise on this topic, see Thomson, E. M. (2012). *Exercises in oral radiography techniques: A laboratory manual* 3rd ed.). Upper Saddle River, NJ: Pearson Education. Chapter 5, "Periapical radiographs—bisecting technique."

REFERENCES

Eastman Kodak Company. (2002). *Successful intraoral radiography*. Rochester, NY: Author.

Rinn Corporation. (1983). *Intraoral radiography with Rinn XCP/BAI instruments*. Elgin, IL: Dentsply/Rinn Corporation.

White, S. C., & Pharoah, M. J. (2008). *Oral radiology: Principles and interpretation* (6th ed.). St. Louis, MO: Elsevier.

CHAPTER OUTLINE

OBJECTIVES

Following successful completion of this chapter, you should be able to:

1. Define the key words.
2. Match the bitewing examination with two ideal uses.
3. Describe the bitewing radiographic technique.
4. List the four sizes of image receptors that can be used for bitewing surveys explaining advantages and disadvantages of each size.
5. Differentiate between horizontal and vertical bitewing radiographs.
6. Identify the type, size, and number of image receptors best suited for a child bitewing survey.
7. Explain the effect of horizontal angulation on the resultant bitewing image.
8. Identify positive and negative vertical angulations.
9. State the recommended vertical angulation for bitewing exposures.
10. Compare methods used for holding the bitewing image receptor in position.
11. Describe the image receptor placement, horizontal and vertical angulation, and point of entry for horizontal and vertical posterior bitewing examinations.
12. Describe the image receptor placement, horizontal and vertical angulation, and point of entry for a vertical anterior bitewing examination.

KEY WORDS

Bitetab	Interproximal radiograph
Bitewing radiograph	Mean tangent
Contact point	Overlap
Embrasure	Point of entry
External aiming device	Proximal surface
Film loop	Vertical angulation
Horizontal angulation	Vertical bitewing
Horizontal bitewing radiograph	radiograph

[handwritten notes:]

BWs → primary xray for diagnosing interproximal decay
Interproximal exposure:
  - open contacts (no overlaps)
  - view alveolar crest height

Introduction

Bitewing radiographs are probably the most frequently performed intraoral dental radiographic technique. Bitewings are most often exposed at the time of regularly scheduled recare or recall appointments. **Bitewing radiographs** image the crowns and alveolar bone of both the maxillary and mandibular teeth on a single radiograph. The name bitewing is descriptive. Traditionally, the bitewing film packet had a tab, or wing, that was either attached to the packet by the manufacturer or attached by the radiographer as a holder (Figures 16-1 and 16-2). The patient bites on this tab to hold the image receptor in place. The purpose of this chapter is to present step-by-step procedures for exposing bitewing radiographs.

Fundamentals of Bitewing Radiography

Bitewing (**interproximal**) **radiographs** may be taken as a series or in conjunction with a full mouth series of periapical radiographs or with a panoramic radiograph. Bitewing radiographs showing the crowns and alveolar bone crests of both the maxillary and mandibular teeth on the same image are ideal for examining dental caries on the **proximal surfaces** of the teeth (where adjacent teeth contact each other in the arch) and periodontal bone levels supporting the teeth (Figure 16-3). The true value of the bitewing radiograph is that it reveals caries in the very early stages when remineralization treatment may be possible. This is particularly important in the premolar and molar regions, where incipient (small) caries are often concealed by the wide bucco-lingual diameters of these teeth. Such caries are frequently unnoticed in a visual inspection. Bitewing radiographs do not image the entire tooth and therefore will not reveal apical conditions or lesions.

To expose a bitewing radiograph, the image receptor is positioned near and almost parallel to the teeth of both arches when

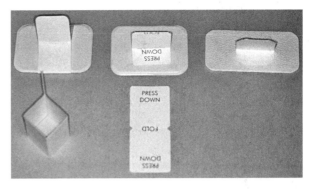

FIGURE 16-1 **Bitewing tabs and loops.** (**A**) Loop tabs; (**B**) Stick-on tabs; (**C**) Size #3 film packet with manufacturer-attached tab.

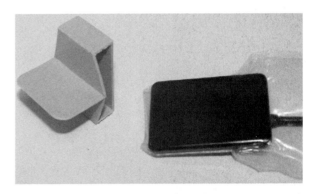

FIGURE 16-2 **Bitewing loop for digital sensor.**

the patient's teeth are occluded (closed). Bitewing image receptor placement is often closer to the teeth, and the central ray of the x-ray beam can be directed at a more ideal angle than for periapical radiographs (Figure 16-4). With this ideal image receptor placement, the bitewing radiograph often images decay and the height

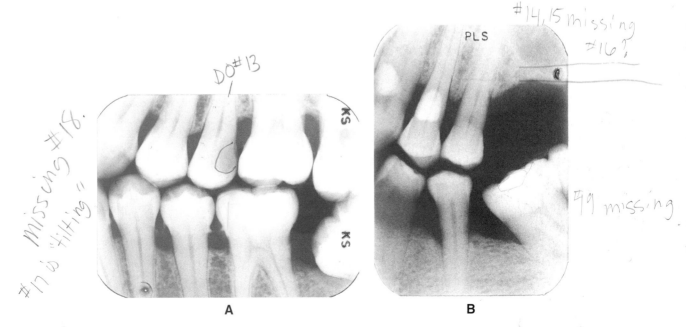

FIGURE 16-3 (**A**) **Horizontal and** (**B**) **vertical bitewing radiographs.** Bitewing radiographs are ideal at imaging the interproximal areas of the teeth to show caries and alveolar bone crests. Note the increased coverage of the alveolar bone imaged on the vertical bitewing radiograph.

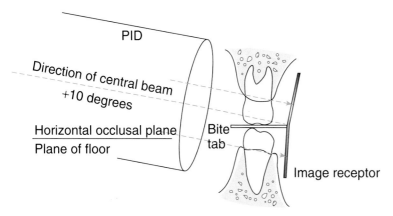

FIGURE 16-4 Bitewing placement. The bitewing image receptor placement, slightly angled to take advantage of the height of the midline of the palate when the patient occludes, is such that the coronal portion of both the maxillary and the mandibular teeth will be recorded on the image. The close relationship between the teeth and the image receptor and the ideal angle of the x-ray beam allow bitewings to accurately image caries and alveolar bone crests.

of the alveolar bone crest better than periapical radiographs. It is because of this improved imaging for these conditions that bitewing radiographs are taken in conjunction with periapical radiographs of the same area when exposing a full mouth series.

The Radiographic Examination

Size, Number, and Placement of Image Receptors

The number and size of image receptors to use depends on the type of survey required and the size and shape of the patient's oral cavity (Table 16-1). Additional factors to be considered when deciding how many and what size image receptor to select is the length and curvature of the arches, which vary in all individuals. A single image receptor placed on each side of the mouth often provides adequate coverage for children, prior to the eruption of the permanent second molars. Although an image receptor size #0 or #1 is usually used for a child with primary teeth, the preferred size for mixed dentition is a #2. However, tissue sensitivity or anatomical limitations must be taken into consideration, so size is often based on the individual patient. The advantage to using the largest size image receptor possible is that the amount of structures imaged, including the developing permanent teeth, will be increased. For most adults, four #2 image receptors (two on each side) are generally preferred.

Size #3 (extra-long) radiographic film packets with preattached tabs are especially made for taking **horizontal bitewing radiographs.** Phosphor plates used for indirect digital imaging

are also available in size #3. (see Figure 9-3) The advantage of these image receptors is that only one image receptor needs to be exposed on each side of the arch to image both premolars and all molars on one image. However, when compared with the standard #2 image receptor, the #3 has two disadvantages. One is that most dental arches curve so that the horizontal angle required to clearly image the proximal surfaces of the premolars is not the same horizontal angle required to clearly image the proximal surfaces of the molars. There are two slightly divergent pathways of the posterior teeth. As the central rays pass through these divergent **embrasures,** it is not likely that all of the interproximal spaces will be imaged clearly without overlapping. The other disadvantage is that the long image receptor is narrower in the vertical dimension than size #2 and may reveal less of the periodontal crestal bone level (Figure 16-5).

As discussed in Chapter 13, the bitewing examination may consist of two to eight images. The posterior bitewing examination consists of either two (one on the left and one on the right) or four (two on the left and two on the right) images (Figure 16-6A,B). The image receptor orientation in the oral cavity may be such that the longer dimension is placed horizontally or vertically. Traditionally, the image receptor has been placed horizontally in the posterior region. This remains the placement of choice for children. However, if there is a need to image more of the supporting bone, as is the case in periodontally involved patients, a **vertical bitewing** is recommended.

TABLE 16-1 Suggested Image Receptor Size and Number to Use for Bitewing Radiographs		
IMAGE RECEPTOR SIZE	RECOMMENDED FOR USE WITH THESE PATIENTS	NUMBER AND ORIENTATION OF IMAGE RECEPTOR
#0	Child with primary dentition 1BW on each side	2 horizontal posterior
#1	Child with primary or mixed dentition	2 horizontal posterior
	Adult for caries detection or the presence of periodontal disease	3 or 4 vertical anterior
#2	Child with mixed dentition, prior to the eruption of the permanent second molars	2 horizontal posterior
	Adolescent after the eruption of the permanent second molars	4 horizontal posterior
	Adult	4 horizontal posterior
	Adult with periodontal disease	4 vertical posterior
#3	Adolescent after the eruption of the permanent second molars	2 horizontal posterior
	Adult	2 horizontal posterior

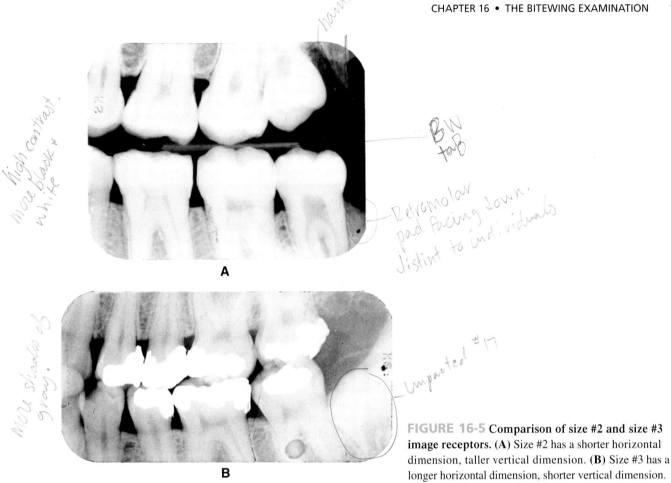

high contrast.
more black +
white

hamulus

BW
tab

Retromolar
pad facing down.
distint to individuals

More shades of
gray.

Impacted #17

FIGURE 16-5 Comparison of size #2 and size #3 image receptors. **(A)** Size #2 has a shorter horizontal dimension, taller vertical dimension. **(B)** Size #3 has a longer horizontal dimension, shorter vertical dimension.

The anterior bitewing examination consists of either three (one just left of center, one centered behind the central incisors, and one just right of center; Figure 16-6C) or four (two just left of center and two just right of center) images. The image receptor orientation in the oral cavity is usually such that the longer dimension is placed vertically. For ease of placement, especially when using rigid digital sensors and to avoid bending the film packet or phosphor plate, the narrow size #1 image receptor is recommended, especially for imaging the lateral-canine region. However, a size #2 may be used for the central incisors when the arch permits. Using a longer bitetab than that used for the posterior exposures may facilitate positioning the image receptor further lingually in the mouth to avoid contact with the lingual gingiva or curvature of the palate when the patient occludes. This may prevent the film or phosphor plate from bending in the middle as the tab is pulled forward when the patient is asked to bite down and may avoid pushing down on or causing the receptor to slant in a way that compromises the vertical angulation. Two stick-on paper bitetabs may be attached to lengthen the bitetab for this purpose (Figure 16-7).

The goal of image receptor placement is to image all contacts (mesial and distal surfaces) of all of the teeth of interest. It is important to remember that each bitewing—molar, premolar, canine, and incisors—has a standard recommended placement. This means that a premolar bitewing taken at one oral health care practice will most likely image the same teeth as a premolar bitewing exposed in every other practice. This standardization is important to learn.

The incisors and canine radiographs instruct the radiographer to center the teeth of interest in the middle of the image receptor. However anatomical considerations prevent centering the premolars and molars. Instead the radiographer should focus on placing the anterior edge of the image receptor and allow the receptor, once in the correct position, to capture the images of the appropriate teeth. For example, when placing the image receptor for a premolar horizontal or vertical bitewing radiograph, the radiographer should not try to center the first and second premolars. Because of the curvature of the arches and the position of the canine, this is not usually possible. The radiographer should focus on placing the anterior edge of the image receptor so that it lines up behind the distal half of the canine, and the rest of the teeth should be imaged correctly.

It is important to visually inspect the patient's occlusion to determine which canine, maxillary, or mandibular, to use to align the image receptor for exposure of premolar bitewing radiographs. The premolar bitewing must image the distal portion of both the maxillary and the mandibular canines to image the mesial surface of the first premolar, one of the teeth of interest for this projection. The radiographer should align the anterior edge of the image receptor behind the canine that is further forward in the mouth (the most mesial canine).

When placing the image receptor to image a molar horizontal or vertical bitewing radiograph, the radiographer should focus on placing the anterior edge of the image receptor so that it lines up behind the distal half of the second premolar. Again, a visual inspection of the patient's occlusion will determine whether to line

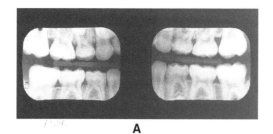

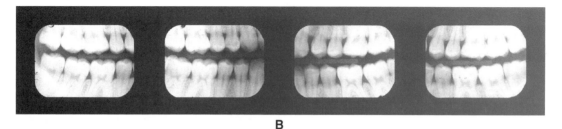

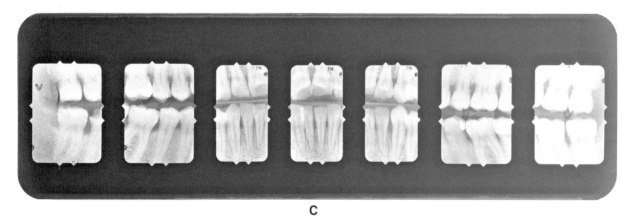

FIGURE 16-6 **Horizontal and vertical bitewing series.** (**A**) Set of two horizontal posterior bitewing radiographs. (**B**) Set of four horizontal posterior bitewing radiographs. (**C**) Set of seven vertical bitewing radiographs, including posterior and anterior images.

up the image receptor with the maxillary or the mandibular second premolar.

Generally, in Class I and III occlusal relationships, the radiographer will choose to align the anterior edge of the image receptor behind the distal half of the mandibular canine for a premolar bitewing radiograph and behind the distal half of the mandibular second premolar for a molar bitewing radiograph. When a Class II occlusal relationship presents, the radiographer will most likely

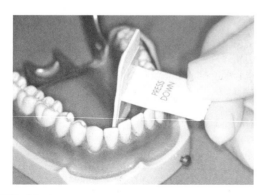

FIGURE 16-7 **Two stick-on bitetabs** lengthen the holder for use in the anterior region.

choose to align the anterior edge of the image receptor behind the distal half of the maxillary canine for a premolar bitewing radiograph and behind the distal half of the maxillary second premolar for a molar bitewing radiograph (Figure 16-8). It should be noted that patients often present with different occlusal relationships on the right and left sides or individual teeth that are malaligned or missing. It is important to perform a visual inspection prior to each placement.

It is important to also position the image receptor well into the oral cavity, a slight distance from the lingual surfaces of the maxillary teeth, taking advantage of the midline where the palate is at its highest to accommodate the image receptor and facilitate correct stabilization and vertical alignment with the x-ray beam. According to the shadow casting principles (see Chapter 13), the image receptor should be positioned as close to the object (tooth) as possible. However, if the image receptor is placed too close to the maxillary teeth, especially in the premolar and anterior regions, the top edge of the receptor may contact the lingual gingiva or curvature of the palate when the patient occludes, pushing down on or causing the receptor to slant away from the correct position (Figure 16-9). A sloping or slanting (tilted) occlusal plane is a frequent reason for having to retake bitewing radiographs.

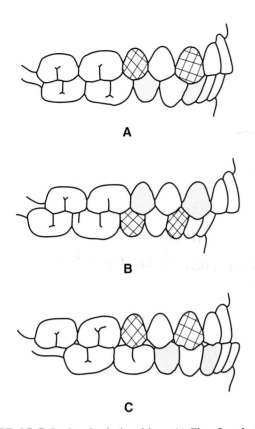

A

B

C

FIGURE 16-8 Occlusal relationships. (A) Class I occlusion demonstrating that the mandibular canine and second premolar (shaded) are located further forward in the oral cavity. **(B) Class II occlusion** demonstrating that the maxillary canine and second premolar (shaded) are located further forward in the oral cavity. **(C) Class III occlusion** demonstrating that the mandibular canine and second premolar (shaded) are located further forward in the oral cavity.

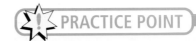

Although contact with the lingual gingiva or curvature of the palate or other obstruction such as tori is the most likely cause of a tilted or slanting occlusal plane, other causes include (1) failure of the patient to maintain a steady pressure occluding on the bitetab, (2) patient swallowing while the exposure is being made, (3) incorrect or slanted placement of the bitetab or image receptor holder. The best corrective action is to position the image receptor far enough away from the lingual surfaces of the maxillary teeth to avoid premature and excessive contact with the palate. Other corrective actions include selecting the appropriately sized image receptor and providing the patient with specific instructions about securely biting on the bitetab and not swallowing during exposure.

Sequence of Placement

It is recommended to always follow a systematic order when taking radiographs to prevent errors and for efficiency (Table 16-2).

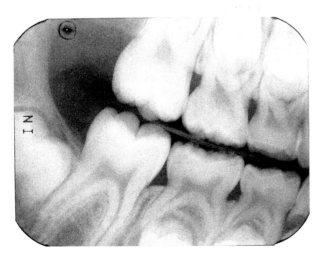

FIGURE 16-9 Tilted image. The slanted occlusal plane observed on this radiograph resulted from a failure to place the image receptor far enough lingually to avoid being pushed down by the palate when the patient occluded onto the bitetab.

TABLE 16-2   Recommended Sequence for Exposing Bitewing Radiographs

BITEWING SERIES	RECOMMENDED SEQUENCE
2 posterior	1st: right* premolar
	2nd: left premolar
4 posterior	1st: right* premolar
	2nd: right molar
	3rd: left premolar
	4th: left molar
7 anterior and posterior	1st: central-lateral incisors
	2nd: left* canine
	3rd: right canine
	4th: right premolar
	5th: right molar
	6th: left premolar
	7th: left molar
8 anterior and posterior	1st: left* canine
	2nd: left central-lateral incisors
	3rd: right central-lateral incisors
	4th: right canine
	5th: right premolar
	6th: right molar
	7th: left premolar
	8th: left molar

*Left-handed radiographers may choose to begin the exposures on the opposite side.

Chapter 13 explained at what point to take bitewing radiographs when exposing a full mouth series. When exposing a set of four posterior bitewings alone, it is recommended that the premolar bitewing on one side be exposed first, followed by the molar bitewing on the same side. Placing the image receptor for exposure of the premolar may be more comfortable for the patient and less likely to excite a gag reflex, gaining the patient's confidence for the molar placements that may sometimes be more difficult. Then the premolar and molar bitewing on the opposite should be exposed. Completing both the premolar and molar bitewing radiographs on one side first will avoid shifting the tube head back and forth across the patient.

Holding the Bitewing Image Receptor in Position

There are many commercially made holders for stabilizing a film packet, phosphor plate, or digital sensor for bitewing exposures. Stick-on paper or plastic **bitetabs** have the most versatility because they can be fastened to the image receptor for both horizontal and vertical bitewings. The paper or plastic **film loop** into which a film packet or digital sensor can be slid is limited to horizontal bitewings. Bitetabs and loops are easy to use, disposable, and readily tolerated by the patient. Bitetabs must be attached to the white unprinted side (front) of the film packet

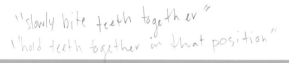

"slowly bite teeth together"
"hold teeth together in that position"

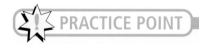

PRACTICE POINT

When using a stick-on tab holder, follow these steps for placement (Figure 16-10).

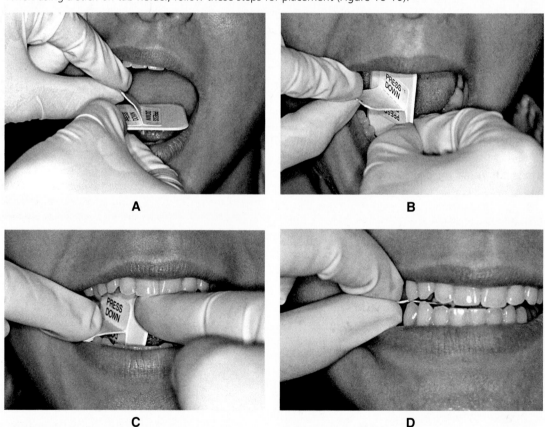

A   **B**

C   **D**

FIGURE 16-10 Bitewing placement using a stick-on tab. (A) Insert the image receptor completely into the patient's mouth. **(B)** Rotate until the image receptor is in a vertical position. Inserting in this manner allows the image receptor to move the tongue out of the way. **(C)** Using the index finger of one hand, hold the bitetab firmly against the occlusal surface of the mandibular teeth while the index finger of the other hand angles the top edge of the image receptor into the midline of the palate. **(D)** Instruct the patient to close so that the teeth occlude normally. Failure to hold the tab firmly may lead to a drift lingually and distally and increase the possibility that the tongue will move the image receptor out of the correct position.

or the plain side of the phosphor plate or digital sensor (over the plastic infection control barrier; see Chapter 10) so that this side will face the PID (x-rays) when placed intraorally.

Generally the bitetab or loop is visible extraorally after the patient bites down to stabilize the image receptor. This extension of the tab serves as a guide for directing the central rays toward the center of the image receptor. Without a significantly visible **external aiming device,** some operators find it difficult to determine the correct horizontal and vertical angulations and centering of the image receptor within the x-ray beam.

Many holders (including the Dentsply Rinn XCP® and Flow Dental RAPD® introduced in Chapter 14) designed for positioning the image receptor for periapical radiographs include a bitewing biteblock that can be used with the metal positioning arm and plastic external aiming ring to assist with locating correct angles and points of entry, making errors less likely (Figure 16-11). The external aiming device also eliminates the need to position the patient's head precisely. Biteblock image receptor holder attachments are available for both horizontal and vertical bitewings. It should be noted that the plastic biteblock on some holders is wider than paper/plastic bitetabs and loops and may prevent the patient from biting down far enough to image the greatest amount of alveolar bone (Figure 16-12). This is especially important when periodontal disease is suspected or present. To overcome this disadvantage, the vertical bitewing biteblock attachment can be substituted.

Regardless of the holder used, care should be taken to ensure that the image receptor is positioned in such a manner that it is evenly divided between the maxillary and mandibular teeth. Once the image receptor is satisfactorily positioned, the patient must close down on the tab or biteblock in an edge-to-edge relationship and hold it there for the duration of the exposure.

It is important to note that if an image receptor holder with an external aiming device is not positioned correctly, the aiming device will indicate directing the x-ray beam to the wrong place. For this reason, it is important that the radiographer develop the skills necessary to evaluate placement of the image receptor for correctness, regardless of the holder used.

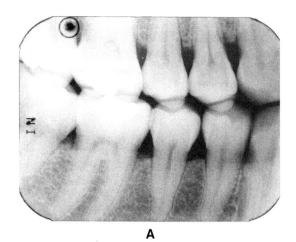

A

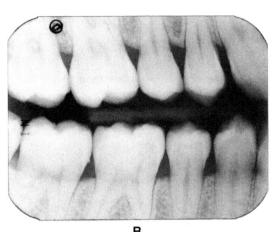

B

FIGURE 16-12 Holder comparison. (A) Bitewing radiograph taken using a disposable paper stick-on bitetab. **(B)** Bitewing radiograph taken using a thicker plastic, autoclavable image receptor holding device. Notice the wider space between the occlusal surfaces of the maxillary and mandibular teeth.

Horizontal and Vertical Angulation Procedures

The correct horizontal and vertical angulations are critical to producing a quality bitewing radiograph.

Horizontal Angulation is the positioning of the central ray (PID) in a horizontal (side-to-side) plane and is of critical importance when exposing bitewing radiographs. The horizontal angulation for bitewing exposures is the same as that used for periapical radiographs of the same region (see Chapter 14). The central ray (PID) should be directed perpendicular to the curvature of the arch or **mean tangent,** through the **contact points** of the teeth (see Figure 13-8). To rely on the image receptor holder's external aiming ring to accurately direct the central ray perpendicularly (at a right angle) toward the surface of the image receptor in a horizontal plane, the image receptor itself must be positioned parallel to the teeth of interest in the horizontal dimension. The image receptor must be positioned parallel to the interproximal space or **embrasure** of two predetermined teeth. The teeth selected depend on the region being imaged. Table 16-3

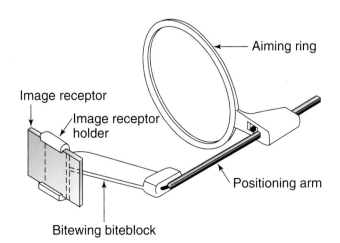

FIGURE 16-11 Bitewing image receptor holder with metal positioning arm and plastic external aiming ring.
(Courtesy of Dentsply Rinn.)

TABLE 16-3 Summary of Steps for Acquiring Bitewing Radiographs

BITEWING RADIOGRAPH	PLACEMENT	VERTICAL ANGULATION*	HORIZONTAL ANGULATION	POINT OF ENTRY*
Central incisors (vertical) (image receptor size #1 or size #2) (Figure 16-17)	Center the image receptor to line up behind the central and lateral incisors; if using a size #2 image receptor, include the mesial halves of the canines. Align the image receptor parallel to the long axes of the incisors and parallel to the left and right central incisor embrasure.	+10	Direct the central ray perpendicular to the image receptor through the left and right central incisor embrasure.	Center the image receptor within the x-ray beam by directing the central ray at the center of the image receptor at a spot on the maxillary and mandibular central incisors.
Canine (vertical) (image receptor size #1 or size #2) (Figure 16-18)	Center the image receptor to line up behind the maxillary and mandibular canines; include the lateral incisor and the first premolar Align the image receptor parallel to the long axes of the canines and parallel to the mesial and distal line angles of the canines.	+10	Direct the central ray perpendicular to the image receptor at the center of the canine. To minimize distal overlap of the canine with the lingual cusp of the first premolar shift the PID no more than 10 degrees toward the distal.	Center the image receptor within the x-ray beam by directing the central ray at the center of the image receptor at a spot on the incisal plane between the maxillary and mandibular canines.
Premolar (horizontal or vertical) (image receptor size #2) (Figure 16-19)	Align the anterior edge of the image receptor to line up behind the distal half of the maxillary or mandibular canine. Choose the most mesially positioned canine; include the first and second premolars and mesial half of the first molar. Align the image receptor parallel to the long axes of the premolars and parallel to the first and second premolar embrasure.	+10	Direct the central ray perpendicular to the image receptor through the first and second premolar embrasure.	Center the image receptor within the x-ray beam by directing the central ray at the center of the image receptor at a spot on the occlusal plane between the maxillary and mandibular second premolars.

Molar (horizontal or vertical) (image receptor size #2) (Figure 16-20)	+10	Align the anterior edge of the image receptor to line up behind the distal half of the maxillary or mandibular second premolar. Choose the most mesially located second premolar; include the first, second, third molars (horizontal placement); include the first, second molars (vertical placement) Align the image receptor parallel to the long axes of the molars and parallel to the first and second molar embrasure.	Direct the central ray perpendicular to the image receptor through the first and second molar embrasure.	Center the image receptor within the x-ray beam by directing the central ray at the center of the image receptor at a spot on the occlusal plane between the maxillary and mandibular first molars.
Premolar-molar (image receptor size #3)	+10	Align the anterior edge of image receptor to line up behind the distal half of the maxillary or the mandibular canine. Choose the most mesially located canine; include all premolars and molars on the image.	Direct the central ray perpendicular to the image receptor through the second premolar and first molar embrasure.	Center the image receptor within the x-ray beam by directing the central ray at the center of the image receptor at a spot on the occlusal plane between the maxillary and mandibular second premolars.
Molar (child) (horizontal) (image receptor size #1 or size #2)	+5 to +10	Align the anterior edge of the image receptor to line up behind the distal half of the maxillary or the mandibular canine. Choose the most mesially located canine; include the remaining erupted teeth on the image.	Direct the central ray perpendicular to the image receptor through the first and second primary molar embrasure; or, if erupted, the first and second premolar embrasure.	Center the image receptor within the x-ray beam by directing the central ray at the center of the image receptor at a spot on the occlusal plane between the primary maxillary and mandibular first molars; or, if erupted, the maxillary and mandibular second premolars.

*The patient must be seated in the correct position, with the occlusal plane parallel to the floor and the midsaggital plane perpendicular to the floor.

lists the embrasure to align the image receptor behind and through which to direct the central ray for each projection. The central ray must be directed appropriately to avoid **overlapping** adjacent teeth on the resultant image (Figure 16-13). The contact points should appear open or separate from each other on the resultant radiograph. When the horizontal angulation is directed obliquely from the mesial, the overlapping will be more severe in the distal or posterior region of the image; when the horizontal angulation is directed obliquely from the distal, the overlapping will be more severe in the mesial or anterior region of the image (Figure 16-14). Because bitewing radiographs are taken to reveal information about the interproximal areas of the teeth, radiographs with overlapping error are undiagnostic.

It is important to note that even with correct horizontal angulation, the canine bitewing will often exhibit significant overlap of the distal portion of the canines with the mesial portions of the first premolars. The anatomical positions of the canines, which are anterior teeth, and the premolars, which are posterior teeth, is such that the lingual cusp of the first premolar is often superimposed over the distal edge of the canine. To minimize this occurrence the horizontal angulation should first be aligned correctly to direct the central ray of the x-ray beam perpendicular to the image receptor at the center of the canine and then shift the PID no more than 10 degrees toward the distal (see Chapter 28).

VERTICAL ANGULATION The correct **vertical angulation** for bitewing radiographs is +10 degrees. (A +5 degree vertical angulation is sometimes recommended for children. See Chapter 26.) Positioning the PID at this slightly downward position will more likely match the vertical slant of the image receptor when it is correctly placed into the oral cavity (Figure 16-4). Because bitewing radiographs are placed to image both the maxillary and the mandibular teeth on one image, consideration is given to the

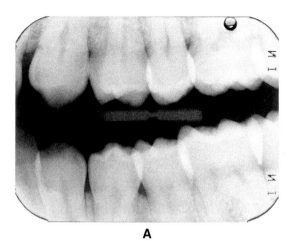

A

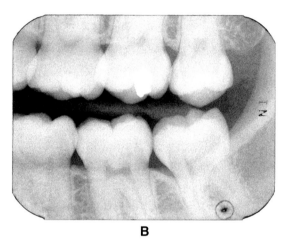

B

FIGURE 16-14 **Horizontal overlap error. (A)** When the PID is directed obliquely from the mesial (mesiodistal projection of the x-ray beam), the overlapping will be more severe in the distal or posterior region of the image. **(B)** When the horizontal angulation is directed obliquely from the distal (distomesial projection of the x-ray beam), the overlapping will be more severe in the mesial or anterior region of the image.

anatomic positions of the teeth in both arches. In the posterior region, the maxillary teeth have a slight buccal inclination, whereas the mandibular teeth often have a slight lingual inclination. This anatomical relationship allows a slight +10 degree slant to the image receptor. Positioning the PID to match this angle will produce the best image. In addition, adjusting the vertical angulation of the PID to +10 degrees will match the slight angle the image receptor takes on when the patient closes and the palate pushes down against the receptor in both the posterior and the anterior regions. If using an image receptor holder with an external aiming device, it is important that the patient occludes fully on the biteblock so that the aiming ring will direct the operator to the correct vertical angle.

Incorrect vertical angulation results in an unequal distribution of the arches on the radiograph. A quality bitewing radiograph should image an equal portion of the maxillary and mandibular teeth plus a portion of the supporting bone. When the vertical angulation is excessive (greater than +10°), more

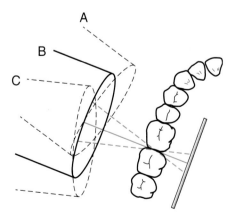

FIGURE 16-13 **Horizontal angulation. (A)** Mesiodistal projection of the x-ray beam shown here deviates from a right angle by about 15°, resulting in greater overlap of the contacts in the posterior region of the radiograph. **(B)** Correct horizontal projection of the x-ray beam produces no overlapping. **(C)** Distomesial projection of the x-ray beam shown here deviates from a right angle about 15°, resulting in greater overlap of the contacts in the anterior region of the radiograph.

To avoid molar overlap follow these steps for placement (Figure 16-15).

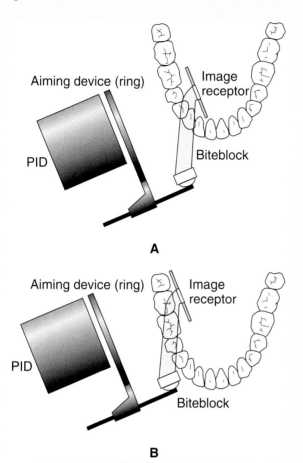

A

B

FIGURE 16-15 Avoiding molar overlap when using a holder with external aiming device. (Courtesy of Dentsply Rinn.) (**A**) Note the recommended premolar bitewing placement positions the image receptor slightly diagonal with the front edge of the image receptor farther from the lingual of the teeth than the back part. (**B**) Because the proximal surfaces of the molar teeth are in a mesiodistal relationship to the sagittal plane, it is recommended that the image receptor be positioned perpendicularly to the embrasures, resulting in a diagonal placement similar to the premolar position.

maxillary teeth and bone are imaged, cutting off a portion of the mandibular structures. When the vertical angulation is inadequate (less than +10°), more mandibular teeth and bone are imaged, cutting off a portion of the maxillary structures (Figure 16-16).

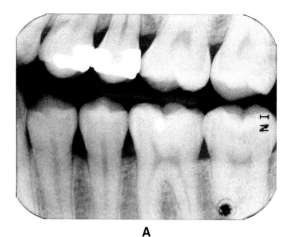

A

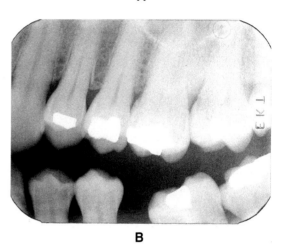

B

FIGURE 16-16 **Vertical angulation error.** (**A**) Inadequate vertical angulation results in imaging more of the mandible. (**B**) Excessive vertical angulation results in imaging more of the maxilla.

Point of Entry

The **point of entry** for the central ray for all bitewing exposures is on the level of the incisal or occlusal plane (near the lip line) at a point opposite the center of the image receptor and through the interproximal spaces of the teeth of interest (Figure 16-4). An image receptor holder with an external aiming device will assist with determining the accurate point of entry. Incorrect point of entry, or not centering the image receptor within the x-ray beam, will result in conecut error, where the portion of the image receptor that was not in the path of the x-ray beam will be clear or blank on the resultant radiograph (see Figures 18-7 and 18-8).

The Bitewing Technique

Figures 16-17 through 16-20 illustrate the precise image receptor positions and required angulations for each of the horizontal and vertical bitewing radiographs discussed in this chapter. See Table 16-3 for a summary of the four basic steps of the technique—placement, vertical angulation, horizontal angulation, and point of entry.

BITEWING TECHNIQUE
Central Incisors Bitewing Exposure

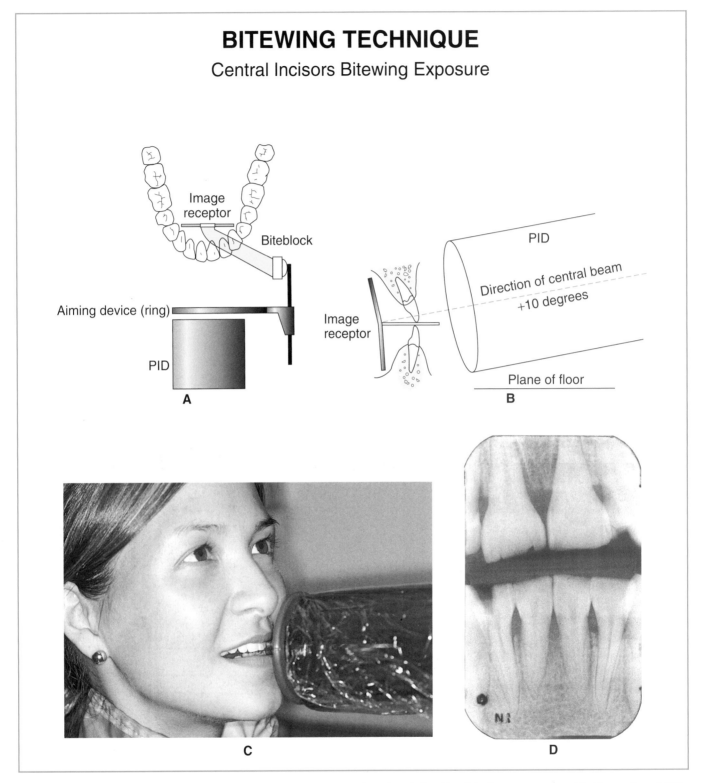

FIGURE 16-17 Central incisors bitewing exposure. (A) Diagrams show the relationship of the image receptor and holder, teeth, and PID. **(B)** Vertical angulation is directed perpendicular to the image receptor at approximately +10° with the PID tilted downward. Central ray is directed at the center of the image receptor at a spot on the incisal plane between the maxillary and mandibular teeth. **(C)** Patient showing position of image receptor holder and 12-in. (30-cm) circular PID. **(D)** Central incisor bitewing radiograph. In the anterior region, the image receptor is positioned with the long dimension vertical.

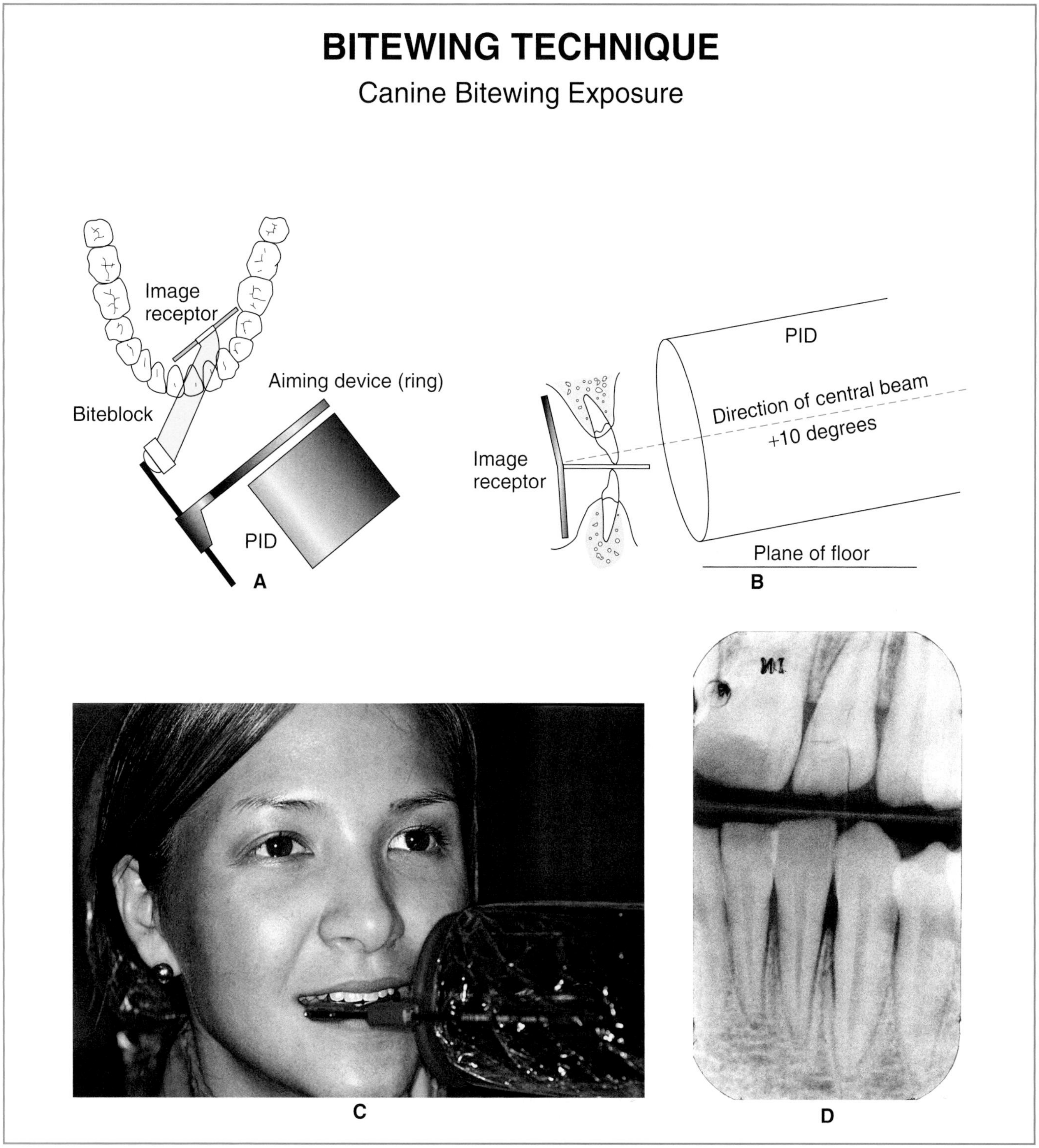

BITEWING TECHNIQUE
Canine Bitewing Exposure

FIGURE 16-18 Canine bitewing exposure. (A) Diagrams show the relationship of the image receptor and holder, teeth, and PID. **(B)** Vertical angulation is directed perpendicular to the image receptor at approximately +10° with the PID tilted downward. Central ray is directed at the center of the image receptor at a spot on the incisal plane between the maxillary and mandibular teeth. **(C)** Patient showing position of image receptor holder and 12-in. (30-cm) circular PID. **(D)** Canine bitewing radiograph. In the anterior region, the image receptor is positioned with the long dimension vertical.

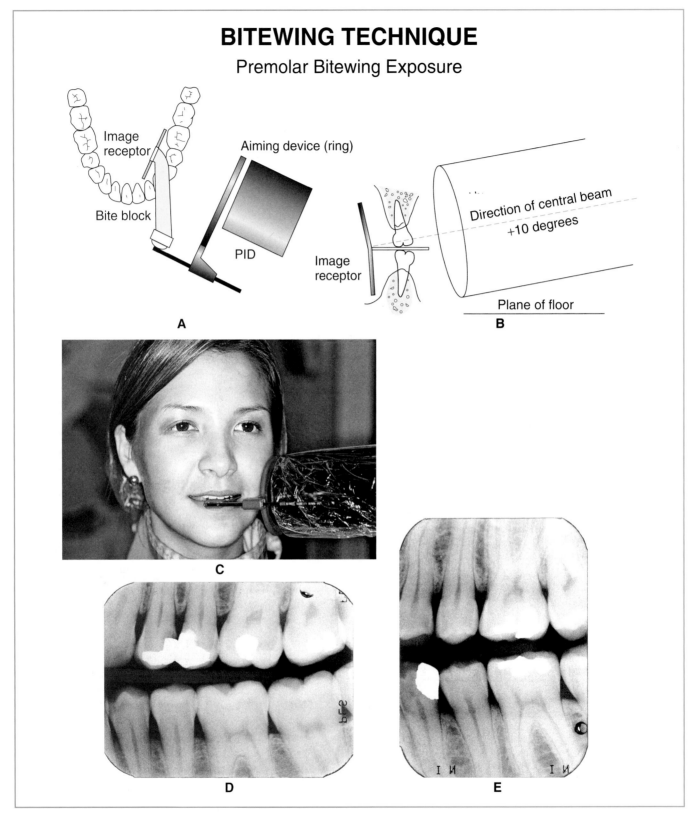

BITEWING TECHNIQUE
Premolar Bitewing Exposure

FIGURE 16-19 Premolar bitewing exposure. (**A**) Diagrams show the relationship of the image receptor and holder, teeth, and PID. (**B**) Vertical angulation is directed perpendicular to the image receptor at approximately +10 degrees with the PID tilted downward. Central ray is directed at the center of the image receptor at a spot on the occlusal plane between the maxillary and mandibular teeth. (**C**) Patient showing position of image receptor holder and 12-in. (30-cm) circular PID. (**D**) Horizontal premolar bitewing radiograph. (**E**) Vertical premolar bitewing radiograph. In the posterior region, the image receptor may be positioned with the long dimension horizontal or vertical.

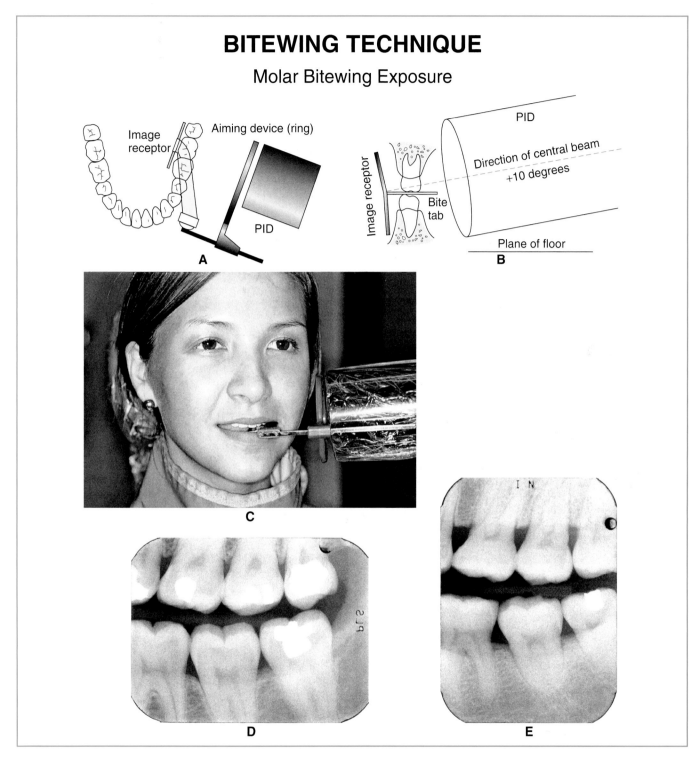

BITEWING TECHNIQUE
Molar Bitewing Exposure

A

B

C

D

E

FIGURE 16-20 Molar bitewing exposure. (**A**) Diagrams show the relationship of the image receptor and holder, teeth, and PID. (**B**) Vertical angulation is directed perpendicular to the image receptor at approximately +10 degrees with the PID tilted downward. Central ray is directed at the center of the image receptor at a spot on the occlusal plane between the maxillary and mandibular teeth. (**C**) Patient showing position of image receptor holder and 12-in. (30-cm) circular PID. (**D**) Horizontal molar bitewing radiograph. (**E**) Vertical molar bitewing radiograph. In the posterior region, the image receptor may be positioned with the long dimension horizontal or vertical.

REVIEW—Chapter summary

Bitewing radiographs image the coronal portion of both maxillary and mandibular teeth on one image receptor. Bitewing radiographs supplement and complete the full mouth survey because of their improved ability to image incipient caries in the tooth contact areas and early resorptive changes in the alveolar bony crest.

The size and number of images to expose depend on the type of survey required and the size and shape of the patient's oral cavity. The image receptor may be positioned with the long dimension horizontally or vertically. Traditionally posterior bitewing radiographs have been positioned horizontally. Anterior bitewing radiographs are positioned vertically. Vertical positioning in the posterior regions image more periodontal bone. The patient's occlusal relationship should be used to determine which arch the radiographer should focus on during placement of the image receptor. Positioning the image receptor a slight distance away from the lingual surfaces of the maxillary teeth of interest will help avoid contact with the curvature of the palate and avoid producing a sloping or slanted image that may result in a retake. Using a systemic order of sequence in exposing bitewing radiographs will help avoid errors.

Image receptor holders/positioners include stick-on or loop bitetabs and instruments with external aiming devices that assist with determining the correct horizontal and vertical angulations and the points of entry. If a holder without an external aiming device is used, the horizontal angulation is determined by directing the central ray of the x-beam perpendicular to the recording plane of the image receptor through the mean tangent of the embrasures between the teeth of interest, and the vertical angulation for all bitewing radiographs is +10 degrees. When the horizontal angulation is directed obliquely from the mesial, overlapping will be more severe in the distal or posterior region of the image; when the horizontal angulation is directed obliquely from the distal, overlapping will be more severe in the mesial or anterior region of the image. When the vertical angulation is excessive (greater than +10°), more maxillary teeth and bone are imaged, cutting off a portion of the mandibular structures. When the vertical angulation is inadequate (less than +10°) more mandibular teeth and bone are imaged, cutting off a portion of the maxillary structures. Directing the central ray of the x-ray beam at the level of the incisal/occlusal plane (at the lip line) will assist with directing the central ray of the x-ray beam to the center of the image receptor to avoid conecut error.

The four basic steps to exposing a bitewing radiograph are placement, vertical angulation, horizontal angulation, and point of entry. Step-by-step illustrated instructions for exposing anterior and posterior bitewing radiographs are presented.

RECALL—Study questions

1. Which of these conditions would NOT be visible on a bitewing radiograph?
   a. Proximal surface caries
   b. Overhanging restoration
   c. Apical abscess
   d. Alveolar crest resorption

2. How many standard-sized #2 image receptors are recommended for a posterior horizontal bitewing survey of an adult patient?
   a. 2
   b. 4
   c. 7
   d. 8

3. In which of the following situations would using a size #3 image receptor be acceptable?
   a. Horizontal bitewings on a child patient who presented a need for them
   b. Horizontal bitewings on an adult patient for caries detection
   c. Horizontal bitewings on an adult patient with periodontal disease
   d. Vertical bitewings on any patient who presented with a need for them

4. In which of the following conditions would vertical bitewing radiographs be recommended over horizontal bitewing radiographs?
   a. Child with rampant caries
   b. Adolescent with suspected third molar impactions
   c. Adult with malaligned teeth
   d. Adult with periodontal disease

5. Which size image receptor is used, and how is it positioned for exposure of an anterior bitewing radiograph of a small and narrow adult arch?
   a. Size #3 placed vertically
   b. Size #2 placed horizontally
   c. Size #1 placed vertically
   d. Size #0 placed horizontally

6. When taking a premolar horizontal bitewing radiograph, the anterior edge of the image receptor should be positioned behind the distal edge of the maxillary canine when presented with which occlusal relationship?
   a. Class I
   b. Class II
   c. Class III

7. When taking a set of eight vertical bitewing radiographs, which of the following should be exposed first?
   a. Left molar bitewing
   b. Left premolar bitewing
   c. Right canine bitewing
   d. Right premolar bitewing

8. Which of the following best fits this description: "Disposable, may be used for placing both horizontal and vertical bitewings, and provides increased imaging of the alveolar bone"?
   a. Stick-on bitetabs
   b. Manufacturer preattached bitetabs
   c. Bite loops
   d. Holder with external aiming device

9. An error in which of these results in overlapping?

   a. Placement of image receptor
   b. Point of entry
   c. Vertical angulation
   d. Horizontal angulation

10. What is the approximate vertical angulation for adult bitewing radiographs?

   a. −10 degrees
   b. 0 degrees
   c. +10 degrees
   d. +20 degrees

11. An error in vertical angulation will result in

   a. unequal distribution of the arches.
   b. overlapping.
   c. overexposure to the patient.
   d. conecut.

12. The image receptor placement for an adult horizontal molar bitewing is to align the receptor so that the

   a. central and lateral incisors are centered.
   b. canine is centered.
   c. anterior portion of the receptor lines up behind the distal half of the canine.
   d. anterior portion of the receptor lines up behind the distal half of the second premolar.

13. The image receptor placement for an adult vertical pre-molar bitewing is to align the receptor so that the

   a. central and lateral incisors are centered.
   b. canine is centered.
   c. anterior portion of the receptor lines up behind the distal half of the canine.
   d. anterior portion of the receptor lines up behind the distal half of the second premolar.

14. Through which interproximal space should the central ray of the x-ray beam be perpendicularly directed when exposing a molar bitewing on a child with primary teeth?

   a. Between the central and lateral incisors
   b. Between the lateral incisor and canine
   c. Between the canine and first molar
   d. Between the first and second molars

15. Through which interproximal space should the central ray of the x-ray beam be perpendicularly directed when exposing a premolar bitewing on an adolescent with permanent teeth?

   a. Between the central and lateral incisors
   b. Between the lateral incisor and canine
   c. Between the canine and first premolar
   d. Between the first and second premolars

REFLECT—Case study

Study the dental chart and patient record that follows. Note the dentist's written prescription for a radiographic examination. Decide the following:

1. What type of bitewings will most likely be exposed?
2. What size image receptor will best fit this patient?
3. How many image receptors will be required to complete the exam?
4. Write out a detailed procedure for exposing each of the required radiographs. Include:

   a. Specific image receptor placements
   b. The vertical angulation required
   c. How the horizontal angulation will be determined
   d. What the point of entry will be

Case:	New patient to your practice.
Age/Gender:	40-year-old male.
Medical History:	Hypertension.
Dental History:	Has had extensive dental treatment in the past as evidenced by several extractions and restored teeth.
Social History:	Appears nervous of dental treatment.
Chief Complaint:	Thinks he has "gum disease."
Current Oral Hygiene Status:	Generalized 4–6 mm pockets; Generalized moderate gingivitis.
Initial Treatment:	Take a set of bitewing radiographs.

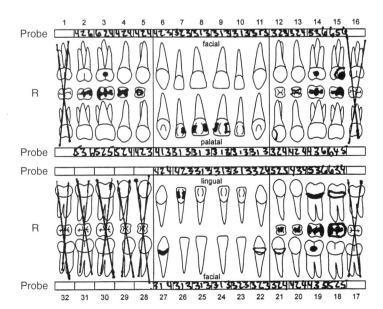

 Clinically visible restoration

 Clinically visible carious lesion

 Clinically missing tooth

RELATE—Laboratory application

For a comprehensive laboratory practice exercise on this topic, see Thomson, E. M. (2012). *Exercises in oral radiography techniques: A laboratory manual* (3rd ed.). Upper Saddle River, NJ: Pearson. Chapter 2, "Bitewing radiographic technique."

REFERENCES

Eastman Kodak Company. (2002). *Successful intraoral radiography.* Rochester, NY: Author.

Rinn Corporation. (1989). *Intraoral radiography with Rinn XCP/BAI instruments.* Elgin, IL: Dentsply/Rinn Corporation.

White, S. C., & Pharoah, M. J. (2008). *Oral radiology: Principles and interpretation* (6th ed.). St. Louis, MO: Elsevier.

Wilkins, E. M. (2010). *Clinical practice of the dental hygienist* (10th ed.). Philadelphia: Lippincott Williams & Wilkins.

The Occlusal Examination

OBJECTIVES

Following successful completion of this chapter, you should be able to:

1. Define the key words.
2. State the purpose of the occlusal examination.
3. List the indications for occlusal radiographs.
4. Match the topographical and cross-sectional techniques with the condition to be imaged.
5. Compare the patient head positions for the topographical and the cross-sectional techniques.
6. Demonstrate the steps for the maxillary and mandibular topographical surveys.
7. Demonstrate the steps for the mandibular cross-sectional survey.

KEY WORDS

Cross-sectional technique
Occlusal radiograph

Topographical technique

Introduction

The purpose of the occlusal examination is to view large areas of the maxilla (upper jaw) or the mandible (lower jaw) on one radiograph. The image receptor is placed in the mouth between the occlusal surfaces of the maxillary and mandibular teeth. The patient occludes (bites) lightly on the image receptor to stabilize it.

The purpose of this chapter is to discuss the use and explain the procedures for the occlusal examination.

Types of Occlusal Examinations

Occlusal radiographs are either topographical or cross-sectional.

Topographical Technique

The **topographical technique** produces an image that looks like a large periapical radiograph (Figure 17-1). The topographical occlusal technique is similar to the bisecting technique used to produce periapical radiographs (see Chapter 15). Topographical occlusal radiographs may be exposed in any area of the oral cavity, the anterior and posterior regions of both the maxilla and the mandible. Topographical occlusal radiographs are best used to image conditions of the teeth and supporting structures when a larger area than that imaged by a periapical radiograph is required. Topographical occlusal surveys generally yield a greater amount of information in the alveolar crest and apical areas than periapical radiographs.

Cross-sectional Technique

The **cross-sectional technique** produces an image much like its name implies (Figure 17-1). The circular or elliptical appearance of the teeth on the radiograph and the increased coverage of the sublingual area (under the tongue) allow the cross-sectional occlusal radiograph to yield more information about the location of tori and impacted or malpositioned teeth and calcifications of soft tissues.

Fundamentals of Occlusal Radiographs

The occlusal examination may be made alone or to supplement periapical or bitewing radiographs. The large size #4 occlusal image receptor is useful for recording information that cannot be adequately recorded on the smaller periapical image receptors. **Occlusal radiographs** are used to:

- Locate supernumerary, unerupted, or impacted teeth (especially impacted canines and third molars)
- Locate retained roots of extracted teeth
- Detect the presence, locate, and evaluate the extent of disease and lesions (cysts, tumors, etc.)
- Locate foreign bodies in the jaws
- Reveal the presence of salivary stones (sialoliths) in the ducts of the sublingual and submandibular glands
- Aid in evaluating fractures of the maxilla or mandible
- Show the size and shape of mandibular tori

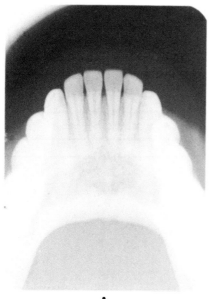
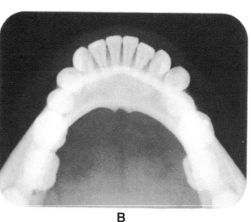

A   **B**

FIGURE 17-1 **A comparison of topographical and cross-sectional occlusal radiographs. (A)** The topographical occlusal radiograph of the anterior mandible closely resembles a periapical radiograph. Note how the large occlusal film images a larger portion of the region. **(B)** The cross-sectional occlusal radiograph of the mandibular anterior region reveals more information about the sublingual area (under the tongue) and conditions of the soft tissue than about the teeth and the supporting bone.

- Aid in examining patients with trismus who can open their mouths only a few millimeters
- Evaluate the borders of the maxillary sinus
- Examine cleft palate patients
- Substitute for a periapical examination on young children who may not be able to tolerate periapical image receptor placement (see Chapter 26)

Occlusal radiographs may be taken in any region of the oral cavity. This chapter focuses on five of the most common standard placements:

1. Maxillary topographical (anterior)
2. Maxillary topographical (posterior)
3. Mandibular topographical (anterior)
4. Mandibular topographical (posterior)
5. Mandibular cross-sectional

Image Receptor Requirements

The large $3 \times 2\ 1/4$ in. (7.7×5.8 cm) #4 film or phosphor plate is used for occlusal radiographs on most adult patients. Currently this larger size #4 is not available as a digital sensor. Smaller size #2 intraoral image receptors may also be used, depending on the area to be examined. The standard #2 periapical film or sensor is frequently used with children, either to image labiolingual or buccolingual unerupted tooth positions or in place of periapical radiographs when needed.

Orientation of the Image Receptor

An image receptor holder is not used for occlusal radiographs. The image receptor is held in place during the exposure by slight pressure of the teeth of the opposite jaw.

When using a size #4 film, the packet is positioned with the white unprinted side (front side) against the arch of interest. When using a phosphor plate, the plain side is positioned against the arch of interest. When imaging the mandibular arch, the white, unprinted side of the image receptor will face the mandible. When imaging the maxillary arch, the white, unprinted side of the image receptor will face the maxilla. The image receptor may be placed into the mouth with the long dimension positioned horizontally or vertically, centered over one small region of interest or over the entire right or left sides of the dental arches. The position used will depend on the type of occlusal radiograph needed and the area to be imaged.

In the correct position, the image receptor should be placed well back into the mouth, but with at least 1/4 in. (1/2 cm) protruding outside the mouth to avoid cutting off part of the image. Because the embossed identification dot (on the film packet) should be positioned away from the area of interest, positioning it toward the anterior should leave it outside the mouth and therefore prevent it from interfering with the image.

Patient Positioning

Because predetermined vertical angulations and points of entry are utilized in taking occlusal radiographs (just as

they are for periapical radiographs using the bisecting technique), it is very important that the patient be seated with the head in the correct position for the area to be imaged. For occlusal radiographs taken on the maxilla, the patient should be seated with the occlusal plane parallel to the plane of the floor and the midsagittal plane perpendicular to the plane of the floor (see Figure 13-14). The head position for the mandibular exposures will depend on the type of occlusal radiograph to be produced. Topographical occlusal radiographs of the mandible may be taken with the head positioned the same as for maxillary exposures, with the occlusal plane parallel to the floor and the midsagittal plane perpendicular to the floor. Mandibular cross-sectional occlusal radiographs are taken with the patient reclined in the chair so that the head is tipped back, positioning the occlusal plane perpendicular to the plane of the floor (Figure 17-2).

Exposure Factors

The exposure factors (kVp, mA, and time) used for occlusal radiographs are usually the same as those settings used for periapical and bitewing radiographs of the same region.

Horizontal and Vertical Angulation Procedures

Horizontal Angulation

The correct horizontal angulation for topographical occlusal radiographs is determined in the same manner as for periapical and bitewing radiographs; by directing the central rays at the image receptor perpendicularly through the teeth embrasures (spaces). When exposing anterior topographical occlusal radiographs, direct the central rays of the x-ray beam perpendicular to the image receptor through the interproximal embrasures of the anterior teeth. When exposing posterior topographical occlusal radiographs, direct the central rays of the x-ray beam perpendicular to the image receptor through

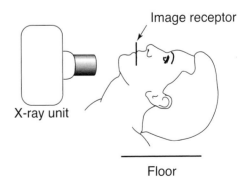

FIGURE 17-2 Patient positioning for mandibular cross-sectional occlusal radiographs. Patient reclined in the chair so that the head is tipped back, positioning the occlusal plane perpendicular to the plane of the floor. The central rays of the x-ray beam are directed toward the image receptor perpendicularly.

the interproximal spaces or embrasures of the posterior teeth. The horizontal angulation for the mandibular cross-sectional is also such that the central rays will intersect the image receptor perpendicularly. This alignment is best determined by positioning the open end of the PID parallel to the image receptor.

Vertical Angulation

The vertical angulation for topographical radiographs follows the rules of the bisecting technique used for periapical radiographs, where the central rays of the x-ray beam are directed through the apices of the teeth perpendicularly toward the bisector (Figure 17-3). To determine the correct vertical angulation when taking a topographical occlusal radiograph, the radiographer must observe the plane of the image receptor, locate the long axes of the teeth of interest, and estimate the imaginary bisector of these two planes. If the patient's head is in the correct position, the radiographer can use predetermined vertical angulation settings (Table 17-1).

The vertical angulation for the mandibular cross-sectional occlusal radiograph of the mandible is such that the central rays of the x-ray beam are directed toward the image receptor perpendicularly (Figure 17-2). To achieve a perpendicular relationship between the plane of the image receptor and the central rays of the x-ray beam, the patient's head position must be such that the occlusal plane is perpendicular to the plane of the floor. In other words, the patient should be reclined and the chin tipped upward. In this position, the vertical angulation will most likely be set at 0°, allowing the x-rays to strike the image receptor perpendicularly.

Cross-sectional occlusal radiographs of the maxilla are sometimes needed to assess the maxillary sinus, edentulous ridges, or other specific needs. However, the significant amount of bony structures located here make cross-sectional occlusal radiographs of the maxilla difficult to image with clarity. Therefore maxillary cross-sectional occlusal radiographs are exposed less frequently.

Points of Entry

If the patient's head is in the correct position, predetermined points of entry may be used (Table 17-2). Essentially, the central rays of the x-ray beam should strike the middle of the image receptor. The open end of the PID must be aligned as close as possible to the patient's skin at the correct point of entry. Although occlusal radiographs can be made with any length position indicating device (PID), the shorter 8-in. (20.5-cm) length may be easier to position into the increased vertical angulation positions required for this technique. In addition, because of the angular relationship between the object (teeth) and the central ray of the x-ray beam, a longer PID length (16-in./41-cm) will likely add to the dimensional distortion of the image.

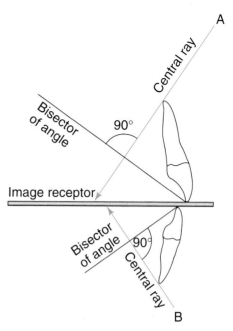

FIGURE 17-3 Angulation theory of topographical occlusal radiographs. The image receptor placement for occlusal radiographs is not parallel to the long axes of the teeth being imaged. Based on the bisecting technique, vertical angulation for (**A**) maxillary and (**B**) mandibular topographical radiographs is determined by directing the central rays of the x-ray beam perpendicular to the imaginary bisector between the plane of the image receptor and the long axes of the teeth of interest.

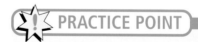

PRACTICE POINT

When exposing an occlusal radiograph on the mandible, it may be necessary to modify placement of the lead/lead equivalent thyroid collar. Although it is very important to use ALARA (as low as reasonably achievable) practices and use the lead/lead equivalent thyroid collar to protect radiation-sensitive tissues in the head and neck region, the thyroid collar may be in the path of the primary beam during mandibular topographical and/or cross-sectional techniques.

You should place the lead/lead equivalent apron and thyroid collar on the patient in the usual manner. After adjusting the patient's head position and placing the image receptor, align the PID and check to be sure that the thyroid collar is not in the path of the x-ray beam. If the thyroid collar is in a position that will block the x-rays from reaching the image receptor, adjust the collar position. Failure to remove the thyroid collar from in front of the open end of the PID will most likely result in a retake of the radiograph.

TABLE 17-1 Recommended Vertical Angulation Settings for Occlusal Radiographs

OCCLUSAL RADIOGRAPH	VERTICAL ANGLE SETTING*
Maxillary topographical (anterior)	+65°
Maxillary topographical (posterior)	+45°
Mandibular topographical (anterior)	−55°
Mandibular topographical (posterior)	−45°
Mandibular cross-sectional	0°**

*The patient must be seated in the correct position, with the occlusal plane of the arch being imaged parallel to the floor and the midsaggital plane perpendicular to the floor.

**The patient must be seated in the correct position, with the occlusal plane of the mandible perpendicular to the floor and the midsaggital plane parallel to the floor.

The Occlusal Examination

Figures 17-4 through 17-8 illustrate the image receptor positions and required angulations for each of the topographical and cross-sectional occlusal radiographs discussed in this chapter. See Table 17-2 for a summary of the technique.

TABLE 17-2 A Summary of Occlusal Radiographic Technique

OCCLUSAL RADIOGRAPH	PLACEMENT	VERTICAL ANGULATION*	HORIZONTAL ANGULATION	POINT OF ENTRY*
Maxillary topographical (anterior) (Figure 17-4)	Long dimension across the mouth (buccal-to-buccal). White unprinted film side toward the maxillary teeth.	Perpendicular to the imaginary bisector between the long axes of the teeth and image receptor in the vertical dimension, +65°.	Perpendicular to the image receptor through the maxillary central incisor embrasure.	Through a point near the bridge of the nose toward the center of the image receptor
Maxillary topographical (posterior) (Figure 17-5)	Long dimension along the midline (front-to-back). White unprinted film side toward the maxillary teeth.	Perpendicular to the imaginary bisector between the long axes of the teeth and the image receptor in the vertical dimension, +45°.	Perpendicular to the image receptor through the maxillary posterior embrasures.	Through a point on the ala–tragus line below the outer cantus of the eye (see Figure 15-7) toward the center of the image receptor
Mandibular topographical (anterior) (Figure 17-6)	Long dimension across the mouth (buccal-to-buccal). White unprinted film side toward the mandibular teeth.	Perpendicular to the imaginary bisector between the long axes of the teeth and the image receptor in the vertical dimension, −55°.	Perpendicular to the image receptor through the mandibular central incisor embrasure.	Through a point on the middle of the chin toward the center of the image receptor
Mandibular topographical (posterior) (Figure 17-7)	Long dimension along the midline (front-to-back). White unprinted film side toward the mandibular teeth.	Perpendicular to the imaginary bisector between the long axes of the teeth and the image receptor in the vertical dimension, −45°	Perpendicular to the image receptor through the mandibular posterior embrasures.	Through a point on the inferior border of the mandible directly below the second mandibular premolar toward the center of the image receptor
Mandibular cross-sectional (Figure 17-8)	Long dimension across the mouth (buccal-to-buccal). White unprinted side toward the mandibular teeth.	Perpendicular to the image receptor; 0°.**	Align the open end of the PID parallel to the plane of the image receptor	Through a point 2 in. (5 cm) back from the tip of the chin toward the center of the image receptor**

*The patient must be seated in the correct position, with the occlusal plane of the arch being imaged parallel to the floor and the midsaggital plane perpendicular to the floor.

**The patient must be seated in the correct position, with the occlusal plane of the mandible perpendicular to the floor and the midsaggital plane parallel to the floor.

OCCLUSAL TECHNIQUE
Maxillary Topographical Occlusal Radiograph (Anterior)

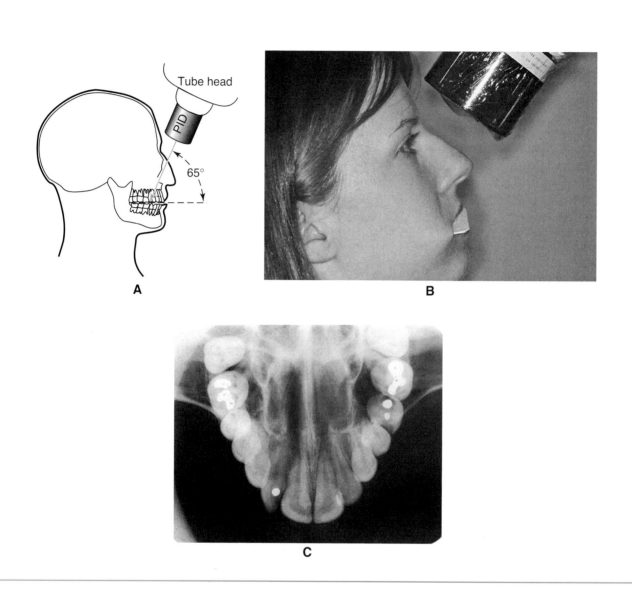

FIGURE 17-4 Maxillary topographical occlusal radiograph (anterior). (A) Diagram showing relationship of tube head and PID to image receptor and patient. Exposure side of the image receptor faces the maxillary arch with longer dimension buccal-to-buccal (across the arch). The central ray is directed perpendicular in the horizontal dimension to the patient's midsagittal plane through the maxillary central incisor embrasure. The vertical angulation is directed approximately +65° through a point near the bridge of the nose toward the center of the image receptor. **(B)** Patient showing position of image receptor and 8-in. (20.5-cm) circular PID. **(C)** Anterior maxillary topographical occlusal radiograph.

OCCLUSAL TECHNIQUE
Maxillary Topographical Occlusal Radiograph (Posterior)

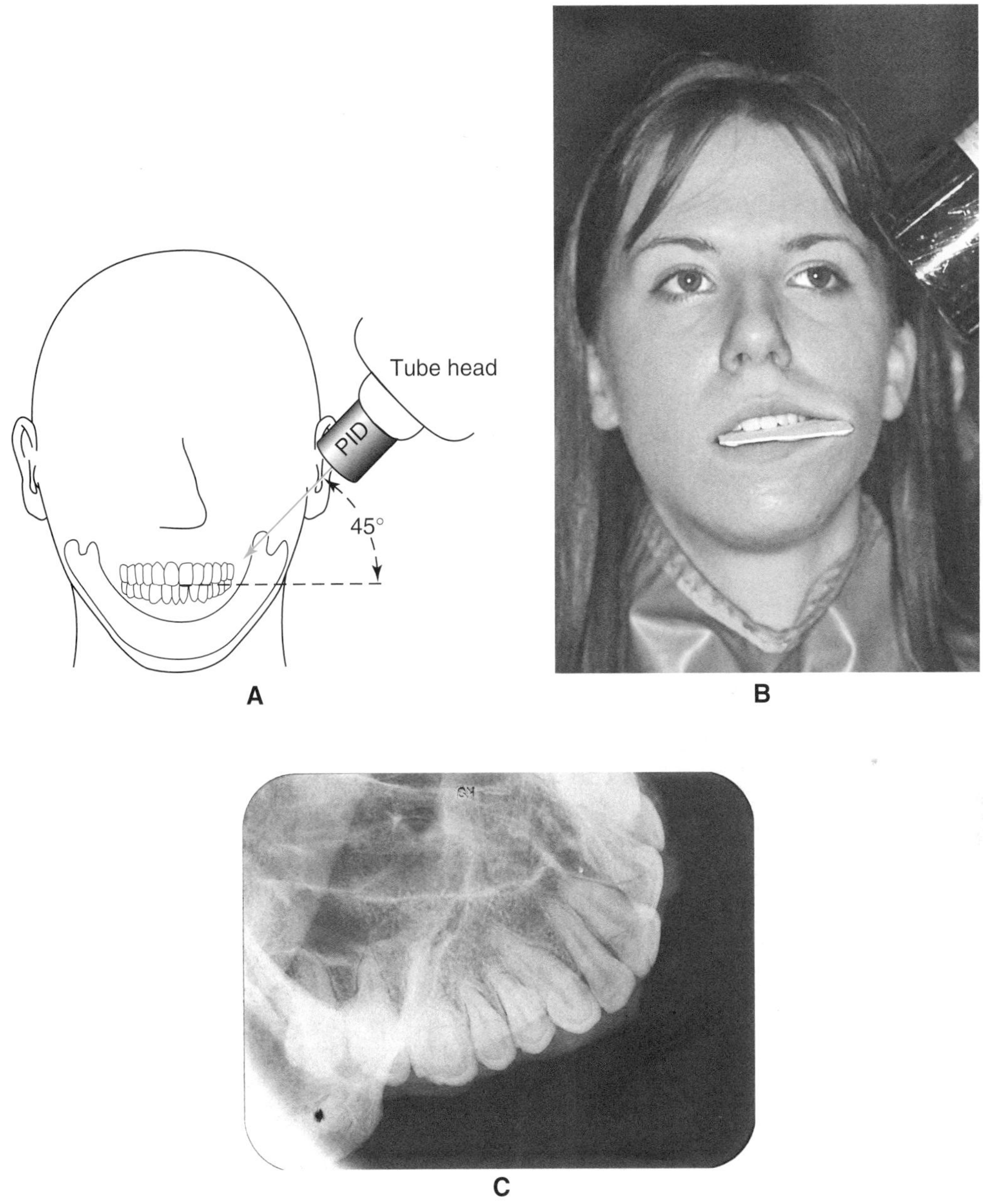

FIGURE 17-5 Maxillary topographical occlusal radiograph (posterior). (A) Diagram showing relationship of tube head and PID to image receptor and patient. The image receptor is positioned over the left or right side, depending on the area of interest. Exposure side of the image receptor faces the maxillary arch with longer dimension along the midline (anterior-to-posterior). The central ray is directed perpendicular in the horizontal dimension to patient's midsagittal plane through the maxillary posterior embrasures. The vertical angulation is directed approximately +45° through a point on the ala–tragus line below the outer canthus of the eye toward the center of the image receptor. **(B)** Patient showing position of image receptor and 8-in. (20.5-cm) circular PID. **(C)** Posterior maxillary topographical occlusal radiograph.

OCCLUSAL TECHNIQUE
Mandibular Topographical Occlusal Radiograph (Anterior)

A

B

C

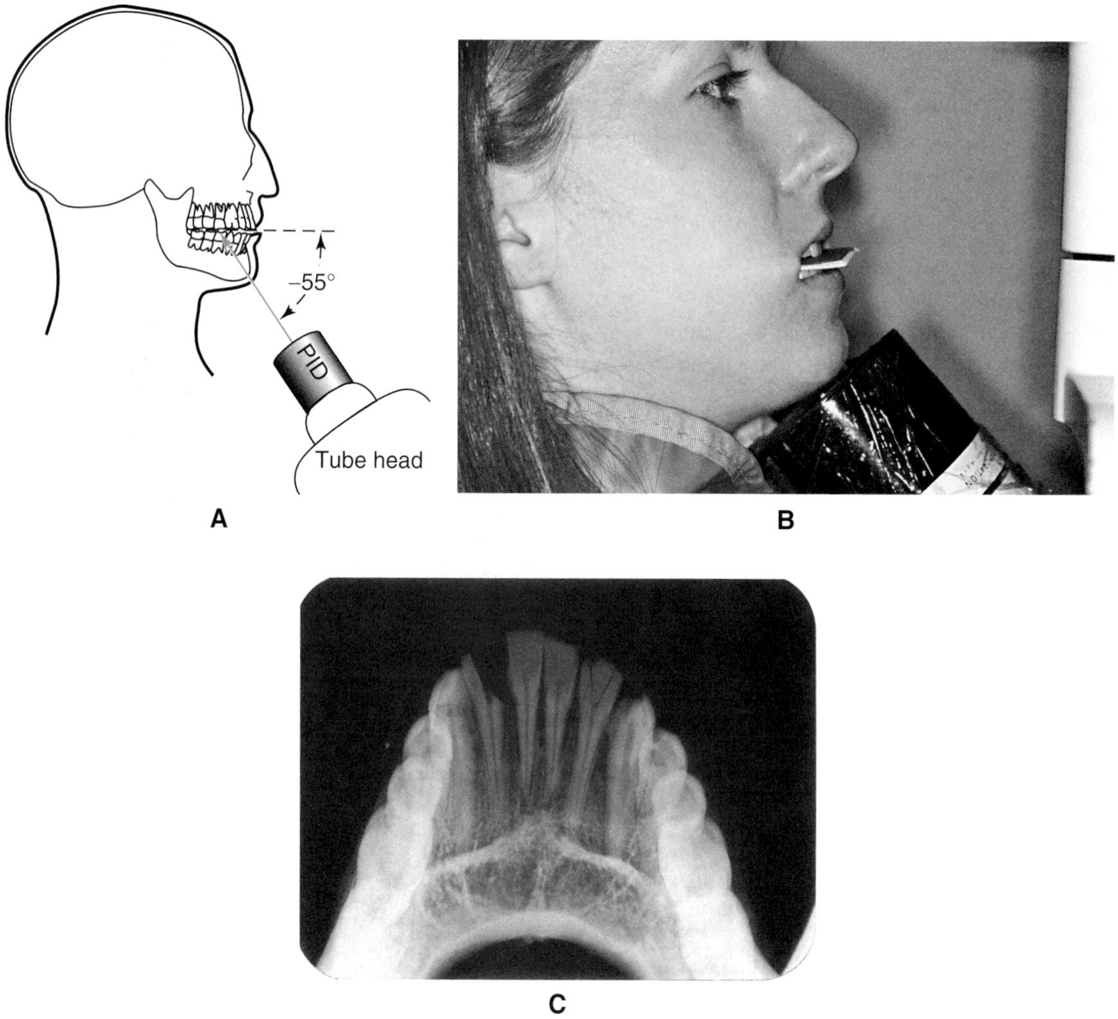

FIGURE 17-6 **Mandibular topographical occlusal radiograph (anterior).** (**A**) Diagram showing relationship of tube head and PID to image receptor and patient. Exposure side of the image receptor faces the mandibular arch with longer dimension buccal-to-buccal (across the arch). The central ray is directed perpendicular in the horizontal dimension to patient's midsaggittal plane through the mandibular central incisor embrasure. The vertical angulation is directed approximately −55° through a point in the middle of the chin toward the center of the image receptor. (**B**) Patient showing position of image receptor and 8-in. (20.5-cm) circular PID. (**C**) Anterior mandibular topographical occlusal radiograph.

OCCLUSAL TECHNIQUE
Mandibular Topographical Occlusal Radiograph (Posterior)

A

B

C

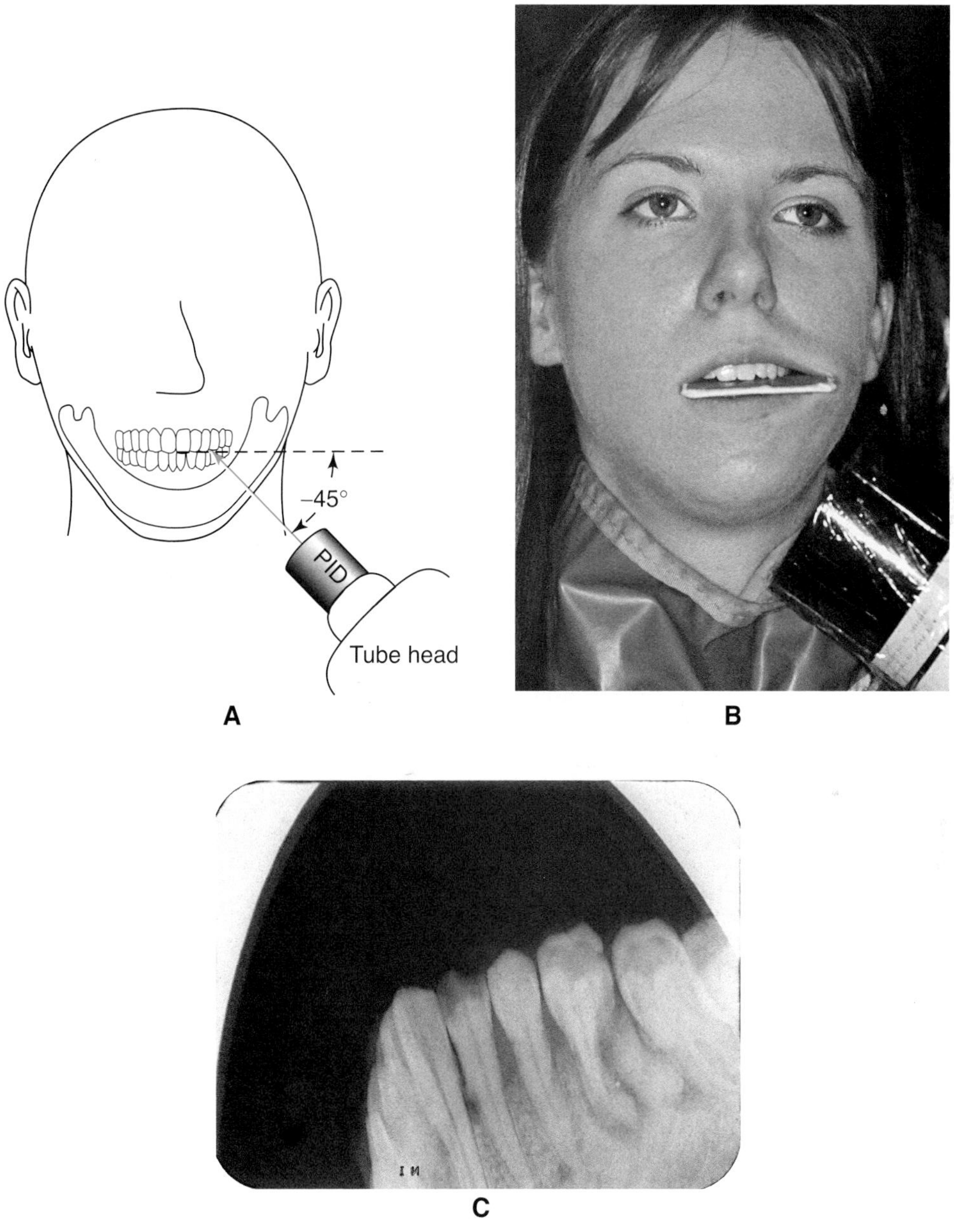

FIGURE 17-7 **Mandibular topographical occlusal radiograph (posterior).** (**A**) Diagram showing relationship of tube head and PID to image receptor and patient. The image receptor is positioned over the left or right side, depending on the area of interest. Exposure side of the image receptor faces the mandibular arch with longer dimension along the midline (anterior-to-posterior). The central ray is directed perpendicular in the horizontal dimension to patient's midsagittal plane through the mandibular posterior embrasures. The vertical angulation is directed approximately −45° through a point on the inferior border of the mandible directly below the second mandibular premolar toward the center of the image receptor. (**B**) Patient showing position of image receptor and 8-in. (20.5-cm) circular PID. (**C**) Posterior mandibular topographical occlusal radiograph.

OCCLUSAL TECHNIQUE
Mandibular Cross-Sectional Occlusal Radiograph

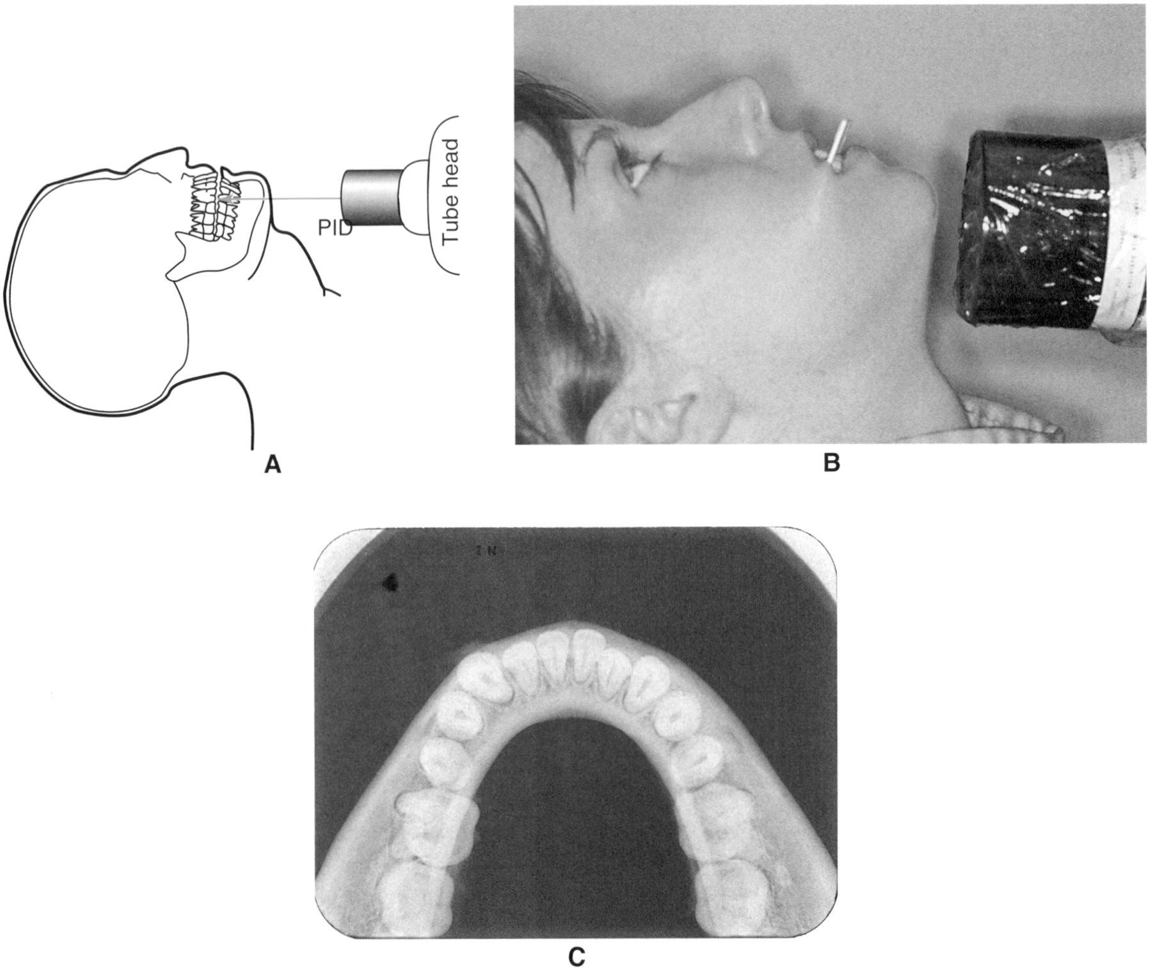

FIGURE 17-8 Mandibular cross-sectional occlusal radiograph. (A) Diagram showing relationship of tube head and PID to image receptor and patient. The exposure side of the image receptor faces the mandibular arch with the longer dimension buccal-to-buccal (across the arch). The central ray is directed perpendicular in both the horizontal and vertical dimensions toward the image receptor. Positioning the open end of the PID parallel to the image receptor achieves the required perpendicular alignment. The vertical angulation is directed approximately 0° through a point 2 in. (5 cm) back from the tip of the chin toward the center of the image receptor. **(B)** Patient showing position of image receptor and 8-in. (20.5-cm) circular PID. **(C)** Mandibular cross-sectional occlusal radiograph.

REVIEW—Chapter summary

The purpose of occlusal radiographs is to image a larger area than that produced on a periapical radiograph. The topographical occlusal teachnique is based on a modification of the bisecting technique used to expose periapical radiographs. The x-ray beam is directed perpendicularly toward the image receptor in both the horizontal and vertical dimensions when exposing a cross-sectional occlusal radiograph. Occlusal radiographs are used to view conditions of the teeth and supporting structures such as impactions, large apical lesions, calcifications in soft tissue, and fractures.

Size #4 image receptor is used for adult examinations. If indicated, a size #2 or smaller image receptor may be used with the occlusal technique, especially for children. An image receptor holder is not required; the patient lightly bites down on the image receptor to hold it in place. The image receptor may be positioned with the long dimension horizontal or vertical with at least 1/4 in. (1/2 cm) protruding outside the mouth.

The patient's head should be positioned with the occlusal plane parallel and the midsaggital plane perpendicular to the floor when exposing maxillary and mandibular topographical occlusal radiographs. The patient's head should be tipped back into a position with the occlusal plane perpendicular to the plane of the floor and the midsaggital plane parallel to the floor when exposing a mandibular cross-sectional occlusal radiograph.

The horizontal angulation used to produce a topographical occlusal radiograph is determined in the same manner as for periapical and bitewing radiographs, where the central rays of the x-ray beam are directed perpendicularly to the image receptor through the embrasures of the teeth of interest. Aligning the open end of the PID parallel to the image receptor will assist in determining the correct horizontal angulation to produce a cross-sectional occlusal radiograph. The vertical angulation used to produce a topographical occlusal radiograph is determined in a similar manner to the bisecting technique used to produce periapical radiographs, where the central rays of the x-ray beam are directed perpendicularly to the bisector between the long axes of the teeth and the plane of the image receptor. Determining the vertical angulation for exposure of a cross-sectional occlusal radiograph is assisted by positioning the open end of the PID parallel to the plane of the image receptor. Correct points of entry position are determined by directing the central rays of the x-ray beam at the center of the image receptor. If the patient's head is in correct position, predetermined vertical angulations and points of the entry may be used. Step-by-step illustrated instructions for exposing five of the most common occlusal radiographs are presented

RECALL—Study questions

1. Each of the following is an indication for exposing occlusal radiographs EXCEPT one. Which one is the EXCEPTION?
   a. Evaluate periodontal disease
   b. Examine sinus borders
   c. Locate foreign bodies
   d. Reveal sialoliths

2. Which of the following will a mandibular cross-sectional occlusal radiograph best image?
   a. Cleft palate
   b. Fractured jaw
   c. Large periapical cyst
   d. Sublingual swelling

3. Which of these sizes is known as the occlusal image receptor?
   a. #1
   b. #2
   c. #3
   d. #4

4. The image receptor should be placed with the long dimension along the midline (front to back) for which of these occlusal radiographs?
   a. Maxillary topographical anterior
   b. Maxillary topographical posterior
   c. Mandibular topographical anterior
   d. Mandibular cross-sectional

5. Where should the embossed dot be positioned when placing an occlusal film packet intraorally?
   a. Toward the apical
   b. Toward the occlusal
   c. Toward the anterior
   d. Toward the posterior

6. The ideal patient head position when exposing a maxillary topographical occlusal radiograph is to position the occlusal plane _____ to the plane of the floor and the midsaggital plane _____ to the plane of the floor.
   a. parallel; perpendicular
   b. perpendicular; parallel
   c. parallel; parallel
   d. perpendicular; perpendicular

7. The ideal patient head position when exposing a mandibular cross-sectional occlusal radiograph is to position the head rest so that the chin is tipped _____ and the occlusal plane is _____ to the plane of the floor.
   a. down; perpendicular
   b. up; perpendicular
   c. down; parallel
   d. up; parallel

8. Assuming that the patient's head is in the correct position, which of the following is the correct vertical angulation setting for a maxillary anterior topographical occlusal radiograph?
   a. +65 degrees
   b. +45 degrees
   c. 0 degrees
   d. −55 degrees

9. Assuming that the patient's head is in the correct position, which of the following is the correct vertical angulation setting for a mandibular cross-sectional occlusal radiograph?

   a. +65 degrees

   b. +45 degrees

   c. 0 degrees

   d. −55 degrees

10. What is the point of entry for correctly exposing a posterior mandible topographical occlusal radiograph?

    a. The middle of the chin

    b. A point 2 in. (5 cm) back from the tip of the chin

    c. A point on the ala–tragus line below the outer cantus of the eye

    d. A point on the inferior border of the mandible directly below the second mandibular premolar

REFLECT—Case study

Consider the following cases. After determining the radiographic assessment for each of these three cases, write out a detailed procedure chart that a radiographer can follow to obtain the needed radiographs. Begin with patient positioning. Be sure to include the steps for determining the correct placement of the image receptor, x-ray beam angles, and landmarks for determining points of entry.

1. An adult patient presents with a sublingual swelling indicating the possibility of a blocked salivary gland. What type of occlusal radiograph will this patient most likely be assessed for?

2. An adult patient presents with severe pain in the mandibular left posterior region, indicating the possibility of an impacted third molar. The pain and swelling in this region is preventing the patient from opening more than a few millimeters. What type of occlusal radiograph will this patient most likely be assessed for?

3. A child patient presents with trauma to the maxillary anterior teeth after a fall off her bicycle. What type of occlusal radiograph will this patient most likely be assessed for?

RELATE—Laboratory application

For a comprehensive laboratory practice exercise on this topic, see Thomson, E. M. (2012). *Exercises in oral radiography techniques: A laboratory manual* (3rd ed.). Upper Saddle River, NJ: Pearson Education. Chapter 10 "Occlusal Radiographic Technique."

REFERENCES

Carroll, M. K. (1993). *Advanced oral radiographic techniques: Part I, occlusal and lateral oblique projections* (videorecording). Jackson, MS: Health Sciences Consortium, Learning Resources, University of Mississippi Medical Center.

Eastman Kodak Company. (2002). *Successful intraoral radiography.* Rochester, NY: Author.

White, S. C., & Pharoah, M. J. (2008). *Oral radiology: Principles and interpretation* (6th ed.). St. Louis, MO: Elsevier.

Identifying and Correcting Undiagnostic Radiographs

OBJECTIVES

Following successful completion of this chapter, you should be able to:

1. Define the key words.
2. Recognize errors caused by incorrect radiographic techniques.
3. Apply the appropriate corrective actions for technique errors.
4. Recognize errors caused by incorrect radiographic processing.
5. Apply the appropriate corrective actions for processing errors.
6. Recognize errors caused by incorrect radiographic image receptor handling.
7. Apply the appropriate corrective actions for handling errors.
8. Identify five causes of film fog.
9. Apply the appropriate actions for preventing film fog.

KEY WORDS

Artifacts	Herringbone error
Conecut error	Mesiodistal overlap
Dead pixel	Overdevelopment
Distomesial overlap	Overexposure
Double exposure	Overlapping
Electronic noise	Static electricity
Elongation	Underdevelopment
Film fog	Underexposure
Foreshortening	

Introduction

Although radiographs play an important role in oral health care, it should be remembered that exposure to radiation carries a risk. The radiographer has an ethical responsibility to the patient to produce the highest diagnostic quality radiographs, in return for the patient's consent to undergo the radiographic examination. Less-than-ideal radiographic images diminish the usefulness of the radiograph. When the error is significant, a radiograph will have to be retaken. In addition to increasing the patient's radiation exposure, retake radiographs require additional patient consent and may reduce the patient's confidence in the operator and in the practice.

> *No radiograph should be retaken until a thorough investigation reveals the exact cause of the error and the appropriate corrective action is identified and can be implemented.*

It is important that the radiographer develop the skills needed to identify radiographic errors. Identifying common mistakes and knowing the causes will help the knowledgeable operator avoid these pitfalls. Being able to identify the cause of an undiagnostic image will allow the radiographer to apply the appropriate corrective action for retaking the exposure.

The purpose of this chapter is to investigate common radiographic errors, identify probable causes of such errors, and present the appropriate corrective actions.

Recognizing Radiographic Errors

To recognize errors that diminish the diagnostic quality of a radiograph, the radiographer must understand what a quality image looks like (Table 18-1). First and foremost, the radiograph must be an accurate representation of the teeth and the supporting structures. The image should not be magnified, elongated, foreshortened, or otherwise distorted. Image density and contrast should be correct for ease of interpretation: not too light, or too dark, or fogged. The radiograph should be free of errors.

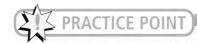

PRACTICE POINT

All errors reduce the quality of the radiograph. However, not all errors create a need to re-expose the patient. Two examples of this are when the error does not affect the area of interest and when the error affects only one image in a series (bitewings or full mouth), where the area of interest can be viewed in an adjacent radiograph. For example, a radiograph may have a conecut error, cutting off part of the image. If the conecut error does not affect the area of interest, a retake would not be required. Consider this situation, where a periapical radiograph is exposed to image a suspected apical pathology in the posterior region. If the conecut error occurs in the anterior portion, cutting off the second premolar, but an abscess at the root apex of the first molar is adequately imaged, the radiograph would most likely not have to be retaken.

When exposing a set of radiographs such as a vertical bitewing or full mouth series, if an error prevents adequate imaging of a condition, adjacent radiographs should be observed for the possibility that the condition may be adequately revealed in another image. For example, if one radiograph in a set of bitewings is overlapped, it should be determined if the adjacent radiograph images the area adequately. If so, a retake would most likely not be indicated. Determining when a retake is absolutely necessary will keep radiation exposure to a minimum.

Recognizing the cause of radiographic errors is important in being able to take corrective action. Errors that diminish the diagnostic quality of radiographs may be divided into three categories:

1. Technique errors
2. Processing errors
3. Handling errors

TABLE 18-1 Characteristics of a Quality Radiograph	
BITEWING RADIOGRAPH	**PERIAPICAL RADIOGRAPH**
• Image receptor placed correctly to record area of interest	• Image receptor placed correctly to record area of interest
• Equal portion of the maxilla and mandible recorded	• Entire tooth plus at least 2 mm beyond the incisal/occlusal edges of the crowns and beyond the root apex recorded
• Occlusal/incisal plane of the teeth is parallel to the edge of the image receptor	• Occlusal/incisal plane of the teeth is parallel with the edge of the image receptor
• Occlusal plane straight or slightly curved upward toward the posterior	• Embossed dot positioned toward the incisal/occlusal edge
• Most posterior contact point between adjacent teeth recorded	• In a full mouth survey, each tooth should be recorded at least once, preferably twice

It is important to note that errors in any of these categories may produce the same or a similar result. For example, it is possible that a dark radiographic image may have been caused by **overexposure** (a technique error) or by **overdevelopment** (a processing error), or by exposing the film to white light (a handling error). For the purpose of defining the more common radiographic errors, we will discuss the errors according to these three categories.

Technique Errors

Technique errors include mistakes made in placement of the image receptor, positioning of the PID (vertical and horizontal angulations), and setting exposure factors. Additional technical problems include movement of the patient, the image receptor, or the PID.

Incorrect Positioning of the Image Receptor

The most basic technique error is not imaging the correct teeth. The radiographer must know the standard image receptor placements for all types of projections and must possess the skills necessary to achieve these correct placements.

NOT RECORDING ANTERIOR STRUCTURES

- **Probable causes:** The image receptor was placed too far back in the patient's oral cavity. Due to the curvature and narrowing of the arches in the anterior region, it is sometimes difficult to place the image receptor far enough anterior without impinging on sensitive mucosa. This is especially likely when tori are present. When using a digital sensor, the wire and/or plastic barrier may further compromise fitting the image receptor into the correct position.
- **Corrective actions:** To avoid placing a corner of the image receptor uncomfortably in contact with the soft tissues lingual to the canine, position the receptor in toward the midline of the oral cavity, away from the lingual surfaces of the teeth of interest. When positioning the image receptor for a premolar radiograph, the anterior edge of the receptor may be positioned to contact the canine on the opposite side to achieve the correct position (Figure 18-1).

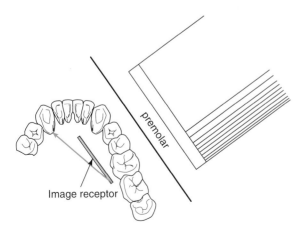

FIGURE 18-1 Tip for positioning the image receptor for exposure of a premolar radiograph. Positioning the anterior edge of the image receptor against the canine on the opposite side places the image receptor into the correct anterior position.

NOT RECORDING POSTERIOR STRUCTURES

- **Probable causes:** The image receptor was placed too far forward in the patient's oral cavity. The beginning radiographer is sometimes hesitant about placing the image receptor far enough posterior to record diagnostic information about the third molar region. This is especially true when the patient presents with a small oral cavity or a hypersensitive gag reflex.

- **Corrective actions:** Communicate with the patient to gain acceptance and assistance with placing the image receptor. Use tips for working with an exaggerated gag reflex. (See Chapter 27.)

NOT RECORDING APICAL STRUCTURES (FIGURE 18-2)

- **Probable causes:**

  1. Image receptor was not placed high enough (maxillary) or low enough (mandibular) in the patient's oral cavity to image the root apices. This often occurs when the patient does not occlude completely and securely on the image receptor holder biteblock or tab.

  2. Inadequate (not steep enough) vertical angulation will result in less of the apical region being recorded onto the radiograph.

- **Corrective actions:** *(In a paralleling technique)*

  1. Ensure that the image receptor is positioned correctly into the holding device and that the patient is biting down all the way. Tip the image receptor in toward the middle of the oral cavity where the midline of the palatal vault is the highest to facilitate the patient biting all the way down on the holder biteblock. When placing the image receptor on the mandible, using an index finger, gently massage the sublingual area to relax and move the tongue out of the way while positioning the image receptor low enough to record the mandibular teeth root apices.

  2. Increase vertical angulation. If correctly directing the central rays perpendicular to the image receptor when using the paralleling technique (see Chapter 14) and perpendicular to the imaginary bisector when using the bisecting technique (see Chapter 15) does not record enough apical structures, increase the vertical angulation slightly. An increase of no greater than 15 degrees will still produce an acceptable radiographic image.

NOT RECORDING CORONAL STRUCTURES (FIGURE 18-3)

- **Probable causes:** Because this error appears to be the opposite of not recording the apical structures, it would seem logical to assume that the image receptor was placed too high (maxillary) or too low (mandibular) in the patient's oral cavity to image the entire crowns of these teeth. However, the use of image receptor holders will almost always eliminate this error. When noted, the cause is more often the result of excessive vertical angulation.

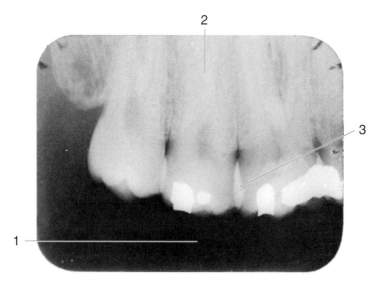

FIGURE 18-2 Radiograph of maxillary molar area. Not recording the apical structures most likely resulted from a combination of not placing the image receptor correctly and inadequate vertical angulation. (**1**) The patient did not occlude completely and securing on the image receptor biteblock causing the image receptor to be placed too low in the mouth. (**2**) Inadequate (not steep enough) vertical angulation resulted in not recording the apical structures and a stretching out of the image called elongation. (**3**) Overlapped contacts results from incorrect horizontal angulation. In this example, the overlapping is more severe in the anterior (mesial) region and less severe in the posterior (distal) region, indicating distomesial projection of the x-ray beam toward the image receptor.

- **Corrective actions:** Decrease vertical angulation. If correctly directing the central rays perpendicular to the image receptor when using the paralleling technique (see Chapter 14) and perpendicular to the imaginary bisector when using the bisecting technique (see Chapter 15) does not record enough coronal structures, decrease the vertical angulation slightly. A decrease of no greater than 15 degrees will still produce an acceptable radiographic image.

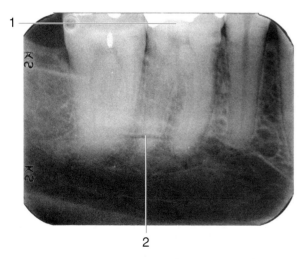

FIGURE 18-3 Radiograph of mandibular molar area.
(**1**) Not recording the entire occlusal structures most likely resulted from excessive (too steep) vertical angulation.
(**2**) Note the radiolucent artifact (horizontal line) that resulted from bending the image receptor, in this case a film packet.

SLANTING OR TILTED INSTEAD OF STRAIGHT OCCLUSAL PLANE (FIGURE 18-4)

- **Probable causes:** The edge of the image receptor was not parallel with the incisal or occlusal plane of the teeth, or the image receptor holder was not placed flush against the occlusal surfaces. This error often results when the top edge of the image receptor contacts the lingual gingiva or the curvature of the palate; and when the image receptor is placed on top of the tongue.
- **Corrective actions:** Straighten the image receptor by positioning away from the lingual surfaces of the teeth. Place the image receptor in toward the midline of the palate. Utilize this highest region of the palatal vault to stand the image receptor up parallel to the long axes of the teeth. For mandibular

⭐ PRACTICE POINT

The misuse of a cotton roll to help stabilize the image receptor holder is often the cause of the root tips being cut off the resultant radiographic image. A cotton roll is sometimes utilized to help the patient bite down on the holder's biteblock to secure it in place (see Chapter 14). This practice is appropriate when used correctly. Correct placement of the cotton roll is on the opposite side of the biteblock from where the teeth occlude. Placing the cotton roll on the same side as the teeth will prevent the image receptor from being placed high enough (maxillary) or low enough (mandibular) in the mouth.

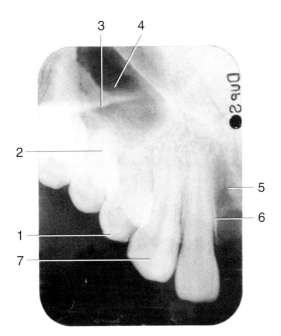

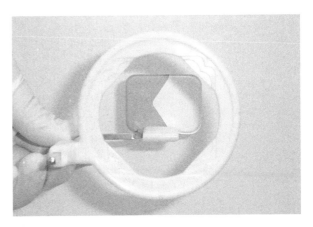

FIGURE 18-6 Incorrect reversed film packet. An examination through the ring of this image receptor holder assembly reveals that the back of the film packet will be positioned incorrectly toward the teeth and the x-ray source.

FIGURE 18-4 Radiograph of maxillary canine area. (**1**) Slanting or diagonal occlusal plane caused by incorrect position of the image receptor. (**2**) Foreshortened images caused by a combination of excessive vertical angulation and incorrect image receptor position. (**3**) Distortion caused by bending the image receptor. (**4**) Maxillary sinus, (**5**) recent extraction site, (**6**) lamina dura, and (**7**) image of the canine is distorted.

placements, slide the image receptor in between the lingual gingiva and the lateral surface of the tongue. Ensure that the patient is biting down securely on the biteblock of the holder.

REVERSED IMAGE ERROR (HERRINGBONE ERROR)

- **Probable causes:** The image receptor film packet was positioned so that the back side was facing the teeth and the radiation source. The first thing that the radiographer will notice is that the radiograph will be significantly underexposed (too light). However, when placed on a view box and examined closely, a pattern representing the embossed lead foil that is in the back of a film packet can be detected. Historically film makers used a herringbone pattern, and therefore some practitioners still call this **herringbone error.** Most films currently available have a pattern resembling a tire track or diamond pattern (Figure 18-5).

- **Corrective actions:** Determine the front side of the film packet prior to placing into the image receptor holder. When in doubt, read the printed side of the film packet for direction. Once attached, examine the film and holder assembly to ensure that the tube side faces toward the teeth and the radiation source (Figure 18-6). Due to the composition of phosphor plates and digital sensors, positioning the incorrect side of these image receptors toward the radiation source will result in failure to produce an image.

INCORRECT POSITION OF FILM IDENTIFICATION DOT

- **Probable cause:** Embossed identification dot positioned in apical area where it can interfere with diagnosis.
- **Corrective actions:** Pay attention when placing the film packet into the film holding device to position the dot toward the incisal or occlusal region, where it is less likely to interfere with interpretation of the image. Some practitioners use the phrase "dot in the slot" to remind them to place the edge of the film packet where the dot is located into the slot of the film holding device. Placing the dot in the slot of a film holder will automatically position the dot toward the occlusal or incisal edges of the teeth and away from the apical regions.

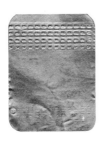
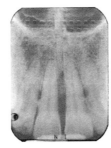
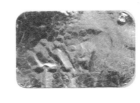
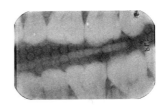

FIGURE 18-5 Reversed film packet error. These embossed patterns will be recorded on the image when the lead foil faces the x-ray beam. Note the different patterns depending on the manufacturer and the film size.

Incorrect Positioning of the Tube Head and PID

Included in this category are the errors that result from incorrect vertical and horizontal angulations and centering of the x-ray beam over the image receptor. We have already discussed that incorrect vertical angulation can result in not recording the apices or the occlusal/incisal edges of the teeth. Elongation (images that appear stretched out) and foreshortening (images that appear shorter than they are), with or without cutting off the apices or the occlusal/incisal edges of the teeth, are dimensional errors that result from incorrect vertical angulation when using the bisecting technique. It is important to remember that it is impossible to create images that are elongated or foreshortened when the image receptor is positioned parallel to the teeth, as is the case when using the paralleling technique. If elongation or foreshortening errors result, it is important that the corrective action be to first try to position the image receptor parallel to the teeth of interest. Correctly positioning the image receptor parallel to the teeth will most likely prevent dimensional errors. If parallel placement of the image receptor to the teeth is not possible, then the bisecting technique must be carefully applied to avoid elongation and foreshortening of the image.

ELONGATION/FORESHORTENING OF THE IMAGE (BISECTING TECHNIQUE ERROR)

- **Probable causes:** Insufficient vertical angulation with the PID not positioned steep enough away from zero degrees results in **elongation** (Figure 18-2). Excessive vertical angulation with the PID positioned too steep enough away from zero degrees results in **foreshortening** (Figure 18-4).
- **Corrective actions:** To correct elongation, increase the vertical angulation. To correct foreshortening, decrease the vertical angulation. Direct the central rays perpendicular to the imaginary bisector between the long axes of the teeth and the plane of the image receptor (see Chapter 15). If relying on predetermined vertical angulation settings, check the position of the patient's head to ensure that the occlusal plane is parallel and that the midsaggital plane is perpendicular to the floor.

OVERLAPPED TEETH CONTACTS (FIGURE 18-2)

- **Probable causes:**
  1. Incorrect rotation of the tube head and PID in the horizontal plane. Superimposition of the proximal surfaces occurs when the central ray of the x-ray beam is not directed perpendicular through the interproximal spaces to the image receptor. Overlapped contacts result when the central ray of the x-ray beam is directed obliquely toward the image receptor from the distal or from the mesial. When the angle of the x-ray beam is directed obliquely from mesial to distal (**mesiodistal overlap**), the **overlapping** contacts are more severe in the posterior part of the image. Conversely, when the angle of the x-ray beam is directed obliquely from distal to mesial (**distomesial overlap**), the overlapping contacts are more severe in the anterior part of the image.

  2. Not positioning the image receptor parallel to the interproximal spaces of the teeth of interest will prevent the central ray of the x-ray beam from being directed perpendicular through the contacts and perpendicular to the image receptor.

- **Corrective actions:**
  1. Examine the image to determine where the overlap is most severe. To correct mesiodistal overlap, rotate the tubehead and PID to a more distomesial angle. Physically move the tubehead toward the posterior of the patient while rotating the PID toward the anterior so that the central ray of the x-ray beam will enter the patient from the distal (or posterior). To correct distomesial overlap, rotate the tubehead and PID to a more mesiodistal angle. Physically move the tubehead toward the anterior of the patient while rotating the PID toward the posterior so that the central ray of the x-ray beam will enter the patient from the mesial (or anterior.). It should be noted that there are cases when mesiodistal and distomesial overlap cannot be distinguished from one another. When this happens, closely examine the teeth of interest to determine the precise contact points through which to perpendicularly direct the central rays of the x-ray beam.

  2. Examine the teeth of interest to determine the contact points prior to positioning the image receptor. Place the image receptor parallel to the contact points of interest so that the central rays of the x-ray beam will intersect the image receptor perpendicularly through those contacts (see Figure 28-2).

> ⚡ **PRACTICE POINT**
>
> Use the phrase *"Move toward it to fix it"* when correcting mesiodistal or distomesial overlap error. If the overlapping appears more severe in the posterior region (mesiodistal overlap), shift the tube head toward the posterior while rotating the PID to direct the x-ray beam from the distal. If the overlapping appears more severe in the anterior region (distomesial overlap), shift the tube head toward the anterior while rotating the PID to direct the x-ray beam from the mesial.

CONECUT ERROR (FIGURES 18-7 AND 18-8)

- **Probable causes:** The primary beam of radiation was not directed toward the center of the image receptor and did not completely expose the entire surface area of the receptor. Image receptor holders with external aiming rings help prevent this error. However, assembling the image receptor holding instrument incorrectly will cause the operator to direct the central ray of the x-ray beam to the wrong place, resulting in **conecut error.**

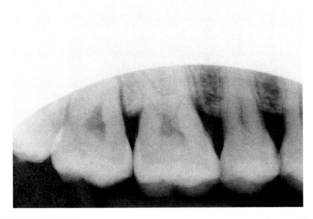

FIGURE 18-7 Conecut error. Results when the central ray of the x-ray beam is not directed toward the middle of the image receptor. The white (clear) circular area was beyond the range of the x-ray beam, and therefore received no exposure. This radiograph illustrates conecut error that resulted from incorrect assembly of a posterior image receptor holder.

- **Corrective actions:** While maintaining correct horizontal and vertical angulation, move the tube head up, down, posteriorly, or anteriorly, depending on which area of the radiograph shows a clear, unexposed region. Check to see that the image receptor holder is assembled correctly, and direct the central ray of the x-ray beam to the center (middle) of the receptor.

Incorrect Exposure Factors

Insufficient knowledge regarding the use of the control panel settings and exposure button will result in less-than-ideal radiographic images.

LIGHT (THIN)/DARK IMAGES (FIGURES 18-9 AND 18-10)

- **Probable causes:** It has already been pointed out that underexposed images result when a film packet is positioned reversed, or backward, in the oral cavity. The presence of an

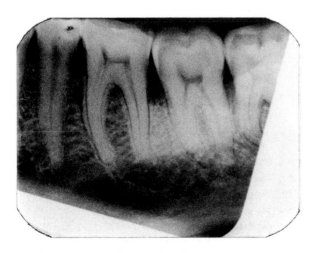

FIGURE 18-8 Conecut error. Can also occur when using rectangular collimation.

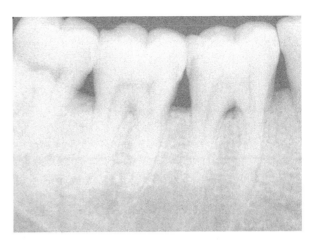

FIGURE 18-9 Light (thin) image. Underexposed or underdeveloped radiograph.

embossed pattern or herringbone error will indicate why the **underexposure** occurred. If a pattern is not noted in a light image, an error with the selection of exposure factors should be suspected. Insufficient exposure time in relation to milliamperage, kilovoltage, and PID length selected by the operator all result in light images, whereas excessive exposure time in relation to these parameters results in overexposure. Inappropriately exposing a phosphor plate to bright light prior to the laser processing step will result in a light or faded image. Under- or overexposure may rarely occur as a result of equipment malfunction. Light/dark images that result from processing errors will be discussed later in this chapter.

- **Corrective actions:** An exposure chart posted near the control panel for easy reference can assist with preventing incorrect exposures. Increasing the exposure time, the milliamperage, the kilovoltage, or a combination of these factors will correct underexposures, whereas decreasing these parameters will correct overexposures. If the PID length is switched, then a cooresponding adjustment in the exposure time must be made. Exposed phosphor plates should be placed with the front side down on the counter or within a containment box until ready for the laser processing step. (see Chapter 9) The exposure button must be depressed for

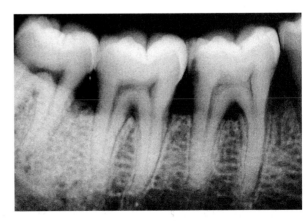

FIGURE 18-10 Dark image. Overexposed or overdeveloped radiograph.

the full cycle. The operator must watch for the red exposure light and the audible signal to end to indicate that the exposure button may be released. If the problem persists, check the accuracy of the timer or switch for possible malfunction.

CLEAR OR BLANK IMAGE

- **Probable causes:** No exposure to x-rays, that results from failure to turn on the line switch to the x-ray machine or to maintain firm pressure on the exposure button during the exposure or, if using digital imaging, exposing the back side of a phosphor plate or digital sensor. Alternate causes: electrical failure, malfunction of the x-ray machine or processing errors (which will be discussed later).
- **Corrective actions:** Turn on the x-ray machine and maintain firm pressure on the exposure button during the entire exposure period. Watch for the red exposure light and listen for the audible signal indicating that the exposure has occurred. Be familiar with digital image receptors to determine the correct exposure side.

DOUBLE IMAGE   Film

- **Probable cause:** Double exposure resulting from accidentally exposing the same film or phosphor plate twice.
- **Corrective actions:** Maintain a systematic order to exposing radiographs. Keep unexposed and exposed image receptors organized.

Miscellaneous Errors in Exposure Technique

POOR DEFINITION

- **Probable causes:** Movement caused by the patient, slippage of the image receptor, or vibration of the tube head.
- **Corrective actions:** Place the patient's head into position against the head rest of the treatment chair and ask him/her to hold still throughout the duration of the exposure. Explain the procedure and gain the patient's cooperation, to maintain steady pressure on the image receptor holder and not to move. Do not use the patient's finger to stabilize the image receptor in the oral cavity. Steady the tube head before activating the exposure.

ARTIFACTS   Artifacts are images other than anatomy or pathology that do not contribute to a diagnosis of the patient's condition (Figures 18-11 and 18-12). Artifacts may be radiopaque or radiolucent.

- **Probable causes:** The presence of foreign objects in the oral cavity during exposure (e.g., appliances such as removable bridges, partial or full dentures, orthodontic retainers, patient glasses, and facial jewelry used in piercings). There may be occasions when the lead/lead equivalent thyroid collar could be in the path of the x-ray beam. These metal objects will result in radiopaque artifacts.

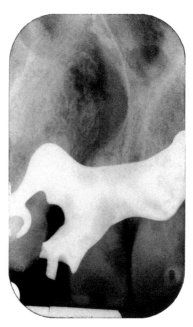

FIGURE 18-11 Radiopaque artifact. Partial denture left in place during exposure.

- **Corrective actions:** Perform a cursory examination of the oral cavity to check for the presence of appliances. Ask the patient to remove any objects that may be in the path of the primary beam. Ensure that the lead/lead equivalent apron and thyroid collar do not block the x-rays from reaching the image receptor.

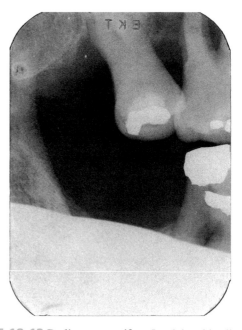

FIGURE 18-12 Radiopaque artifact. Lead thyroid collar got in the way of the primary beam during exposure.

Processing Errors

Processing errors that result in retake radiographs also increase patient radiation dose, add time to a busy day's schedule, and waste money. Processing errors occur with both manual and automatic processing. Processing errors include under- and overdevelopment, incorrectly following protocols, and failure to maintain an ideal darkroom setting.

Development Error

LIGHT/DARK IMAGE (FIGURES 18-9 AND 18-10)

- **Probable causes: Underdevelopment** results when a film is not left in the developer for the required time. Overdevelopment results when a film is left in the developer too long. The colder the developer, the longer the time required to produce an image of ideal density, and the warmer the developer, the less developing time required. Images may be too light or too dark as a result of incorrectly mixing developer from concentrate. A weak developer mix produces light images; a strong mix produces dark images. Light images also result when the developer solution is old, weakened, or contaminated. A low solution level in the developer tank of an automatic processor that does not completely cover the rollers may also produce a light image.

- **Corrective actions:** When processing manually, check the temperature of the developer and consult a time–temperature chart before beginning processing. Ensure that the automatic processor indicates that the solutions have warmed up and the correct timed cycle is used. If weakened or old solutions are suspected, change the solutions. Maintain good quality control to replenish solutions to keep them functioning at peak conditions and at the appropriate levels in the tanks.

Processing and Darkroom Protocol Errors

BLANK/CLEAR IMAGE

- **Probable causes:** It has already been discussed that no exposure to x-rays will produce a blank or clear radiograph. Film that is accidentally placed in the fixer before being placed in the developer will also result in a blank or clear image. If allowed to remain in warm rinse water too long the emulsion may dissolve also resulting in a clear image.

- **Corrective actions:** When processing manually, and when filling automatic processor tanks during solution changes and cleaning procedures, the operator must have knowledge of which tank contains the developer and which tank contains the fixer. Labelling the tanks prevents confusion. To prevent the emulsion from separating from the film base, promptly remove the film at the end of the washing period.

PARTIAL IMAGE

- **Probable causes:** A manual processing error—when the level of the developer is too low to cover the entire film, the emulsion in the section of the film that remains above the solution level will not be developed. Once in the fixer, the emulsion in this section will be removed leaving a blank or clear section.

- **Corrective actions:** Replenish the processing solutions to the proper level or attach the films to lower clips on the film hanger to ensure that they will be submerged completely in the solution.

GREEN FILMS

- **Probable causes:** When films stick together in the developer the solution is prevented from reaching the (green) emulsion. The most common causes include failure to separate double film packets, placing additional films into the same intake slot of an automatic processor too close together resulting in overlapping of the two films, and attaching two films to one clip used in manual processing, or allowing films on adjacent film racks to contact each other.

- **Corrective actions:** The operator must be skilled at separating double film packets under safelight conditions. Use alternating intake slots or wait 10 seconds before loading subsequent films into the automatic processor. Carefully handle manual film hangers and clips to avoid placing films in contact with each other.

Chemical Contamination

BLACK/WHITE SPOTS (FIGURE 18-13)

- **Probable causes:** Premature contact with developing chemicals—drops of developer or fixer that splash onto the work area may come in contact with the undeveloped film. Developer contamination will produce black spots. Fixer contamination will produce white spots. Excessive wetting of phosphor plates during the disinfecting step can damage the plate and result in a digital image with missing information in the form of white or clear spots.

- **Corrective actions:** Maintain a clean and orderly darkroom and work area. Consult manufacturer recommendations to properly disinfect digital image receptors.

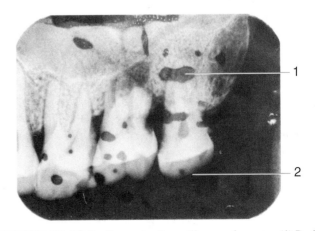

FIGURE 18-13 Radiograph of maxillary molar area. (1) Dark spots caused by premature contact of film surface with developer. **(2)** Uneven occlusal margin resulted because the patient did not occlude all the way down on the image receptor biteblock.

BROWN IMAGES

- **Probable cause:** Insufficient or improper washing. It is important to note that films that have not been washed completely will appear normal immediately after drying. Films will turn brown over a period of several weeks after processing as the chemicals that remain on the surface of the film erode the image.
- **Corrective actions:** When processing manually, rinse films in circulating water for at least 20 minutes. Always return a film to complete the fixing and washing steps after a wet-reading. When processing automatically, ensure that the main water supply to the unit is turned on and that the water bottles of closed systems are full.

STAINS

- **Probable causes:** Iridescent, gray, and yellow stains can result when processing chemicals become exhausted or contaminated.
- **Corrective actions:** Maintain quality control with regular replenishment and replacing of the processing solutions.

Handling Errors

The manner in which the image receptor is handled contributes to its ability to record a diagnostic quality image. Bending the film produces artifacts and significantly reduces the quality of the radiographic image. Bending a phosphor plate will damage the surface. Exposing the image receptor to conditions such as static electricity and the potential for scratching the emulsion will further compromise diagnostic quality.

BLACK IMAGE

- **Probable cause:** Film was accidentally exposed to white light.
- **Corrective actions:** Turn off all light in the darkroom except the proper safelight before unwrapping the film packet. Lock the door or warn others not to enter. Use an "in-use" sign to prevent others from opening the door. When using an automatic processor, ensure that the film has completely entered the light-protected processor before turning on the white overhead light or removing hands from the daylight loader baffles.

BLACK PRESSURE MARKS (BENT FILM; FIGURES 18-3 AND 18-14)

- **Probable cause:** Bending the film or excessive pressure to the film emulsion can cause the emulsion to crack. Accidentally bending the film often occurs when the radiographer is placing the film packet into the image receptor holder. Although not recommended, a corner of the film packet is sometimes purposely bent by the radiographer to fit comfortably into position.
- **Corrective actions:** Use caution when loading the film packet into the image receptor holding device. Films should

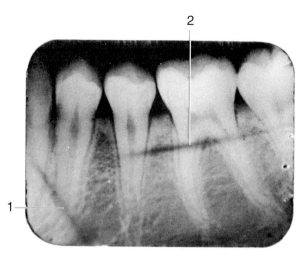

FIGURE 18-14 Radiograph of mandibular premolar area. (**1**) Purposely bending the lower left film corner to make the receptor fit the oral cavity resulted in distortion and a pressure mark (thin radiolucent line). (**2**) Long radiolucent pressure mark caused by bending or by careless handling with excessive force.

not be bent to fit the oral cavity. Instead, use a smaller-sized film, the occlusal technique (see Chapter 17), or an extraoral procedure (see Chapter 29).

THIN BLACK LINES, STAR-BURSTS, DOTS, LIGHTNING PATTERN (SEE FIGURE 29-6)

- **Probable causes: Static electricity** may be produced when the film is pulled out of the packet wrapping too fast. Static electricity creates a white light spark that exposes (blackens) the film.
- **Corrective actions:** Follow infection control protocols for opening film packets (see Chapter 10). Reduce the occurrence of static electricity by increasing humidity in the darkroom. Use antistatic products on protective clothing to prevent the buildup of static electricity.

WHITE LINES OR MARKS OR BLANK IMAGE (FIGURE 18-15)

- **Probable causes:** The film emulsion is soft and can be easily scratched by a sharp object such as the film clip used for manual processing or when trying to separate double film packets. Scratching removes the emulsion from the base. Damaged digital sensors also result in images with missing information in areas of **dead** (damaged) **pixels.** Damage to the digital sensor wire attachment can result in complete failure of the device to record an image.
- **Corrective actions:** Carefully handle all types of radiographic image receptors. Avoid contacting the film with other films or hangers. Mount dried radiographs promptly and enclose in a protective envelope. Care should be taken to store wired digital sensors without crimping or folding the sensitive wire attachment.

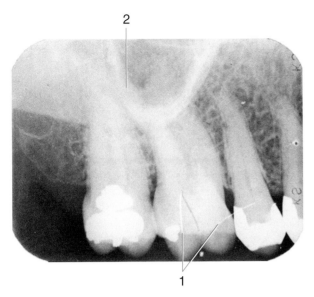

FIGURE 18-15 Radiograph of maxillary posterior area.
(**1**) White streak marks show where the softened emulsion has been scratched off. (**2**) U-shaped radiopaque band of dense bone shows the outline of the zygoma.

SMUDGED FILM (FIGURE 18-16)

- **Probable causes:** Handling the film with damp fingers or latex treatment gloves, or with residual glove powder on the fingers will leave black smudges.
- **Corrective actions:** Avoid contact with the surface of the film. Handle all radiographs carefully and by the edges only. Hands should be clean and free of moisture or glove powder.

BLACK PAPER STUCK TO FILM

- **Probable causes:** A tear or break in the outer protective wrapping of the film packet by rough handling enables saliva to penetrate to the emulsion. Moisture softens the emulsion, causing the black paper to stick to the film.
- **Corrective actions:** Careful handling prevents a break in the seal of the film packet. Always blot excess moisture from the film packet after removing it from the patient's mouth.

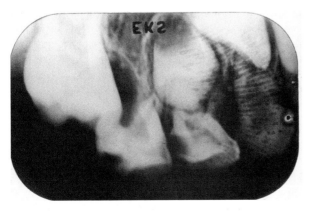

FIGURE 18-16 Radiograph of primary molar area showing fingerprint.

Fogged Images

Another cause of undiagnostic radiographs is the formation of a thin, cloudy layer that compromises the clarity of the image. This **film fog** and **electronic noise** (digital images) diminishes contrast and makes it difficult and often impossible to interpret the radiograph (Figure 18-17). Fogged images are produced in many ways and can occur before, during, or after exposure or during processing (Box 18-1). Most fogged radiographs have a similar appearance, making it difficult to pinpoint the cause. Careful attention to the exposure techniques and processing method used and darkroom and image receptor handling protocols will help reduce the occurrence of fogged images.

RADIATION FOG

- **Probable cause:** Not properly protecting film from stray radiation before or after exposure.
- **Preventive measures:** Store film in its original package at a safe distance from the source of x-rays. Exposing a film increases its sensitivity; therefore, it is very important that once a film has been exposed, it should be protected from the causes of film fog until processed.

WHITE LIGHT FOG

- **Probable causes:** White light leaking into the darkroom from around doors or plumbing pipes. White light leaking into the film packet through a tear in the outer wrapping.

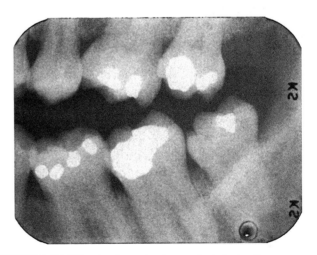

FIGURE 18-17 Film fog. Film fog results in lack of image contrast.

BOX 18-1   Causes of Film Fog
- Radiation - Light - Heat - Humidity - Chemical fumes - Aging

- **Preventive measures:** Check the darkroom for white light leaks. Handle the film packet carefully to prevent tearing the light-tight outer wrapping.

SAFELIGHT FOG

- **Probable cause:** A safelight will fog film if the wattage of the safelight bulb is stronger than recommended; the distance the safelight is located over the work space area is too close; the filter is the incorrect type or color for the film being used; or the filter is scratched or otherwise damaged, allowing white light through. Even when adequate, prolonged exposure to the safelight will fog film.
- **Preventive measures:** Perform periodic quality control checks on the darkroom and safelight. Follow film manufacturer's guidelines when choosing filter color. Check the bulb wattage, check the distance away from the work space, and examine the filter for defects. The radiographer should develop skills necessary to open film packets aseptically within a two- to three-minute period to minimize the time films are exposed to the safelight.

MISCELLANEOUS LIGHT FOG

- **Probable causes:** Glowing light that reaches the film such as that from watches with fluorescent faces, indicator lights on equipment stored in the darkroom, and cells phone carried into the darkroom in a radiographer's pocket have the potential to create fog. This is especially true when processing sensitive extraoral films.
- **Preventive measures:** Watches with fluorescent faces should not be worn in the darkroom while processing film unless covered with the sleeve of the operator's protective barrier gown or lab coat. Luminous dials of equipment located in the darkroom that glow in unsafe light colors should be masked with opaque tape. Cell phones should be powered off to avoid accidental illumination by an incoming call or message.

STORAGE FOG (HEAT, HUMIDITY, AND CHEMICAL FUMES)

- **Probable causes:** Film fog will result when film is stored in a warm, damp area or in the vicinity of fume-producing chemicals.
- **Preventive measures:** Store film unopened, in its original package in a cool, dry area. Many practices store film in a refrigerator until ready to use. Film should not be stored in the darkroom unless protected from heat, humidity, and fume-producing processing solutions.

CHEMICAL FOG

- **Probable causes:** Developing films too long, at too high a temperature, or in contaminated solutions will produce film fog.
- **Preventive measures:** Develop at the recommended time–temperature cycle. Avoid contamination of processing chemicals. Always replace the manual tank cover in the same position, with the side over the developer remaining over the developer and the side over the fixer remaining over the fixer to prevent contamination of the solutions. Thoroughly rinse films to remove developer before moving the film hanger into the fixer.

AGED FILM FOG

- **Probable causes:** Film emulsion has a shelf life with an expiration date (see Figure 7-9). As film ages, it can become fogged.
- **Preventive measures:** Watch the date on film boxes. Rotate film stock so that the oldest film is used before newer film. Do not overstock film. Thoroughly research a supplier before purchasing film, especially when buying in bulk or from a source found on the Internet.

DIGITAL RADIOGRAPHIC NOISE

- **Probable causes:** Exposure settings that are extremely low. When switching from film-based radiography to digital imaging, there is a tendency to set the exposure factors too low resulting in radiographic electronic noise.
- **Preventive measures:** Use correct exposure settings. After setting at manufacturer's recommendations, evaluate the images to determine the need for varying the settings to eliminate radiographic noise and obtain the desired image clarity and contrast.

REVIEW—Chapter summary

The dental radiographer should know what a quality diagnostic radiograph should look like and be able to identify when errors occur. No radiograph should be retaken until a thorough investigation reveals the exact cause of the error and the appropriate corrective action is identified and can be implemented. Although radiographic errors may be classified as technique errors, processing errors, and handling errors, undiagnostic radiographs are traceable to many causes. Different errors can often produce similar-looking results.

Technique errors include mistakes made in placement of the image receptor, positioning the tube head and the PID, and choosing the correct exposure factors. Processing errors include development mistakes, not following protocols for processing and darkroom use, and chemical contamination. Handling errors include black images, and bent, scratched, damaged, and fogged images.

Examples of probable causes and corrective actions were given for not recording the entire tooth and supporting structures, for creating a slanted occlusal plane, for producing herringbone error, and for incorrectly positioning the embossed identification dot. Examples of probable causes and corrective actions were given for elongation and foreshortening, overlapping teeth contacts, and conecut error. Examples of probable causes and corrective actions were given for light/dark, clear/blank, and double-exposed images and images with poor definition, the presence of artifacts such as static electricity, black/white spots and lines, and pressure marks. Examples of probable causes and corrective actions were given for over- and underdevelopment; partial images; and green, brown, stained, and fogged images. Fogged radiographs result from exposure to stray radiation, light, heat, humidity, chemical fumes, and contamination. Film has a shelf life, and aging may produce film fog. Electronic noise, the digital equivalent of film fog, results when radiation exposure settings are set extremely low. Measures to prevent fogged images include controlling these causes.

RECALL—Study questions

1. What is the appropriate corrective action for a periapical radiograph of the maxillary molar region that did not image the third molar?
   a. Position the image receptor higher in the oral cavity.
   b. Position the image receptor lower in the oral cavity.
   c. Move the image receptor forward in the oral cavity.
   d. Move the image receptor back further in the oral cavity.

2. Each of the following will result in not recording the apices of the maxillary premolar teeth on a periapical radiograph EXCEPT one. Which one is the EXCEPTION?
   a. Image receptor not placed high enough in relation to the teeth.
   b. Image receptor not placed in toward the midline of the palate.
   c. Patient not occluding all the way down on the image receptor holder biteblock.
   d. Vertical angulation was excessive.

3. What does herringbone error indicate?
   a. Embossed dot was positioned incorrectly.
   b. Lead foil was processed with the film.
   c. Film packet was placed in the oral cavity backwards.
   d. Temperatures of the processing chemicals were not equal.

4. When using the bisecting technique, which of these errors results from inadequate vertical angulation?
   a. Elongation
   b. Foreshortening
   c. Conecut
   d. Overlapping

5. What error results in overlapped contacts being more severe between the first and second molar than between the first and second premolar?
   a. Excessive vertical angulation
   b. Inadequate vertical angulation
   c. Mesiodistal projection of horizontal angulation
   d. Distomesial projection of horizontal angulation

6. Overlapped teeth contacts renders a bitewing radiograph undiagnostic. The overlap appears more severe in the anterior region. What corrective action is needed?
   a. Increase the vertical angulation.
   b. Decrease the vertical angulation.

   c. Shift the horizontal angulation toward the mesial.
   d. Shift the horizontal angulation toward the distal.

7. Which of these conditions results from a failure to direct the central ray toward the middle of the image receptor?
   a. Overlapping
   b. Conecut
   c. Elongation
   d. Foreshortening

8. Which of these indicates an overexposed radiograph?
   a. Clear image
   b. Light image
   c. Dark image
   d. Double image

9. Each of the following will result in radiographs that are too light EXCEPT one. Which one is the EXCEPTION?
   a. Hot developer solution
   b. Old, expired film
   c. Underexposing
   d. Underdeveloping

10. Each of the following will result in radiographs that are blank (clear) EXCEPT one. Which one is the EXCEPTION?
    a. No exposure to x-rays
    b. Placing films in the fixer first
    c. Extended time in warm water rinse
    d. Accidental white light exposure

11. If two films become overlapped together because they were inserted into the automatic processor too quickly, what is the result?
    a. Green films
    b. Brown films
    c. Light films
    d. Black films

12. Which of these indicates that a film was not properly washed?
    a. Image appears light
    b. Fogging results
    c. Film turns brown
    d. White spots form

13. Each of the following will result in black artifacts on the radiograph EXCEPT one. Which one is the EXCEPTION?
    a. Static electricity
    b. Bent film
    c. Glove powder
    d. Fixer splash

14. Static electricity appears radiographically as black
    a. thin lines.
    b. starbursts.
    c. dots.
    d. Any of the above

15. Each of the following is a cause of film fog EXCEPT one. Which one is the EXCEPTION?
    a. Exposure to scatter radiation
    b. Use of old, expired film
    c. Double exposing the film
    d. Chemical fume contamination

REFLECT—Case study

You have just finished taking a full mouth series of periapical and bitewing radiographs. After processing and mounting the films, you notice the following:

1. The maxillary right molar periapical radiograph did not image the third molar.
2. The maxillary right canine periapical radiograph appears elongated, and the image of the root tip is not recorded.
3. The teeth contacts in the right premolar bitewing radiograph are overlapped. The overlapping appears most severe in the posterior portion of the image and less severe in the anterior region.
4. The left molar bitewing film was bent when it was placed into the image receptor holder.
5. The mandibular central incisors periapical radiograph appears very light, with a hint of a diamondlike pattern superimposed over the image of the teeth.
6. The film that should have been a left mandibular molar periapical radiograph is blank, with no hint of an image.
7. The left maxillary premolar periapical radiograph appears to have been double exposed.

Consider these seven radiographs with the errors noted and answer the following questions:

a. What is the most likely cause of this error? How did you arrive at this conclusion?

b. Could there be multiple causes for this error? What other errors would produce this result?
c. Why do you think this error occurred?
d. What corrective action would you take when retaking this radiograph? Be specific.
e. What are you basing your decision to reexpose the patient on?
f. What steps or actions would you recommend to prevent this error from occurring in the future?

RELATE—Laboratory application

For a comprehensive laboratory practice exercise on this topic, see Thomson, E. M. (2012). *Exercises in oral radiography techniques: A laboratory manual* (3rd ed.). Upper Saddle River, NJ: Pearson Education. Chapter 7, "Identifying and correcting radiographic errors."

REFERENCES

Carestream Health, Inc. (2007). *Kodak Dental Systems:Exposure and processing for dental film radiography.* Pub. N-414, Rochester, NY: Author.

Eastman Kodak Company. (2002). *Successful intraoral radiography.* N-418 CAT No. 103. Rochester, NY: Author.

Thomson, E. M. (2012). *Exercises in oral radiographic techniques: A laboratory manual* (3rd ed.,). Upper Saddle River, NJ: Pearson Education.

White, S. C., & Pharoah, M. J. (2008). *Oral radiology: Principles and interpretation* (6th ed.). St. Louis, MO: Elsevier.

Quality Assurance in Dental Radiography

OBJECTIVES

Following successful completion of this chapter, you should be able to:

1. Define the key words.
2. Explain the relationship between quality assurance and quality control.
3. List the steps of a quality assurance program.
4. Explain the role a competent radiographer plays in quality assurance.
5. List the four objectives of quality control tests.
6. Make a step-wedge with cardboard and lead foil and demonstrate how to use it.
7. List two tests the radiographer can use to monitor a dental x-ray machine.
8. Explain the use of the coin test to monitor darkroom safelighting.
9. Describe how to test for light leaks in the darkroom.
10. Explain the use of a reference film to test processing chemistry.
11. Explain the use of the fresh-film test to monitor the quality of a box of film.
12. Describe quality control tests for radiographic viewing equipment.
13. Advocate the use of quality assurance to produce diagnostic-quality radiographs with minimal radiation exposure.

KEY WORDS

Coin test
Fresh-film test
Light-tight
Quality assurance

Quality control
Reference film
Step-wedge

Introduction

Quality assurance is defined as the planning, implementation, and evaluation of procedures used to produce high-quality radiographs with maximum diagnostic information (yield) while minimizing radiation exposure. Establishing a quality control program for radiographic procedures helps to increase the quality of radiographs produced and decrease the incidence of retake radiographs. Quality assurance includes both quality administration procedures and quality control techniques (Table 19-1).

The purpose of this chapter is to present quality control tests that are used to monitor operator competency, the dental x-ray machine, the darkroom and x-ray processing systems, film and equipment used to view the images, and documentation and administrative maintenance.

Quality Administration Procedures

Quality administration refers to conducting a quality assurance program in the oral health care practice. A quality assurance program should include an assessment of current practices, where and how the problems seem to be occurring, a written plan that identifies who is responsible and what training the personnel need to be able to carry out the quality control tests, record-keeping, and periodic evaluations of the plan.

Needs Assessment

Periodically the oral health care team should review patient radiographs for quality. Problems that occur should be documented and then periodically reviewed to look for areas where a change in policy, maintenance schedules, or other area is noted.

Written Plan

The oral health care team should develop a written plan that will guide quality control. The plan should include, but not be limited to, the purpose of the quality assurance program, assignment of authority and responsibilities, a list of equipment that requires monitoring, a list of tests that will be performed and at what time intervals (Table 19-2), a log of all quality assurance test results, a log of retake radiographs, documentation of training, and evaluation interval and report.

TABLE 19-1 Quality Assurance Includes Both Quality Administration and Quality Control

QUALITY ADMINISTRATION	QUALITY CONTROL
Assess needs	Operator competence
Develop a written plan	X-ray machines
Assign authority and responsibility	Darkroom
Provide training	Processing equipment
Monitor maintenance schedule	Processing chemistry
Document actions and keep records/log	X-ray film and storage
Perform periodic evaluation	Image viewing

TABLE 19-2 Suggested Time Intervals for Performing Quality Control Tests

QUALITY CONTROL TEST	SUGGESTED TIME INTERVAL
Output consistency	Annually
Tube head stability	Monthly
Darkroom safelighting	Annually
Automatic processor	Daily
Processing solutions	Daily
Cassettes and screens	Annually
Viewboxes	Monthly

Careful planning and thoroughly carrying out a quality assurance program increases the likelihood of producing the highest quality radiographs while minimizing radiation exposure.

Authority and Responsibilities

Although the dentist is ultimately responsible for the overall quality care that his/her practice provides the patient, each oral health care team member can be given authority to carry out specific aspects of the quality control program. Assigning authority and clearly defining specific tasks and/or maintenance procedures helps to ensure that the procedures are being carried out. Each oral health care team member must be informed of how and why the tasks are to be performed and provided with training opportunities to ensure compentency in performing in this capacity.

Monitoring and Maintenance Schedules

A monitoring schedule listing all the quality control tests, identification of the person responsible for each test, and the frequency of testing should be generated and posted. Checkoff lists can be used to record maintenance and inspections.

Logs and Periodic Evaluation

A log should be kept of all quality control tests. Include the date, the specific test, the results, action taken if any, and the name of the person who conducted the test. Also, a log of all radiographs retaken should be recorded to identify recurring problems. The oral healthcare team should meet periodically to evaluate the logs and the quality assurance program.

Competency of the Radiographer

Essential to a quality assurance program is the ability of the radiographer. Operator errors that result in undiagnostic radiographs generate the need for retake radiographs. Retakes result in unnecessary radiation exposure to the patient and lost time for both the patient and the practice. The radiographer must be competent not only in exposing, processing, and mounting dental radiographs, but also in identifying when errors occur. Even competent radiographers encounter situations where less-than-ideal radiographic images result. It is important, therefore, that the radiographer be able to recognize poor quality, identify the cause, and apply the appropriate corrective action.

Operator errors and retakes should be recorded to identify recurring problems. Each exposure may be recorded in a log that can be reviewed periodically to monitor for problems and the application of the appropriate corrective actions. This will also help monitor the skills of the radiographer. To aid in operator competency, opportunities such as continuing education courses or on-the-job-training can assist the radiographer in brushing up on skills, improving in an area of deficiency, and/or staying apprised of the newest technology and treatment recommendations.

Quality Control

Quality control is defined as a series of tests to ensure that the radiographic system is functioning properly and that the radiographs produced are of an acceptable level of quality. The objectives of quality control include the following:

1. Maintain a high standard of image quality.
2. Identify problems before image quality is compromised.
3. Keep patient and occupational exposures to a minimum.
4. Reduce the occurrence of retake radiographs.

Examples of quality control measures include tests to evaluate dental x-ray machine output; tests to evaluate safelighting of the darkroom, processing chemistry testing and replenishing, evaluation of safe film storage, view box inspections, calibrations of computer monitors used to view digital images, documentation such as records of when processing chemistry needs changing, posted technique factors near x-ray machines, and a maintenance log of retakes to keep track of common errors and find solutions for avoiding them in the future.

Dental X-ray Machine Monitoring

Periodic comprehensive testing of the x-ray machine is essential to a quality assurance program. These tests include radiation output, timer accuracy, accuracy of milliamperage and kilovoltage settings, focal spot size, filtration (beam quality), collimation, beam alignment, and tube head stability (Box 19-1). State and local health departments may provide or require x-ray machine

testing as part of their registration or licensing programs. In this case, a qualified health physicist will conduct most of these tests prior to renewing registration or license. However, the radiographer who uses the equipment on a daily basis should also play a role in monitoring the x-ray machine. Additionally, a working knowledge of the quality control tests available will help the radiographer identify when the equipment is not functioning at peak performance.

OUTPUT CONSISTENCY TEST (PROCEDURE BOXES 19-1 AND 19-2)   Radiation output may be monitored by the radiographer using a step-wedge. A **step-wedge** is a device of layered metal steps of varying thickness used to determine image density and contrast. A step-wedge may also be used to test the strength of the processing chemicals, which will be discussed later.

A step-wedge may be obtained commercially or be made using several pieces of lead foil from intraoral film packets (Figure 19-1). To perform the radiation output test, the step-wedge is placed on a size #2 intraoral image receptor on the counter or exam chair and then exposed with set exposure factors. This film is put aside, protected from stray radiation, heat and humidity, and other potential causes of film fog (see Chapter 18). The process is repeated with a new film at intervals determined by the practice. For example, the first exposure may be made in the morning, followed by a second exposure at midday and a third exposure at the end of the day. At the end of the desired time frame, all the exposed films are processed at the same time and evaluated. Consistency in radiation output will produce three radiographs with images of the step-wedge that are identical in densities and contrast. A failed test will produce images that are different from each other, indicating that the radiation output varied over the course of the day (Figure 19-2). A failed test would indicate that a qualified health physicist should examine the x-ray machine.

TUBE HEAD STABILITY   Another test the radiographer should make regularly on the dental x-ray machine is tube head stability. A drifting tube head must not be used until the support arm and yoke are properly adjusted to prevent movement of the tube head during exposure. To test for drift, the radiographer should position the tube head in various positions that will likely be needed for radiographic exposures to evaluate stability in each

---

BOX 19-1   Quality Control Tests for Dental X-ray Machines

1. Radiation output
2. Timer accuracy
3. Milliamperage accuracy
4. Kilovoltage accuracy
5. Focal spot size
6. Filtration (beam quality)
7. Collimation
8. Beam alignment
9. Tube head stability

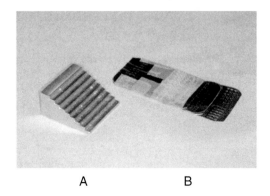

A   B

FIGURE 19-1 Step-wedge. (A) Commercially made step-wedge. **(B)** Step-wedge made from discarded sheets of lead foil from intraoral film packets.

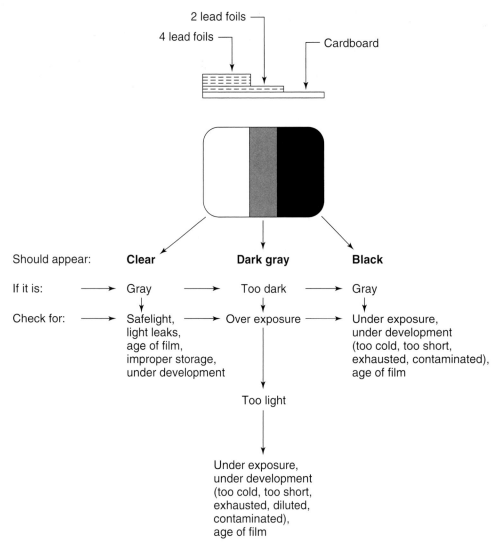

FIGURE 19-2 **Sketch of a step-wedge.** A step-wedge is useful in making visual comparisons for quality control.

of the positions. When not in use, the support arm should be folded into a closed position with the PID pointing down to prevent weight stress from loosening the support arm and causing drift (Figure 19-3).

Darkroom Monitoring

The darkroom should be evaluated for the presence of conditions that create film fog and compromise image quality. The darkroom should be checked to determine that it is adequately ventilated, free from chemical fumes, within the prescribed temperature and humidity range recommended by the film manufacturer, beyond the reach of stray radiation, and **light-tight.** The key to a safe darkroom is an appropriate safelight.

SAFELIGHT TEST As you will recall from Chapter 8, the safelight must have a bulb of the proper wattage, have a filter color

---

PROCEDURE 19-1
Assembling a step-wedge

1. Divide a piece of cardboard the size of a #2 x-ray film into thirds.
2. Leave the first third uncovered, and cover the remaining two-thirds with two pieces of lead backing from a discarded film packet. Tape into place.
3. Cover the final third with four additional pieces of lead backing, taping them into place.

PROCEDURE 19-2
Procedure for x-ray machine output consistency test

1. Prepare a step-wedge or use a commercially made device (see Procedure Box 19-1).
2. Obtain three (or desired number) size #2 intraoral film packets from the same package.
3. Place two of the films in a safe place, protected from film fog–causing elements (stray radiation, heat, humidity, chemical fumes).
4. Place one of the film packets on the counter or exam chair within reach of the x-ray tube head.
5. Place the step-wedge on top of the film packet.
6. Position the x-ray tube head over the film packet and step-wedge, and direct the central rays of the x-ray beam perpendicularly toward the film packet. Place the open end of the PID exactly 1 in. (2.5 cm) above the film packet. Use a ruler for accuracy.
7. Set the exposure factors to those utilized for an adult patient maxillary anterior periapcial radiograph.
8. Make the exposure.
9. Place the exposed film in a safe place, protected from film fog–causing elements (stray radiation, heat, humidity, chemical fumes).
10. Some time after the first exposure (at the desired time interval), retrieve one of the stored size #2 intraoral film packets.
11. Repeat steps 4 through 9.
12. Some time after the first two exposures (at the desired time interval), retrieve the other stored size #2 intraoral film packet.
13. Repeat steps 4 through 9.
14. When ready, process all three of the films at the same time.
15. When processing is complete, observe all three of the films for consistency in density and constrast.
16. A failed test will show a difference in density or contrast among the three images.
17. Call a qualified health physicist to examine the x-ray machine if needed.

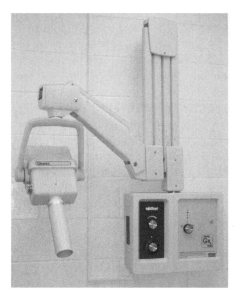

FIGURE 19-3 Correct position of tube head when not in use. Extension arm folded, tube head and PID aimed at the floor.

PROCEDURE 19-3
Coin test for safelight adequacy

1. Obtain a size #2 intraoral film packet and a coin.

2. Place the film packet on the counter or exam chair within reach of the x-ray tube head.

3. Position the x-ray tube head over the film packet. Direct the central rays of the x-ray beam perpendicularly toward the film packet. Place the open end of the PID about 12 in. (30 cm) above the film packet.

4. Set the exposure factors to the lowest possible setting.

5. Make the exposure.

6. Take the slightly exposed film and a coin to the darkroom. Turn off the overhead white light and turn on the safelight.

7. Unwrap the film packet and place the film on the counter where you would normally process patient films.

8. Place the coin on top of the unwrapped film.

9. Wait approximately two or three minutes.

10. Remove the coin from the film and process the film in the usual manner.

11. When processing is complete, observe the film for any outline of the coin. (The film will have an overall gray appearance or slight fogging from the slight radiation exposure in step 5. However, you are looking for a distinguishable outline of the coin.)

12. A failed test will show an outline of the coin.

13. Examine the safelight for correct bulb wattage, filter color, scratches or cracks, and distance away from working area. Perform additional tests to check for possible white light leaks or the presence of other light sources.

deemed safe for the film being processed, and be located a safe distance from the working area where films will be unwrapped. The coin test can be used to test the safelight for adequacy.

The **coin test** uses a coin and a slightly exposed film to determine safelight adequacy (Procedure Box 19-3). Because films that have already been exposed are more sensitive to conditions that cause film fog, a true test of the safelight uses a film that is preexposed to a small amount of radiation. After the test film has been slightly exposed, it is unwrapped in the darkroom under safelight conditions and placed on the counter where patient films will normally be unwrapped. A coin is placed on top of the unwrapped film for two or three minutes. This period simulates the approximate time required to aseptically unwrap a full mouth series of films and load them into the processor. It is assumed that while the film is on the counter, the portion of the film that remains under the metal coin would be protected from possible light exposure, while the rest of the area would receive exposure if the light was unsafe.

When the time is up, the film is processed as usual. After processing, the film is examined. An image of the outline of the coin would indicate a failed test, suggesting that the safelight conditions in the darkroom are fogging the film. A failed test should

prompt the radiographer to check to be sure that the safelight bulb wattage is correct and that the filter color is appropriate for the film used. The distance away from the working area should be checked, and the safelight filter should be visually inspected for scratches or cracks in the filter that would allow white light to escape.

TEST FOR LIGHT LEAKS Whether the darkroom is light-tight can be determined by closing the door and turning off all lights, including the safelight. Light leaks, if present, become visible after about five minutes when the eyes become accustomed to the dark. Possible sources of light leaks include around the entry door or around the pipes leading into the darkroom. Drop ceiling tiles and ventilation screens may also allow white light to enter the darkroom. While eyes are still adjusted to the dark, white light leaks may be marked with tape or chalk to allow the radiographer to find them when the white overhead lights are turned back on. Light leaks should be sealed with tape or weather stripping.

Additional sources of inappropriate light include illuminated dials or fluorescent objects worn or carried into the darkroom by personnel. Illuminated dials on equipment located in the darkroom must be red or may be masked with tape if necessary.

Fluorescent wristwatch faces should not be worn in the darkroom unless covered by the sleeve of the operator's lab coat. Operators who carry a cell phone in a pocket must completely shield any light or shut off the phone to prevent accidental illumination should there be an incoming call.

Processing System Monitoring

Processing equipment and chemistry need to be monitored, and quality control tests should be performed on a periodic basis.

AUTOMATIC PROCESSOR   The key to peak performance of an automatic processor is maintenance. Often the unit manufacturer will recommend daily, weekly, monthly, and quarterly maintenance and cleaning procedures to ensure quality performance. A schedule of set maintenance procedures, and a log of when those procedures need to be performed, should be posted with the maintenance scheduling.

These two tests are helpful in daily monitoring of the automatic processor:

1. Begin by processing an unexposed film under safelight conditions. The film should come out of the return chute of the automatic processor clear (slightly blue tinted) and dry.
2. Then process a film that has been exposed to white light. This film should come out of the return chute of the automatic processor black and dry after processing.

A failed test should prompt the operator to check the solutions, the water supply, and film dryer. The solution levels should be checked and must be replenished and changed on a regular basis. The processor should maintain the correct temperature. The water supply must be turned on and the dryer operating correctly to produce a clear, dry film.

PROCESSING SOLUTIONS   As explained in Chapter 8, chemical manufacturers recommend extending the life of processing solutions with regular replenishment and changing out expired solutions with fresh chemicals at regular intervals. Therefore it is important to monitor the strength of the processing solutions on a daily basis, before undiagnostic film images result.

The developer solution is the most critical of the processing solutions and demands careful attention. When the developer solution deteriorates and loses strength, the underdeveloped radiographic images lighten. Commercially available instruments are available that can be utilized to monitor the developer. (Figure 19-4) These

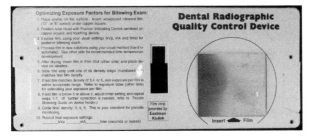

FIGURE 19-4 Dental radiographic quality control device.
Available from Xray QC [formerly Dental Radiographic Devices], www.xrayqc.com.

devices utilize a filmstrip with several density steps for comparison to a test film.

The radiographer may prepare a step-wedge from discarded lead foil from intraoral film packets, discussed earlier, to monitor the developer as well (Procedure Box 19-4). Using the step-wedge, several films are exposed at the same settings, all at the same time. At the beginning of the day, immediately after fresh chemistry has been prepared, one of the exposed films is processed. This becomes the **reference film,** with the ideal image density and contrast. The remaining exposed films should be stored in a cool, dry place protected from stray radiation and other conditions that produce film fog. At the beginning of each day, one of the previously exposed films is processed and compared to the reference film. Each subsequent film should match the reference film in density and contrast. A failed test would indicate that the processing chemicals, particularly the developer, is losing strength and needs to be changed (Figure 19-2).

X-ray Film Monitoring

Only fresh x-ray film should be used for exposing dental radiographs. Film manufacturers use a series of quality control tests to ensure dental x-ray film quality. Film should be properly stored, protected, and used before the expiration date. Check the expiration date on the x-ray film box and always use the oldest film first.

The **fresh-film test** can be used to monitor the quality of each box of film. When a new film box is opened for use, immediately process one of the films without exposing it. If the film is fresh, it will appear clear with a slight blue tint. If the film appears fogged, the remaining films in the box should not be used.

Equipment Used to View Radiographic Images Monitoring

VIEWBOX   If functioning properly, the viewbox should give off a uniform, subdued light. Flickering light may indicate bulb failure. The surface of the viewbox should be wiped clean as needed.

COMPUTER MONITOR   As discussed in Chapter 9, all types of monitors perform equally well at displaying digital radiographs for interpretation and diagnosis. Periodically performing quality control calibrations on the monitor will keep the image displayed at the proper resolution and gray scale. The manufacturer's recommendations should be followed

The location of the monitor where images are viewed should be evaluated to ensure that bright ambient light is not producing glare off the monitor surface that will compromise viewing the images. With the computer turned off, take the usual operator position in front of the monitor, either seated or standing. Observe the monitor for reflected images indicating that the monitor should be moved to a position that eliminates glare.

Extraoral Equipment Monitoring

CASSETTES AND INTENSIFYING SCREENS   Quality control procedures include periodically examining cassettes and intensifying

PROCEDURE 19-4
Reference film to monitor processing solutions

1. Prepare a step-wedge or use a commercially made device (see Procedure Box 19-1).
2. Obtain several size #2 intraoral film packets from the same package.
3. Place one of the film packets on the counter or exam chair within reach of the x-ray tube head.
4. Place the step-wedge on top of the film packet.
5. Position the x-ray tube head over the film packet and step-wedge, and direct the central rays of the x-ray beam perpendicularly toward the film packet. Place the open end of the PID exactly 1 in. (2.5 cm) above the film packet. Use a ruler for accuracy.
6. Set the exposure factors to those utilized for an adult patient maxillary anterior periapcial radiograph.
7. Make the exposure.
8. Place the exposed film in a safe place, protected from film fog–causing elements (stray radiation, heat, humidity, chemical fumes).
9. Immediately repeat steps 3 through 8 with the rest of the films.
10. Following a complete solution change of the processing chemistry, process one of the exposed films. This film is the reference film.
11. Mount the reference film on the viewbox.
12. Each day immediately after replenishing the processing chemistry, retrieve one of the stored exposed films and process as usual.
13. Compare the film processed on this day to the reference film processed when the chemistry was changed. Look for similar density and contrast indicating that the processing solutions are functioning at peak levels.
14. Repeat steps 12 and 13 each day. The solutions are exhausted and need to be changed when the density and contrast of the just-processed film does not match the reference film.

screens. Extraoral cassettes should be checked for warping and light leaks that can result in fogged radiographs. Defective cassettes should be repaired or replaced.

Intensifying screens should be examined for cleanliness and scratches. Any specks of dirt, lint, or other material will absorb the light given off by the screen crystals and produce white or clear artifacts on the resultant radiographic image. Dirty screens should be cleaned as needed with solutions recommended by the screen manufacturer. However, overuse of chemical cleaning should be avoided. Any scratched or damaged screen should be repaired or replaced.

Benefits of Quality Assurance Programs

Everyone benefits from a well-organized quality assurance program. The time required to assess, plan, implement, and evaluate a quality assurance program is made up in the time saved and the benefits gained avoiding the production of poor-quality radiographs and retakes.

Periodic evaluation of the program will allow for flexibility as changes in recommended protocols or new techniques come into being. The ultimate goal of quality assurance is to produce radiographs with the greatest amount of diagnostic yield using the smallest amount of radiation exposure.

REVIEW—Chapter summary

Quality assurance is defined as the planning, implementation, and evaluation of procedures used to produce high-quality radiographs with maximum diagnostic information (yield) while minimizing radiation exposure. Quality assurance includes both quality administration procedures and quality control techniques.

Quality administration refers to conducting a quality assurance program in the oral health care practice. The five steps to a quality administration program are (1) assess needs, (2) develop a written plan, (3) assign authority and responsibilities, (4) develop monitoring and maintenance schedules, and (5) utilize a log and evaluations to check on the program.

The key to producing the highest quality diagnostic radiographs with the lowest possible radiation exposure is operator competence.

Quality control is defined as a series of tests to ensure that the radiographic system is functioning properly and that the radiographs produced are of an acceptable level of quality.

These tests include the monitoring of the dental x-ray machine, the darkroom, processing system, and x-ray film. A step-wedge is a valuable tool that can be used in a variety of tests.

Quality control tests for monitoring dental x-ray machines include the output consistency test and tube head stability. Quality control tests for monitoring the darkroom include the coin test for checking the safelight and for checking for light leaks. Quality control tests for monitoring the processing system include monitoring the processing solutions with the use of a reference film or a commercial device. The fresh film test is used to monitor dental x-ray film.

Everyone, the oral health care team and the patients, benefits from a well-organized quality assurance program.

RECALL—Study questions

1. The goal of quality assurance is to achieve maximum diagnostic yield from each radiograph.
   Quality control means using tests to ensure quality.
   a. The first statement is true. The second statement is false.
   b. The first statement is false. The second statement is true.
   c. Both statements are true.
   d. Both statements are false.

2. On-the-job training and continuing education courses contribute to radiographic competence.
   Competent radiographers are key to a quality assurance program.
   a. The first statement is true. The second statement is false.
   b. The first statement is false. The second statement is true.
   c. Both statements are true.
   d. Both statements are false.

3. List the four objectives of quality control.
   a. _____
   b. _____
   c. _____
   d. _____

4. The step-wedge can be used to test each of the following EXCEPT one. Which one is the EXCEPTION?
   a. Dental x-ray machine output consistency
   b. Processing chemistry strength
   c. Density and contrast of the image
   d. Adequacy of the safelight

5. Each of the following is a quality control test for monitoring the dental x-ray machine EXCEPT one. Which one is the EXCEPTION?
   a. Tube head stability test
   b. Coin test
   c. Output consistency test
   d. Timer, milliamperage, and kilovoltage setting accuracy test

6. The use of the coin test will monitor darkroom safelight conditions.
   When an image of the coin appears on the radiograph, the safelight is adequate.
   a. The first statement is true. The second statement is false.
   b. The first statement is false. The second statement is true.
   c. Both statements are true.
   d. Both statements are false.

7. A film processed under ideal conditions and used to compare subsequent radiographic images is a
   a. fresh film.
   b. fogged film.
   c. periapical film.
   d. reference film.

8. When the automatic processor is functioning properly, an unexposed film will exit the return chute dry and
   a. black.
   b. clear.
   c. green.
   d. with the image of a coin.

9. In addition to the dentist, who is responsible for planning, implementing, and evaluating a quality assurance plan?
   a. Dental assistant
   b. Dental hygienist
   c. Practice manager
   d. All of the above

REFLECT—Case study

The practice where you work needs to update their radiographic quality control plan. Currently the basic plan mentions the need to test the x-ray machine and monitor the darkroom and processing systems. Applying what you have learned in this chapter, develop a quality control plan for your practice. Include the following:

1. List of equipment you think the practice should be testing
2. The name of the test needed
3. Recommended time interval for performing the test
4. Name of the person assigned to perform the test
5. A description of what a failed test and a successful test would look like
6. The action required if a failed test results

Then prepare the following documents that your practice would use to assist the quality assurance plan:

1. A detailed, step-by-step procedure that someone could follow to perform each of the tests you have recommended
2. Forms to keep a log of the outcomes for each of the tests you recommended

RELATE—Laboratory application

For a comprehensive laboratory practice exercise on this topic, see Thomson, E. M. (2012). *Exercises in oral radiography techniques: A laboratory manual* (3rd ed.). Upper Saddle River, NJ: Pearson Education. Chapter 13, "Radiographic quality assurance."

REFERENCES

American Academy of Dental Radiology Quality Assurance Committee. (1983). Recommendations for quality assurance in dental radiography. *Oral Surgery, 55,* 421–426.

Eastman Kodak. (1998). *Quality assurance in dental radiography.* Rochester, NY: Author.

National Council of Radiation Protection and Measurements. (1988). *Quality assurance for diagnostic imaging equipment: Recommendations of the National Council on Radiation Protection and Measurements.* NCRP Report no. 99. Bethesda, MD: NCRP Publications.

Thomson, E. M. (2012). *Exercises in oral radiographic techniques. A laboratory manual,* (3rd ed.). Upper Saddle River, NJ: Pearson Education.

Safety and Environmental Responsibilities in Dental Radiography

OBJECTIVES

Following successful completion of this chapter, you should be able to:

1. Define the key words.
2. Identify agencies responsible for regulations regarding safe handling of hazardous radiographic products.
3. Use MSDSs to identify proper handling and disposal of chemicals and materials associated with radiographic procedures.
4. List the requirements of the OSHA Hazard Communication Standard.
5. Identify radiographic wastes that are considered hazardous to personnel and harmful to the environment.
6. Advocate the need for safe handling and proper disposal of radiographic chemicals and materials.
7. Demonstrate effective use of an eyewash station.

KEY WORDS

Alkaline
Biodegradable
Caustic
Eyewash station
Hazardous waste
Material Safety and Data Sheets (MSDSs)
Neoprene gloves
Nitrile gloves
pH
PPE (personal protective equipment)
Silver thiosulphate complex
Waste stream

Introduction

To work safely with and around ionizing radiation, dental assistants and dental hygienists study the characteristics and properties of x-ray energy. Competence in dental radiation safety results from a thorough understanding of the appropriate uses and the potential effects of x-radiation. It is equally important that oral health care professionals understand the properties and actions of the chemicals and materials that are used in the production of dental radiographs. Radiographic chemicals and materials that require careful handling and special disposal considerations include silver in radiographic film emulsions and silver thiosulphate complexes in used fixer chemistry; the lead used in intraoral film packets, lead aprons and thyroid collars, and older film storage boxes; and broken or obsolete digital imaging systems. Safe handling of these materials and other products used in dental radiography will help prevent errors that may lead to retake radiographs for the patient; avoid injury to the radiographer; and reduce the potential harm to the environment. Although the individual oral health care practice generates a small amount of these hazardous wastes, collectively the potential exists for a significant impact on the environment. A heightened awareness of the impact of these wastes on our environment is changing the way we manage their disposal.

Requirements for Safety and Environmental Health

Two agencies responsible for recommendations and regulations regarding safe handling of chemicals and other potentially harmful materials and for the management of **hazardous wastes** used in dental radiography are:

- **Occupational Safety and Health Administration (OHSA)** Introduced in Chapter 10, we learned that OHSA sets and enforces regulations that protect the radiographer from infection in the oral health care setting. OHSA also develops standards for workplace safety regarding the handling of radiographic chemicals.
- **U.S. Environmental Protection Agency (EPA)** We learned in Chapter 10 that the EPA plays a role in the regulation of disinfectants used in radiographic infection control practices. The EPA's primary responsibility is to establish and enforce national standards that protect humans and the environment.

OSHA requires that manufacturers of chemical products such as developer and fixer supply **Material Safety Data Sheets (MSDSs)** to the oral health care practices that purchase these products (Figure 20-1). MSDS provide the oral health care professional with information regarding the properties and the potential health effects of the product. MSDSs include the following information:

- Chemical ingredients and common name
- Potential hazards of working with the product
- An explanation of the product's stability and reactivity
- Requirements for safe handling and storage
- Exposure controls and personal protection required when using the product
- Disposal considerations
- Regulatory information

Dentists are required by OHSA to obtain and keep on file an MSDS for every chemical product used in the practice. The MSDS should be reviewed by all personnel who will work with the product and kept for easy reference and periodic review to ensure safe handling. All personnel should receive training and practice with safe handling of the product and appropriate emergency exposure responses.

Chemical product manufacturers must also provide warning labels. Labeling products assists the radiographer in safe management of these products (Figure 20-2). Product labels should be designed according to the OSHA Hazard Communication Standard that states that oral health care employees have a right to know the identities of, and the potential hazards of, the chemicals they will be working with (Box 20-1). Radiographers also need to know what protective measures to take to prevent adverse effects that might result when working with the product. This information will assist the radiographer in establishing proper work practices and in taking steps to reduce exposure and the occurrence of work-related illnesses and injuries caused by the products. All containers must be labeled. This includes the developer and fixer tanks, even those inside an automatic processor, tubs used to clean the processor rollers, and any containers used for disposing absorbent towels used to clean up a spill.

MSDSs and product labels must be obtained from the manufacturer for all chemicals used in radiographic procedures. These include:

- Fixer
- Developer
- Disinfectants
- Cleaners used on processing equipment

Safe Handling of Radiographic Chemicals and Materials

Safe handling and appropriate exposure emergency responses when working with the chemicals used in radiographic procedures can be found on the MSDSs for the specific product being used. The following are general safe handling instructions. Because the chemical makeup of products will vary depending on the manufacturer, the radiographer must be familiar with the

---

BOX 20-1   Requirements of OSHA Hazard Communication Standard

- Develop a written hazard communication program.
- Maintain an inventory list of all hazardous chemicals present in the oral health care facility.
- Obtain and have accessible MSDSs for all chemicals.
- Label containers of hazardous chemicals.
- Train all personnel in safe handling of the hazardous chemicals.

MATERIAL SAFETY DATA SHEET

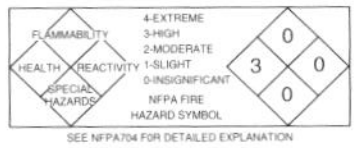

1. CHEMICAL PRODUCT AND COMPANY IDENTIFICATION

PRODUCT NAME: FORMULA 2000 PLUS COMPONENT 1
PRODUCT TYPE: Special cleaner for removal of oxidation/
           reduction products from X-ray film developers

IMPORTER/
DISTRIBUTOR: Air Techniques, Inc.
         1295 Walt Whitman Road
         Melville, NY 11747, USA
         Phone: 516-433-7676

PRIMARY EMERGENCY
CONTACT: CHEMTREC Phone: 1-800-424-9300

2. COMPOSITION/INFORMATION ON INGREDIENTS

Component	CAS#	% By Wt.	Exposure Limits
1-Hydroxyethane-1, 1-diphosphonic acid	**2809-21-4**	1 - 5	**N/A**
Thiourea	62-56-6	1 - 5	OSHA 1 mg/kg
Water	7732-18-5	60 - 95	N/A

3. HAZARD IDENTIFICATION

POTENTIAL HEALTH EFFECTS:
ROUTE(S) OF ENTRY: Skin and eye contact
HUMAN EFFECTS AND SYMPTOMS OF OVEREXPOSURE:
1-Hydroxyethane-1,1-diphosphonic acid is a severe eye irritant and a skin irritant. Thiourea is toxic by ingestion or inhalation. It is an irritant to skin, eyes and respiratory passages. It may cause sensitization.

CARCINOGENICITY:
NTP: Yes thiourea listed as "reasonably anticipated to be a human carcinogen"
IARC: Yes thiourea group 2B, "possibly carcinogenic to humans"
OSHA: No
California Prop. 65 thiourea listed as "Chemicals known to the State to cause cancer"

4. FIRST AID MEASURES

SKIN: Remove contaminated clothing and shoes. Flush affected area with large amounts of water. Do not use solvents or thinners. Get immediate medical attention.
EYES: Hold eyes open and flush for at least 15 minutes with large amounts of water. Get immediate medical attention.
INGESTION: Do not induce vomiting. Give two glasses of water to dilute stomach contents. Never give anything by mouth to an unconscious person. Get immediate medical attention.
INHALATION: Remove to fresh air immediately. If breathing is difficult administer oxygen. Get immediate medical attention.

5. FIRE FIGHTING MEASURES

FLASH POINT:. N/A
EXTINGUISHING MEDIA: Use extinguishing media suitable for surrounding fire.
SPECIAL FIRE FIGHTING PROCEDURES: Product is not flammble. However, overheating of containers will produce toxic fumes. Use self contained breathing apparatus and full protective clothing.

6. ACCIDENTAL RELEASE MEASURES

SPILL AND LEAK PROCEDURES: Wear appropriate personal protective equipment; contain spills onto inert absorbent and place in suitable containers.

7. HANDLING AND STORAGE

STORAGE: Store closed containers in an area away from heat. Do not store at temperatures below 5°C.
HANDLING: Use with adequate ventilation. Avoid skin and eye contact. Do not eat, drink or smoke in application area.

8. EXPOSURE CONTROLS/PERSONAL PROTECTION

RESPIRATORY PROTECTION: If airborne concentration exceeds recommended limits, use a NIOSH approved respirator in accordance with OSHA Respirator Protection requirements under 29 CFR 1910.134.
SKIN PROTECTION: Clothing suitable to avoid skin contact. Use neoprene, nitrile or natural rubber gloves. Check suitability recommendations by protective equipment manufacturers, especially towards chemical breakthrough resistance.
EYE PROTECTION: Safety goggles with side shields.

9. PHYSICAL AND CHEMICAL PROPERTIES

PHYSICAL FORM: Clear Colorless Liquid
ODOR: Characteristic
PH: 1.0 - 2.0
BOILING POINT: -212°F (100°C)
AUTOIGNITION: N/A
VAPOR PRESSURE: N/A
SOLUBILITY IN WATER: Completely
DENSITY: 1.02 -1.04 g/cm^3

10. STABILITY AND REACTIVITY

CHEMICAL STABILITY: Stable
HAZARDOUS DECOMPOSITION PRODUCTS: Sulfur dioxide.
POLYMERIZATION: Hazardous polymerization will not occur.
INCOMPATIBILITIES: Strong acids and alkaline materials.

11. TOXICOLOGICAL INFORMATION

See Section 3 - Human Effects and Symptoms of Overexposure

12. ECOLOGICAL INFORMATION

Avoid contamination of ground water or waterways. Do not discharge into sewers.

13. DISPOSAL CONSIDERATIONS

Dispose of in accordance with Federal, State or Local regulations.

14. TRANSPORT INFORMATION

DOT SHIPPING NAME: NOT REGULATED.

15. REGULATORY INFORMATION

All components of this product are on the TSCA Inventory.
SARA Title III:
Thiourea is subject to the supplier notification requirements of Section 313 of the Superfund Amendments and Reauthorization Act (SARA/EPCRA) and the requirements of 40 CFR Part 372.
Note: Entries under this section cover only those regulations typically addressed in the MSDS generating process, such as TSCA, and EPCRA/SARA Title III.

16. OTHER INFORMATION

HAZCOM LABEL: DANGER! CAUSES EYE BURNS. MAY CAUSE SKIN IRRITATION. POSSIBLE CANCER HAZARD. CONTAINS INGREDIENT THAT CAUSED CANCER IN ANIMALS.
To the best of our knowledge, the information contained in this MSDS is accurate. It is intended to assist the user in his evaluation of the product's hazards, and safety precautions to be taken in its use. The data on this MSDS relate only to the specific material designated herein. We do not assume any liability for the use of, or reliance on this information, nor do we guarantee its accuracy or completeness.

Printed in Germany

2009-21-01

(Continued)

FIGURE 20-1 Sample MSDS. (Courtesy of Air Techniques, Inc.)

FIGURE 20-1 (Continued)

MATERIAL SAFETY DATA SHEET

1. CHEMICAL PRODUCT AND COMPANY IDENTIFICATION

PRODUCT NAME: FORMULA 2000 PLUS COMPONENT 2
PRODUCT TYPE: Special cleaner for removal of oxidation/
reduction products from X-ray film developers

IMPORTER/
DISTRIBUTOR:
Air Techniques, Inc.
1295 Walt Whitman Road
Melville, NY 11747, USA
Phone: 516-433-7676

PRIMARY EMERGENCY
CONTACT: CHEMTREC   Phone: 1-800-424-9300

2. COMPOSITION/INFORMATION ON INGREDIENTS

Component	CAS#	% By Wt.	Exposure Limits
Sodium persulfate	7775-27-1	45 - 55	0.1 mg/m³ TWA ACGIH
Sodium sulfate	7757-82-6	45 - 55	N/A

3. HAZARD IDENTIFICATION

POTENTIAL HEALTH EFFECTS:
ROUTE(S) OF ENTRY: Inhalation, skin and eye contact
HUMAN EFFECTS AND SYMPTOMS OF OVEREXPOSURE:
Sodium persulfate is a severe irritant to skin, eyes and respiratory passages. May
cause sensitization by inhalation or skin contact.

CARCINOGENICITY:
NTP: No
IARC: No
OSHA: No

4. FIRST AID MEASURES

SKIN: Remove contaminated clothing and shoes. Flush affected area with large
amounts of water. Do not use solvents or thinners. Get immediate medical attention.
EYES: Hold eyes open and flush for at least 15 minutes with large amounts of
water. Get immediate medical attention.
INGESTION: Do not induce vomiting. Give two glasses of water to dilute stomach
contents. Never give anything by mouth to an unconscious person. Get immediate
medical attention.
INHALATION: Remove to fresh air immediately. If breathing is difficult administer
oxygen. Get immediate medical attention.

5. FIRE FIGHTING MEASURES

FLASH POINT: N/A
EXTINGUISHING MEDIA: Alcohol foam, carbon dioxide, dry powder, or water
spray.
SPECIAL FIRE FIGHTING PROCEDURES: Product is not flammable. However, overheating of containers will produce toxic fumes. Use self contained breathing apparatus and full protective clothing.

6. ACCIDENTAL RELEASE MEASURES

SPILL AND LEAK PROCEDURES: Wear appropriate personal protective equipment;
collect and place in suitable containers.

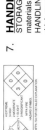

7. HANDLING AND STORAGE

STORAGE: Store closed containers in an area away from heat and combustible
materials.
HANDLING: Use with adequate ventilation. Avoid skin and eye contact. Do not eat,
drink or smoke in application area.

8. EXPOSURE CONTROLS/PERSONAL PROTECTION

RESPIRATORY PROTECTION: If airborne concentration exceeds recommended
limits, use a NIOSH approved respirator in accordance with OSHA Respirator
Protection requirements under 29 CFR 1910.134.
SKIN PROTECTION: Clothing suitable to avoid skin contact. Use neoprene, nitrile
or natural rubber gloves. Check suitability recommendations by protective equipment
manufacturers, especially towards chemical breakthrough resistance.
EYE PROTECTION: Safety goggles with side shields.

9. PHYSICAL AND CHEMICAL PROPERTIES

PHYSICAL FORM: White powder
ODOR: Odorless
pH: N/A
AUTOIGNITION: N/A
VAPOR PRESSURE: N/A
SOLUBILITY IN WATER: Completely
BULK DENSITY: 1100 kg/m³

10. STABILITY AND REACTIVITY

CHEMICAL STABILITY: Stable.
HAZARDOUS DECOMPOSITION PRODUCTS: Oxides of Sulfur.
POLYMERIZATION: Hazardous polymerization will not occur.
INCOMPATIBILITIES: Will oxidize organic substances. Keep away from alkalis,
metals, reducing agents and combustible substances.

11. TOXICOLOGICAL INFORMATION

See Section 3 Human Effects and Symptoms of Overexposure

12. ECOLOGICAL INFORMATION

Avoid contamination of ground water or waterways. Do not discharge into sewers.
May be toxic to aquatic organisms.

13. DISPOSAL CONSIDERATIONS

Dispose of in accordance with Federal, State or Local regulations.

14. TRANSPORT INFORMATION

DOT SHIPPING NAME: NOT REGULATED.

15. REGULATORY INFORMATION

All components of this product are on the TSCA Inventory.
SARA Title III:
To the best of our knowledge this product contains no toxic chemicals subject to
the supplier notification requirements of Section 313 of the Superfund Amendments
and Reauthorization Act (SARA/EPCRA), and the requirements of 40 CFR Part 372.
Note: Entries under this section cover only those regulations typically addressed in
the MSDS generating process, such as, TSCA, and EPCRA/SARA Title III.

16. OTHER INFORMATION

HAZCOM LABEL: WARNING! CAUSES SKIN AND EYE IRRITATION. MAY
CAUSE SENSITIZATION BY INHALATION AND SKIN CONTACT.
To the best of our knowledge, the information contained in this MSDS is accurate.
It is intended to assist the user in his evaluation of the product's hazards, and safety
precautions to be taken in its use. The data on this MSDS relate only to the specific
material designated herein. We do not assume any liability for the use of, or
reliance on this information, nor do we guarantee its accuracy or completeness.

Printed in Germany   2009-21-01

KODAK GBX Developer and Replenisher

WHEN DILUTED FOR USE AS RECOMMENDED

Contains:	CAS Reg. #
Water	7732-18-5
Hydroquinone	123-31-9
Diethylene glycol	111-46-6
Potassium sulfite	10117-38-1

*Principal hazardous components.
Warning: causes skin and eye irritation. May
cause allergic skin reaction. Wash thoroughly after handling.   (see MSDS)

Concentrates (not diluted solution) made by: This label is for use only with
Eastman Kodak Company   the indicated product.
Rochester, New York 14650   TM: KODAK
(716)722-5151

Attach these labels directly to the proper chemical tanks or containers, or on the protective cover of the processor near the chemicals.

List Price $1.00

KODAK GBX Fixer and Replenisher

WHEN DILUTED FOR USE AS RECOMMENDED

Contains:	CAS Reg. #
Water	7732-18-5
Ammonium thiosulfate	7783-18-8
Sodium bisulfite	7631-90-5

LOW HAZARD FOR RECOMMENDED HANDLING   (see MSDS)

Concentrates (not diluted solution) made by: This label is for use only with
Eastman Kodak Company   the indicated product.
Rochester, New York 14650   TM: KODAK
(716)722-5151

These labels are provided to assist you in complying with the U.S. Federal OSHA Hazard Communication Standard – 29 CFR 1910. 1200

CIESSL10

FIGURE 20-2 Sample label that meets OSHA Hazard Communication Standard. (Courtesy Carestream Health.)

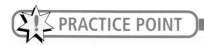

PRACTICE POINT

Although OSHA requires manufacturers of chemical products to provide users with an MSDS that lists the specific chemicals found in the product, there is sometimes a reluctance to disclose a chemical when it is considered a trade secret or special ingredient that the manufacturer considers unique to their product. A trade secret can help the manufacturer advertise their product as better, or having an advantage over competitors. OSHA allows leeway for ingredients considered a trade secret, provided that the secret ingredient must be disclosed immediately on the occurrence of an emergency. For example, if a reaction occurs following contact with a chemical that the oral health care professional then seeks medical attention for, the product manufacturer will be contacted, and they must disclose the identity of the chemical to the medical professional so that appropriate treatment can occur.

specific requirements for safe handling of the specific brand of product being used at his/her facility. The following are general guidelines for safe handling of these chemicals and materials.

Fixer

Safe handling begins with a well-ventilated darkroom and the use of **PPE (personal protective equipment;** see Chapter 10), including protective clothing, mask, eyewear, and impervious gloves (that do not permit liquid penetration), especially when cleaning the processing equipment or changing or replenishing chemistry (Box 20-2). Strong chemicals may penetrate latex medical examination gloves that are used for patient treatment.

Nitrile or **neoprene** (rubber) utility **gloves** provide the radiographer with better protection. The radiographer should avoid prolonged breathing of fixer chemical vapors. Under normal conditions, fixer should not cause respiratory difficulty in most individuals. If heated sufficiently or an accidental contact with developer occurs, an irritating sulphur dioxide gas may be released. Close, prolonged contact with this gas may cause some hypersensitive or asthmatic individuals discomfort. If uncomfortable symptoms occur, move to a well-ventilated area. If symptoms persist, seek medical attention.

Avoid inhaling mist or vapors when pouring fixer liquid from bottles or when mixing concentrated chemicals with water. If fixer contacts skin, immediately wash off with soap and water. If fixer splashes in eyes, flush immediately with water. A sink and **eyewash station** should be available in the darkroom or in close proximity to where processing equipment and chemistry is handled (Figure 20-3). The radiographer must know how to use the eye wash equipment so that it can be appropriately operated in an emergency. (Procedure Box 20-1) Regular training and practice in responding to a potential exposure can help the radiographer react quickly and appropriately in an emergency. Minor contact with a small amount of fixer is not likely to cause irritation, or an allergic reaction. If irritating symptoms persist as a result of inhaling sulphur dioxide gas or from repeated, prolonged skin or eye contact, the radiographer should seek medical attention.

Fixer chemistry should be stored in the original container. The container must remain unopened or tightly capped until ready for use to prevent oxidation and the buildup of chemical vapors in the storage area. An accidental spill should be absorbed with a disposable towel immediately. A spill can increase the amount of vapors released in the vicinity. The towel used to absorb the spill should be treated as chemical waste and disposed of in the same manner as used fixer. The surface where the spill occurred should then be cleaned thoroughly to remove any trace of the chemical. After handling fixer containers or after wiping up a spill, remove contaminated PPE and wash hands before performing any other task. The impervious gloves should be disinfected and dried before storing. Wash contaminated clothing prior to wearing again.

Developer

Developer requires the same safe handling precautions as fixer, which includes adequate ventilation and avoiding contact (Box 20-2). Developer has a high **pH**, meaning that it is

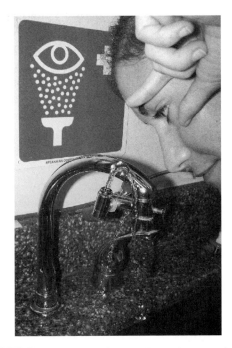

FIGURE 20-3 Eyewash station. Radiographer preparing to use the eyewash station in response to accidental contact with a potentially hazardous chemical. Note the recognizable label on the wall noting the location of the eyewash station.

alkaline or **caustic** and very capable of burning biological tissues on contact. It is this caustic property that makes developer an even more serious eye irritant than fixer. An accidental eye exposure requires an immediate flushing with water at an eyewash station for a minimum of 15 minutes (Procedure Box 20-1). If a contact lens is present, it should be removed if easy to do. The radiographer should seek medical attention following accidental eye contact with developer. If developer contacts skin, immediately wash off with soap and water. Prolonged or

---

BOX 20-2   General Recommendations for Safe Handling of Hazardous Chemicals

- Read MSDS for the specific product being used.
- Provide training on the use of the product.
- Keep container of product tightly closed.
- Store in the original container.
- Do not store product in the same area where food or drinks are stored or consumed.
- Ensure proper labeling of product.
- Wear appropriate PPE.
- Impervious clothing or vinyl apron recommended.
- Use protective eyewear with side shields. Safety goggles recommended.
- Use nitrile or neoprene gloves.
- Avoid breathing mist or vapor.
- Avoid contact with eyes.
- Avoid prolonged or repeated contact with skin.
- Use only with adequate ventilation.
- Wash hands thoroughly after handling.
- Do not consume foods or drink or smoke where chemicals are handled.
- Dispose of container appropriately.
- Do not reuse container.
- Remove and launder clothing if contaminated.
- Periodically check PPE to ensure working condition.

PROCEDURE 20-1
Use of an emergency eyewash station

1. Eyewash station

   a. Must be within 25 feet of where potentially hazardous chemicals are being used.

   b. Personnel must be able to get to the station within 10 seconds from where they are handling potentially hazardous chemicals.

   c. Must be clearly labeled with appropriate signage that is easily recognized.

2. Remove the caps covering the eye wash faucets. Caps should be easy to remove.

3. Turn on the water flow to a rate of about 0.5 gallons per minute.

4. Water temperature should be warm, between 60 to 95 degrees.

5. Hold the eye lids open with an index finger and thumb. Do not touch the eyeballs.*

6. Maintain water contact with the eyes for the recommended rinsing time, 5 to 60 minutes, even if uncomfortable.

7. Consult the product MSDS to determine the recommended rinsing time. Acids such as fixer are easier to rinse away than alkalines such as developer. Truly caustic chemicals that may be used in processor cleaners may require a 60-minute rinse time.

8. Seek medical attention at completion of the recommended rinse time.

*If easy to do, contact lens should be removed. Rinse fingers well. Do not use the same finger to hold open the eyelids unless thoroughly washed of possible chemical contamination.

repeated skin contact may cause irritation that results in drying or cracking and can result in depigmentation.

Accidentally mixing developer with fixer, even in minute droplets, will result in the release of an irritating sulphur dioxide gas. If contamination occurs between developer and fixer, both tanks should be emptied and cleaned, disposing of both solutions appropriately. When cleaning the processing equipment or changing or replenishing chemistry, the radiographer should take care to avoid a splash that would mix developer and fixer (Figure 20-4). If developer is spilled, the same steps taken to contain a fixer spill should be followed. Using a disposable towel, absorb the liquid and then thoroughly clean the surface to remove any trace of the chemical. The towel should be treated as chemical waste and disposed of appropriately. Remove, disinfect, and dry the impervious gloves; remove contaminated PPE; and wash hands before performing any other task.

Disinfectants

The radiographer should be aware of the possible hazards of contact with or inhaling the vapors of the disinfectants that will be used in the radiographic process. (See Chapter 10.) The oral health care facility should have written documentation of what chemicals are used to disinfect radiographic equipment and clinical contact surfaces, where these are stored, and the preparation dates to avoid using expired disinfectants.

Updating the inventory at regular intervals will assist with maintaining only effective disinfectant solutions and knowing when to discard older chemicals. The radiographer must use PPE (personal protective equipment; see Figure 10-2), including protective clothing, mask, eyewear, and impervious gloves when preparing and using any level of disinfectant. Low- or intermediate-level disinfectants are commonly used to prepare clinical contact surfaces prior to radiographic procedures. Although not as corrosive as high-level disinfectants

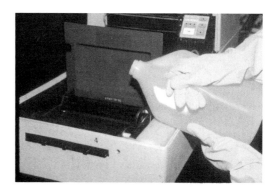

FIGURE 20-4 Barrier placed to separate the developer and fixer tanks when adding chemicals.

or sterilants, the same level of caution should be used when handling any chemical. The radiographer should be familiar with the emergency first aid requirements for the product being used. Regular review of the MSDS and training updates, especially if a new product has been introduced, will prepare the radiographer for the appropriate action in an emergency.

Contact with the disinfectant should be avoided. If eye or skin contact should occur, flush immediately with water. If diluting or mixing of the chemical concentrate is required prior to use, the bottle used for this purpose must be labeled appropriately. Labels should be maintained and checked periodically to be sure that the information remains readable. Never use or reuse a container that was made for another product to prepare disinfectant solutions.

Although the affects of accidental skin and eye contact or inhaling the vapors of the disinfectant will depend on the chemical used in the product, in general, accidental exposures should be handled in the same manner as described previously for fixer or developer contact. If discomfort does not subside after flushing skin or eyes with water or moving to a well-ventilated area, the radiographer should seek medical attention.

Cleaners Used on Processing Equipment

Processing equipment, especially the rollers in the tanks of automatic processors, require cleaning to provide optimal radiographs. Cleaning agents used to remove residue and oxidized chemicals from the reducing agents in developer usually contain strong acids and corrosive agents. As with disinfectants, the radiographer should consult the MSDS on the product to determine the appropriate PPE (personal protective equipment) and to be prepared with the correct action should an accidental exposure occur. Most manufacturers of processing cleaners recommend that PPE (personal protective equipment) cover the skin, especially around the wrists and arms. Puncturing inner safety seals to open bottles of chemicals and mixing, pouring, and/or spraying cleaner products all increase the risk of a splash that could lead to accidental exposure. Most processor cleaners will cause skin irritations and eye burns on contact. An apron made from an impervious material such as vinyl or rubber is recommended. Nitrile or other suitable heavy-duty utility gloves must be used when handling these cleaners. It is recommended that the radiographer check with the manufacturer of the gloves to determine their ability to prevent the chemical cleaner from breaking through the glove material. Safety goggles are the recommended eyewear protection, especially when using a spray bottle to apply the cleaner to rollers (Figure 20-5).

Adequate ventilation will prevent irritation to respiratory tissues. If discomfort results, the radiographer should move to a well-ventilated area. If symptoms persist, seek medical attention. If there is accidental contact with skin, flush with plenty of water. Because of the caustic nature of cleaners of this type, accidentally splashing cleaner in the eyes requires medical attention after flushing the eyes with water for a minimum of 15 minutes. If cleaner contacts the radiographer's

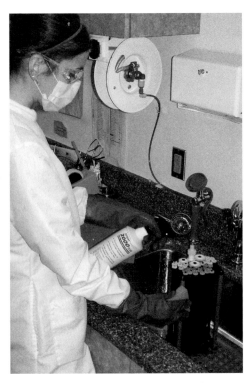

FIGURE 20-5 PPE used when cleaning processing equipment.

clothes or shoes, these should be removed and washed before reusing.

Lead

Normal handling of intact lead foil used in intraoral film packets and lead sealed in aprons and thyroid collars will not present a hazard to the radiographer. In years past, lead-lined containers or film packet dispensers were available in which to store film safely away from stray radiation until ready for use. Improvements made to fast-speed film have made these lead-lined boxes unnecessary. In fact these lead-lined containers should not be used either for storage of film or any other storage or dispensing purpose. The lead lining is subject to flaking off in a powder form with the potential for inhalation or ingestion (Figure 20-6). All old radiographic storage containers suspected of being made

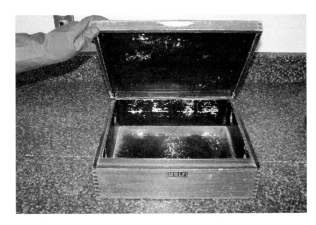

FIGURE 20-6 Old lead-lined storage box showing signs of flaking.

of lead should be appropriately discarded. (See next section on management of radiographic wastes.) All intra- and extraoral film should be stored in original packaging until ready for use.

Management of Radiographic Wastes

Disposal of hazardous wastes generated by the oral health care practice is often mandated by federal law. It is important to note that some state and local waste management regulations are more stringent than federal regulations. In many areas, it is against the law to discard used fixer into the municipal sewer system or to discard lead foil at municipal landfills. The radiographer must know what laws apply in the practice area. Equally important is the ethical responsibility to recycle or properly dispose of wastes that may be harmful to the environment.

The most common way to dispose of the hazardous materials used in dental radiography appropriately is to contract with a waste disposal company. Many practices already employ a waste management company to dispose of biohazard materials. These same companies usually offer a hazardous waste service that can manage radiographic wastes as well.

The MSDS for the product can sometimes be vague in proper disposal of the product, often stating to "dispose of according to state or local regulations." Therefore is it important to know what the regulations are for the practice area. Some of the options for proper management of radiographic wastes are:

- Contract with a waste management company to provide container and pick-up service.
- Contract with a lead or silver reclaiming company for recycling.
- Establish an agreement with the supplier to "take back" used fixer/unused radiographic film.
- Collect the used product and transport it to a designated drop-off center in your community.
- Utilize silver recovery or reclaiming system (for used fixer).

Although it is most important to know what the laws are in the location of the oral health care practice, the following are general guidelines for proper management of radiographic wastes.

Used Fixer Waste

Both developer and fixer are **biodegradable**, meaning that they can be broken down into harmless products by a wastewater treatment facility. In Chapter 7 we learned that the function of fixer is to remove the unexposed and undeveloped silver halide crystals from the emulsion of radiographic film. Compared to photographic processing facilities, which also use fixer to remove silver halides, oral health care practices generate a very small amount of silver waste. The silver found in used fixer of dental radiographic processors is in the form of a very stable **silver thiosulphate complex**. Thus bonded, there are virtually no free silver ions present in used fixer, prompting experts to conclude that used fixer poses very little threat to the environment if discharged into wastewater treatment facilities. However, many state and local municipalities have regulations regarding the amount and/or the concentration of used fixer that can be discharged to a wastewater treatment facility. The oral health care practice has several sound and environmental-friendly options to responsibly dispose of used fixer. Collecting used fixer for the purpose of extracting the silver ions will conserve a resource and prevent adding this metal to the **waste stream**. The easiest way for an oral health care facility to achieve these goals is often to contract with a licensed company that will provide containers for collection and periodic pickup for proper disposal. It is important that the qualifications of the contractor selected for disposal of hazardous wastes or recycling be thoroughly investigated. If materials are disposed of inappropriately, it is possible that the oral health care practice would be partly liable for fines and costs incurred by faulty handling of materials by the disposal service (Box 20-3).

An option that allows for silver recovery in-office at the site of use is to purchase a silver recovery system. Silver recovery or reclaiming systems attach to the automatic processor

---

BOX 20-3   Questions to Ask of a Waste Management Service

- Are you licensed to handle hazardous wastes?
- What types of hazardous wastes do you accept?
- Do you have certifications in the management of certain materials?
- Do you provide a pickup service, or do you accept shipment of wastes at your facility?
- Will containers for collecting the wastes be supplied?
- Is your company the primary recycler?
- What will be the final destination of the materials?
- How do you track the transport of the materials from our practice to the final destination?
- What materials will be recycled? Where will these materials end up?
- Who is responsible for completing EPA or other state-required documentation?
- What is the cost of your service?
- Is there a reimbursement payment for returning silver, lead, or other precious metals (from recycled electronic equipment) for recycling?

fixer and/or rinse water drain line (Figure 20-7). These systems can be adapted for use with manual and chairside processing as well. When attached to an automatic processor, as the processor operates and when the fixer tank is drained for cleaning and changing the chemistry, the used fixer is circulated through the silver recovery unit. Silver recovery systems that use metallic replacement technology remove the hazardous silver ions from the used fixer before allowing the solution to go down the drain. Once the cartridge inside the silver recovery unit is saturated with silver ions, it can be removed by a commercial waste disposal company and replaced with a fresh cartridge.

Lead Waste

Lead foil from inside intraoral film packets should be separated from the outer moisture-proof wrap and black paper to keep it out of the waste stream (Figure 20-8). Many states or local municipal landfills have regulations regarding disposal of this heavy metal. Lead foil waste can be recovered and recycled for another use. Other lead-containing products that are no longer serviceable, such as damaged lead aprons or thyroid collars, or no longer recommended, such as lead-lined film storage boxes or dispensers (Figure 20-6), should also have the lead recovered or recycled prior to disposing of these items into the waste stream. Options for disposal of items containing lead are suggested in Table 20-1. As mentioned previously, when selecting a contractor, it is important that the contractor be licensed to avoid litigation or fines as a result of their faulty handling of materials.

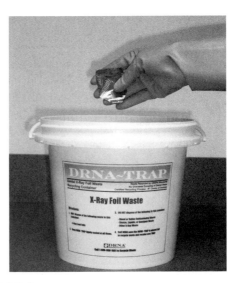

FIGURE 20-8 Lead foil waste. Collecting lead foil from film packets for proper disposal by a licensed waste management contractor.

Discarded Radiographs Waste

Oral health care practices are advised to keep dental radiographs indefinitely. (See Chapter 11.) Legal issues such as malpractice and the varying statutes of limitations between states make this recommendation a good risk management strategy. However, there are times when a practice may have a need to dispose of unwanted or very old radiographs. Unused radiographic film may occasionally need to be discarded, as is the case when it has been damaged or contaminated by exposure conditions that cause fogging or it is past the expiration date (see Figure 7-9). Radiographs contain silver that should be recovered or recycled prior to disposal into the waste stream. The amount of silver remaining in the film will depend on whether it has been processed (old radiographs) or not and also on the density of the radiographic image. Film that has been processed will have had some of the silver ions removed during fixation, and radiographs that are more dense (darker) will have more of the silver ions remaining on the radiograph base material. Options for proper disposal of radiographic film include contacting the company that the product was purchased from to see if they will take back the product or contracting with a licensed waste management company.

Digital Imaging Equipment

The move away from film-based radiography to digital imaging will reduce and may eventually eliminate many of the hazardous wastes associated with dental radiography. However, electronic equipment poses a whole new set of considerations for disposal and recycling. As technology advances, older equipment becomes obsolete. Computers, monitors, solid-state digital sensors, and phosphor plates (see Chapter 9) continue to improve, phasing out older systems. Also, electronic failure of computer equipment, broken sensor wires, and damaged phosphor plates will all need to be disposed of properly. This electronic equipment contains both hazardous materials such as lead, mercury, cadmium, and beryllium and valuable metals such as gold, palladium, platinum, and silver. Computers and monitors also contain glass, plastic, and aluminum that are readily recycled. Proper

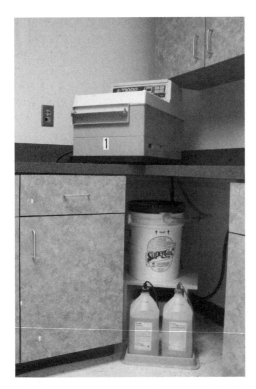

FIGURE 20-7 Silver reclaiming unit. Attached to the drain tube of the automatic processor. Note the appropriately labeled bottles of developer and fixer attached to the unit for automatic chemical replenishment.

TABLE 20-1	Options for Disposal of Radiographic Waste Products	
Fixer	1. Collect for recycling/return to supplier for recovery of silver.
	2. Treat to remove silver before discharge to municipal wastewater treatment.
	3. Contract with hazardous waste disposal company.
Developer	1. Usually acceptable to discharge to municipal wastewater treatment. Check state/local regulations.
Disinfectants	1. Usually acceptable to discharge to municipal wastewater treatment. Check state/local regulations.
	2. Choose disinfectants containing less-hazardous materials.
	3. Use barriers to minimize the need for disinfecting.
Radiographic processor cleaners	1. Choose cleaners containing less-hazardous materials.
	2. Take steps daily, such as the use of a cleaning sheet, to minimize the need for strong chemicals (Figure 20-9).
	3. Use mechanical methods (brush/sponge) instead of chemicals.
Radiographs/unused film	1. Collect for recycling/return to supplier for recovery of silver.
	2. Contract with hazardous waste disposal company.
	3. Send to metal reclaimer.
	4. May be acceptable to discharge to municipal landfills. Check state/local regulations. However, recovery and recycling is recommended.
Lead foils and other lead-containing items (aprons/boxes)	1. Collect for recycling/return to supplier for recovery of lead.
	2. Contract with hazardous waste disposal company.
	3. Send to metal reclaimer.
Digital imaging equipment	1. Collect for recycling/return to supplier for recovery of precious metals and plastics.
	2. Remanufacture and upgrade.
	3. Donate usable equipment. Remove sensitive data regarding patient records before recycling/donating.
	4. Visit EPA Web site eCycle: How to recycle or donate used electronics

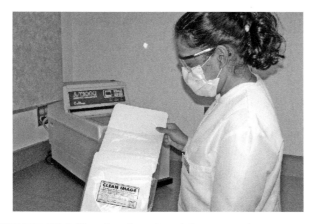

FIGURE 20-9 Cleaning sheet. Run daily or more often, the cleaning sheet can pick up debris from the rollers maintaining the processor for longer intervals between cleanings with a strong chemical.

recycling and disposal of electronic equipment can preserve precious resources and keep hazardous materials out of municipal landfills. Options for reusing older digital imaging equipment include refurbishing and/or upgrading to accommodate new technology or donating still usable equipment for uses that may not require the latest technology. If disposal is required, the same considerations regarding the qualifications of a hazardous waste company previously discussed should be given.

The radiographer must possess a working knowledge of safe handling and safe disposal of the chemicals and materials used in dental radiography. It is important to be familiar with national, state, and local laws regulating the handling and disposal of hazardous wastes. Laws and regulations guide and direct the oral health care practice to handle radiographic chemicals and materials safely, but an ethical responsibility to the environment should also play a role in how the oral health care practice reduces, reuses, and recycles materials to avoid adding to the waste stream.

REVIEW—Chapter summary

Many of the chemicals and materials used in the radiographic process are considered hazardous and require a working knowledge of safe handling and proper disposal. Two agencies responsible for regulations that help to protect and inform the radiographer are the Occupational Health and Safety Administration (OHSA) and the Environmental Protection Agency (EPA). OSHA requires that oral health care practices maintain Material Safety Data Sheets (MSDSs) and product labels for all hazardous chemicals used in the radiographic process. The hazardous chemicals used in the radiographic process that require an MSDS include fixer, developer, disinfectants, and cleaners used on processing equipment.

Safe handling instructions for hazardous chemicals can be found on the MSDSs. The radiographer should be familiar with safe handling and effective emergency responses when working with hazardous chemicals. General safe handling and emergency responses were outlined and include use of PPE, impervious gloves, adequate ventilation, and avoiding inhalation or contact with skin or eyes. However, because the chemical ingredients vary among product manufacturers, the radiographer is responsible for studying the MSDS for the specific product being used.

Emergency responses to skin and eye exposures include immediate flushing with water and seeking medical attention for symptoms that persist. Emergency eyewash stations must be within 25 feet or 10 seconds from where the chemical is being handled. The radiographer should be trained in the use of the emergency eyewash equipment.

Oral health care practices have a legal and ethical responsibility to the environment to properly dispose of hazardous radiographic chemicals and materials. Chemicals and materials that must be given consideration for proper disposal or recycling include used fixer (because it contains silver thiosulphate complexes), lead foils from intraoral film packets, or other sources such as lead aprons and thyroid collars and lead-lined storage boxes. Safe and proper disposal instructions can be found on the product MSDS and by contacting the federal, state, and local agencies responsible for regulation of wastes. Safe disposal options include contracting with a licensed waste disposal company, collecting the waste for recycling, and eliminating or reducing the waste on-site. Although the shift to digital imaging will eventually eliminate most of the hazardous chemicals and materials associated with film-based radiography, electronic equipment will require the development of safe disposal protocols as well.

RECALL—Study questions

1. List two agencies responsible for the development of safe handling standards for hazardous chemicals and materials used in the radiographic process.

    a. _____
    b. _____

2. Each of the following may be found on a Material Safety Data Sheet (MSDS) EXCEPT one. Which one is the EXCEPTION?

    a. Chemical ingredients
    b. Date of manufacture
    c. Requirements for safe handling
    d. Disposal considerations

3. A Material Safety Data Sheet (MSDS) would NOT need to be obtained for which of the following?

    a. Lead foils from intraoral film packets
    b. Radiographic fixer
    c. Radiographic developer
    d. Low-level disinfectant

4. Each of the following is a requirement of the OSHA Hazard Communication Standard EXCEPT one. Which one is the EXCEPTION?

    a. Maintain an inventory of all hazardous chemicals.
    b. Provide training for all personnel who handle the chemicals.
    c. Label all containers that will hold hazardous chemicals.
    d. Store all hazardous chemicals in the same central location.

5. List radiographic wastes that are considered hazardous to personnel and harmful to the environment.

    a. _____
    b. _____
    c. _____
    d. _____
    e. _____

6. Which of the following lists of personal protective equipment (PPE) is the best recommendation for the dental radiographer when cleaning the processing equipment?

    a. Long-sleeve lab coat, eyeglasses, mask, latex gloves
    b. Long-sleeve barrier gown, eyeglasses with side shields, mask, vinyl gloves
    c. Long-sleeve barrier gown with rubber apron, safety goggles, mask, nitrile gloves
    d. Scrubs with rubber apron, safety face shield, respirator mask, neoprene gloves

7. Each of the following will help prevent an accidental exposure to hazardous chemicals EXCEPT one. Which one is the EXCEPTION?

    a. Store the product in the smallest container possible.
    b. Be familiar with the MSDS information regarding the product.
    c. Use the chemical in a well-ventilated area.
    d. Wash hands thoroughly after handling the chemical.

8. In general, what is the emergency recommendation if fixer or developer splashes into the eyes?

    a. If an irritation develops, then move to a well-ventilated area.
    b. Keep eyes securely closed and seek medical attention immediately.
    c. Wait 5 minutes to determine the severity of the exposure. Then seek medical attention.
    d. Immediately flush with a steady stream of warm water for a minimum of 15 minutes.

9. Which of the following is NOT a requirement for an emergency eyewash station?

    a. Must be clearly labeled.
    b. Water temperature must not exceed 60 degrees.
    c. Must be located within 25 feet or 10 seconds of where the chemical is handled.
    d. The flow of water must be easy to activate.

10. Chemicals with what pH would be most likely to cause severe eye irritation?

    a. Low pH (acidic)
    b. Neutral pH
    c. High pH (alkaline)

11. Which of the following is LEAST likely to require special consideration prior to discharging into the waste stream?

    a. Lead foils from intraoral film packets
    b. Used fixer
    c. Used developer
    d. Digital imaging equipment

REFLECT—Case study

Oral health care practices have a legal and an ethical responsibility to the environment to properly dispose of hazardous radiographic chemicals and materials. However, today the focus has shifted from proper disposal and recycling to prerecycling, or reducing the amount of waste generated in the first place. Make a list of all the materials and resources you can think of that are used in the radiographic process. Include the plastic barriers used to cover equipment, the types of image receptor holders available for use, the wash water that circulates when the automatic processor is running, etc. Then using the technique of brainstorming, list ways to reduce the generation of waste and to conserve resources. For example: (1) eliminate the use of image receptors made from polystyrene Styrofoam® and (2) purchase film from a "green" company who has demonstrated environmentally sound operations in manufacturing their product. Combine your ideas with your classmates and consider sharing the list in a presentation at the next meeting of your professional association.

RELATE—Laboratory application

Assess and update the written hazard communication program at your facility. Begin by performing a physical inventory of all chemicals and potentially hazardous products. Make note of where the products are stored. Is the product stored in one location, or in multiple areas throughout the facility? Are the containers labeled appropriately? List the products by their trade name. Next, using the Internet, visit the product manufacturer's Web site to get an up-to-date copy of the MSDS and product labels. Print out and organize the MSDSs into a three-ring binder. A suggested way to organize the MSDSs is:

MSDS Number	Product
1	Kodak READYMATIC Dental Developer and Replenisher
2	Kodak READYMATIC Dental Fixer and Replenisher
3	Birex Disinfectant Wipes
4	Air Techniques Formula 2000 Plus

Print out and attach labels to all containers, including the developer and fixer tanks inside the automatic processor and any tubs used to wash and clean the rollers. Once organized, study the MSDS for each of the products, or assign one or more of the MSDSs to each member of the oral health care team or your class to study. Then schedule a training session for your oral health care team or class where each person will review the steps for safe handling and disposal of the product. Provide the opportunity for everyone to practice safe protocols and simulated emergency responses to exposures.

REFERENCES

American Dental Association. (2007). Best management practices for amalgam waste. Retrieved March 28, 2010, from http://www.ada.org/prof/resources/topics/topics_amalrecyclers.pdf

American Dental Association Council on Scientific Affairs. (2003). Managing silver and lead waste in dental offices. *Journal of the American Dental Association, 134*, 1095–1096.

Carestream Health Inc. (2007). *Kodak dental systems: Exposure and processing for dental film radiography.* Pub. N-414. Rochester, NY: Author.

Carestream Health Inc. (2010). Environmental health and safety support. Health, safety and environment frequently asked questions. Retrieved March 28, 2010, from http://carestreamhealth.com/ehs-faqs.html

DePaola, L. G. (2008). Surface disinfection in the dental office. *The infection control forum. Current infection control insights from The Richmond Institute.* The Richmond Institute for Continuing Education, 6(6).

Eastman Kodak Company. (1990). *Management of photographic wastes in the dental office.* Pub N-414 8–90. Rochester, NY: Author.

Eastman Kodak Company. (1994). *Waste management guidelines.* Pub N-414 6-94-BX revision. Rochester, NY: Author.

Molinari, J. A., & Harte, J. A. (2009). *Cottone's practical infection control in dentistry* (3rd ed.). Philadelphia: Lippincott Williams & Wilkins.

Rockett, W. M. (2009). Revamped recycling. Simple steps to do your part and make the dental practice a more eco-conscious environment. Retrieved March 28, 2010, *DentalProductsReport.com.*

Thomson, E. M. (2012). *Exercises in oral radiographic techniques. A laboratory manual,* (3rd ed.,). Upper Saddle River, NJ: Pearson Education.

Thomson-Lakey, E. M. (1996). Developing an environmentally sound oral health practice. *Access, 10*(4), 19–26.

United States Environmental Protection Agency. (n.d.). eCycling. Retrieved April 3, 2010, from http://www.epa.gov/epawaste/conserve/materials/ecycling/index.htm

Wikipedia. (n.d.). United States Environmental Protection Agency. Retrieved March 28, 2010, from http://en.wikipedia.org/wiki/Epa

CHAPTER

21

Mounting and Introduction to Interpretation

CHAPTER OUTLINE

OBJECTIVES

Following successful completion of this chapter, you should be able to:

1. Define the key words.
2. List at least five advantages of mounting radiographs.
3. Discuss the use and importance of the identification dot.
4. Compare labial and lingual methods of film mounting.
5. Demonstrate mounting radiographs according to the suggested steps presented.
6. List at least five anatomic generalizations that aid in mounting radiographs.
7. Compare interpretation and diagnosis.
8. Describe the roles of the film mount, viewbox, and magnification in viewing radiographs.
9. List considerations for reading digital radiographic images not encountered when reading film-based radiographs.
10. Demonstrate viewing radiographs according to the suggested steps presented.

KEY WORDS

Anatomical order

Diagnosis

Film mount

Film mounting

Identification dot

Interpretation

Labial mounting method

Lingual mounting method

Viewbox

Introduction

Mounting is an important step in the interpretation of dental radiographs. Dental radiographs must be mounted in the correct anatomic order to allow for a thorough and systematic interpretation. A thorough knowledge of the normal anatomy of the teeth and jaws is needed to mount radiographs correctly. Therefore, mounting and interpreting dental radiographs go hand in hand.

The purpose of this chapter is to describe the step-by-step procedures for mounting and viewing dental radiographs. To aid in this process, basic key points regarding anatomic landmarks will be discussed. Chapter 22 provides the detailed radiographic interpretation of normal radiographic anatomy.

Mounting Radiographs

Film mounting is the placement of radiographs in a holder arranged in **anatomical order** (Figure 21-1). The advantages of film mounting are:

- Intraoral radiographs are easier to view and interpret in the correct anatomical position.
- Mounting decreases the chance of error caused by confusing the patient's right and left sides.
- Viewing films side by side allows for easy comparison between different views.
- Less handling of individual radiographs results in fewer scratches and fingerprint marks.
- Film mounts can mask out distracting side light, making radiographs easier to view and interpret.
- Film mounts provide a means for labeling the radiographs with patient's name, date of exposure, name of the practice, etc.
- Mounted films are easy to store.

- Patient education and consultations are enhanced when films are mounted.
- When mounted labially, radiographic findings can be easily transferred to the patient's dental chart.

Film mounting generally refers only to intraoral films. Large extraoral radiographs must be labeled with lead letters or tape that identify the right and left sides and are often placed in an envelope so the patent's name and the date of the exposure can be written on the outside.

Occasionally, single intraoral radiographs are not mounted, but are placed into a small envelope and attached to the patient record. However, it is better to mount even a single or a small group of radiographs. A full mouth series should always be mounted for accurate viewing. In addition, the film mount provides a place to record the patient's name, date, and other pertinent information.

Film Mounts

Film mounts are celluloid, cardboard, or plastic holders with frames or windows for the radiographs (Figure 21-2). Attaching the radiographs to the film mounts is called film mounting. Film mounts are available in many sizes and with numerous combinations of windows or frames to fit films of different sizes. Mounts may be large enough to accommodate a full-mouth series of radiographs or hold only a few or even a single radiograph. Standard commercially made mounts are available, or companies will make custom mounts to suit special needs. Black plastic or gray cardboard mounts are often preferred over clear plastic mounts because these can block out extraneous light from the viewbox, enhancing viewing and interpretation.

Identification Dot

An embossed **identification dot** near the edge of the film appears convex or concave, depending on the side from which the film is

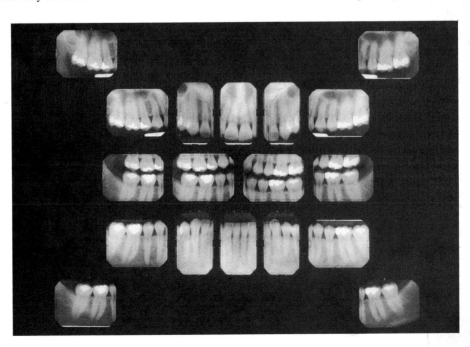

FIGURE 21-1 Full mouth series mounted in an opaque mount.

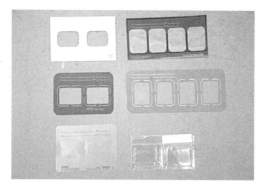

FIGURE 21-2 Examples of various film mounts. Film mounts are available in a variety of sizes and film combinations.

viewed. If the film packet was placed in the patient's oral cavity correctly, the raised portion of the identification dot (the convexity) automatically faces the x-ray tube and the source of radiation. Therefore, when the radiograph is viewed later, the identification dot may be relied on to determine which are the patient's left and right sides. Because the radiograph may be viewed from either side, it is important that the radiographer understand the role the identification dot plays in film orientation.

Film Mounting Methods

Because the radiograph may be viewed from either side, two methods of film mounting have been used. The first method, now obsolete but still used by some dentists, is the lingual method. With the **lingual mounting method,** the radiographs are mounted so that the embossed dot is concave. In this position, the viewer is reading the radiograph as if standing behind the patient (Figure 21-3). Therefore, what the viewer observes on the right side of the radiograph would correspond to the patient's right as well. Essentially, the viewer's right is the patient's right.

The second method, recommended by the American Dental Association and the American Academy of Oral and Maxillofacial Radiology, is the **labial mounting method.** With the labial method of film mounting, the radiographs are mounted so that the embossed dot is convex. In this position, the viewer is reading the radiograph as if standing in front of, and facing, the patient (Figure 21-4). Therefore, what the viewer observes on the right side of the radiograph would correspond to the patient's left side. Essentially, the viewer's right is the patient's left. This also corresponds to the order in which teeth and anatomical structures are drawn on most dental and periodontal charts.

Film Mounting Procedure

Radiographs should be mounted immediately after processing. Handle films by the edges to avoid smudging or scratching them, and label the radiographs to prevent loss or mixing them up with other patient films. An orderly sequence to the mounting procedure is suggested (Procedure Box 21-1). This is especially true for the beginner. Although the sequence for mounting is often a matter of preference, the first step in mounting all radiographs should be to orient the embossed dot the same way for all the films. When mounting using the labial method, orient all the films so that the embossed dot is convex.

When mounting a full mouth series of periapical and bitewing radiographs, it is helpful to use the film sizes and orientation in the oral cavity to help with the mounting process. Size #1 film is often used to radiograph the anterior region. Additionally, anterior periapical radiographs are placed in the oral cavity with the long dimension of the film packet positioned vertically, whereas posterior periapical radiographs are

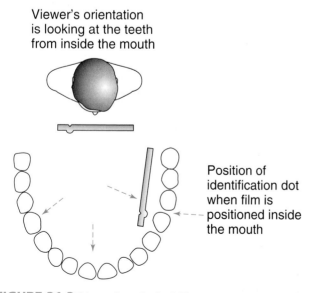

FIGURE 21-3 Lingual method of film mounting. When the identification dot is viewed in the concave position, the viewer's orientation is from behind the patient. The patient's left is the viewer's left.

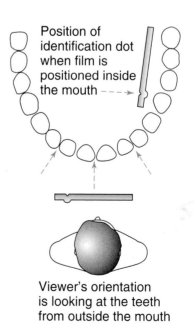

FIGURE 21-4 Labial method of film mounting. When the identification dot is viewed in the convex position, the viewer's orientation is in front of and facing the patient. The patient's left is the viewer's right.

PROCEDURE 21-1
Suggested sequence for mounting a full mouth series of radiographs

1. Place the films on a clean white or light-colored paper towel or tray cover on the counter in front of a viewbox.
2. Wash hands to prevent smudging the films.
3. Orient the embossed dots all the same way.
4. Separate the bitewing from the periapical radiographs.
5. Separate the anterior from the posterior periapical radiographs.
6. Separate the maxillary from the mandible periapical radiographs.
7. Orient the periapical radiographs so that the roots are pointing up for the maxilla and down for the mandible.
8. Orient the bitewing radiographs so that the occlusal plane slants upward in the posterior, producing a slight "smile" appearance.
9. Place the anterior periapical radiographs into the appropriate frame on the left or right side of the film mount.
10. Place the posterior periapical radiographs into the appropriate frame on the left or right side of the film mount.
11. Place the bitewing radiographs into the appropriate frame on the left or right side of the film mount.
12. Label the film mount with the patient's name, date of exposure, facility name, and other pertinent information.
13. Check the mounted films to be sure they are secured in the mount and are mounted appropriately. (Embossed dots all facing the same direction, no films upside down.)
14. Place the mounted radiographs on the viewbox for use during the patient appointment and for interpretation.

placed in the oral cavity with the long dimension of the film packet positioned horizontally. These clues may be utilized to help the radiographer determine where to position the films in the mount.

To mount correctly, the radiographer must have a base knowledge in radiographic anatomy. Chapter 22 covers radiographic anatomy observed on intraoral radiographs, (Table 21-1). However, to aid in the mounting procedure, the following generalizations are offered:

- Roots and crowns of the maxillary anterior teeth are larger and longer than those of the mandibular teeth.

TABLE 21-1 Anatomical Landmarks Distinguishing Maxillary Radiographs from Mandibular Radiographs

AREA	MAXILLARY ANATOMICAL LANDMARKS	MANDIBULAR ANATOMICAL LANDMARKS
Incisor	Incisive foramen	Lingual foramen
	Median palatine suture	Genial tubercles
	Nasal fossa	Nutrient canals
	Nasal septum	Mental ridge
	Anterior nasal spine	Mental fossa
Canine	Inverted Y	
	Lateral fossa	
Premolar	Maxillary sinus	Mental foramen
Molar	Maxillary sinus	Mandibular canal
	Zygomatic process of maxilla	Oblique ridge
	Zygoma	Mylohyoid ridge
	Maxillary tuberosity	Submandibular fossa
	Hamulus	
	Coronoid process of mandible	

- Canine teeth generally have the longest roots when compared to adjacent teeth.
- Maxillary molars generally have three roots. The presence of the palatal root makes it difficult to visual three distinct roots.
- Mandibular molars generally have two divergent roots that are distinctly observed. Bone is visible in between the two roots.
- Most roots curve toward the distal.
- Large radiolucent areas denoting the nasal fossa or the maxillary sinus indicate that the radiograph is of a maxillary area.
- The body of the mandible has a distinct upward curve toward the ramus in the molar area. The film should be oriented so that a slight "smile" appearance is detected.

After the last radiograph has been mounted, the entire film mount should be carefully checked to see that:

- Identification dots all face the same direction.
- All radiographs are arranged in proper anatomical order.
- No radiographs were reversed or mounted upside down.
- The radiographs are firmly attached to the mount.
- The patient's name and date have been recorded on the mount.

Viewing the Radiographs

Proper viewing is essential for the interpretation of dental radiographs. One must be familiar with and understand optimal viewing conditions and the proper sequence of viewing the radiographs.

Interpretation versus Diagnosis

Dental radiographs are viewed by any trained professional (dentist, dental hygienist, or dental assistant) with knowledge of normal anatomic landmarks of the maxilla, mandible, and related structures. Radiographs may be interpreted by all members of the oral health care team, but the dentist is responsible for the final interpretation and diagnosis. **Interpretation** is explanatory and may be defined as reading the radiograph and explaining what is observed in terms the patient understands. Items that a dental hygienist or dental assistant may interpret are radiographic errors such as overlapped contacts or elongated images; artifacts that may have appeared on the radiograph such as the image of a film holder; and normal radiographic anatomy such as the absence of a developing permanent tooth under a primary tooth or the presence radiographically of unerupted third molars. **Diagnosis** is defined as the determination of the nature and the identification of an abnormal condition or disease. An example of interpretation would be showing the patient the image of the developing third molar on the radiograph, whereas diagnosis would be the dentist determining that the third molar is impacted. Referring a patient to the dentist for evaluation of a radiolucent finding on the proximal surface of a tooth that appears on a bitewing is interpretation. Dental hygienists and dental assistants are trained to identify this deviation from normal-appearing enamel and can point out these deviations for further evaluation by the dentist. Telling the patient that the radiolucency is caries and requires treatment is diagnosis, a responsibility of the dentist.

The dental hygienist and dental assistant play a valuable role in the preliminary diagnosis, by interpreting deviations from normal radiographic anatomy and calling these to the attention of the dentist. The more pairs of eyes evaluating the radiographs, the more benefit to the patient.

Viewing Equipment

A **viewbox** and a magnifying glass are required for optimal film viewing (Figure 21-5). Holding radiographs up to the overhead room light will not provide adequate conditions in which to observe detailed, subtle changes often revealed by radiographs.

- **Viewbox.** Many types of viewboxes are available. The viewbox lighting must be of uniform intensity and be evenly diffused. The viewing surface should be large enough to accommodate a full set of intraoral radiographs as well as typical dental extraoral radiographs (i.e., panoramic radiographs). The film mount or a cardboard template should be used to mask out distracting light around the mount. Blocking out excess sidelight reduces glare and facilitates viewing. The use of gray or black cardboard or frosted plastic film mounts helps to reduce glare and enhances the detail of the images. Always use subdued room lighting to allow the eyes to adapt to the light level of the radiographs.
- **Magnifying glass.** Some viewboxes are equipped with a magnifying device (Figure 21-6). Otherwise, a handheld magnifying glass should be used to aid the radiographer.
- **Computer monitor.** Transferring the ability to read film-based radiographs to the ability to read digital images on a computer monitor requires practice for radiographers who are new to digital imaging. Instead of utilizing a viewbox, digital images are read directly off the computer monitor. Considerations not encountered when reading film-based radiographs include the possibility of not being able to view an entire full mouth series of images on one screen without switching between views and the multiple mouse clicks that may be needed to view images side by side, especially when viewing radiographs taken on different days and stored in different files on the computer. Additionally, viewing digital images will be restricted to the area where the computer and monitor

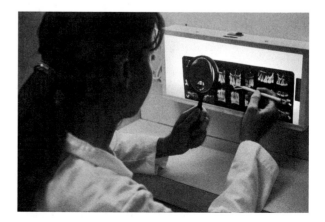

FIGURE 21-5 Radiographer viewing radiographs.
Radiographs should be viewed in subdued room lighting, using a viewbox and a magnifying glass. Note the black film mount that blocks distracting light around the films.

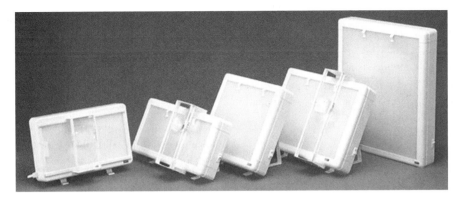

FIGURE 21-6 Viewboxes come in many varieties. Note the attached magnifying device on three of these viewboxes. (Courtesy of Dentsply Rinn.)

are located. Coping with overhead room lighting reflecting off the monitor screen is another consideration the radiographer will have to manage. Setting up the monitor in a position to minimize reflections from overhead room lighting or ambient lighting entering the room through windows will assist with reducing glare that can interfere with interpretation.

The radiographer can utilize the computer software features to magnify images and enhance gray scale levels to assist with interpretation. (See Chapter 9.)

Depending on the radiographer's training and responsibility, the individual may now proceed to make a preliminary interpretation and discuss it with the dentist, who will make the final diagnosis regarding any findings. A thorough examination is best accomplished when a specific sequence of analysis is used (Procedure Box 21-2 and Figure 21-7). The mounted radiographs must be viewed in a systematic order to prevent errors in interpretation. All available radiographs should be examined for a specific condition, and then the

PROCEDURE 21-2
Suggested sequence for viewing a full mouth series of radiographs

1. Place the mounted radiographs on the viewbox.

2. Dim the overhead lights and turn on the viewbox light.

3. Using a magnifying glass, begin the examination in the patient's maxillary right posterior region (Figure 21-7).

4. Proceed horizontally to the anterior region and continue to the patient's maxillary left posterior region.

5. Next, move down to the patient's mandibular left posterior region.

6. Proceed horizontally to the anterior region and continue to the patient's mandibular right posterior region.

7. Next, move up to the bitewing radiographs, starting with the right molar bitewing radiograph on the left side of the film mount. Proceed horizontally, examining each bitewing radiograph until you finish with the left molar bitewing radiograph on the right side of the film mount.

8. Repeat steps 3 through 7 for the following conditions:

    a. Presence or absence of teeth

    b. Tooth morphology and eruption patterns

    c. Deviations from normal and/or suspected pathology

    d. Presence, type, and condition of dental materials

    e. Caries

    f. Periodontal conditions and risk factors

9. Document all findings on a preliminary radiographic interpretative form.

10. Collaborate with the dentist regarding findings.

11. After confirmation and diagnosis of findings by the dentist, record findings on the patient's permanent record.

12. Assist the dentist in explaining findings and treatment plan to the patient using the radiographs.

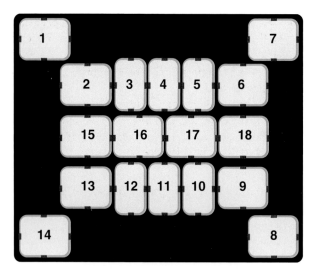

FIGURE 21-7 Proper sequence for viewing radiographs. The radiographer should view the radiographs in the sequence illustrated. Start with number 1 and proceed clockwise through number 18.

examination process should be repeated for the next condition. For example, the radiographs may be examined first for the presence or absence of teeth and other development anomalies. A second examination could concentrate on detecting caries, and the third examination would look for periodontal conditions. Interpreting these conditions is discussed in Chapters 23, 24, and 25.

When interpreting more than one radiograph, such as a set of bitewings or a full mouth series, the teeth and the supporting structures are often imaged more than once. While maintaining a systematic order of interpretation, it is helpful to compare each area in all of the views. For example, a suspected periodontal condition may be observed on a maxillary periapical radiograph, whereas the bitewing radiograph may possibly image the level of bone with more detail. Comparing adjacent films will add to a thorough interpretation.

All radiographic findings must be noted in the patient's record after confirmation by the dentist. Although all professionals may record findings, the final interpretation and diagnosis is the responsibility of the dentist.

Using Mounted Radiographs

Radiographs should be developed and mounted as soon as possible and placed on the viewbox during the patient's appointment for easy reference during treatment. At each subsequent appointment the latest radiographs should be placed on the viewbox, where they can be easily accessed as needed.

After the appointment, all radiographs should be thoroughly interpreted during time set aside for this purpose. Unless only one or two radiographs were taken, there may not have been enough time during the patient's appointment to thoroughly review each film for all possible conditions. Once the interpretation is complete, the radiographs should be filed appropriately and kept indefinitely as part of the patient's permanent record.

(See Chapter 11.) Although radiographs often lose value after more than six months to one year due to changes in the patient's oral conditions, they are valuable for comparing present with previous conditions. The need for an orderly filing system cannot be overstressed. Misplaced radiographs can result in inappropriate treatment being rendered, may cause risk management problems, and may have legal implications. All radiographs should be handled with care to prevent smudging or scratching. Radiographs should be protected from heat damage by storage in cool, well-ventilated areas.

REVIEW—Chapter summary

A thorough knowledge of normal radiographic anatomical landmarks is needed for mounting and interpreting radiographs. Mounting films is recommended for its many advantages. Film mounts vary in size and number of frames, but all have space for documenting information such as the patient's name and date of exposure. Each film has an embossed identification dot used to determine the patient's left and right sides. Lingual mounting places the identification dot in a concave position, so that the patient's left side is the viewer's left side. Labial mounting places the identification dot in a convex position, so that the patient's left side is the viewer's right side. Labial mounting method is the recommended method.

To aid in fast and accurate mounting of radiographs, a systematic procedure should be followed. The first step in film mounting is to orient the embossed identification dot the same way (convex) for all radiographs. Several generalizations regarding the teeth and oral cavity anatomy can be used to aid in mounting radiographs correctly.

Interpretation is explanatory, as is the reading of radiographs. Diagnosis uses radiographs to determine the nature and identification of the disease or abnormality. Dental radiographs may be interpreted by the dentist, dental hygienist, or dental assistant. The dentist is responsible for the final diagnosis.

Viewing radiographs is facilitated with the use of a viewbox and magnification. Mounted radiographs must be viewed in a systematic order to prevent errors in interpretation. Locating the computer monitor away from the glare of ambient lighting will assist the radiographer in viewing digital radiographic images.

Radiographs should be interpreted thoroughly during or after the patient's appointment. Radiographs should be accurately labeled, used to compare present with previous conditions, and kept indefinitely.

RECALL—Study questions

1. List four advantages of mounting intraoral radiographs.
   a. _____
   b. _____
   c. _____
   d. _____

2. A desirable film mount should be
   a. made of cardboard.
   b. made of plastic.
   c. translucent, to allow light to reach the film.
   d. black, to block out light transmission and prevent glare.

3. Which of these helps to determine whether the radiograph is the patient's left or right side?
   a. Slight "smile" appearance
   b. Distally curved roots
   c. Large crowns
   d. Identification dot

4. Labial method film mounting positions the identification dot concave.

   The labial method is the recommended film mounting method.
   a. The first statement is true. The second statement is false.
   b. The first statement is false. The second statement is true.
   c. Both statements are true.
   d. Both statements are false.

5. Lingual method film mounting positions the identification dot convex.

   When utilizing the lingual method, the viewer's right is the patient's left.
   a. The first statement is true. The second statement is false.
   b. The first statement is false. The second statement is true.
   c. Both statements are true.
   d. Both statements are false.

6. Mounting is the placement of radiographs in a holder arranged in anatomical order.

   All radiographs should be handled with care to prevent smudging or scratching.
   a. The first statement is true. The second statement is false.
   b. The first statement is false. The second statement is true.
   c. Both statements are true.
   d. Both statements are false.

7. Which of the following should be done first when mounting radiographs?
   a. Orient the identification dot the same way.
   b. Separate bitewing from periapical films.
   c. Separate the anterior from the posterior films.
   d. Orient the teeth roots to point in the correct direction.

8. Each of the following will aid the radiographer in correctly mounting radiographs EXCEPT one. Which one is the EXCEPTION?
   a. Anterior films are positioned with the long dimension vertically.
   b. Canine teeth generally have the longest roots.
   c. Maxillary molars usually have three roots.
   d. Roots and crowns of mandibular teeth are usually larger than maxillary teeth.

9. Reading and explaining radiographic images is
   a. diagnosing.
   b. interpreting.
   c. viewing.
   d. mounting.

10. The final responsibility to diagnose the radiograph rests with the
    a. dental assistant.
    b. dental hygienist.
    c. dentist.
    d. patient.

11. Viewing mounted radiographs in a systematic sequence can help prevent errors in interpretation.

    Mounted radiographs may be thoroughly viewed by holding the mount up to overhead room lighting.
    a. The first statement is true. The second statement is false.
    b. The first statement is false. The second statement is true.
    c. Both statements are true.
    d. Both statements are false.

12. Which of these is NOT a consideration when viewing digital radiographic images?
    a. Glare off the computer monitor must be managed to enhance interpretation.
    b. Radiographic images must be utilized where a computer monitor is located.
    c. Multiple mouse clicks may be required to view a full mouth series of radiographs.
    d. A magnifying glass will be required for optimal viewing and interpretation.

13. In which region is it best to begin the interpretation process when viewing radiographs mounted using the labial method?
    a. Maxillary left posterior
    b. Maxillary right posterior
    c. Mandibular left posterior
    d. Mandibular right posterior

14. Following diagnosis by the dentist, the radiographic findings must be recorded on the patient's record by the

a. dental assistant.
b. dental hygienist.
c. dentist.
d. Any of the above

REFLECT—Case study

These four radiographs have just exited the automatic processor. Based on what you learned in this chapter, correctly "mount" each of these four radiographs by writing the corresponding number in the correct frame of the film mount. Assuming the identification dots are all positioned convex, label the film mount indicating the left and right sides. Then address the following:

1. Describe how you determined which side was the left and which side was the right.
2. List the steps you followed to mount these radiographs correctly.
3. List three generalizations you used to mount these films.

4. List three final checks you would make to double-check your mounting procedure.

RELATE—Laboratory application

For a comprehensive laboratory practice exercise on this topic, see Thomson, E. M. (2012). *Exercises in oral radiography techniques: A laboratory manual* (3rd ed.). Upper Saddle River, NJ: Pearson. Chapter 6, "Film mounting and radiographic landmarks."

REFERENCES

Horner, K., Drage, N., & Brettle, D. (2008). *21st century imaging.* London: Quintessence Publishing Co.

Langland, O. E., & Langlais, R. P. (2002). *Principles of dental imaging* (2nd ed.). Philadelphia: Lippincott Williams & Wilkins.

White, S. C., & Pharoah, M. J. (2008). *Oral radiology: Principles and interpretation* (6th ed.). St. Louis, MO: Elsevier.

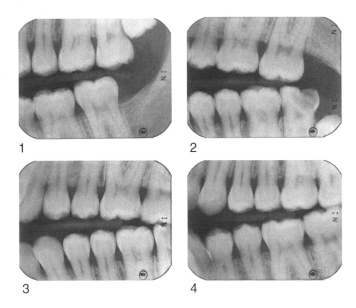

1

2

3

4

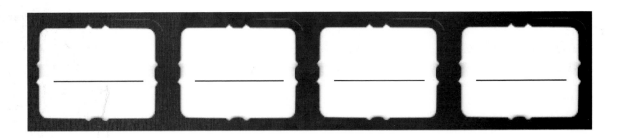

Recognizing Normal Radiographic Anatomy

OBJECTIVES

Following successful completion of this chapter, you should be able to:

1. Define the key words.
2. Provide three rationales for why it is important to recognize and identify normal anatomical landmarks of the face and head.
3. Describe and identify the facial and cranial bones.
4. Differentiate between the lamina dura and the periodontal ligament space.
5. Describe and identify the radiographic appearance of all structures of the teeth.
6. Name significant anatomical landmarks of the maxilla and mandible.
7. Identify significant anatomy normally seen on intraoral radiographs of the maxilla and mandible.

KEY WORDS

Alveolar bone
Alveolar process
Alveolus
Angle of mandible
Anodontia
Anterior nasal spine
Apical foramen
Cancellous bone
Cementum
Condyle
Coronoid process of the mandible
Cortical bone
Dentin
Dentition
Enamel
Exfoliation
External auditory meatus (foramen)
Frontal bone

Genial tubercles
Hamulus
Impacted teeth
Incisive (anterior palatine) foramen
Inferior border
Inverted Y
Lamina dura
Lateral fossa
Lingual foramen
Mandible
Mandibular canal
Mandibular foramen
Mandibular notch
Mastoid process
Maxilla
Maxillary sinus
Maxillary tuberosity
Median palatine suture

Introduction

Learning to read radiographic images and to recognize normal radiographic anatomy, the radiographer begins to develop an appreciation for precise placement of the image receptor and accurate techniques. Before the radiographer can identify a deviation from the normal, a solid base knowledge of what is normal is required. The importance of learning to identify normal radiographic anatomy may be summarized as follows:

1. To evaluate the image receptor for correct positioning so that the areas of interest and anatomical structures are clearly visible, enhancing the diagnostic value of the radiograph

2. To assist with determining into which frame of the x-ray mount each radiograph is to be mounted

3. To assist in interpreting radiographs and recognizing a deviation from the normal that would require referral to the dentist for evaluation

The purpose of this chapter is to review the anatomy of the head and neck region and to describe these anatomical structures as they often appear on dental radiographs.

Significant Normal Anatomical Landmarks

Although most anatomical landmarks observed on intraoral radiographs are located on the maxilla or the mandible, the radiographer should also be able to recognize and identify the major bones and anatomical structures of the cranium and face. This knowledge is particularly useful when reading extraoral radiographs such as a panoramic radiograph.

Some of the cranial and facial bones that may be imaged on dental radiographs are illustrated in Figures 22-1 and 22-2. These include the **frontal bone;** the right and left parietal bones; the **occipital bone;** the right and left **temporal bones;** the right and left **zygomas** (zygomatic bone, also called malar bone or cheekbone); the **zygomatic arch,** which is made up of

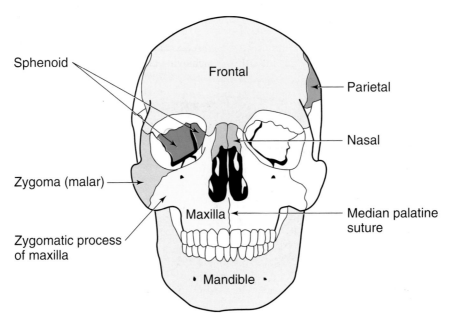

FIGURE 22-1 Frontal view of the skull.

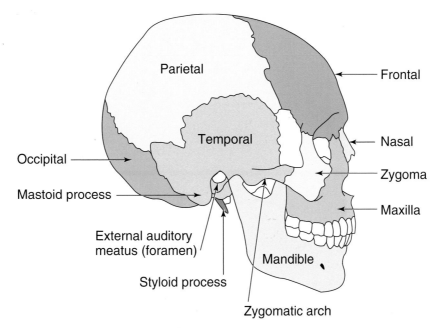

FIGURE 22-2 Lateral view of the skull.

the temporal process of the zygoma and the zygomatic process of the temporal bone; the **sphenoid bone;** the right and left **nasal bones;** the **external auditory meatus (foramen);** the **styloid process;** the **mastoid process** of the temporal bone; the right and left **maxilla;** and the **mandible.**

The teeth are located within the alveolar processes of the maxillae and the mandible; thus most dental radiographs include portions of these bones. The maxillae are actually two bones, a right and left maxilla, whereas the mandible is a single bone. Generally, but not always, the same landmarks appear on both right and left sides.

It is helpful to consider the overall location of these features prior to learning how and where each will appear on an intraoral radiograph. Figure 22-3 shows the **nasal septum** and the **anterior nasal spine.** Figure 22-4 illustrates the location of the **median palatine suture,** the **maxillary tuberosity** area, and the **incisive (anterior palatine) foramen.** The **maxillary sinus** is an empty space within the maxilla.

Figures 22-5 and 22-6 illustrate the structures of the mandible: body; **ramus; inferior border; alveolar process; angle of the mandible; condyle; coronoid process; mandibular notch; mandibular foramen; mental foramen; mandibular canal,** which is located within the mandible between the mandibular foramen and the mental foramen; **mental ridge; symphysis; lingual foramen; genial tubercles; oblique ridge; mylohyoid ridge;** and the **submandibular fossa.**

Some of these landmarks are visible only on larger occlusal and extraoral radiographs. Depending on the placement of the image receptor, patient positioning and the angle of the x-ray beam, certain landmarks may or may not be imaged. Furthermore, the angle of the x-ray beam may distort the appearance of the structure so that it may not always appear exactly as illustrated in this textbook. However, a working knowledge of what structures are likely to be imaged will assist the radiographer in achieving competence in this skill.

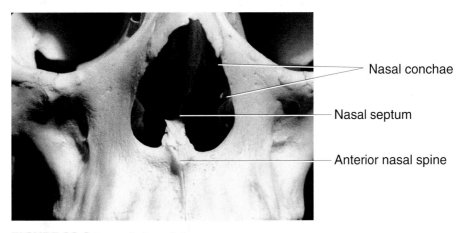

FIGURE 22-3 Frontal view of the nose.

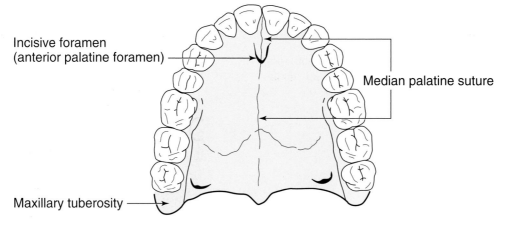

FIGURE 22-4 Palatal view of maxilla.

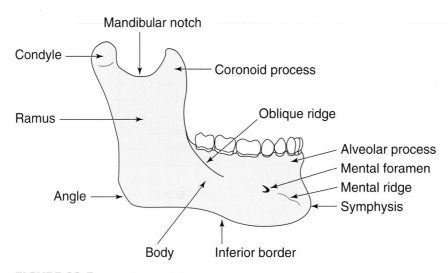

FIGURE 22-5 Lateral view of detached mandible.

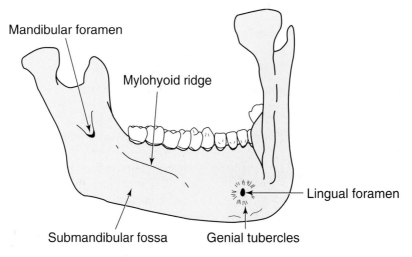

FIGURE 22-6 Lingual view of detached mandible.

Radiographic Appearance of the Alveolar Bone and Tooth Area

Before considering the appearance of these specific bones and their features on a full mouth series of radiographs, it is important to recognize and identify the normal appearance of the **alveolar bone** and the structures of the teeth. Compare the drawing in Figure 22-7 with a radiograph of the same area shown in Figure 22-8.

Bone

Although bones appear solid, they are solid only on the outside and are honeycombed within. Bone is classified as **cortical bone,** a compact or dense form of bone, such as what lines the outside layers of the maxillae and the mandible, and **cancellous** or spongy **bone,** which forms the bulk of the inner bone.

Small, interconnected **trabeculae** (bars or plates of bone) form a multitude of various-sized compartments that account for the honeycomb appearance. These **trabecular bone** spaces are usually filled with fat, blood, or bone cells, which accounts for the difference in the radiographic appearance of bone.

All bone tissues appear radiopaque. The compact or cortical outside layer appears extremely radiopaque (white), whereas the cancellous bone varies in radiopacity (shades of gray) according to the size and number of the trabecular spaces. The area may even appear almost radiolucent (black) if these spaces are very large or if the bone is thin, as is the case in the area of the submandibular fossa.

By definition, the **alveolar process** is that portion of the maxilla or mandible that surrounds and supports the teeth. It is composed of the **lamina dura** and the supporting bone.

LAMINA DURA The lamina dura is the hard, cortical bone that lines the **alveolus** (the tooth socket). On radiographs, the lamina dura appears as a thin radiopaque (white) border that outlines the shape of the alveolus (the root of the tooth). The supporting bone is cancellous and varies in density in the different parts of the alveolar process.

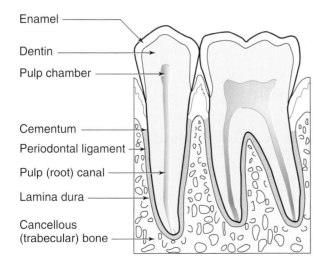

FIGURE 22-7 Drawing of mandibular premolar–molar area.

Labels in figure:
Enamel
Dentin
Pulp chamber
Cementum
Periodontal ligament
Pulp (root) canal
Lamina dura
Cancellous (trabecular) bone

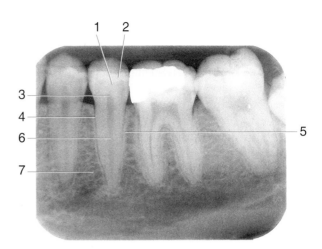

FIGURE 22-8 Radiograph of mandibular premolar area showing (**1**) dentin, (**2**) enamel, (**3**) pulp chamber, (**4**) periodontal ligament space, (**5**) lamina dura, (**6**) pulp (root) canal, and (**7**) cancellous (trabecular) bone. Note that because only a very thin layer of cementum covers the root, it is radiographically indistinguishable from the underlying dentin.

PERIODONTAL LIGAMENT SPACE The teeth are attached to the lamina dura by the fibers of the **periodontal ligament (PDL).** The PDL itself is made up of soft tissues and therefore will not be imaged on a radiograph. However, the space in which the PDL lies is often visible as a thin radiolucent (dark) border between the lamina dura and the roots of the teeth.

NUTRIENT CANALS Nutrient canals are thin radiolucent lines of fairly uniform width that sometimes exhibit radiopaque borders. They contain blood vessels and nerves that supply the teeth, bone, and gingivae. Nutrient canals are most often visualized in the anterior of the mandible and in edentulous areas. When nutrient canals open at the surface of the bone, they often appear radiographically as a tiny radiolucent dot called the **nutrient foramen.**

Teeth

The tooth structures are enamel, dentin, cementum, and pulp. **Enamel,** the hardest body structure, covers the crown and is very radiopaque. The underlying **dentin** is not as dense and appears less radiopaque. The **cementum** that covers the roots is even less dense. Because only a thin layer of cementum covers the root, it is generally indistinguishable radiographically from the underlying dentin (Figure 22-8). Although all three highly calcified tooth structures vary in radiopacity in direct proportion to the thickness of each structure in the path of the x-ray beam, for descriptive purposes enamel, dentin, and cementum are considered radiopaque.

The tooth pulp that occupies the **pulp chamber** and the root canals is the only noncalcified tooth tissue. As this soft tissue offers only minimal resistance to the passage of x-rays, it appears radiolucent. The end of the root canal is called the **apical foramen.** This foramen permits the passage of nerves and blood vessels that nourish the tooth structures.

DENTITION To correctly identify and interpret radiographs, one needs to understand the **dentition.** Young children have 20 **primary teeth** that are gradually lost as they grow older. During the transition years a mixed dentition—that is, both primary and permanent teeth—may be present. A radiograph may show the primary teeth with partially resorbed roots, which are in a process of **exfoliation,** as well as permanent teeth whose roots are not yet fully formed, which are in the process of eruption. This is a normal phenomenon and is often observed in radiographs of children between 6 and 12 years old (Figure 22-9). There are 32 **permanent teeth,** including all four of the third molars (wisdom teeth).

Occasionally, teeth form but are unable to erupt. These are described as **impacted teeth.** Some people have one or more extra teeth, called **supernumerary teeth.** Another deviation is the congenital absence of certain teeth, described as **anodontia.** These conditions occur so frequently that, although not normal, they are not considered pathologic.

Anatomy Basics, Intraoral Radiographs

Learning to identify anatomical structures and their specific landmarks takes practice. Radiographs provide a two-dimensional image of three-dimensional structures. When imaging the head and neck region, multiple structures may be imaged superimposed on top of each other, adding to the difficulty of correctly identifying these structures. The first step in becoming competent at this skill is to understand what basic anatomy may be in the

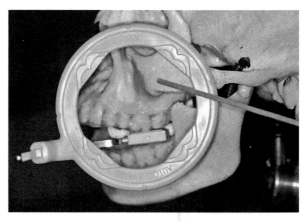

FIGURE 22-10 **Facial bones recorded on radiographs.** Note the position of the PID when exposing a maxillary posterior periapical radiograph. The zygomatic arch will most likely be recorded on this radiograph.

path of the x-ray beam. This will assist the radiographer in distinguishing what will be recorded on the radiograph (Figure 22-10).

It is helpful to be aware of which structures appear radiopaque and radiolucent. As you will recall from Chapter 4, structures that are dense and absorb or resist the passage of x-rays will appear light or white on the radiograph. Structures that permit the passage of x-rays with little or no resistance will appear dark or black. Bone and its dense features such as a ridge, spine, or tubercle will appear radiopaque, whereas less dense features such as a foramen, canal, or **suture** will appear radiolucent. To aid the radiographer in learning the radiographic appearance of anatomy, it is helpful to remember that a landmark called the oblique *ridge* will be a radiopaque structure, and a landmark called the mental *foramen* will appear radiolucent (Table 22-1).

Just as it is helpful to follow a systematic order when mounting and interpreting films, the radiographer will benefit from organizing the identification of anatomical landmarks into specific steps. Because memorizing the structures that make up the head and neck region can be an overwhelming task, the following system is offered to assist the beginning radiographer in learning to identify structures commonly imaged on intraoral radiographs (Figure 22-11).

As illustrated by the flowchart in Figure 22-11, differentiating among which structures will most likely be imaged on intraoral radiographs of the maxilla and which structures will

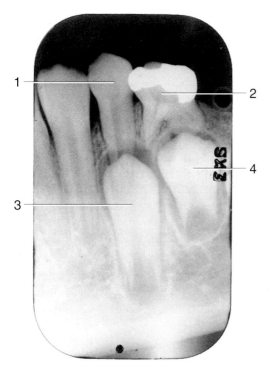

FIGURE 22-9 **Radiograph of mixed dentition in mandibular canine area** showing (**1**) primary canine, (**2**) primary first molar with partially resorbed roots, (**3**) permanent canine, and (**4**) permanent first premolar with incomplete root formation.

TABLE 22-1	Radiopaque and Radiolucent Features
RADIOPAQUE	RADIOLUCENT
• Bone	• Canal
• Border (wall)	• Foramen
• Process	• Fossa
• Ridge	• Meatus
• Spine	• Sinus
• Tubercles	• Space (PDL)
• Tuberosity	• Suture

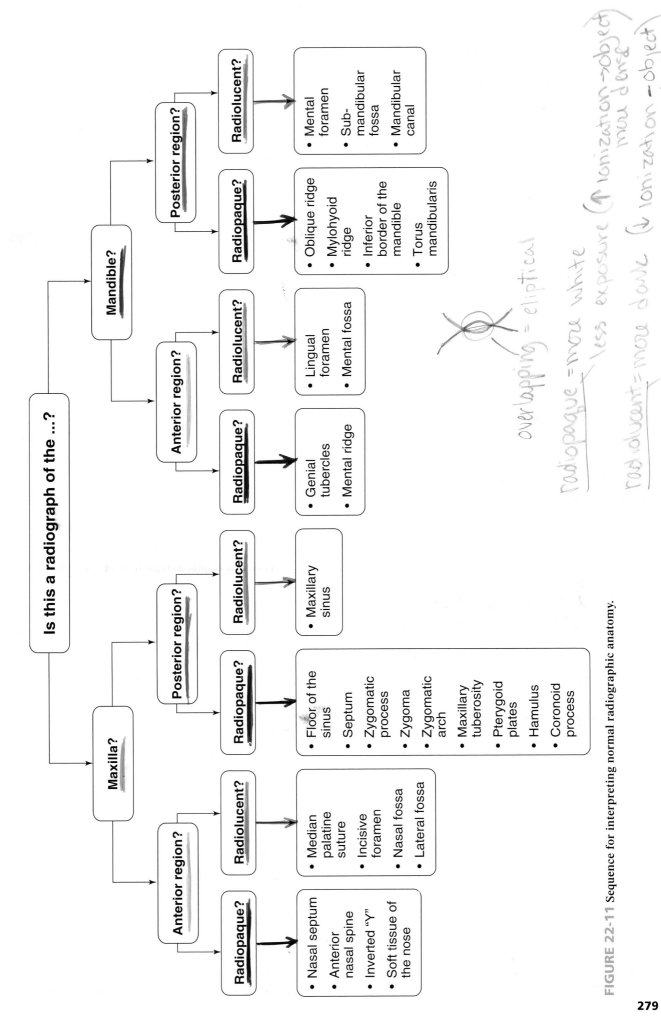

FIGURE 22-11 Sequence for interpreting normal radiographic anatomy.

Is this a radiograph of the ...?

Maxilla?
- Anterior region?
  - Radiopaque?
    - Nasal septum
    - Anterior nasal spine
    - Inverted "Y"
    - Soft tissue of the nose
  - Radiolucent?
    - Median palatine suture
    - Incisive foramen
    - Nasal fossa
    - Lateral fossa
- Posterior region?
  - Radiopaque?
    - Floor of the sinus
    - Septum
    - Zygomatic process
    - Zygoma
    - Zygomatic arch
    - Maxillary tuberosity
    - Pterygoid plates
    - Hamulus
    - Coronoid process
  - Radiolucent?
    - Maxillary sinus

Mandible?
- Anterior region?
  - Radiopaque?
    - Genial tubercles
    - Mental ridge
  - Radiolucent?
    - Lingual foramen
    - Mental fossa
- Posterior region?
  - Radiopaque?
    - Oblique ridge
    - Mylohyoid ridge
    - Inferior border of the mandible
    - Torus mandibularis
  - Radiolucent?
    - Mental foramen
    - Sub-mandibular fossa
    - Mandibular canal

[Handwritten notes:]

↑ ionization →object more dense

↓ ionization →object less dense

overlapping = eliptical

radiopaque = more white — less exposure

radiolucent = more dark — more exposure

be imaged on intraoral radiographs of the mandible will help the radiographer organize the anatomy terms and narrow the possible choices. When beginning the interpretation process, first determine if the intraoral radiograph you are looking at is a maxillary view or a mandibular view. See Chapter 21 for generalizations that aid in determining whether or not a radiograph is of the maxilla or the mandible. Once the correct arch is identified, determine whether the view is of the anterior or the posterior region. As you will recall, in the anterior regions, the image receptor is usually positioned with the long dimension vertically, whereas in the posterior regions the image receptor is placed with the long dimension positioned horizontally. Certain anatomical structures are more likely to be visible on radiographs of the anterior region, whereas others are more likely to be visible in the posterior region. Prior to deciding which anatomical structure is being observed, the radiographer should determine whether or not the structure is radiopaque or radiolucent. A radiopaque appearance indicates a structure that is dense, eliminating structures such as a foramen or fossa or other feature that would not present as radiopaque. Likewise, a radiolucent appearance indicates a structure that is less dense, so the terms *process* or *ridge* would not apply to radiolucent observations.

Organizing the interpretation of normal radiographic anatomy in this manner (Figure 22-11) will assist the beginning radiographer by providing a framework on which to learn the terms associated with head and neck radiography and will continue to be a basis for building on these basic interpretative skills. A working knowledge of the radiographic appearance of normal anatomy must be mastered to develop the skills needed to recognize deviations from the normal such as periodontal disease, caries, and growth and development anomalies.

In keeping with the system laid out in Figure 22-11, anatomical landmarks in this chapter are separated into the regions where they are most likely to be observed on intraoral radiographs:

1. Maxillary anterior region
2. Maxillary posterior region
3. Mandibular anterior region
4. Mandibular posterior region

Depending on the manner in which the image receptor was positioned, and the angle at which the exposure was made, the expected anatomical landmark may or may not be visible. Sometimes the landmark is visible on only the right or only the left side. Keeping this in mind, the following descriptions offer guidance for learning these structures.

Maxillary Anterior Region (Figures 22-12 through 22-15)

RADIOPAQUE FEATURES

1. **Nasal septum.** A dense cartilage structure that separates the right **nasal fossa** from the left. Usually appears as a vertical radiopaque line separating the paired radiolucencies of the nasal cavity.

2. **Anterior nasal spine.** A V-shaped projection from the floor of the nasal fossa in the midline. Usually appears as a triangle-shaped radiopacity.

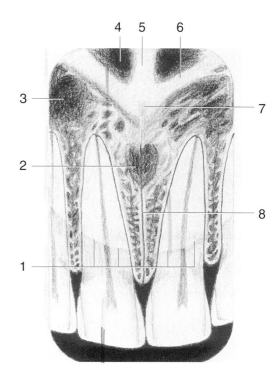

FIGURE 22-12 Drawing of maxillary midline area illustrating (**1**) outline of nose, (**2**) incisive foramen (anterior palatine foramen), (**3**) lateral fossa, (**4**) nasal fossa, (**5**) nasal septum, (**6**) border of nasal fossa, (**7**) anterior nasal spine, and (**8**) median palatine suture.

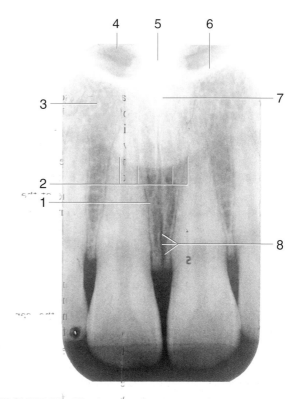

FIGURE 22-13 Radiograph of maxillary midline area showing (**1**) incisive (anterior palatine) foramen, indicated by an irregularly shaped, rounded radiolucent area, (**2**) outline of the nose, (**3**) lateral fossa, (**4**) nasal fossa (radiolucent), (**5**) nasal septum, (**6**) border of nasal fossa, (**7**) anterior nasal spine, and (**8**) median palatine suture.

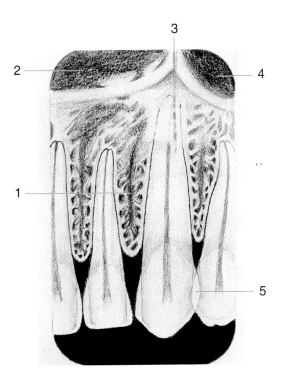

FIGURE 22-14 Drawing of maxillary canine area illustrating (**1**) lateral fossa, (**2**) nasal fossa, (**3**) inverted Y (intersection of the borders of nasal fossa and maxillary sinus), and (**4**) maxillary sinus. (**5**) Note the dense radiopaque area caused by overlapping of the mesial surface of the first premolar over the distal surface of the canine. This overlapping is common in this region of the oral cavity because of the curvature of the arch.

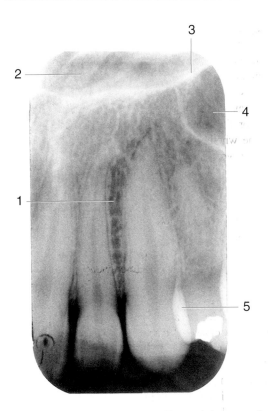

FIGURE 22-15 Radiograph of maxillary canine area showing (**1**) lateral fossa, (**2**) nasal fossa, (**3**) inverted Y (intersection of the borders of the nasal fossa and maxillary sinus), (**4**) maxillary sinus, and (**5**) dense radiopaque area caused by overlapping of the mesial surface of the first premolar over the distal surface of the canine. This overlapping is common in this region of the oral cavity because of the curvature of the arch.

3. **Inverted Y.** An important landmark seen in the canine–premolar area, made up of the lateral wall of the nasal fossa and the anterior–medial wall of the maxillary sinus. The intersection of these two radiopaque lines often criss-cross each other in the form of the letter Y. This Y shape often appears upside down or turned on its side.

4. **Soft tissue of the nose.** Sometimes an outline of the soft tissue of the nose may be shadowed onto anterior intraoral radiographs (Figures 22-16 and 22-17).

RADIOLUCENT FEATURES

1. **Median palatine suture.** A radiolucent thin line that delineates the midline of the palate and the junction of the right and left maxillae. Frequently seen between the central incisors, this structure should not be mistaken for a fracture.

2. **Incisive foramen (anterior palatine foramen).** A round or pear-shaped radiolucent opening that varies greatly in size serves for the passage of nerves and blood vessels. It is often visible near or between the apices of the central incisors. (This foramen should not be mistaken for an abscess, cyst, or other pathological condition.)

3. **Nasal fossa (cavity).** A large air space divided into two paired radiolucencies by the radiopaque nasal septum, often visible above the roots of the incisors. The radiolucency of

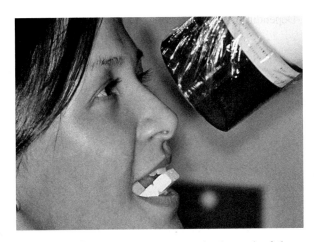

FIGURE 22-16 Soft tissue of the nose in the path of the x-ray beam. Note that the soft tissue of the nose will be in the path of the x-ray beam in this exposure. The resultant radiograph will most likely show an image of the soft tissue, outlining the tip of the nose.

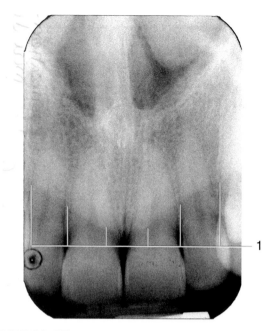

FIGURE 22-17 Soft tissue image of the nose. (1) The resultant image of the soft tissue of the nose is often magnified to a large size. According to the rules of shadow casting (see Chapter 4), the further an object is from the image receptor, the more likely that object will appear magnified. The tip of the nose is at an increased distance from the intraoral image receptor, resulting in a magnification of the size of the nose.

the nasal cavities will vary in dark appearance, depending on the angle of the x-ray beam. At times, the x-ray beam may have to penetrate the **nasal conchae,** thin bony extensions of the nasal wall, and result in a less radiolucent appearance of the nasal fossa itself. (Figure 22-3)

4. **Lateral fossa.** A radiolucency between the maxillary lateral incisor and the maxillary canine representing the decreased thickness in bone in this area.

Maxillary Posterior Region (Figures 22-18 through 22-22)

RADIOPAQUE FEATURES

1. **Floor** or inferior border of the sinuses. A thin, dense bone indicating the walls of the maxillary sinuses, whereas the sinus cavities themselves are referred to as radiolucent. The term *radiopaque* is used when referring to the sinus walls. The anterior extent of the maxillary sinus is often visible on an intraoral radiograph of the canine region as well.

2. **Septum.** A radiopaque wall (or partition) may be seen separating the maxillary sinus into two or more compartments. Septa (plural) are not always visible on all patients.

3. **Zygomatic process** of the maxilla. Appearing as a broad U-shaped band often seen above or superimposed over the roots of the first and second molars.

4. **Zygoma** (malar or cheekbone). Extends laterally and distally from the zygomatic process of the maxilla.

5. **Zygomatic arch.** Is continuous with the zygoma and extends distally. Because radiographs are a two-dimensional

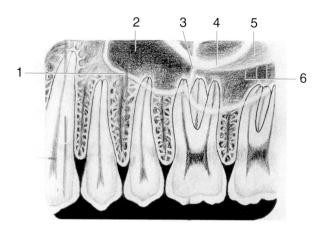

FIGURE 22-18 Drawing of maxillary premolar area illustrating (**1**) border (floor) of maxillary sinus, (**2**) maxillary sinus, (**3**) septum in maxillary sinus dividing the sinus into two compartments, (**4**) zygomatic process of maxilla, (**5**) zygoma, and (**6**) lower border of zygomatic arch.

picture of three-dimensional structures, it is difficult to distinguish radiographically where the zygomatic process, zygoma, and zygomatic arch end and begin.

6. **Maxillary tuberosity.** The extension of the alveolar bone behind the molars marking the posterior limits of the maxillary arch. The maxillary tuberosity is usually referred to as radiopaque; however, depending on the size of the trabeculae located here, the radiopacity will vary.

7. **Pterygoid plates** of the sphenoid will usually appear only on the most posterior intraoral radiograph. To distinguish this structure from the maxilla, look for the posterior outline of the maxilla, distal to the maxillary tuberosity. A radiolucent suture may be detected separating the lateral ptyergoid plate from the maxilla, or the pterygoid plate may appear to overlap onto the maxilla.

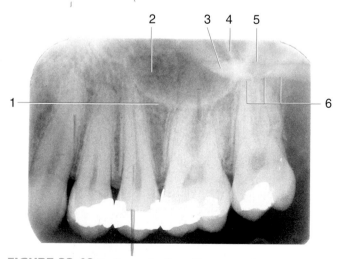

FIGURE 22-19 Radiograph of maxillary premolar area showing (**1**) border (floor) of maxillary sinus, (**2**) maxillary sinus, (**3**) zygomatic process of maxilla, (**4**) septum in maxillary sinus dividing the sinus into two compartments, (**5**) zygoma, and (**6**) inferior border of the zygomatic arch.

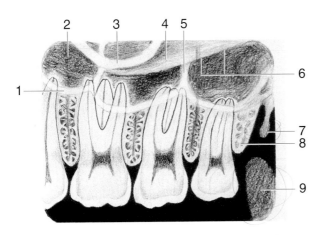

FIGURE 22-20 Drawing of maxillary molar area illustrating (**1**) border (floor) of maxillary sinus, (**2**) maxillary sinus, (**3**) zygomatic process of maxilla, (**4**) zygoma, (**5**) septum in maxillary sinus, (**6**) lower border of zygomatic arch, (**7**) hamulus (hamular process), (**8**) maxillary tuberosity, and (**9**) coronoid process (mandible).

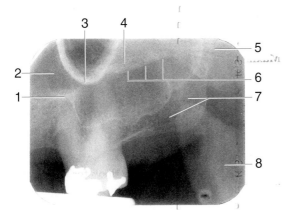

FIGURE 22-21 Radiograph of maxillary molar area showing (**1**) border (floor) of maxillary sinus, (**2**) maxillary sinus, (**3**) zygomatic process of maxilla, (**4**) zygoma, (**5**) lateral pterygoid plate, (**6**) lower border of zygomatic arch, (**7**) maxillary tuberosity, and (**8**) coronoid process of the mandible.

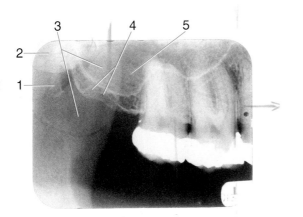

FIGURE 22-22 Radiograph of maxillary molar area showing (**1**) hamulus (hamular process), a downward projection of the medial pterygoid plate, (**2**) lateral pterygoid plate, (**3**) coronoid process of the mandible, (**4**) maxillary tuberosity, and (**5**) maxillary sinus.

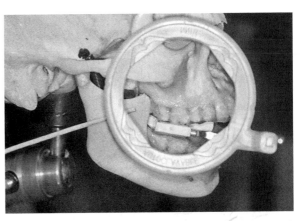

FIGURE 22-23 Coronoid process of the mandible may be recorded on intraoral radiographs of the maxillary posterior region. Note the position of the image receptor holder when exposing a maxillary posterior periapical radiograph. The coronoid process of the mandible will most likely be recorded on this radiograph.

8. **Hamulus** (hamular process). A downward projection of the medial pterygoid plate. It appears as a radiopaque pointed, sometimes hooklike, structure that serves as a muscle attachment. The hamulus is usually observed on only the most posterior intraoral radiographs.

9. **Coronoid process** of the mandible is sometimes seen as a triangle or large pointed radiopacity superimposed over the maxillary tuberosity. Although this structure is technically a feature of the mandible, it is often in the path of the x-ray beam when positioning the PID for images of the maxillary posterior region (Figure 22-23).

RADIOLUCENT FEATURES

1. **Maxillary sinus.** This large air chamber inside the maxilla is visible in almost all periapical radiographs from the region of the canines posterior to the molars. The thin, radiopaque sinus wall can be observed outlining the radiolucent sinus.

Mandibular Anterior Region (Figures 22-24 through 22-27)

RADIOPAQUE FEATURES

1. **Genial tubercles.** Are made up of four small, bony crests on the lingual surface of the mandible that serve for muscle attachments. Generally visible as a round radiopaque "doughnut" at the midline below the apices of the central incisors.

2. **Mental ridge.** Located on the lateral surface of the mandible, the mental ridge appears as a horizontal radiopaque line extending from the premolar region to the symphysis (the midline of the mandible where the left and right sides of bone are fused together).

RADIOLUCENT FEATURES

1. **Lingual foramen.** A very small circular radiolucency in the middle of the radiopaque genial tubercles. May not be recorded on the radiograph because of its small size.

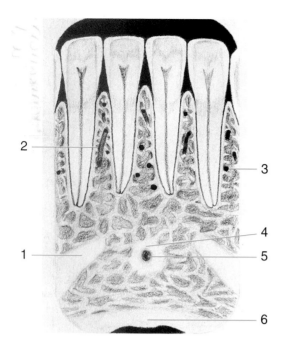

FIGURE 22-24 Drawing of mandibular midline area illustrating (**1**) mental ridge, (**2**) nutrient canal, (**3**) nutrient foramen, (**4**) genial tubercles surrounding the (**5**) lingual foramen, and (**6**) inferior border of mandible.

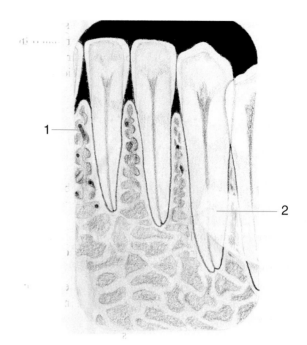

FIGURE 22-26 Drawing of mandibular canine area illustrating (**1**) nutrient canal, and (**2**) torus mandibularis (lingual torus).

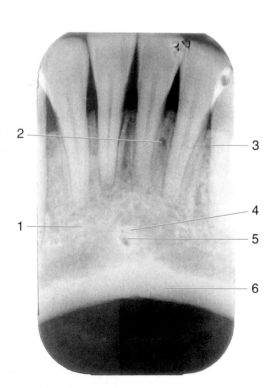

FIGURE 22-25 Radiograph of the mandibular midline area showing (**1**) mental ridge, (**2**) nutrient canal, (**3**) nutrient foramen, (**4**) genial tubercles surrounding the (**5**) lingual foramen, and (**6**) inferior border of the mandible (radiopaque band of dense cortical bone).

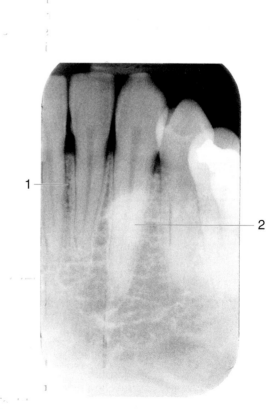

FIGURE 22-27 Radiograph of mandibular canine area showing (**1**) nutrient canal, (**2**) torus mandibularis (lingual torus).

2. **Mental fossa.** A depression on the labial aspect of the mandibular incisor area, representing an accentuated thinness of the mandible. On a mandibular incisor radiograph, the mental fossa appears as a generalized radiolucent area around the incisor apices.

Mandibular Posterior Region (Figures 22-28 through 22-32)

RADIOPAQUE FEATURES

1. **Oblique ridge.** A continuation of the anterior border of the ramus that extends downward and forward on the lateral surface of the mandible. The oblique ridge (sometimes called the external oblique ridge) appears as a radiopaque horizontal line of varied width superimposed across the molar roots.

2. **Mylohyoid ridge** is an irregular crest of bone for muscle attachments on the lingual surface of the mandible in the molar region. The mylohyoid ridge appears as a horizontal radiopaque line parallel and always inferior to (below) the oblique ridge. The mylohyoid ridge will most likely be imaged apical to (below) the teeth roots.

3. **Inferior border of the mandible** is a heavy layer of cortical bone that is imaged only if the radiograph is deeply depressed in the floor of the mouth or the vertical angle of the x-ray beam is excessive. The inferior border of the mandible will appear as a distinct, thick radiopaque border.

4. **Torus mandibularis (lingual torus).** This bony growth extending out from the lingual surface of the mandible is a frequently encountered form of benign tumor. Depending on the size of the torus, the increased thickness in the bone will appear as a radiopaque fuzzy cotton ball imaged over or apical to the roots of posterior teeth.

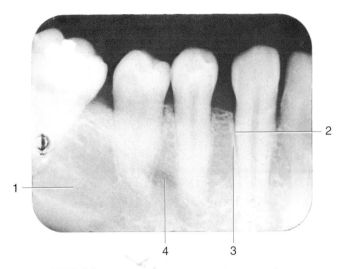

FIGURE 22-29 Radiograph of mandibular premolar area showing (**1**) submandibular fossa, (**2**) thin radiolucent line indicating the periodontal ligament space, (**3**) thin radiopaque line representing the lamina dura, and (**4**) the mental foramen.

RADIOLUCENT FEATURES

1. **Mental foramen.** A small opening on the lateral side of the body of the mandible, often seen near the apices of the premolars. This foramen should not be mistaken for an abscess, cyst, or other pathological condition.

2. **Submandibular fossa.** A large irregular-shaped area below the mylohyoid ridge and the roots of the mandibular molars, where the bone is thin, allowing more x-rays to penentrate this area and reach the image receptor. The submandibular fossa should not be mistaken for pathology.

3. **Mandibular canal.** A canal for the passage of the mandibular nerve and blood vessels, it is outlined by two paired, thin, barely visible, parallel radiopaque lines, which represent thin layers of cortical bone. The mandibular canal is often imaged in the premolar–molar areas below the apices of the teeth.

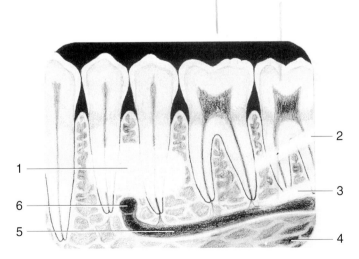

FIGURE 22-28 Drawing of mandibular premolar area illustrating (**1**) torus mandibularis, (**2**) oblique ridge, (**3**) mylohyoid ridge, (**4**) submandibular fossa, (**5**) mandibular canal, and (**6**) mental foramen.

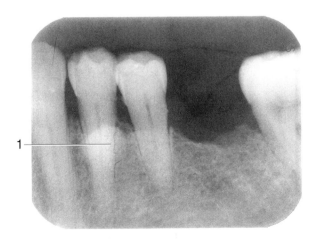

FIGURE 22-30 Radiograph of mandibular premolar area showing (**1**) small torus mandibularis (lingual torus).

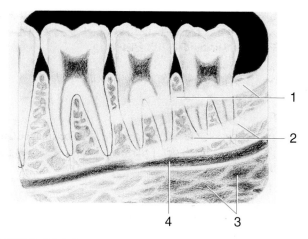

FIGURE 22-31 Drawing of mandibular molar area illustrating (**1**) oblique ridge, (**2**) mylohyoid ridge, (**3**) submandibular fossa, and (**4**) mandibular canal.

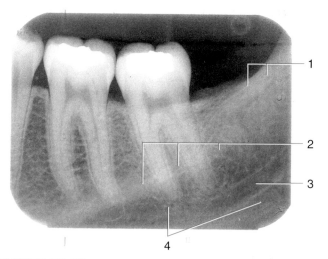

FIGURE 22-32 Radiograph of mandibular molar area showing (**1**) oblique ridge, (**2**) mylohyoid ridge, (**3**) mandibular canal (note the thin, parallel radiopaque lines representing the canal walls), and (**4**) submandibular fossa.

REVIEW—Chapter summary

Knowledge of the anatomical landmarks of the face and skull is needed to properly position the image receptor to clearly image the area of interest, to assist in mounting intraoral radiographs, and to develop the ability to interpret radiographs and recognize deviations from normal.

The radiographer should be able to identify cranial and facial bones as well as the specific landmarks and features of the maxilla and mandible. The radiographic appearance of the alveolar bone and the structures of the teeth were presented.

For the purpose of organizing anatomical structures for learning, landmarks are divided into the following categories, depending on where they would be most likely to appear: maxillary anterior region, maxillary posterior region, mandibular anterior region, and mandibular posterior region. Anatomical landmarks are further separated into radiopaque images or radiolucent images. A systematic procedure is helpful to the beginning radiographer in learning to identify normal radiographic anatomy.

RECALL—Study questions

1. A competent dental hygienist and dental assistant must be able to identify which of the following radiographically?
   a. Caries
   b. Periodontal abcess
   c. Normal anatomy
   d. Periapical pathology

2. Which of the following facial bones would most likely appear on a periapical radiograph?
   a. Occipital
   b. Parietal
   c. Frontal
   d. Zygoma

3. Bone sometimes has a mixed radiopaque-radiolucent appearance due to the nature of the
   a. cortical plates.
   b. trabeculae patterns.
   c. alveolar process.
   d. genial tubercles.

4. Which of the following will most likely appear as a radiopacity outlining the tooth root?
   a. PDL space
   b. Lamina dura
   c. Nutrient canal
   d. Cementum

5. When nutrient canals open at the surface of the bone, they often appear radiographically as
   a. small radiolucent dots.
   b. large radiopaque lines.
   c. small radiolucent lines.
   d. small radiopaque dots.

6. Which of these structures appears radiolucent?
   a. Enamel
   b. Cementum
   c. Dentin
   d. Pulp

7. A periapical radiograph of a 10-year-old will most likely reveal developing permanent dentition.

   Evidence of a congenitally missing permanent tooth is called an impaction.
   a. The first statement is true. The second statement is false.
   b. The first statement is false. The second statement is true.
   c. Both statements are true.
   d. Both statements are false.

8. On a periapical radiograph of the maxillary molars, which of the following structures may be recorded superimposed over the roots of the teeth?
   a. Mastoid process
   b. Maxillary tuberosity
   c. Zygomatic process
   d. Mylohyoid ridge

9. Each of these features will appear radiolucent EXCEPT one. Which one is the EXCEPTION?
   a. Foramen
   b. Suture
   c. Canal
   d. Spine

10. Each of these features will appear radiopaque EXCEPT one. Which one is the EXCEPTION?
    a. Ridge
    b. Sinus
    c. Tubercles
    d. Process

11. Which of the following is the best recommended sequence for learning to identify normal radiographic anatomy?
    a. 1. Determine if radiograph is of the maxilla or mandible.
       2. Determine if radiograph is of the anterior or posterior region.
       3. Determine if the structure is radiopaque or radiolucent.
    b. 1. Determine if radiograph is of the anterior or posterior region.
       2. Determine if the structure is radiopaque or radiolucent.
       3. Determine if radiograph is of the maxilla or mandible.
    c. 1. Determine if the structure is radiopaque or radiolucent.
       2. Determine if radiograph is of the maxilla or mandible.
       3. Determine if radiograph is of the anterior or posterior region.
    d. 1. Determine if radiograph is of the maxilla or mandible.
       2. Determine if the structure is radiopaque or radiolucent.
       3. Determine if radiograph is of the anterior or posterior region.

12. Each of the following may appear on a periapical radiograph of the maxillary anterior region EXCEPT one. Which one is the EXCEPTION?
    a. Nasal septum
    b. Median palatine suture
    c. Maxillary tuberosity
    d. Inverted Y

13. Each of the following may appear on a periapical radiograph of the maxillary posterior region EXCEPT one. Which one is the EXCEPTION?
    a. Maxillary sinus
    b. Incisive foramen
    c. Zygomatic arch
    d. Hamulus

14. A mandible landmark feature that may be imaged on a periapical radiograph of the maxillary posterior region is the
    a. mandibular canal.
    b. submandibular fossa.
    c. inferior border of the mandible.
    d. coronoid process.

15. Each of the following may appear on a periapical radiograph of the mandibular anterior region EXCEPT one. Which one is the EXCEPTION?
    a. Genial tubercles
    b. Mental ridge
    c. Coronoid process
    d. Lingual foramen

16. Each of the following may appear on a periapical radiograph of the mandibular posterior region EXCEPT one. Which one is the EXCEPTION?
    a. Mental foramen
    b. Pterygoid plate
    c. Mandibular canal
    d. Mylohyoid ridge

17. The inverted Y landmark is composed of the intersection of which two structures?
    a. Lateral wall of the nasal cavity and anterior border of the maxillary sinus
    b. Anterior border of the maxillary sinus and inferior border of the mandible
    c. Lateral wall of the nasal cavity and soft tissue shadow of the nose
    d. Inferior border of the zygomatic process and the anterior nasal spine

REFLECT—Case study

Your colleague is viewing a full mouth series of radiographs that he just finished mounting. As he is describing the following features, see if you can tell him the name of the anatomic landmark.

1. A dense, vertical radiopacity separating two paired oval radiolucencies observed in the maxillary anterior region.
2. Large, paired oval radiolucencies separated by a dense, vertical radiopacity observed in the maxillary anterior region.
3. A thin radiolucent line resembling a fracture observed between the maxillary central incisors.

4. A round or pear-shaped radiolucency observed between the maxillary central incisors.

5. A broad, U-shaped radiopacity observed superimposed over the maxillary posterior teeth roots.

6. A radiopaque downward projection of bone that appears pointed or hooklike observed in the far posterior region of the maxilla.

7. A large triangular-shaped radiopacity observed superimposed over the maxillary tuberosity region.

8. A large radiolucency outlined by a thin radiopaque border that is observed in almost all the periapical radiographs of the maxilla, from the canine posteriorly.

9. A very small, round radiolucency observed in the midline apical (below) the mandibular incisors.

10. A horizontal radiopaque line extending from the premolar region to the symphysis.

11. A round radiolucency that resembles an abscess observed near the apex of the mandibular second premolar.

12. A horizontal radiopaque line observed in the mandibular posterior region, superimposed across the molar roots.

13. Another horizontal radiopaque line observed in the mandibular posterior region, but inferior to (below) the line described in #12 above. This line is observed inferior to the molar roots.

14. A large, irregularly shaped radiolucency observed inferior to the line described in #13 above.

RELATE—Laboratory application

Developing the ability to recognize, identify, and describe radiographic anatomy of the head and neck region takes practice. Using the illustrations in this chapter, compare the appearance of the structures labeled with how they appear on a dry skull. Looking at a skull, point out each of the landmarks in the figures. To make it easier to locate these bones or structures, turn the skull so that it is oriented in the same direction as the illustration at which you are looking. Many structures can be seen readily; others may only be seen from one specific direction.

REFERENCES

Farman, A. G., Nortje, C. J., & Wood, R. E. (1993). *Oral and maxillofacial diagnostic imaging.* St. Louis, MO: Mosby.

White, S. C., & Pharoah, M. J. (2008). *Oral radiology: Principles and interpretation* (6th ed.). St. Louis, MO: Elsevier.

Recognizing Deviations from Normal Radiographic Anatomy

OBJECTIVES

Following successful completion of this chapter, you should be able to:

1. Define the key words.
2. Identify the radiographic appearance of dental materials.
3. Identify the radiographic appearance of developmental anomalies.
4. Identify the radiographic appearance of periapical abscesses, cysts, and granulomas.
5. Identify the radiographic appearance of external and internal tooth resorption.
6. Identify the radiographic appearance of calcifications and ossifications.
7. Identify the radiographic appearance of odontogenic tumors.
8. Identify the radiographic appearance of nonodontogenic tumors.
9. Identify the radiographic appearance of fractures.

KEY WORDS

Abscess
Amalgam
Amalgam tattoo
Ameloblastoma
Anodontia
Anomaly
Base material
Benign
Carcinoma
Composite
Condensing osteitis
Crown
Cyst
Dens in dente
Dentigerous cyst

Dilaceration
Exostosis
External resorption
Follicular (eruptive) cyst
Foreign body
Fracture line
Fusion
Gemination
Globulomaxillary cyst
Granuloma
Gutta percha
Hypercementosis
Idiopathic resorption
Incisive canal cyst
Internal resorption

KEY WORDS (*Continued*)		
Malignant	Phleboliths	Sarcoma
Mesiodens	Post and core	Sclerotic bone
Nonodontogenic cyst	Pulp stone	Sialolith
Odontogenic cyst	Radicular cyst	Silver point
Odontoma	Residual cyst	Supernumerary tooth
Ossification	Resorption	Taurodontia
Osteosclerosis	Retained root	Torus
Overhang	Retention pin	Tumor
Periapical cemental dysplasia (PCD)	Rhinoliths	

Introduction

The most important skill in interpreting radiographs that a dental hygienist and dental assistant can possess is the ability to recognize deviations from normal radiographic anatomy. Although the dentist is responsible for the final diagnosis and treatment of dental disease, all members of the oral health care team should be able to recognize radiographic deviations from the normal. Patient care is enhanced when the entire team views and interprets the radiographs.

Interpretation is a skill that requires a great deal of practice. The beginning radiology student is often frustrated by not being able to "see" what the expert easily identifies. To help develop this skill, a solid working knowledge of normal radiographic anatomy is needed. The radiographer should first identify normal radiographic anatomy, then systematically progress through a sequence of evaluation, naming each radiopaque and radiolucent structure observed.

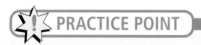

PRACTICE POINT

The rule follows that when viewing radiographs, you should *give everything you see a name.* Every radiopaque and radiolucent object observed on the radiograph should be identified as an anatomical landmark. Is the observation in question the mental foramen, the submandibular fossa, or the periodontal ligament space? When you have exhausted all possibilities of what a finding could be, it then becomes a deviation from the normal, requiring the attention of the dentist.

The purpose of this chapter is to help build on the skills acquired in Chapter 22 and to begin to identify common radiographic features that patients often present with (Procedure Box 23-1). These include the radiographic appearance of restorative materials, developmental anomalies, periapical pathology and other common pathological conditions of the teeth and the jaws, and the effects of trauma.

Prior to the discussion of the radiographic appearance of these materials and conditions, it should be noted that interpretation of radiographic findings is enhanced when the patient is present, allowing the practitioner to compare the radiographic findings with the clinical examination of the patient. Attempting to determine what a particular finding is from the radiograph alone may sometimes be difficult; for example, a radiolucency observed in the otherwise radiopaque enamel of a maxillary central incisor may give the appearance of caries. However, a clinical examination of this tooth may reveal the presence of a composite restoration, which can sometimes mimic decay radiographically. In addition, the dentist will always use radiographs in conjunction with the patient's clinical examination, medical and dental histories, and physical signs and symptoms, together with other necessary diagnostic tests to make a final diagnosis.

Radiographic Appearance of Dental Restorative Material

It is important to observe restorative materials radiographically for the presence of recurrent decay, defective margins that contribute to periodontal disease, and other potential problems. Restorative materials may appear radiopaque or radiolucent, and some can be differentiated by their relative degree of radiopacity or radiolucency (Table 23-1). Others are better identified by their size and contour or by their probable location on the tooth. However, because radiographs are a two-dimensional image of three-dimensional objects, the image of a restoration on one surface may be superimposed on the image of another large restoration on the same tooth, giving the appearance of only one restoration instead of two, or even more. Often, there is more than one type of material superimposed. For example, the appearance of a base material may be observed apical to a metallic restoration, or the presence of metallic retention pins may be detected apical to a crown. In addition, it is not always possible to determine on which tooth surface the restoration is located. A restoration looks the same whether it is on the facial (buccal) or lingual surface of the tooth.

TABLE 23-1   Metallic and Nonmetallic Restorations

METALLIC DENTAL MATERIALS	NONMETALLIC DENTAL MATERIALS	
RADIOPAQUE	LESS RADIOPAQUE	SOMETIMES RADIOLUCENT
Amalgam	Composite	Composite
Gold	Porcelain	Acrylic resins
Stainless steel	Acrylic resins	Silicate
Retention pin	Silicate	
Post and core	Base	
Silver point	Cement	
Orthodontic appliance	Temporary filling	
Implants	Gutta percha	
	Sealants	

Metallic Restorations

The images of all metallic restorations of approximately equal density appear extremely radiopaque. Therefore, it is impossible to determine whether the material is gold, silver, or a base metal alloy. Only by looking at the size and contour of the restoration is it possible to make an educated guess based on what materials are generally used in such circumstances. For example, metal crowns will most often appear to have smooth

PROCEDURE 23-1
Sequence for interpreting a full mouth series for deviations from normal radiographic anatomy

1. See Procedure Box 21-2, Suggested Sequence for Viewing a Full Mouth Series of Radiographs.

2. Examine one anatomic structure at a time. Compare each finding with its appearance in adjacent radiographs.

3. First, examine the supporting structures (the bones of the head and neck).

   a. Identify each landmark (see Chapter 22).

   b. Determine whether the landmark is in the appropriate region.

   c. Determine whether the landmark is of accurate size and shape.

   d. Examine the trabecular spaces and cortical plate of the bones.

4. Second, examine the teeth.

   a. Determine if each tooth is present or absent.

   b. Examine the shape and morphology of the crowns and roots.

   c. Look for developmental stages and/or abnormalities.

   d. Examine the pulp chamber and root canals.

5. Third, observe any dental restorations and the presence of dental materials.

   a. Check for shape and contour.

   b. Check for appropriate placement.

   c. Look for radiolucencies that suggest recurrent decay (see Chapter 24).

6. Fourth, examine the teeth for possible carious lesions (see Chapter 24).

7. Fifth, examine the supporting alveolar bone and the periodontal ligament space for evidence of periodontal disease (see Chapter 25).

8. Present a preliminary interpretation for the dentist's review.

9. Following confirmation by the dentist, document all findings on the patient's permanent record.

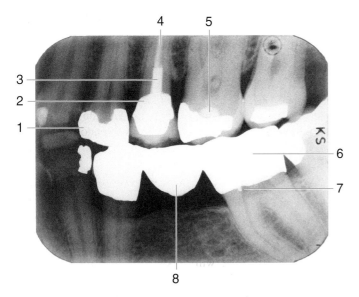

FIGURE 23-1 **Dental materials.** (**1**) Amalgam. (**2**) Porcelain-fused-to-metal crown. (**3**) Post and core. (**4**) Gutta percha. (**5**) Base material. (**6**) Full metal crown, which is the posterior abutment of a three-unit bridge. (**7**) Retention pin. (**8**) Metal pontic (part of the three-unit bridge).

margins, whereas amalgam restorations have irregular margins (Figure 23-1).

Nonmetallic Restorations

Aesthetic materials, such as **composites,** porcelain, silicate, and acrylic resins (plastics), may appear radiopaque or radiolucent and may be barely visible or not detected at all. Radiolucent dental materials have a tendency to mimic decay radiographically, so some manufacturers add radiopaque particles to their product so that the viewer will not mistake it for caries (Figure 23-2).

Other restorative materials such as **base material** (calcium hydroxide pastes; Figure 23-1) and cements (Figure 23-2) exhibit about the same degree of radiopacity as dentin. Sealants may appear very slightly radiopaque, or not at all.

Identification of Common Restorative Materials

• **Amalgam.** The most common restorative material; appears radiopaque with irregular margins and varies in size and shape. The amalgam radiopacity observed will most likely not cover the entire crown of the teeth; the less radiopaque enamel cusps are often still visible. Radiographs help to image the contours of amalgam restorations and can reveal poorly contoured margins called **overhangs** (Figure 23-3).

Radiographs sometime reveal particles of amalgam in the soft tissue. Often found in edentulous areas of the mandible, amalgam that fractures during an extraction and falls into the root socket or under the gingival tissue may impart a bluish-purple color to the tissue, called an **amalgam tattoo** (Figure 23-4).

• **Composite.** Varies in appearance from radiopaque to radiolucent. When radiolucent, composite may mimic caries

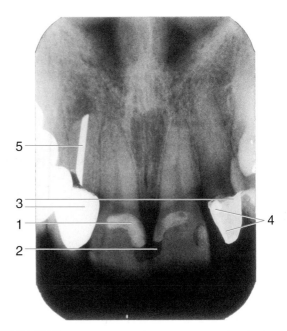

FIGURE 23-2 **Comparision of radiopaque and radiolucent appearance of composite.** (**1**) Radiopaque composite. (**2**) Radiolucent composite (or acrylic resin or silicate). (**3**) Porcelain-fused-to-metal crowns. Overexposure (darkness) of this radiograph makes it especially difficult to view the porcelain on the left lateral incisor. (**4**) However, the overexposure made it possible to image the cement under this crown. (**5**) Silver point endodontic filler.

(Figure 23-2). To help distinguish composite from caries, look for the restoration to appear to have straight margins and a prepared look, whereas the radiolucency of caries appears more diffuse (see Figure 24-17). A clinical examination may be needed to determine definitively whether caries or composite is present.

• **Crown (full metal).** Appears radiopaque and is distinguished from amalgam by its smooth margins. Full metal **crowns** usually cover the entire crown of the tooth and will be contoured to resemble the correct shape of the cusps of the tooth (Figure 23-1).

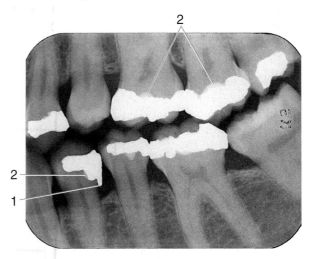

FIGURE 23-3 Overhang. (**1**) Amalgam overhang. (**2**) Base material. Note the many shapes and sizes of the amalgam restorations.

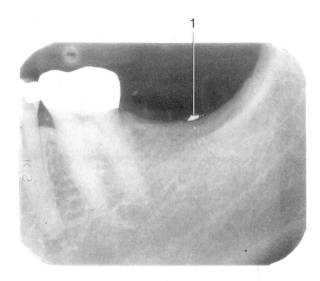

FIGURE 23-4 Amalgam fragment (1) embedded in the soft tissue, probably left after an extraction. Clinically called an amalgam tattoo because the amalgam fragment produces a bluish-purple spot on the gingiva.

- **Crown (porcelain-fused-to-metal).** The metal core of the crown appears radiopaque, whereas the porcelain appears less radiopaque. The radiopaque shape of the metal core will be more rounded than a full metal crown and is not contoured to resemble the correct shape of the cusps of the tooth. Instead, the porcelain will take the shape of the cusps (Figure 23-1).

- **Crown (porcelain jacket).** Appears less radiopaque than a full metal crown because no metal is present. The porcelain material will appear to be about the same radiopacity as dentin.

- **Crown (stainless steel).** As a temporary restoration, this metal is less dense and will allow the passage of more x-rays, giving the material a "see-through" appearance. These crowns are prefabricated and do not appear to fit the tooth very well (Figure 23-5).

- **Retention pin.** A metal pin used to support a restoration. **Retention pins** appear radiopaque in a very easy-to-identify

shape (Figures 23-1 and 23-6). Because another restorative material such as an amalgam, composite, or crown will be placed over the retention pin, it may not be recorded on the radiograph. It should be noted that retention pins will only be located in the dentin and will not be observed penetrating the pulp. A retention pin should not be confused with a post and core restoration, which penetrates the pulp chamber and must be observed in conjunction with an endodontic filling material (Figures 23-1 and 23-7). These materials are described later.

- **Base material (calcium hydroxide pastes).** Base materials are used to line the cavity preparation to protect the tooth's pulp. Because another restorative material such as an amalgam or composite will be placed over the base, it may not be recorded on the radiograph. When recorded, the base material will appear very slightly radiopaque (Figure 23-1 and Figure 23-3).

- **Endodontic fillers.** Radiopacities observed within the pulp chamber may be either **silver points** (Figure 23-2), a very radiopaque metal root canal filling, **or gutta percha,** a less radiopaque filling (Figures 23-1 and 23-7).

- **Post and core.** A metal restoration that builds up a tooth so that it can support a crown; appears radiopaque. The core section penetrates the pulp chamber, so the presence of endodotic filler will be observed along with a post and core. It should be noted that in addition to location, a post and core restoration can be distinguished from a retention pin by its significantly larger size (Figure 23-7).

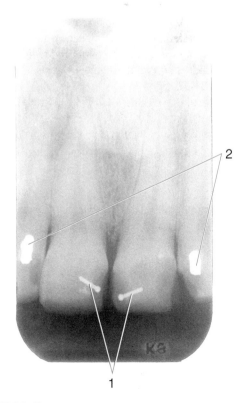

FIGURE 23-6 Retention pins. (1) Radiopaque pins help retain the radiolucent composite restorations. (**2**) Small radiopaque amalgam restorations.

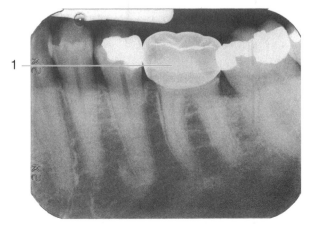

FIGURE 23-5 Stainless steel crown (1). Note the "see-through" appearance.

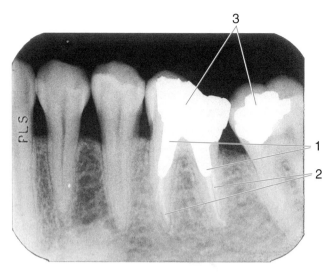

FIGURE 23-7 Endodontic treatments. (1) Post and core within the root canals. **(2)** Gutta percha. Endodontic filling material will also be present when a post and core restoration is observed. **(3)** Amalgam restorations.

- **Implant.** Appears as a distinct radiopacity. The implant is located in an area of a missing tooth (Figure 23-8).
- **Orthodontic and surgical materials.** Metal orthodontic bands, wires, and brackets and surgical wires, pins, and screws all appear as distinct radiopacities (Figures 23-9 and 23-10).

Radiographic Appearance of Developmental Anomalies

An **anomaly** is defined as any deviation from normal. Dental anomalies are numerous, so it is important that the dental hygienist and the dental assistant be skilled at identifying the more common of these. Such anomalies include the following:

- **Anodontia.** Absence of the teeth (may be complete or partial). The third molars are the most common congenitally missing teeth, followed by the premolars (Figure 23-11) and the maxillary lateral incisors. It is important when viewing

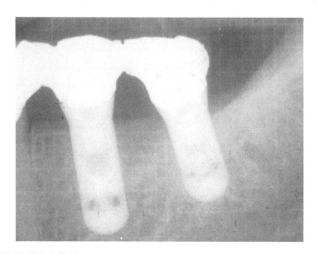

FIGURE 23-8 Implants take the shape of the missing teeth roots.

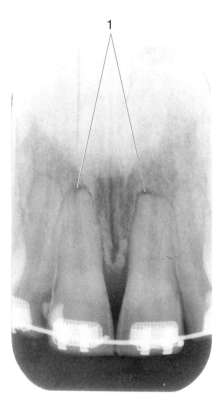

FIGURE 23-9 Orthodontic appliance. (1) Note the root-end external resorption caused by trauma of orthodontic treatment.

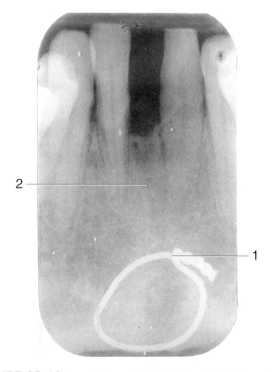

FIGURE 23-10 Surgical materials. (1) Surgical wire used to treat a fractured mandible. **(2)** Mandibular fracture indicated by the radiolucent line.

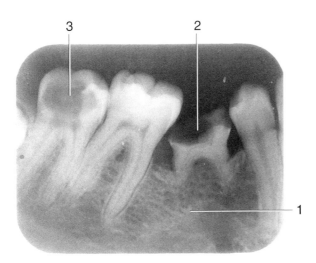

FIGURE 23-11 Congenitally missing tooth. (**1**). Second premolar did not develop under this primary molar. (**2**) Severe caries. (**3**) Severe caries.

radiographs of children that the presence of the developing permanent teeth be noted.

- **Supernumerary teeth (extra teeth).** It is equally important that the presence of **supernumerary teeth** be detected. (Figure 23-12) Often there is not a space for these extra teeth to erupt into, or the radiopacities may be deformed and not resemble normal tooth form. Complications caused by supernumerary teeth include the possibility of cyst formation and the malposition, noneruption, or both of the normal teeth.

- **Mesiodens.** A supernumerary tooth located in the maxillary midline (Figure 23-13).

- **Dens in dente** (dens invaginatus). Literally, a tooth within a tooth, an invagination of the enamel within the body of the tooth. This anomaly occurs most frequently in the maxillary lateral incisor (Figure 23-14).

- **Hypercementosis.** Usually appears radiopaque and is caused by excessive cementum formation. The excessive cementum on the roots often causes a bulbous enlargement along the root surface, with the area near the apex appearing most bulbous (Figure 23-15). **Hypercementosis** is

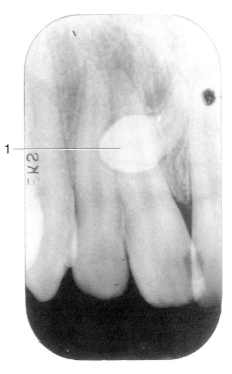

FIGURE 23-13 Mesiodens. (**1**) A small supernumerary tooth, located in the midline between the central incisors.

distinguished from radiopacities surrounding or near the tooth roots by the outline of the periodontal ligament (PDL) space. When observing hypercementosis, the PDL contains the radiopacity and separates it from the bone.

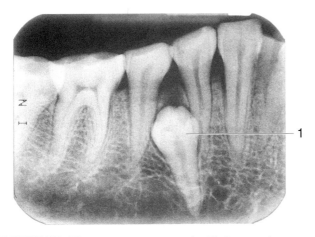

FIGURE 23-12 Supernumerary tooth. (**1**). Impacted supernumerary premolar.

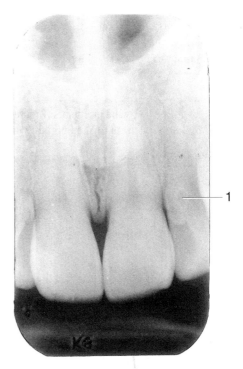

FIGURE 23-14 Dens in dente. (**1**) An invagination of the enamel within the body of the lateral incisor.

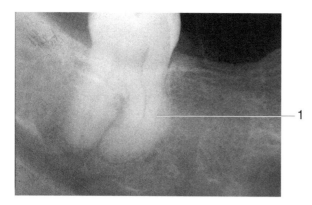

FIGURE 23-15 **Hypercementosis.** (**1**) Overgrowth of cementum on the roots of the molar.

This distinction will help to avoid mistaking hypercementosis for sclerotic bone, explained later.

- **Dilaceration.** When the tooth root is misshapen with a sharp bend. (Figure 23-16).
- **Taurodontia.** Characterized by an elongated pulp chamber and very short roots.
- **Gemination (twinning).** A single tooth bud that divides and forms two joined teeth. The presence of adjacent teeth helps to distinguish this condition from fusion.
- **Fusion.** A condition where the dentin and one other dental tissue of adjacent teeth are united (Figure 23-17). In this case, two adjacent teeth will be involved, distinguishing fusion from gemination.

Radiographic Appearance of Apical Disease

Radiolucencies surrounding the apices or root tips of the teeth indicate pathological changes in the hard (bony) tissues. These radiolucenies cannot usually be distinguished from each other

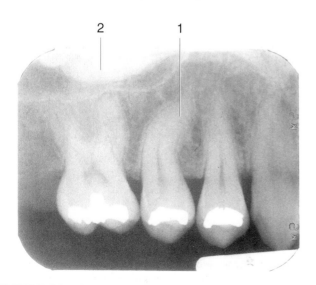

FIGURE 23-16 **Dilaceration.** (**1**) A sharp bend in the root of the second premolar. (**2**) Torus palatinus, a radiopaque benign overgrowth of bone on the midline of the palate.

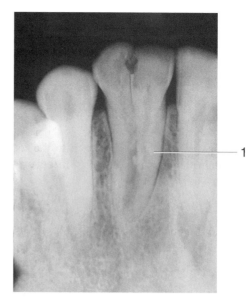

FIGURE 23-17 **Fusion.** (**1**) Two joined adjacent incisors.

based on the radiographic image alone. The appearance of apical pathology on a radiograph must be carefully correlated with other assessment information before a diagnosis can be made. The three most common periapical lesions observed on radiographs are **abscess, granuloma,** and **cyst** (Figure 23-18).

- **Periapical abscess.** Periapical infections usually result from pulpal inflammation. Bacteria from caries infect the pulp and gain access to the periapical bone by way of the root canals. As a rule, an acute abscess (early stage of pulpal or periapical infection) is barely discernible

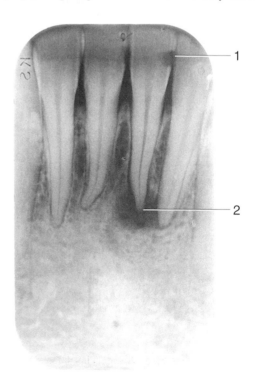

FIGURE 23-18 **Periapical pathology.** (**1**) Caries on the distal surface of the left central incisor. (**2**) Round radiolucent lesion that may be a periapical abscess, a granuloma, or a cyst.

radiographically, becoming more radiolucent as it becomes chronic. In fact, in the very early acute stage there may be no radiographic evidence at all. The earliest sign may be a break, or loss of radiopacity, in the lamina dura. A chronic abscess may appear as a circular radiolucency around the root apices and eventual turn into a granuloma.

- **Granuloma.** A mass of granulation tissue usually surrounded by a fibrous sac continuous with the periodontal ligament space that appears attached to the root apices. Under certain conditions, epithelial elements may proliferate to form a cyst.

- **Cyst.** Epithelium-lined sac filled with fluid or semisolid material. The periapical cyst (also known as a **radicular cyst**) is a cyst around the end of the tooth root. Unless the cyst is completely removed at the time of the extraction or surgery, it will remain and is then called **a residual cyst.** Because of osmotic imbalance within a cyst, pressure is exerted in all directions; therefore, cysts tend to be spherical unless unequal resistance is encountered. Although usually unilocular (made up of one compartment), cysts may also be multilocular (made up of several compartments). Radiographically, a cyst may appear as a fairly uniform radiolucent cavity within the bone and surrounded by a well-defined radiopaque border that resembles the lamina dura.

A **dentigerous** or **follicular cyst** (Figure 23-19) is associated with impacted or unerupted teeth—most often third molars and supernumerary teeth—and is always associated with the crown only of the involved tooth. If the tooth causing the cyst continues to develop and is able to erupt, the cyst is often destroyed by natural means (Figure 23-20).

Periapical, residual, and dentigerous cysts are categorized as **odontogenic cysts,** which means of tooth origin. **Nonodontogenic cysts** arise from epithelium other than that associated with tooth formation. Two types of nonodontogenic cysts are the **incisive canal** (nasopalatine) cyst (Figure 23-21), located within the incisive canal, and the rare **globulomaxillary cyst** (Figure 23-22), which arises between the maxillary lateral incisor and the canine.

Radiographic Appearance of Tooth Resorption

Evidence of tooth **resorption** is a common finding on dental radiographs. Natural physiologic resorption, such as when the roots of primary teeth resorb in response to the erupting permanent teeth, is considered normal (Figure 23-20). Other resorptive processes, however, are the result of infection, trauma, or some unusual condition. Tooth resorption may be external or internal. **External resorption** is most often characterized by root-end resorption, where the roots of the teeth appear shorter than normal (Figure 23-23). External resorption is not limited to the root end, but can occur anywhere along the tooth root. Other examples of external resorption include the resorption caused by pressure from an adjacent impacted or unerupted tooth; resorption caused by slowly growing tumors; or trauma, such as when teeth are moved too rapidly during orthodontic treatment (Figure 23-9). When the resorption cause is unknown, it is called **idiopathic resorption.**

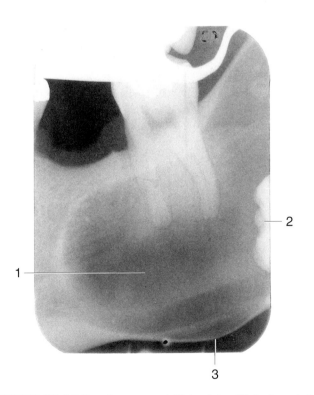

FIGURE 23-19 Dentigerous cyst (1) involving (**2**) the impacted third molar. (**3**) Note the expansion and thinning of the cortical bone of the mandible in response to the cyst. (The image receptor was purposely placed in a vertical position instead of the usual horizontal position to better record this condition.)

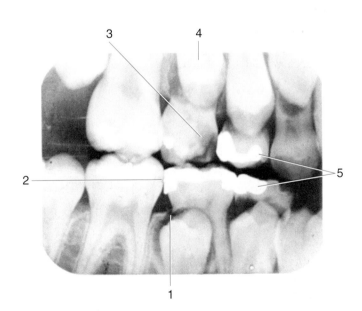

FIGURE 23-20 Follicular cyst (1) surrounds the crown of the unerupted second premolar. (**2**) Incipient caries on the first permanent molar. (**3**) Advanced caries on the primary second molar. (**4**) Erupting second premolar. (**5**) Primary first molars about to be exfoliated. Note the physiologic external resorption of the primary roots.

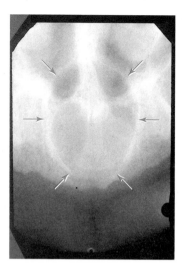

FIGURE 23-21 Incisive canal cyst. Arrows outline an incisive canal (nasopalatine) cyst in an edentulous maxilla.

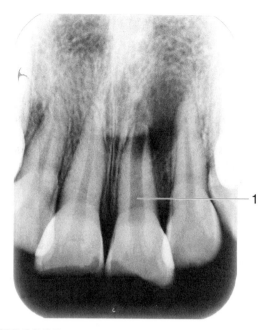

FIGURE 23-24 Internal resorption. (1) Idiopathic resorption noted as the widening of the pulp chamber.

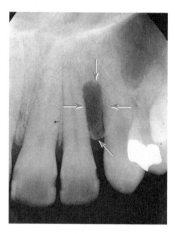

FIGURE 23-22 Globulomaxillary cyst. Arrows outline a globulomaxillary cyst between the maxillary lateral incisor and the canine.

Internal resorption typically appears as a radiolucent widening of the root canal, representing the resorption process taking place from the inside out (Figure 23-24).

Although not classified as resorption, but often undergoing a resorption process, are **retained root** fragments that may be observed on radiographs of an edentulous area (Figure 23-25). These structures may have broken off the tooth and were left behind following extraction or remain as the result of severe decay or trauma that broke off the crown of the tooth, leaving behind the root. The patient did not seek dental tratment for the condition, and the root tip remained. Retained root tips may be clearly visible radiographically or less so, depending on their size and degree of resorption.

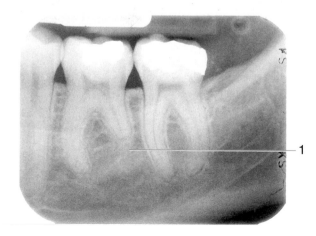

FIGURE 23-23 External resorption. (1) Idiopathic resorption of the distal root of the first molar.

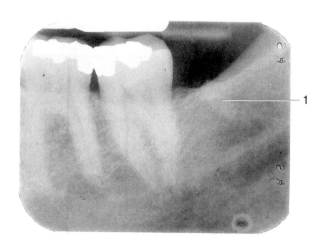

FIGURE 23-25 Retained root (1) fragment in an extraction site.

Radiographic Appearance of Calcifications and Ossifications

Calcifications in the dental pulp occur in the form of small nodules called **pulp stones** (Figure 23-26). These appear as radiopaque ovoid structures of varied size. Pulp stones are very common but of little significance, unless root canal therapy is needed on the affected tooth.

Other less frequently encountered calcifications are **sialoliths,** depositions of calcium salts in the salivary glands and ducts (Figure 23-27); **rhinoliths,** stones within the maxillary sinuses; and **phleboliths** or calcified thrombi, calcified masses that are observed as round or oval bodies in the soft tissues of the cheeks.

Two forms of **ossification** (the conversion of structures into hardened bone) are often imaged on radiographs. **Condensing osteitis** occurs when **sclerotic** (hardened) **bone** is formed as a result of infection (Figure 23-28). The increased radiopacity of the bone is often accompanied by an increased widening (radiolucency) of the periodontal ligament space. **Osteosclerosis** occurs when regions of abnormally dense bone form, but not as a direct result of infection (Figure 23-29). Although the cause is unknown, osteosclerosis commonly occurs in the interseptal premolar area and may be associated with fragments of retained primary roots.

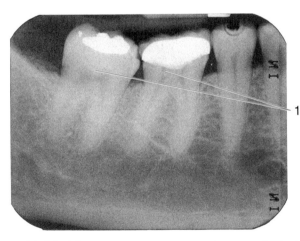

FIGURE 23-26 Pulp stones. (1) Ovoid radiopaque calcifications observed in the pulp chambers.

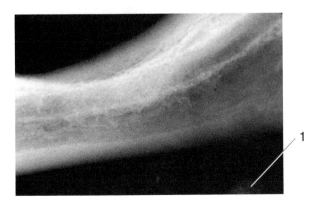

FIGURE 23-27 Sialolith (1) in a salivary gland. Note the edentulous mandible.

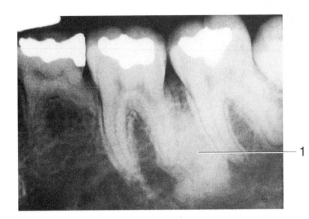

FIGURE 23-28 Condensing osteitis. (1) Radiopaque, sclerotic (hardening of) bone.

Radiographic Appearance of Odontogenic Tumors

Odontogenic tumors result from abnormal proliferation of cells and tissues involved in odontogenesis (the formation of the teeth). The three types occasionally seen on radiographs are **ameloblastomas, odontomas,** and **periapical cemental dysplasia (PCD).** Ameloblastomas have the greatest potential for serious implications for the patient. These appear as large radiolucencies of enamel origin. Radiographically, ameloblastomas may be monolocular (one compartment) or multilocular (many compartments). The monolocular form closely resembles a dentigerous cyst (Figure 23-30). The multilocular form has a characteristic "soap bubble" appearance.

Odontomas are the most common ondontogenic tumors (Figure 23-31). These are tumors of small misshaped teeth whose number in each odontoma varies widely. These toothlike structures appear radiopaque and are located within a radiolucent fibrous capsule that often resembles a cyst.

Periapical cemental dysplasia (PCD), sometimes called cementomas, is a bone dysplasia derived from the periodontal

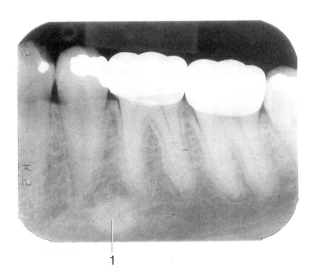

FIGURE 23-29 Osteosclerosis. (1) Diffuse idiopathic osteosclerosis.

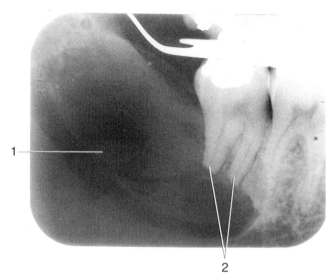

FIGURE 23-30 **Ameloblastoma.** (**1**) Large radiolucency. (**2**) Resorption of the molar roots caused by pressure of the tumor.

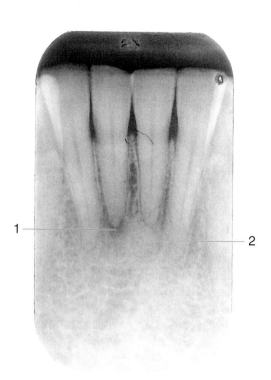

FIGURE 23-32 **Periapical cemental dysplasia (PCD).** (**1**) Early PCD (radiolucent). (**2**) Late stage of development (radiopaque). The teeth are vital.

ligaments of fully developed and erupted teeth. Early PCD is radiolucent and appears identical to radicular cysts. In the later stages of development, PCD appears as radiopaque masses surrounded by a radiolucent line (Figure 23-32). PCD occurs more frequently in middle-aged females than males. The teeth are vital, and the condition needs no treatment.

Radiographic Appearance of Nonodontogenic Tumors

The majority of tumors found in the head and neck region do not have a characteristic radiographic appearance that enables a diagnosis from the radiograph alone. In fact, a diagnosis of a **tumor** cannot be made until the dentist, the pathologist, and the radiologist have combined their findings. However, the oral health care professional may be the first to detect the presence of a lesion and make the appropriate referral.

Tumors are classed as **benign** (doing little or no harm) and **malignant** (very dangerous or life threatening). Fortunately, most tumors detected in the oral health care practice are benign. Careful examination of the radiograph can often help to differentiate benign from malignant lesions.

Benign tumors may be either radiolucent or radiopaque, with well-defined margins. Malignant tumors tend to have irregular margins and are less distinct, blending into the adjacent bone.

Exostoses and tori are the most frequently encountered forms of benign tumors. An **exostosis** is a localized overgrowth of bone. The term **torus** (plural tori) is often used to describe an exostosis that occurs near the midline of the palate (torus palatinus; Figure 23-16) and on the lingual surface of the mandible (torus mandibularis; see Figures 22-26 and 22-27). Radiographically, both appear as an area of increased radiographic density (radiopaque).

The two main types of oral malignancies are **carcinoma** and **sarcoma.** Both grow rapidly and spread into adjacent tissues. Carcinomas are malignant tumors of epithelial origin, and sarcomas are malignant tumors of connective tissue origin. The

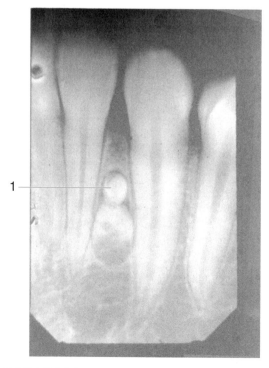

FIGURE 23-31 **Odontoma.** (**1**) Consisting of small, misshaped teeth located within a radiolucent fibrous capsule.

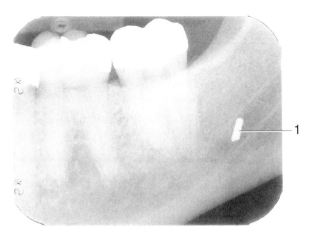

FIGURE 23-33 **Foreign object.** (**1**) Broken dental bur, which probably lodged here when it was used during removal of the third molar.

radiographic appearance of these tumors is radiolucent, with irregular and poorly defined borders. Sarcomas often have a "patchy" appearance with no demarcation from normal surrounding bone. Radiographs are vitally important in early detection because sarcomas produce changes in bone early in their development.

Radiographic Appearance of Trauma

The two most common injuries observed on dental radiographs are fractures of facial bones and teeth. **Fracture lines** are thin radiolucent lines that demarcate the region of bone or tooth separation (Figure 23-10). Fractures may on occasion have a similar appearance to the nutrient canals described in Chapter 22.

Radiographs will sometimes reveal the presence of **foreign bodies.** Note the broken dental instrument imaged in Figure 23-33.

REVIEW—Chapter summary

The dental hygienist and dental assistant should possess the ability to recognize deviations from the normal. Developing this skill requires practice. Although identifying deviations from the normal radiographically is important, a diagnosis cannot be made from the radiograph alone. Common radiographic observations that the dental hygienist and dental assistant should be able to identify radiographically include the appearance of restorative materials, developmental anomalies, periapical pathology and other pathological conditions, and the effects of trauma.

Metallic restorative materials such as amlagam, metal crowns, retention pins, post and core, and silver points appear radiopaque and are distinguished from each other by their size and shape. Nonmetallic restorative materials such as composite, porcelain, base material, and gutta percha appear less radiopaque than metal. Composite materials, may appear slightly radiopaque or radiolucent.

Developmental anomalies that may be recorded on radiographs include anodontia, supernumerary teeth, mesiodens, dens in dente, hypercementosis, dilaceration, taurodontia, gemination, and fusion.

Periapical abscesses, granulomas, and cysts all appear radiolucent and cannot be distinguished from each other radiographically.

Radiographs may record external and internal tooth resorption. Radiographic evidence of calcifications and ossifications include pulp stones, sialoliths, rhinoliths, phleboliths, condensing osteitis, and osteosclerosis.

Although tumors may not be diagnosed from radiographs alone, the presence of ameloblastomas, odontomas, periapical cemental dysplasia (PCD), and benign and malignant tumors may be detected radiographically.

Fractures of the tooth and bone and foreign objects may be detected radiographically.

RECALL—Study questions

1. Amalgam and a full metal crown can be distinguished from each other radiographically by their
   a. degree of radiopacity.
   b. shape and margins.
   c. location in the mouth.
   d. use of retention pins.

2. Which of these dental restorative materials appears most radiopaque?
   a. Amalgam
   b. Porcelain
   c. Silicate
   d. Acrylic resin

3. Which of these dental restorative materials is most likely to mimic decay radiographically?
   a. Gold
   b. Stainless steel
   c. Amalgam
   d. Composite

4. Dens in dente appears radiographically as a
   a. Tiny tooth.
   b. Large tooth.
   c. Twin tooth.
   d. Tooth within a tooth.

5. A sharp bend in the tooth root is called
   a. taurodontia.
   b. hypercementosis.
   c. dilaceration.
   d. exostosis.

6. Radiographically, it is not possible to accurately differentiate between a periapical abscess, a granuloma, and a cyst.
   Radiographically, it is not possible to accurately differentiate between carcinoma and sarcoma.
   a. The first statement is true. The second statement is false.
   b. The first statement is false. The second statement is true.
   c. Both statements are true.
   d. Both statements are false.

7. Which of these appears radiolucent on a radiograph?
   a. Sialolith
   b. Abscess
   c. Torus
   d. Odontoma

8. A large radiolucency surrounding the crown only of an unerupted tooth is most likely what type of cyst?
   a. Dentigerous
   b. Radicular
   c. Residual
   d. Periapical

9. The evidence of resorption that appears to shorten the tooth root is called
   a. internal resorption.
   b. external resorption.
   c. primary resorption.
   d. secondary resorption.

10. The radiographic appearance of a small ovoid radiopacity within the pulp chamber of the tooth is called a
    a. rhinolith.
    b. phlebolith.
    c. pulp stone.
    d. pulp cap.

11. Which of the following appears radiolucent in its early stages and as a radiopaque mass in later stages?
    a. Condensing osteitis
    b. Periapical granuloma
    c. Osteosclerosis
    d. Periapical cemental dysplasia (PCD)

12. Which of the following tumors appears radiolucent radiographically?
    a. Torus palatinus
    b. Odontoma
    c. Sarcoma

13. Radiographic evidence of a bone fracture appears as a radiolucent line that may resemble a
    a. nutrient canal.
    b. cyst.
    c. tumor.
    d. retained root tip.

REFLECT—Case study

You have just accepted a position in a large oral health care clinic at a university-based dental school, where your primary role will be to process, mount, and prepare a preliminary interpretation of full mouth series of radiographs taken on incoming patients. You know how valuable it is to follow a systematic order when mounting films, so you decide to apply an orderly system to interpreting the radiographs as well.

Design a form that will guide you and other radiographers through the interpretive process. Your form should include the following:

1. A place to record basic information (the patient's name, date the radiographs were exposed, name of the person interpreting the radiographs, date of interpretation, etc.).
2. A step-by-step guide for where to begin and end the interpretive process.
3. A list of common conditions or deviations from normal that you will be looking for. (Organize the conditions you will be interpreting logically.)
4. Organize the conditions according to what you will examine the radiographs for first, second, third, etc.
5. Prepare columns, rows of boxes, or whatever your design requires as a place to record or list the condition.
6. Label the columns, rows of boxes, or whatever your design uses, with the appropriate headings.
7. Prepare a place to document that the condition needs a referral to the dentist.
8. Prepare your form in such a manner that other professionals may be able to utilize the form. Prepare written instructions for utilizing the form as needed.

RELATE—Laboratory application

For a comprehensive laboratory practice exercise on this topic, see Thomson, E. M. (2012). *Exercises in oral radiography techniques: A laboratory manual* (3rd ed.). Upper Saddle River, NJ: Pearson. Chapter 14, "Radiographic interpretation."

REFERENCES

Farman, A. G., Nortje, C. J., & Wood, R. E. (1993). *Oral and maxillofacial diagnostic imaging.* St. Louis, MO: Mosby.

Hatrick, C. D., Eakle, W. S., & Bird, W. F. (2010). *Dental materials: Clinical applications for dental assistants and dental hygienists* (2nd ed.). St. Louis, MO: Elsevier.

Langlais, R. P. (2003). *Exercises in oral radiology and interpretation* (4th ed.). Philadelphia: Saunders.

Langlais, R. P., Langland, O. E., & Nortje, C. J. (1995). *Diagnostic imaging of the jaw.* Philadelphia: Williams & Wilkins.

White, S. C., & Pharoah, M. J. (2008). *Oral radiology: Principles and interpretation* (6th ed.). St. Louis, MO: Elsevier.

The Use of Radiographs in the Detection of Dental Caries

OBJECTIVES

Following successful completion of this chapter, you should be able to:

1. Define the key words.
2. Explain why caries appear radiolucent on radiographs.
3. Define the role radiographs play in detecting caries.
4. Identify the ideal type of projection, technique, and exposure factors that enhance a radiograph's ability to image caries.
5. List and describe the four categories of the caries depth grading system.
6. List the four locations of dental caries and identify their radiographic appearance.
7. Define and identify the radiographic appearance of recurrent dental caries.
8. List three conditions that resemble dental caries radiographically and discuss how to distinguish these from caries.

KEY WORDS

Advanced caries
Arrested caries
Buccal caries
Caries
Cemental (root) caries
Cementoenamel junction (CEJ)
Cervical burnout
Dentinoenamel junction (DEJ)
Incipient (enamel) caries
Interproximal

Interproximal caries
Lingual caries
Mach band effect
Moderate caries
Nonmetalic restoration
Occlusal caries
Proximal caries
Rampant caries
Recurrent (secondary) caries
Severe caries

Introduction

The detection of caries (tooth decay) is probably the most common reason for exposing dental radiographs. The dental hygienist or dental assistant who is skilled in identifying normal radiographic anatomy should be able to differentiate between the appearance of normal tooth structures and dental caries on a radiograph.

The purpose of this chapter is to describe the radiographic appearance of dental caries, identify a caries depth grading system, and offer some tips that may influence caries interpretation (Procedure Box 24-1).

Dental Caries

Description

Dental caries, or tooth decay, is a pathological process consisting of localized destruction of dental hard tissues by organic acids produced by microorganisms. The caries process is one of demineralization of tooth structure (enamel, dentin, cementum). This demineralization of tooth density allows more x-rays to pass through the tooth and darken the image. Therefore, **caries** appear radiolucent on the radiograph (Figure 24-1).

Detection

Radiographs reveal carious lesions that may go undetected clinically, especially caries on the proximal surfaces (in between the teeth; Table 24-1). To be a useful diagnostic aid, the radiographs must be precisely exposed and meticulously processed. Improper angulation can render a radiograph worthless for caries detection. Incorrect vertical angulation may prevent the radiograph

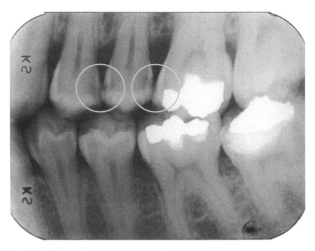

FIGURE 24-1 Proximal surface caries found just apical to the contact area between two adjacent teeth.

from imaging caries (Figure 24-2). The horizontal angulation is particularly important. Overlapping of the contact areas between the teeth will make it impossible to detect caries in these areas (Figure 24-3).

The bitewing radiograph, described in Chapter 16, is the radiograph of choice for the evaluation of caries due to the precise parallelism established between the tooth and the plane of the image receptor. However, a precisely placed periapical radiograph exposed using the paralleling technique will adequately image dental caries (Figure 24-4).

Although the exposure factors (mA, kVp, and time) used will depend on the patient and the area to be exposed, some

---

PROCEDURE 24-1
Radiographic interpretation for caries

1. See Procedure Box 21-2, Suggested Sequence for Viewing a Full Mouth Series of Radiographs.
2. View all surfaces of each tooth.
3. Examine the contact points and just apical to the estimated gingival margin (soft tissue will not be imaged on the radiograph) for radiolucencies indicating proximal caries.
4. Examine the dentin just apical to the occlusal enamel for radiolucencies indicating occlusal caries.
5. Examine the dentin in the middle of the tooth for a round radiolucency indicating buccal/facial or lingual caries.
6. If there is bone loss and evidence that cementum is exposed in the oral cavity, examine the cervical region of the tooth for an ill-defined, radiolucent crescent-shaped area below the cementoenamel junction (CEJ) indicating cemental (root) caries.
7. Examine existing restorations for recurrent decay.
8. Confirm findings and/or clarify uncertain interpretations with a clinical examination of the patient.
9. Consult the patient's chart for confirmation or clarification of findings as needed.
10. Present a preliminary interpretation for the dentist's review.
11. Following confirmation by the dentist, document all findings on the patient's permanent record.

TABLE 24-1   Radiographic Appearance of Caries

GRADE	SEVERITY	PROXIMAL	OCCLUSAL	BUCCAL/LINGUAL	CEMENTAL
C-1	Incipient	Radiolucent notch in the enamel only. Radiolucency is less than halfway through the enamel.	Not evident radiographically.	Not evident radiographically.	Not applicable.
C-2	Moderate	Radiolucent triangle with the apex pointing toward the DEJ. Radiolucency is more than halfway through the enamel, but does not invade the DEJ.	Not evident radiographically.	Not evident radiographically.	Not applicable.
C-3	Advanced	Radiolucency takes on a double triangle shape, first through the enamel with the apex pointing toward the DEJ and a second triangle base spreading along the DEJ with the apex pointing toward the pulp. Radiolucency is less than halfway through the dentin toward the pulp.	Flat radiolucent line, often with no or little change detected in the enamel. Radiolucency is less than halfway through the dentin toward the pulp.	Not possible to distinguish advanced from severe. Both appear as a round radiolucency in the middle of the tooth with well-defined borders.	Although enamel is not involved in this type of caries, at this stage an ill-defined, radiolucent, cresent-shaped area below the cementoenamel junction (CEJ) may be observed. Bone loss must be evident.
C-4	Severe	Radiolucency may retain a double triangle shape, or be so severe as to appear as a large diffuse radiolucency. Radiolucency is more than halfway through the dentin toward the pulp.	Large radiolucency detected in the dentin below the occlusal enamel. Depending on the extent of destruction, radiolucent breaks in the occlusal enamel may be imaged. Radiolucency is more than halfway through the dentin toward the pulp.	Not possible to distinguish advanced from severe. Both appear as a round radiolucency in the middle of the tooth with well-defined borders.	Although enamel is not involved in this type of caries, at this stage an ill-defined, radiolucent, crescent-shaped area below the cementoenamel junction (CEJ) may be observed. Bone loss must be evident.

practitioners prefer to use a lower kVp to best image caries. A low setting, such as 60 kVp (with direct current x-ray equipment), will result in a high-contrast image: black and white with few shades of gray in between. Because caries appear radiolucent against a radiopaque enamel (or lesser radiopaque dentin), a high-contrast image is preferred by some practitioners for imaging carious lesions.

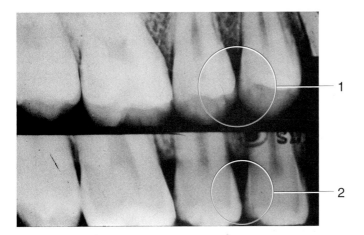

FIGURE 24-2 Vertical angulation. (**1**) Excessive vertical angulation prevents viewing this proximal surface carious lesion. (**2**) Proper vertical angulation shows the proximal surface caries. Note the difference in alveolar bone crest heights between the two radiographs indicating a change in the vertical angulation.

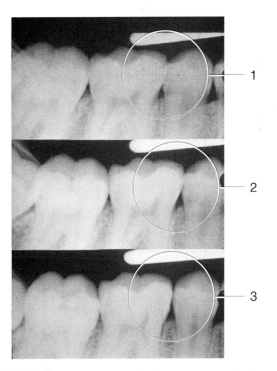

FIGURE 24-3 Horizontal angulation. (**1**) Incorrect horizontal angulation causes overlapping between adjacent teeth, which prevents viewing for interproximal caries. (**2**) Improved horizontal angulation, but caries difficult to view. (**3**) Correct horizontal angulation clearly images caries.

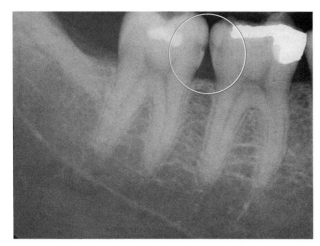

FIGURE 24-4 Periapical radiograph records proximal surface caries.

Interpreting Dental Caries

Dental caries is a process of decalcification and requires 40 to 50 percent loss of calcium and phosphorus before the decreased density can be seen on a radiograph. For this reason, the depth of penetration of a carious lesion is deeper clinically than it appears on the radiograph. Also, because the proximal surfaces of posterior teeth are broad, the loss of small amounts of mineral from incipient lesions may be difficult to see on the radiograph (Figure 24-5).

Caries Depth Grading System

Several systems are used to grade the depth of penetration of caries. This text will use a grading system suggested by Hauge-jorden and Slack, 1977 (Figure 24-6). The advantage of this system is that it allows one to accurately grade the penetration of caries (establish a baseline) and to track the progression

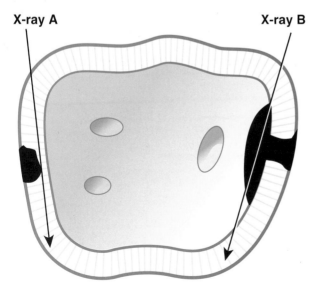

FIGURE 24-5 Drawing showing ratio of caries to enamel. **X-ray A** passing through a small ratio of caries to enamel, resulting in the caries being difficult to view. **X-ray B** passing through a large ratio of caries to enamel, results in the caries being easier to view.

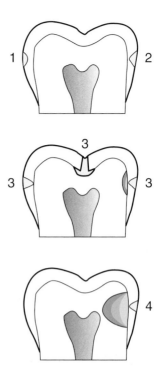

FIGURE 24-6 Diagram of classification of dental caries recommended by Haugejorden and Slack. (**1**) **C-1 caries.** Less than halfway through the enamel (incipient caries). (**2**) **C-2 caries.** Penetrate over halfway through the enamel (moderate caries). (**3**) **C-3 caries.** At or through the dentinoenamel junction (DEJ), but less than halfway through the dentin toward the pulp (advanced caries). (**4**) **C-4 caries.** Penetrate over halfway through the dentin toward the pulp (severe caries).

and/or remineralization of the carious lesions at future appointments. These grades may also be called incipient, moderate, advanced, or severe.

- **C-1: Enamel caries,** also called **incipient caries** (meaning the first stage of existence), penetrate less than halfway through the enamel of the tooth toward the **dentinoenamel junction (DEJ)** (Figure 24-6, 1).
- **C-2: Moderate caries,** penetrating over halfway through the enamel toward the dentinoenamel junction (DEJ), but not reaching the DEJ. Moderate caries are only seen in the enamel (Figure 24-6, 2).
- **C-3: Advanced caries** are of enamel and dentin at or through the dentinoenamel junction (DEJ), but less than halfway through the dentin toward the pulp (Figure 24-6, 3). Advanced caries are seen in both the enamel and dentin.
- **C-4: Severe caries** are of enamel and dentin penetrating over halfway through the dentin toward the pulp (Figure 24-6, 4). Severe caries are seen in both the enamel and the dentin.

Classification of the Radiographic Appearance of Caries

The radiographic appearance of caries may be classified according to their location on the tooth.

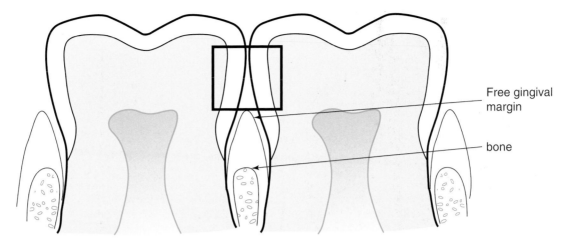

FIGURE 24-7 Drawing indicating the area to examine for interproximal caries. View the area where two adjacent teeth contact, and apical down to where the gingival margin would most likely be (boxed area). Avoid mistaking caries in the region apical to the gingival margin, where the optical illusion cervical burnout is most likely to be appear.

There are four locations on the tooth that caries occur:

1. Proximal (mesial and distal)
2. Occlusal
3. Buccal/lingual
4. Cemental (root surface)

Caries may be categorized as recurrent, rampant, or arrested.

Radiographs are often prescribed to detect proximal surface caries. Occlusal, buccal/lingual, and cemental caries are more readily detected clinically than with radiographs. In fact, early (incipient and moderate) occlusal, buccal/lingual, and cemental caries often do not show up on radiographs, even though these may be detected clinically. However, moderate and severe occlusal, buccal/lingual, and cemental caries will appear radiographically, so it is important that the radiographer recognize these.

Proximal Caries

Interproximal means between two adjacent surfaces. On dental radiographs, **proximal surface caries,** often referred to as **interproximal caries,** are located on the tooth surface that contacts the adjacent tooth. The interproximal is an area that is almost impossible to examine clinically, making the use of radiographs vitally important in caries detection. The tooth surface should be examined for caries at the point of contact and just apical to this point of contact to the gingival margin (Figure 24-7). The location of the height of the gingival margin, which is soft tissue, is not imaged on the radiograph. So the gingival margin location is estimated based on where the alveolar bone crest height is imaged. Assume that the gingival margin will be located at least 1 mm above the level of bone imaged on the radiograph.

The shape of proximal caries begins as a radiolucent notch on the enamel (C-1; Figure 24-6, 1). As the demineralization of enamel progresses, caries takes on a triangular shape (like a pyramid) with the apex pointing toward the dentinoenamel junction (DEJ) and the base toward the outer surface of the

tooth (C-2; Figure 24-6, 2). At the DEJ the caries spreads, undermining normal enamel, and again takes on a triangular shape as it penetrates toward the pulp (C-3; Figure 24-6, 3). The base of this second triangle is along the DEJ and the apex points toward the pulp (C-4; Figure 24-6, 4).

Occlusal Caries

Occlusal caries are located on the chewing surface of the posterior teeth. Because of the superimposition of the buccal and lingual cusps, occlusal caries in early stages (incipient and moderate) may not be imaged on a radiograph (Figure 24-6, 3, and Figure 24-8), even when a clinical examination does detect incipient or moderate occlusal caries.

After occlusal caries has reached the DEJ (advanced caries), it may be imaged on the radiograph (Figures 24-9 and 24-10). At the DEJ occlusal caries will appear as a flat radiolucent line. Often no or little change is detected in the enamel radiographically at this stage. As demineralization progresses, the size of the radiolucency increases. It is important to note that when examining radiographs for occlusal caries, the area of interest is below

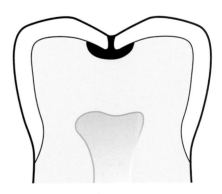

FIGURE 24-8 Drawing of occlusal caries, early stage. Early occlusal caries (C-1 and C-2) extend along the dentinoenamel junction (DEJ) and may not be seen on the radiograph, even though the lesion may be detected clinically.

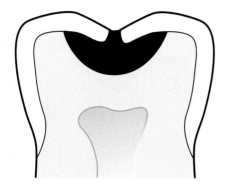

FIGURE 24-9 **Drawing of advanced occlusal caries.** Advanced (up to halfway toward the pulp) or severe occlusal caries (more than halfway toward the pulp) will most likely be imaged radiographically.

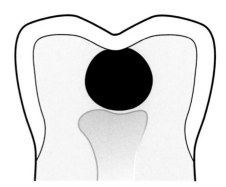

FIGURE 24-11 **Drawing of buccal or lingual caries.** Advanced buccal or lingual caries have well-defined borders.

the occlusal enamel, in the area of the dentin, and not from the top of the tooth. The irregularity of the cusps and occlusal surface pits and fissures do not usually indicate the presence of caries. Changes (radiolucencies) in the dentin below the occlusal enamel are indicative of occlusal caries. As advanced caries progress to a severe stage, changes in the occlusal enamel are more likely to be imaged as the crown of the tooth begins to break down.

Buccal and Lingual Caries

Buccal caries involves the buccal or facial surface of a tooth, and **lingual caries** involves the lingual surface (Figure 24-11). Buccal and lingual caries are best detected clinically. Early buccal and lingual carious lesions are almost impossible to detect radiographically. This is due to the superimposition of the normal tooth structures over the caries. As the demineralization becomes severe, the caries appears as a radiolucency characterized by well-defined borders, often described as looking into a hole on the radiograph (Figure 24-12). However, because the radiograph is a two-dimensional image of three-dimensional structures, it is

impossible to tell the depth of buccal or lingual caries or the relationship to the pulpal tissue.

Cemental (Root) Caries

Cemental caries (also known as **root caries**) develop between the enamel border and the free margin of the gingiva on the cemental surface (Figure 24-13). Bone loss and recession of the gingival tissue are necessary for the caries' process to start on the root surfaces. Cemental caries may appear on the buccal, lingual, mesial, or distal surface of the tooth.

Radiographically, cemental caries appear as an ill-defined, radiolucent, crescent-shaped area just below the **cementoenamel junction (CEJ;** Figure 24-14). Cemental caries may at times be misinterpreted as cervical burnout (discussed later in this chapter), an optical illusion of the radiographic image. Cemental caries are more easily detected clinically than radiographically.

Recurrent (Secondary) Caries

Recurrent or **secondary caries** is decay that occurs under a restoration or around its margins. Recurrent caries often occur

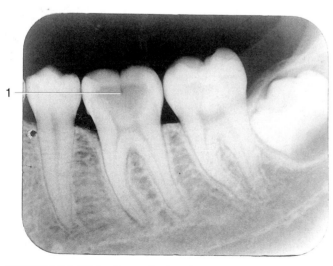

FIGURE 24-10 **Radiograph of occlusal caries. (1)** Severe occlusal caries appearing as a large radiolucent lesion in the first molar.

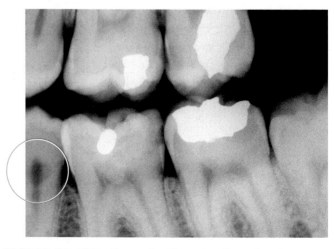

FIGURE 24-12 **Radiograph of buccal or lingual caries** on this mandibular second premolar appears as a round radiolucency (superimposed over the pulp chamber).

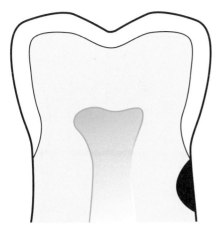

FIGURE 24-13 Drawing of cemental (root) caries illustrates involvement of only the roots of teeth. Gingival recession and bone loss precede the demineraliztion process to expose the root surfaces.

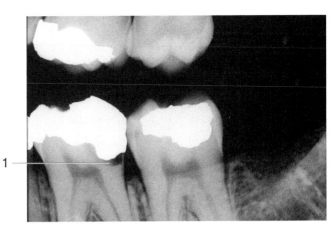

FIGURE 24-15 Radiograph of recurrent caries. (1) Radiolucent caries under the metallic restoration.

because of poor cavity preparation, defective margins of the restoration, or incomplete removal of the caries prior to the placement of the restoration. Recurrent caries appears on a radiograph as a radiolucent area beneath a restoration or apical to the interproximal margin of a restoration (Figure 24-15).

Rampant Caries

The term *rampant* means growing rapidly or spreading unchecked. **Rampant caries** are severe, unchecked caries that affect multiple teeth (Figure 24-16).

Arrested Caries

The term *arrested* means stopped or inactive. **Arrested caries** are caries that are no longer active. Carious lesions may become arrested if there is a significant shift in the oral environment from factors that cause caries to those that slow down the caries' process. Incipient enamel caries (C-1) can

Demineralization ~~proces~~ exceeded remineralization

remain dormant for long periods of time. Some carious lesions may even be reversed by remineralization. It is important that radiographic exams continue to monitor arrested caries.

Conditions Resembling Caries

Three conditions that resemble caries are **nonmetallic restorations, cervical burnout,** and **mach band effect.**

Nonmetallic Restorations

Nonmetallic esthetic restorations may mimic decay radiographically (Figure 24-17). Nonmetallic restorations such as composite, silicate, and acrylic resin, discussed in Chapter 23, may mimic decay when they appear radiolucent. To aid in distinguishing a restoration from caries, look for the restoration to have straight borders, or a prepared look, with an overall even

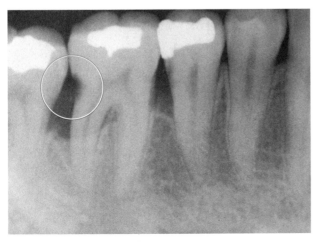

FIGURE 24-14 Radiograph of cemental (root) caries. The large radiolucency on the distal surface of the distal root of the first mandibular molar is cemental caries. Note the bone loss exposing the root surface.

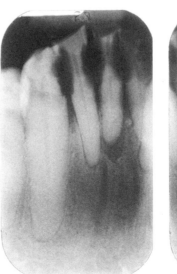
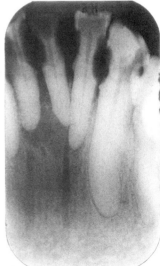

FIGURE 24-16 Radiographs of rampant caries. Multiple teeth affected by severe cemental caries.

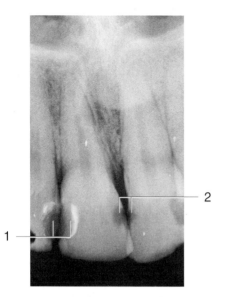

FIGURE 24-17 Radiograph of nonmetalic restorations and carious lesions in anterior teeth. (**1**) Radiolucent nonmetallic restorations on the mesial surface of the lateral incisor and distal surface of the central incisor. Note that under both restorations is a base of radiopaque material. (**2**) The radiolucencies on the mesial surfaces of both central incisors are carious lesions.

radiolucency. A radiopaque base material may also be present under the radiolucent nonmetallic restoration. Caries tend to have more diffuse borders and an uneven radiolucency that takes on a triangular shape, with the apex pointing toward the DEJ or pulp. A clinical examination may be required to make a final determination.

Cervical Burnout

Cervical burnout is an optical illusion created when the eye must distinguish between a very light (white) area and a very

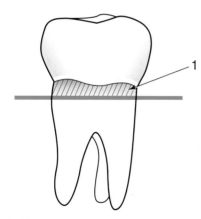

FIGURE 24-18 Drawing of cervical burnout. (**1**) Thin cervical root surface between dense crown and alveolar bone crest allows more x-rays to pass and reach the image receptor. This cervical area of the teeth will most likely be imaged at an increased radiolucency.

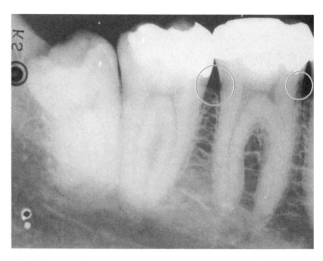

FIGURE 24-19 Radiograph demonstrating cervical burnout. Note the radiolucent optical illusion of cervical burnout on the mesials and distals between the enamel and restorations and the alveolar crest of bone.

dark (black) area on the radiograph. The area of the tooth most likely to produce this optical illusion is the cervical root, or neck of the tooth. In this region, the concavity of the root surfaces allows greater penetration by the x-rays (Figure 24-18). This region will appear especially dark next to radiopaque structures. When the radiopaque enamel on one side and the radiopaque lamina dura on the other side sandwich the radiolucent cervical of the tooth in between, the effect is an increased darkness called cervical burnout. Cervical burnout often appears as an irregularly shaped radiolucent area with a fuzzy outline seen on the mesial and/or the distal surfaces of the tooth along the cervical line (Figure 24-19). To assist in distinguishing cervical burnout from caries, remember to focus caries detection only in the area of the contact point of adjacent teeth and apical to the gingival margin (Figure 24-7). Cervical burnout appears more apical, apparently under the gingival margin.

Mach Band Effect

Another optical illusion is a radiolucency caused by overlapping images of the teeth. When two proximal surfaces overlap (caused either by natural overlap of misaligned teeth or by improper horizontal angulation of the x-ray beam), the result is a dense radiopaque area surrounded by radiolucent lines. These radiolucent lines represent an optical illusion called the **mach band effect,** resulting from the high contrast between the normal enamel and the dense overlapped enamel (Figure 24-20). The ability of these overlapped structures to produce this optical illusion illustrates how important it is to produce radiographs that do not have angulation errors.

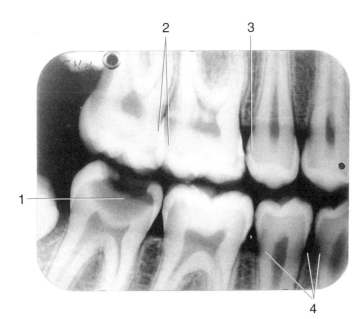

FIGURE 24-20 Caries and optical illusions that mimic decay.
(**1**) Severe occlusal caries. (**2**) Radiolucent lines creating a mach band effect caused by overlapped enamel. (**3**) Incipient distal surface caries. (**4**) Cervical burnout.

REVIEW—Chapter summary

The detection of caries is often the most common reason for taking dental radiographs. Caries appear radiolucent because the demineralization of the tooth allows more x-rays to pass through to reach the image receptor. Only precisely exposed and meticulously processed radiographs are useful in detecting caries.

Detecting proximal surface caries is the main purpose of bitewing radiographs. Carefully positioned periapical radiographs, exposed using the paralleling technique, are also valuable in detecting proximal surface caries. Some practitioners prefer a high-contrast image (produced with a low kVp) for detecting caries. Radiographs detect more proximal surface caries than a clinical exam alone. A clinical exam is better at detecting early occlusal, buccal/lingual, and cemental caries. The depth of the caries penetration is deeper clinically than it appears on the radiograph.

An example of a caries depth grading system is presented. These grades may also be referred to as incipient, moderate, advanced, and severe caries.

The radiographic appearance of caries may be classified according to their location on the tooth: proximal, occlusal, buccal/lingual, and cemental (root surface). Three conditions that resemble caries are nonmetallic restorations, cervical burnout, and mach band effect.

RECALL—Study questions

1. Caries appear radiopaque, *because* more radiation is passing through the demineralization than the surrounding tissues.
   - a. The first part of the statement is true, but the second part of the statement is false.
   - b. The first part of the statement is false, but the second part of the statement is true.
   - c. Both parts of the statement are true.
   - d. Both parts of the statement are false.

2. Each of the following will produce an ideal radiographic image for detecting caries EXCEPT one. Which one is the EXCEPTION?
   - a. Bitewing radiographs
   - b. Periapical radiographs
   - c. Horizontal angulation that avoids overlapping
   - d. Excessive vertical angulation

3. Caries in the earliest stage is called
   - a. incipient.
   - b. moderate.
   - c. advanced.
   - d. severe.

4. Radiographs are best at detecting incipient caries of which of these locations on the tooth?
   - a. Occlusal
   - b. Proximal
   - c. Buccal/lingual
   - d. Cemental

5. The key to successfully interpretating radiographs for proximal surface caries is to examine the contact point between adjacent teeth and just apical to the
   - a. DEJ.
   - b. CEJ.
   - c. estimated gingival margin.
   - d. alveolar bone crest.

6. Proximal surface carious lesions appear
   - a. triangular.
   - b. square.
   - c. round.
   - d. crescent-shaped.

7. Which of the following appears radiographically as a radiolucent notch that is less than half-way through the enamel?
   - a. Incipient proximal caries
   - b. Moderate proximal caries
   - c. Advanced proximal caries
   - d. Severe proximal caries

8. Which of the following appears radiographically as a radiolucent double triangle that is less than halfway through the dentin toward the pulp?

    a. Incipient proximal caries

    b. Moderate proximal caries

    c. Advanced proximal caries

    d. Severe proximal caries

9. The key to successfully interpretating radiographs for occlusal caries is to examine

    a. the occlusal surface for changes in the pits and fissures.

    b. under the occlusal surface for changes in the dentin.

    c. the contact point between adjacent teeth for changes in the enamel.

    d. just apical to the contact point for changes in the DEJ.

10. Which of the following appears radiographically as a round radiolucency in the middle of the tooth with well-defined borders?

    a. Proximal caries

    b. Occlusal caries

    c. Cemental caries

    d. Buccal/lingual caries

11. Which of the following appears radiographically as an ill-defined crescent-shaped radiolucency below the CEJ?

    a. Proximal caries

    b. Occlusal caries

    c. Cemental caries

    d. Buccal/lingual caries

12. Caries that occur under a restoration or around its margins are called

    a. recurrent caries.

    b. cemental caries.

    c. root caries.

    d. buccal caries.

13. Each of the following may mimic caries radiographically EXCEPT one. Which one is the EXCEPTION?

    a. Composite restorations

    b. Stainless stain crowns

    c. Cervical burnout

    d. Mach banding

14. An optical illusion created by an increased radiolucency observed at the cervical area of the tooth is called mach banding.

The mach banding effect increases when overlap error occurs.

    a. The first statement is true. The second statement is false.

    b. The first statement is false. The second statement is true.

    c. Both statements are true.

    d. Both statements are false.

REFLECT—Case study

You are interpreting a full mouth series of radiographs on a patient who had dental hygiene services at your facility this morning. The completed patient's dental examination chart is available, but the patient has been dismissed. As you examine the radiographs, you notice the following:

1. Incipient proximal caries on the distal of the maxillary right first molar.

    a. Describe the radiographic appearance of this lesion.

    b. Indicate why you classified this lesion as incipient.

2. Moderate proximal caries on the mesial of the maxillary left first premolar.

    a. Describe the radiographic appearance of this lesion.

    b. Indicate why you classified this lesion as moderate.

3. Advanced proximal caries on the mesial of the mandibular left second premolar.

    a. Describe the radiographic appearance of this lesion.

    b. Indicate why you classified this lesion as advanced.

4. Severe proximal caries on the distal of the mandibular right first molar.

    a. Describe the radiographic appearance of this lesion.

    b. Indicate why you classified this lesion as severe.

5. Advanced occlusal caries on the maxillary right second molar.

    a. Describe the radiographic appearance of this lesion.

    b. Indicate why you classified this lesion as advanced.

6. Cemental caries on the mesial of the mandibular right first premolar.

    a. Describe the radiographic appearance of this lesion.

    b. Indicate why you classified this lesion as cemental.

7. The patient's chart indicates incipient occlusal caries detected clinically on the maxillary left first and second molars. However, these do not seem to be evident radiographically.

    a. Explain why these caries are not observed on the radiographs.

8. The patient's chart indicates incipient buccal caries detected clinically on the mandibular left first molar. However, this lesion does not seem to be evident radiographically.

    a. Explain why the buccal caries is not observed on the radiographs.

9. The radiographs reveal two radiolucencies resembling cemental (root) caries around the cervical of the mandibular right first and second premolars. However, the patient's chart does not indicate that cemental caries were detected clinically.

    a. Explain the possible cause of these radiolucencies.

10. The periapical radiograph of the maxillary left molar region is overlapped between the maxillary first and second molars.
    a. Explain why detecting caries in this area will be compromised.
    b. What optical illusion will most likely present in this area?
    c. Describe the appearance of this optical illusion.

RELATE—Laboratory application

For a comprehensive laboratory practice exercise on this topic, see Thomson, E. M. (2012). *Exercises in oral radiography techniques: A laboratory manual* (3rd ed.). Upper Saddle River, NJ: Pearson. Chapter 14, "Radiographic interpretation."

REFERENCES

Berry, H. (1983). Cervical burnout and mach band: Two shadows of doubt in radiologic interpretation of carious lesions. *Journal of the American Dental Assocication, 106,* 622.

Langlais, R. P., & Kasle, M. J. (1992). *Exercises in oral radiographic interpretation* (3rd ed.). Philadelphia: Saunders.

Langlais, R. P., Langland, O. E., & Nortje, C. J. (1995). *Diagnostic imaging of the jaws.* Philadelphia: Williams & Wilkins.

Langlais, R. P. (2003). *Exercises in oral radiology and interpretation* (4th ed.). Philadelphia: Saunders.

White, S. C., & Pharoah, M. J. (2008). *Oral radiology: Principles and interpretation* (6th ed.). St. Louis, MO: Elsevier.

The Use of Radiographs in the Evaluation of Periodontal Diseases

CHAPTER OUTLINE

OBJECTIVES

Following successful completion of this chapter, you should be able to:

1. Define the key words.
2. List the uses of radiographs in the assessment of periodontal diseases.
3. Differentiate between horizontal and vertical bone loss.
4. Identify three local contributing factors for periodontal disease that radiographs can help locate.
5. Explain how imaging anatomical configurations aids in the prognosis of periodontally involved teeth.
6. List the limitations of radiographs in the assessment of periodontal diseases.
7. Recognize the role vertical and horizontal angulations play in imaging periodontal diseases.
8. Use the appropriate radiographic techniques to best detect and evaluate periodontal diseases.
9. Describe the radiographic appearance of the normal periodontium.
10. List four American Academy of Periodontology disease classification case types, and describe their radiographic appearance.

KEY WORDS

Alveolar (crestal) bone
Calculus
Cementoenamel junction (CEJ)
Furcation involvement
Generalized bone loss
Gingivitis
Horizontal bone loss
Interdental septa
Lamina dura
Local contributing factor

Localized bone loss
Occlusal trauma
Pathogen
Periodontal diseases
Periodontal ligament space
Periodontitis
Periodontium
Triangulation
Vertical (angular) bone loss
Vertical bitewing series

Introduction

Dental radiographs play a key role in the diagnosis, prognosis, management and evaluation of periodontal diseases. Properly exposed and meticulously processed radiographs are invaluable aids in the diagnosis of periodontal diseases. To get the most diagnostic information from radiographs taken to image periodontal status, radiographers should have an extensive knowledge of the radiographic techniques that will produce quality images. The purpose of this chapter is to introduce the dental radiographer to the radiographic appearance of periodontal diseases, to outline the radiographic examinations and techniques best suited to produce quality radiographs for the purpose of evaluating periodontal diseases, and to describe local contributing factors for the disease that radiographs help to identify.

Radiographic Appearance of Periodontal Diseases

Periodontal diseases are diseases that affect both soft tissues (gingiva) and bone around the teeth. The severity of periodontal disease may range from a simple inflammation of the gingiva to the destruction of supporting bone and the periodontal ligament. The most common periodontal diseases are gingivitis and periodontitis. **Gingivitis** is inflammation of the gingiva and limited to the soft tissue (gingiva). **Periodontitis** is also the result of infection, but includes loss of **alveolar bone.**

The proper diagnosis and evaluation of periodontal diseases must be made with a combination of radiographic and clinical examinations.

Radiographic Examination

Uses (Box 25-1)

Radiographs, along with a thorough clinical examination, allow the dentist and dental hygienist to evaluate and document periodontal diseases. The uses of radiographs in the assessment of periodontal diseases include the following:

1. **Imaging supporting bone.** Radiographs allow the practitioner to evaluate crestal bone irregularities and **interdental septa** changes (alveolar bone changes between the teeth). Radiographs document the amount of bone remaining rather than the amount lost. The amount of bone loss is estimated as the difference between the physiologic bone level and the height of the remaining bone (Figure 25-1).

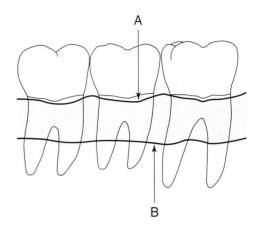

FIGURE 25-1 Drawing illustrating horizontal bone loss. **(A)** Normal (physiologic) level of bone (alveolar bone parallel to the cementoenamel junction) and **(B)** Bone level of patient with periodontal disease. Horizontal bone loss is the difference between **(A)** and **(B)** (shaded area).

Radiographs also allow the practitioner to determine the pattern of bone loss; horizontal or vertical. **Horizontal bone loss** describes height loss around adjacent teeth in a region. In horizontal bone loss, both buccal and lingual plates have been resorbed as well as the intervening interdental bone. Horizontal bone loss occurs in a plane parallel to the **cementoenamel junctions (CEJ)** of adjacent teeth (Figure 25-2). **Vertical bone loss,** sometimes called **angular bone loss,** occurs in a vertical direction where the resorption of one tooth root sharing the interdental septum (bone between the teeth) is greater than the other tooth (Figures 25-3, 25-4, and 25-5).

Radiographs can help the practitioner determine the distribution of bone loss: localized or generalized. **Localized bone loss** occurs in local areas and involves one or only a few teeth. **Generalized bone loss** occurs throughout the entire dental arches.

BOX 25-1   Periodontal Bone Changes Recorded by Radiographs

- Crestal irregularities
- Interdental alveolar bone changes
- Pattern of bone loss (horizontal/vertical)
- Distribution of bone loss (localized/generalized)
- Severity of bone loss (slight, moderate, advanced)
- Furcation involvement

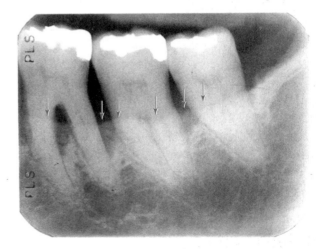

FIGURE 25-2 Horizontal bone loss. Arrows show bone level of patient with periodontal disease. Note that the level of bone loss is parallel to an imaginary line drawn between the cementoenamel junctions of the adjacent teeth.

Vertical bone loss

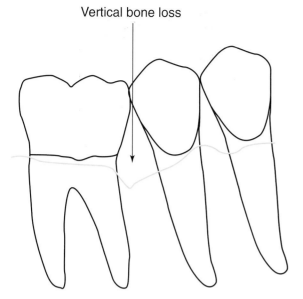

FIGURE 25-3 Drawing illustrating vertical bone loss. Vertical bone loss appears angular where the resorption is greater on the side of one tooth than on the side of the adjacent tooth.

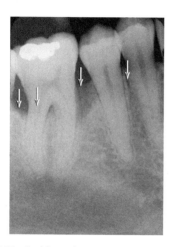

FIGURE 25-4 Vertical bone loss. Arrows show bone level of patient with periodontal disease.

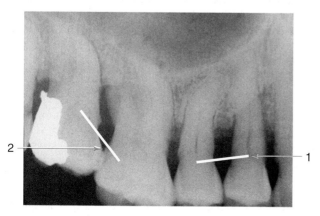

FIGURE 25-5 Comparison of horizontal and verical bone loss. Use the CEJ of adjacent teeth as a guideline. (1) Horizontal bone loss. (2) Vertical bone loss.

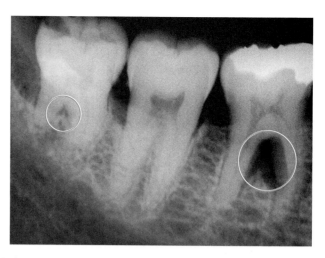

FIGURE 25-6 Furcation involvement. Note the radiolucency in between the roots of these multirooted teeth.

Radiographs can reveal the severity of bone loss—slight, moderate, or advanced—and **furcation involvement** (bone loss between the roots) of multirooted teeth (Figure 25-6).

2. **Imaging local contributing factors.** Radiographs can detect conditions such as amalgam overhangs (see Chapter 23), poorly contoured crown margins, and calculus deposits that act as traps that can lead to the buildup of bacterial **pathogens** that cause periodontal diseases (Figures 25-7 and 25-8). **Calculus,** essentially hardened plaque, appears slightly radiopaque (about the radiopacity of dentin) and must be significantly calcified to be recorded on radiographs. Depending on the density and the amount of the deposit, calculus may appear as pointed or irregular projections on the proximal root surfaces, or as a ringlike radiopacity around the cervical neck of a tooth.

Radiographs often reveal the effects of traumatic occlusion, another contributing factor for periodontal disease. **Occlusal trauma** does not cause periodontal disease, but has been shown to hinder the body's response to the disease. The effects of excessive occlusal forces show up

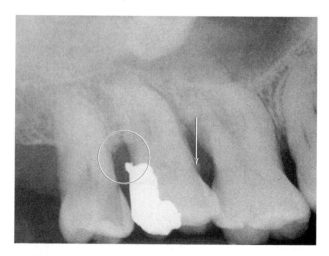

FIGURE 25-7 Local contributing factors. Calculus (arrow) and amalgam overhang (circled) are likely to collect bacterial pathogens that can contribute to the progression of periodontal diseases.

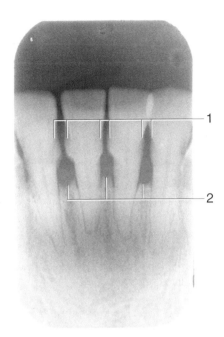

FIGURE 25-8 Calculus. (1) large deposits around the necks of the teeth. **(2)** Height of alveolar bone remaining as a result of periodontal disease.

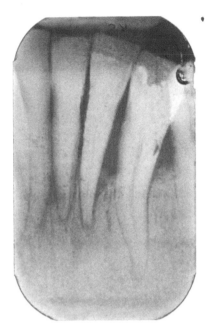

FIGURE 25-10 Root length and root-to-crown ratio. Although the bone loss observed on this radiograph is significant, the longer than normal, dilacerated root improves the prognosis for the canine.

on radiographs as a widening of the periodontal ligament space (Figure 25-9), called **triangulation.** Triangulation is bordered by the lamina dura and the root surface of the tooth, with its base toward the tooth crown.

3. **Imaging anatomical configurations.** Radiographs can reveal information about root morphology and lengths and the presence of dilacerations (see Chapter 23); root shape and width, such as multirooted teeth with ample supporting bone in between the roots; or narrow, close, or fused roots, all of which can help determine the treatment and predict treatment outcomes. For example, a tooth with a shortened root as a result of external resorption (see Chapter 23) will have a poor prognosis, whereas a tooth with a normal or long root may have a better prognosis (Figure 25-10). Additionally, teeth that have ample bone surrounding widely spaced roots will

be more likely to have a better prognosis because of the amount of bone support.

4. **Evaluating the prognosis and treatment intervention needs.** By providing information on the tooth root-to-crown ratio, and adjacent tooth proximity, radiographs help the practitioner plan treatment and predict outcomes.

5. **Serving as a baseline and as a means for evaluating the results of treatment.** Radiographs provide documentation on the progression of disease and provide a permanent record of the condition of the bone throughout the course of the disease and treatment.

Limitations

1. **Radiographs are a two-dimensional image of three-dimensional objects.** Radiographs lack the third dimension of depth, which results in bone and tooth structures being superimposed over each other. This will often hide bone loss on the buccal and lingual surfaces and furcation area, especially in the posterior region of the oral cavity.

2. **Changes in soft tissue not imaged.** Because soft tissue is not recorded on radiographs, gingivitis cannot be detected radiographically. Radiographs do not add any information regarding the location and/or depth of periodontal pockets.

3. **Cannot distinguish treated versus untreated disease.** Radiographs do not indicate the presence or absence of active disease.

4. **Actual destruction more advanced clinically.** Radiographs cannot detect early signs of periodontal diseases. A significant loss of bone density must occur before radiographic changes are detected.

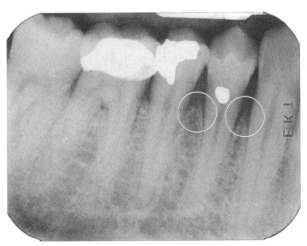

FIGURE 25-9 Triangulation. Widening of the periodontal ligament space indicative of occlusal trauma.

Radiographic Techniques

Bitewings, especially the **vertical bitewing series** of anterior and posterior radiographs described in Chapter 16, are most useful for examining the **periodontium** (Figure 25-11). The precise parallelism established between the tooth and the plane of the image receptor when taking bitewing radiographs makes it possible to image the alveolar crestal bone accurately. To achieve this same degree of accuracy when using periapical radiographs to image the periodontium, the paralleling technique must be used. The image receptor must be placed parallel to the long axis of the teeth to ensure that the images of the bone and teeth on the radiograph are not distorted.

To be a useful diagnostic aid, the radiographs must be precisely exposed and meticulously processed. Incorrect angulation can render a radiograph worthless for evaluating periodontal disease. Excessive vertical angulation may not reveal bone loss, whereas inadequate vertical angulation may result in a radiographic image that falsely indicates bone loss when there is none (Figures 25-12 and 25-13).

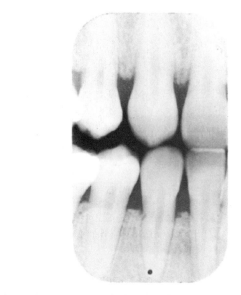

A

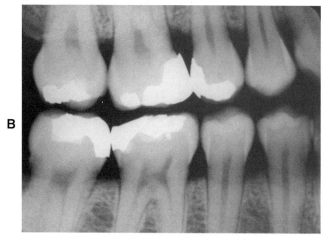

B

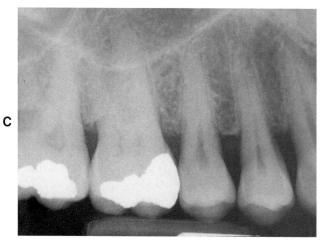

C

FIGURE 25-11 Comparsion of bitewing and periapcial radiographs imaging the periodontium. (A) Vertical bitewing. **(B)** Horizontal bitewing. **(C)** Periapical.

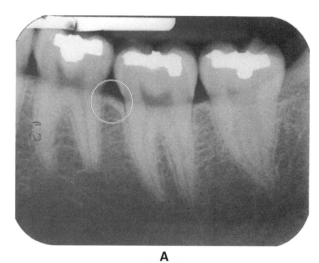

A

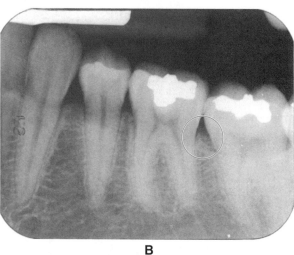

B

FIGURE 25-12 Correct and incorrect vertical angulation. (A) Correct vertical angulation accurately records crestal bone indicating no bone loss between the mandibular first and second molars. **(B)** Incorrect vertical angulation produces a radiolucent, cupping-out appearance of the lamina dura falsely indicating bone loss between these same teeth. (Thomson, E. M., & Tolle, S. L. (1994). A practical guide for using radiographs in the assessment of periodontal diseases. Part 2: Interpretation and future advances. *Journal of Practical Hygiene, 3*(2), 12. Permission from Montage Media.)

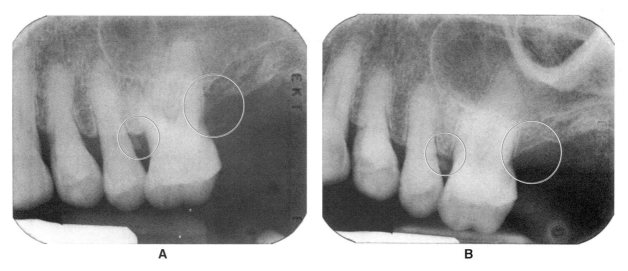

FIGURE 25-13 Correct and incorrect vertical angulation. (A) Correct vertical angulation accurately records crestal bone indicating bone loss mesial and distal to the maxillary first molar,. **(B)** Incorrect vertical angulation produces a false appearance to the level of bone in these same areas. (Thomson, E. M., & Tolle, S. L. (1994). A practical guide for using radiographs in the assessment of periodontal diseases. Part 2: Interpretation and future advances. *Journal of Practical Hygiene, 3*(2), 12. Permission from Montage Media.)

Accurate horizontal angulation is also important in evaluating periodontal disease. Incorrect horizontal angulation results in overlapping of the contact areas between the teeth, making it impossible to determine the condition of interdental bone (bone in between the teeth). Second, varying the horizontal angulation slightly may actually increase the chances of imaging interdental defects and furcation involvement. For example, a bitewing series of seven radiographs (discussed in Chapter 16) and a full mouth series of multiple periapical and bitewing radiographs (discussed in Chapter 14) will contain images that were produced with different horizontal angles. The varying angulations used allow for multiple views of the condition of the periodontium (Figure 25-14).

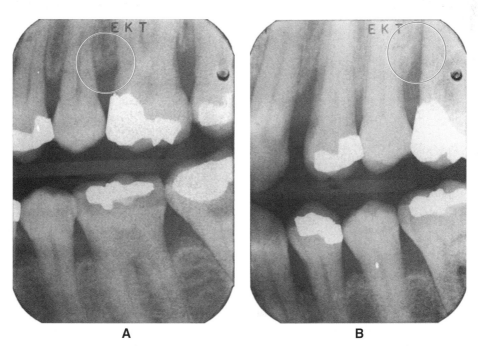

FIGURE 25-14 Example of varying horizontal angulation. (A) Correct horizontal angulation, but image does not reveal the vertical (angular) defect on the mesial of the maxillary first molar. **(B)**. Slightly varied horizontal angulation of the same region now reveals the vertical bony defect. (Thomson, E. M., & Tolle, S. L. (1994). A practical guide for using radiographs in the assessment of periodontal diseases. Part 2: Interpretation and future advances. *Journal of Practical Hygiene, 3*(2), 13. Permission from Montage Media.)

PROCEDURE 25-1
Radiographic interpretation for periodontal disease

1. See Procedure Box 21-2, Suggested Sequence for Viewing a Full Mouth Series of Radiographs.
2. View all surfaces of each tooth.
3. Note the alveolar bone height. Use the CEJ as a reference point. Measure with a probe as needed (see Figure 21-5).
4. Examine the periodontal ligament space, following it around the entire tooth. Note widening, triangulation.
5. Examine the furcation area of multirooted teeth.
6. Identify local contributing factors such as restoration overhangs and calculus.
7. Confirm findings and/or clarify uncertain interpretations with a clinical examination of the patient.
8. Consult the patient's chart for confirmation or clarification of findings as needed.
9. Present a preliminary interpretation for the dentist's review.
10. Following confirmation by the dentist, document all findings on the patient's permanent record.

Although the exposure factors (mA, kVp, and time) used will depend on the patient and the area to be exposed, some practitioners prefer to use a higher kVp to best image subtle bone changes. A higher setting, such as 90 kVp, will result in an image that has a low contrast: black and white with many shades of gray in between. Because bone changes that accompany periodontal diseases appear as a radiolucency within the radiopaque bone, a low-contrast image is preferred by some practitioners for imaging these early signs of bone destruction.

Radiographic Interpretation of Periodontal Diseases

The dental radiographer should be familiar with the radiographic appearance of the normal periodontium to be able to identify deviations from normal that may indicate possible periodontal diseases (Procedure Box 25-1). The American Academy of Periodontology classifies periodontal disease based on etiologic factors of the disease and tissue response to treatment. Four classifications of periodontal disease are described, based on changes in the periodontium as seen on radiographs (Table 25-1).

Case Type I: Gingivitis

Radiographs do not image soft tissue, and therefore the radiographic appearance of the periodontium in all types and severities of gingivitis appears the same as normal bone. The **lamina dura** (dense cortical plate of the bony tooth socket) appears as an unbroken, dense radiopaque line around the roots of the teeth. The alveolar crest is located 1.5 to 2.0 mm apical to the cementoenamel junctions (CEJ) of the teeth (Figure 25-15). In the anterior region of the oral cavity, the

TABLE 25-1   American Academy of Periodontal Disease Classification

CLASSIFICATION	RADIOGRAPHIC APPEARANCE[a]
Case Type I: Gingivitis	*Alveolar crest:* Unbroken, radiopaque at a level 1.5–2.0 mm below and parallel to the CEJ
	Anterior: Pointed *Posterior:* Flat, smooth
Case Type II: Slight Chronic Periodontitis	*Alveolar crest:* Loss of density with slight radiolucencies evident; triangulation observed
	Anterior: Blunted *Posterior:* Fuzzy, cupping-out appearance
Case Type III: Moderate Chronic or Aggressive Periodontitis	*Alveolar crest:* Level greater than 2.0 mm below the CEJ, indicating 30–50 percent bone loss
	Anterior and posterior: Horizontal and/or vertical patterns of bone loss observed
	Posterior: Furcation radiolucencies evident
Case Type VI: Advanced Chronic or Aggressive Periodontitis	*Alveolar crest:* Easily identified with level of bone loss greater than 50 percent
	Anterior and Posterior: Evidence of tooth position changes, drifting

[a]*Source:* Perry, D. A., Beemsterboer, P., & Taggart, E. J. (2007). *Periodontology for the dental hygienist* (3rd ed.). St. Louis, MO: Elsevier.

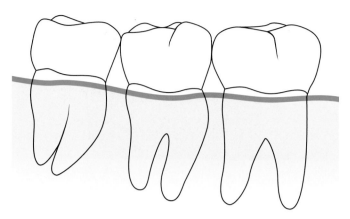

FIGURE 25-15 Drawing illustrating Case Type I: Gingivitis. Alveolar crest located 1.5 to 2.0 mm apical to the cementoenamel junctions (CEJ) of the teeth.

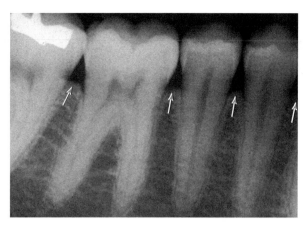

FIGURE 25-17 Case Type I: Gingivitis-posterior region. Note the normal radiopaque flat appearance of the lamina dura and thin radiolucent line of the periodontal ligament space.

alveolar crest appears pointed and sharp (Figure 25-16). In the posterior region of the oral cavity, the alveolar crest is more flat, smooth, and parallel to an imaginary line drawn between adjacent CEJ (Figure 25-17). The **peridontal ligament space** appears as a thin radiolucent line between the lamina dura and the root of the tooth.

Case Type II: Slight Chronic Periodontitis

Early bone loss up to 30 percent is evident (Figure 25-18). Loss of crestal bone density that often appears as a fuzzy cupping-out of the alveolar crest is the first radiographic indication of periodontal disease (Figure 25-19). The alveolar crest appears blunted in the anterior region of the oral

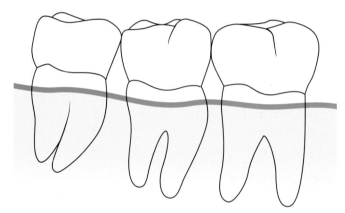

FIGURE 25-18 Drawing illustrating Case Type II: Slight Chronic Periodontitis.

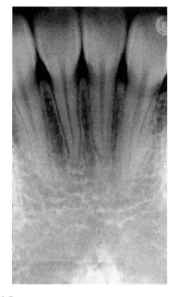

FIGURE 25-16 Case Type I: Gingivitis-anterior region. Note the normal pointed radiopaque appearance of the lamina dura and thin radiolucent line of the periodontal ligament space.

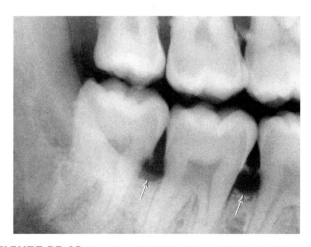

FIGURE 25-19 Case Type II: Slight Chronic Periodontitis-posterior region. Note the slight radiolucent cupping-out of the lamina dura, especially visible between the mandibular first and second molars. Radiopaque calculus is visible on the proximal surfaces of the teeth.

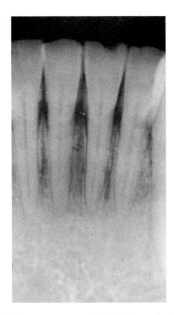

FIGURE 25-20 Case Type II: Slight Chronic Periodontitis-anterior region. Note the blunting of the lamina dura and slight radiolucent widening of the periodontal ligament space. Slightly radiopaque calculus is visible.

cavity (Figure 25-20). In the posterior region of the oral cavity triangulation, a widening of the periodontal ligament space becomes evident at the mesial or distal surfaces of the teeth.

Case Type III: Moderate Chronic or Aggressive Periodontitis

Moderate bone loss (30 to 50 percent) may appear in both the horizontal and vertical planes (Figures 25-21 and 25-22). As the bone levels resorb, radiolucencies may appear in the furcations of multirooted teeth. (Figure 25-23).

Case Type IV: Advanced Chronic or Aggressive Periodontitis

The advanced stage of periodontal disease (greater than 50 percent bone loss) is characterized radiographically by severe horizontal and/or vertical bone loss, evidence of furcation

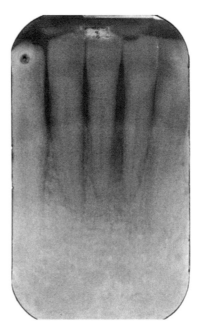

FIGURE 25-22 Case Type III: Moderate Chronic or Aggressive Periodontitis-anterior region. Note the 30–50 percent bone level resorption.

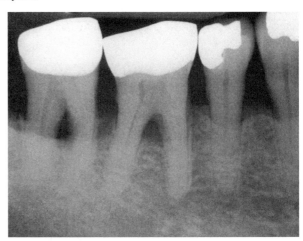

FIGURE 25-23 Case Type III: Moderate Chronic or Aggressive Periodontitis-posterior region. Note the 30–50 percent bone level resorption and radiolucency in the furca of the mandibular molars indicating furcation involvement.

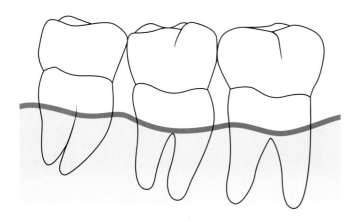

FIGURE 25-21 Drawing illustrating Case Type III: Moderate Chronic or Aggressive Periodontitis.

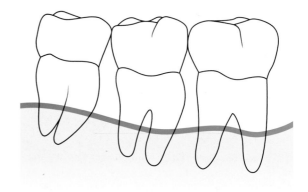

FIGURE 25-24 Drawing illustrating Case Type IV: Advanced Chronic or Aggressive Periodontitis.

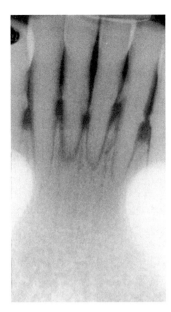

FIGURE 25-25 Case Type IV: Advanced Chronic or Aggressive Periodontitis-anterior region. Note the 50 percent or greater bone level resorption.

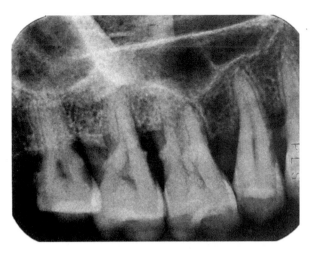

FIGURE 25-26 Case Type IV: Advanced Chronic or Aggressive Periodontitis-posterior region. Note the 50 percent or greater bone level resorption and obvious furcation involvement.

involvement, widened periodontal spaces, and indications of changes in tooth position (Figures 25-24 through 25-26).

REVIEW—Chapter summary

Periodontal diseases are diseases that affect both soft tissues (gingivitis) and bone around the teeth (periodontitis). Properly exposed and meticulously processed radiographs play a key role in the diagnosis and evaluation of periodontal diseases.

The uses of radiographs in the evaluation and treatment of periodontal diseases include imaging the supporting bone, locating local contributing factors, imaging anatomical configurations, evaluating prognosis and treatment intervention needs, and serving as a baseline for identifying and documenting the progression of the disease and the results of treatment. Radiographs are limited in their ability to image periodontal diseases because they are two-dimensional pictures of three-dimensional teeth and supporting bone; changes in soft tissue are not imaged; treated disease cannot be distinguished from untreated disease, and the actual destruction of bone is more clinically advanced than what is revealed on radiographs.

The ideal radiographs for imaging periodontal diseases are bitewings, particularly vertical bitewings, or periapical radiographs exposed by the paralleling technique. Some practitioners prefer low-contrast images produced with a high kVp for detecting subtle changes in the bone.

Radiographs are important aids in identifying changes in the periodontium and can assist in classifying various stages of periodontal disease. The dental hygienist and the dental assistant should possess a working knowledge of normal radiographic appearance of the periodontium to be able to recognize deviations from normal that indicate periodontal disease.

RECALL—Study questions

1. Each of the following may be determined from a dental radiograph EXCEPT one. Which one is the EXCEPTION?
   a. Bone loss
   b. Pocket depth
   c. Furcation involvement
   d. Local contributing factors

2. List four uses of radiographs in the assessment of periodontal diseases.
   a. _____
   b. _____
   c. _____
   d. _____

3. Which of the following terms describes bone loss that occurs in a plane parallel to the cementoenamel junction of adjacent teeth?
   a. Irregular
   b. Vertical
   c. Horizontal
   d. Periapical

4. Significant bone loss that results in a radiolucency observed in the area between the roots of multirooted teeth is called
   a. localized bone loss.
   b. interdental septa.
   c. local contributing factor.
   d. furcation involvement.

5. Radiographs may help to locate each of the following local contributing factors EXCEPT one. Which one is the EXCEPTION?
   a. Calculus
   b. Poorly contoured crown margin
   c. Deep pocket
   d. Amalgam overhang

6. Excessive occlusal force may result in a widening of the periodontal ligament space.

   Widening of the periodontal ligament space is called furcation involvement.

   a. The first statement is true. The second statement is false.
   b. The first statement is false. The second statement is true.
   c. Both statements are true.
   d. Both statements are false.

7. Dental radiographs are important because they document the location and depths of periodontal pockets.

   Dental radiographs may serve as a baseline and as a means for evaluating the outcomes of periodontal treatments.

   a. The first statement is true. The second statement is false.
   b. The first statement is false. The second statement is true.
   c. Both statements are true.
   d. Both statements are false.

8. List four limitations of dental radiographs in the assessment of periodontal diseases.

   a. _____
   b. _____
   c. _____
   d. _____

9. Which of the following would be best for imaging a slight, but generalized periodontal status?

   a. Select periapical radiographs using the bisecting technique.
   b. Select periapical radiographs using the paralleling technique.
   c. Posterior horizontal bitewing radiographs.
   d. Posterior and anterior vertical bitewing radiographs.

10. Correct horizontal angulation is needed to accurately image interdental bone levels.

    Altering the horizontal angulation can reveal additional information regarding interdental bone levels.

    a. The first statement is true. The second statement is false.
    b. The first statement is false. The second statement is true.
    c. Both statements are true.
    d. Both statements are false.

11. Alveolar crests pointed in the anterior region and a radiopaque flat, smooth lamina dura 1.5 to 2.0 mm below the CEJ in the posterior region describes

    a. Case Type I: Gingivitis
    b. Case Type II: Slight Chronic Periodontitis
    c. Case Type III: Moderate Chronic or Aggressive Periodontitis
    d. Case Type IV: Advanced Chronic or Aggressive Periodontitis

12. Radiolucent changes observed on a radiograph such as a fuzzy, cupping-out of the crestal bone and a blunted appearance of the lamina dura in the anterior region describes

    a. Case Type I: Gingivitis
    b. Case Type II: Slight Chronic Periodontitis
    c. Case Type III: Moderate Chronic or Aggressive Periodontitis
    d. Case Type IV: Advanced Chronic or Aggressive Periodontitis

REFLECT—Case study

Describe what radiographic changes in the periodontium you would expect to observe on a seven-image series of vertical bitewing radiographs on the following patients classified according to the American Academy of Periodontology Disease Classification:

1. Case Type I: Gingivitis
2. Case Type II: Slight Chronic Periodontitis
3. Case Type III: Moderate Chronic or Aggressive Periodontitis
4. Case Type IV: Advanced Chronic or Aggressive Periodontitis

RELATE—Laboratory application

For a comprehensive laboratory practice exercise on this topic, see Thomson, E. M. (2012). *Exercises in oral radiography techniques: A laboratory manual* (3rd ed.). Upper Saddle River, NJ: Pearson Education. Chapter 14, "Radiographic interpretation."

REFERENCES

Langlais, R. P. (2003). *Exercises in oral radiology and interpretation* (4th ed.). Philadelphia: Saunders.

Perry, D. A., Beemsterboer, P., & Taggart, E. J. (2007). *Periodontology for the dental hygienist* (3rd ed.). St. Louis, MO: Elsevier.

Thomson, E. M., & Tolle, S. L. (1994). A practical guide for using radiographs in the assessment of periodontal disease, Part 2: Interpretation and Future Advances. *Practical Hygiene 3*, 2.

White, S. C., & Pharoah, M. J. (2008). *Oral radiology: Principles and interpretation* (6th ed.). St. Louis, MO: Elsevier.

Radiographic Techniques for Children

OBJECTIVES

Following successful completion of this chapter, you should be able to:

1. Define the key words.
2. State the basis for prescribing dental radiographs for children.
3. List the conditions that would indicate radiographs be taken on children.
4. Identify suggested exposure intervals for the child patient.
5. List the factors that determine the number and size of image receptors to be exposed on children.
6. List image receptor size and type suggested for use with primary dentition.
7. List image receptor size and type suggested for use with transitional (mixed primary and permanent) dentition.
8. Identify two types of extraoral radiographs that may be acceptable substitutes for children who cannot tolerate intraoral image receptor placement.
9. Identify adaptations or modifications in standard paralleling and bisecting techniques that aid in radiographic procedures for children.
10. Explain the role occlusal radiographs play in imaging children.
11. Appropriately adjust standard adult exposure settings to apply to children.
12. Explain the roles that the patient management techniques show-tell-do and modeling play in assisting the radiographer with child patient management.
13. Interpret radiographs taken on children with primary and transitional (mixed primary and permanent) dentition.

KEY WORDS

ALARA (as low as reasonably achievable)
Anodontia
Exfoliation
Lateral jaw projection (mandibular oblique lateral projection)
Modeling
Panoramic radiograph
Pediatric dentistry
Permanent teeth
Primary teeth
Show-tell-do
Supernumerary teeth
Transitional mixed dentition

Introduction

Children have the same basic needs for oral health care as do adults. In fact, the best time to prevent dental problems is in childhood. Children are at a higher risk for caries that progress more rapidly than in adults. Radiographs play an important role in both detecting disease and assessing growth and development for the child patient.

Radiographic techniques and the types of projections used to image the oral cavity of the child patient do not differ significantly from those used for adult patients. However, the child patient presents with unique characteristics such as a smaller oral cavity and behavioral considerations that often require adaptations to standard procedures. The purpose of this chapter is to discuss ways the radiographer can adapt these standard techniques to best image the child's smaller and sometimes more sensitive oral cavity. These adaptations, along with behavior modification strategies can assist the radiographer in gaining the confidence of the child patient to produce the highest quality diagnostic images using the least amount of radiation exposure.

Assessment of Radiographic Need

The indication to expose dental radiographs on a child patient is based on the individual needs of the patient. The evidence-based selection criteria guidelines, discussed in Chapter 6, have categories for assessing children and adolescents as well as adults (see Table 6-1). Indications for exposing radiographs for the child patient include the detection of caries and periodontal diseases; the assessment of growth and development and the need for orthodontic intervention; the detection of congenital dental abnormalities, such as **anodontia** (absence of teeth) and **supernumerary** (extra) **teeth;** the evaluation of third molars; the diagnosis of pathologic conditions such as an abscess or other infection; and the assessment of the effect of trauma, such as a fall or accident, not only for **primary teeth,** but for the developing, unerupted **permanent teeth** as well.

Suggested Exposure Intervals

The American Academy of Pediatric Dentistry (**pediatric dentistry**—*pedia* is Greek for child—is the branch of dentistry that specializes in providing comprehensive preventive and therapeutic oral health care for children), and other oral health and medical organizations, recommend that a child's first professional oral examination be made within 12 months following the eruption of the first primary tooth, usually between six and twelve months of age. Early prevention is key to preventing tooth loss and developing good oral self-care habits. At this early age the teeth can usually be visually inspected clinically without the need for radiographs. Unless an accident, toothache, or other unusual circumstance causes a need for radiographs, the selection criteria guidelines discussed in Chapter 6 (see Table 6-1) suggest that the first radiographic survey may not be necessary until all the primary teeth have erupted, preventing a visual inspection of the proximal (contact) surfaces via a clinical inspection. Patients without evidence of disease and with open interproximal contacts may not require a radiographic exam. Once the teeth have erupted

in such a manner that the proximal surfaces can no longer be viewed clinically, and caries are suspected, or the patient presents with high risk factors for caries, such as poor oral self-care or inadequate fluoride protection, radiographs may be indicated.

Image Receptor Sizes and Numbers and Types of Projections

Once it has been determined that radiographs are needed, the child's age, size of the oral cavity, and cooperation level must be considered when determining the size and number of radiographs to expose (Box 26-1). Although a size #0 or #1 intraoral image receptor is usually used for radiographs of a child with primary teeth, the preferred size for **transitional mixed dentition,** where the child presents with a mix of both primary and permanent teeth, is a standard size #2 image receptor. The radiographer should use the largest size image receptor that the child can tolerate. The amount of radiation required does not change with different sizes of intraoral image receptors. Using a size #2 image receptor whenever possible instead of a size #0 or size #1 will provide more information due to the coverage of a larger area. This is particularly important when imaging permanent teeth that are developing. The choice of image receptor size should be individualized based on anatomical limitations and tissue sensitivity. To aid with accurate and comfortable positioning, a smaller-size film packet should be selected rather than bending the larger-size film, and a smaller-size digital sensor or phosphor plate would be more likely retained in position for the duration of the exposure.

The number of image receptors required depends on the needs of the individual (see Table 15-1). When exposing bitewing radiographs on a child patient prior to the eruption of the permanent second molar, two horizontal posterior bitewings, one on each side, is recommended. Following eruption of the permanent second molar, four horizontal (or vertical if periodontal disease is suspected) posterior bitewings must be taken to image all proximal contacts of the posterior teeth without overlap.

If conditions exist that require additional exposures, the following radiographic full mouth surveys are offered as suggestions.

BOX 26-1 Considerations for Choosing the Number and Size of Image Receptor to Expose on the Child Patient

- Oral health needs
- Willingness to cooperate
- Attention span and emotional state
- Ability to understand and follow directions
- Ability to hold still throughout the exposure
- Size of the opening to the oral cavity
- Size and shape of the teeth and the dental arches
- Sensitivity of the oral mucosa
- Operator's ability to gain patient's trust
- Operator's ability to position the image receptor
- Operator's knowledge of and skill ability to adapt standard techniques

Primary Dentition

Small oral cavity size, tongue resistance, and gagging can be a problem in small children aged three to six years old. Ideally, it is advisable to expose four radiographs, one anterior occlusal (see Chapter 17) of each arch (maxilla and mandible) and one posterior bitewing on each side (Figure 26-1).

Transitional (Mixed Primary and Permanent) Dentition

At six years, the first permanent teeth have begun to erupt. Ideally, the survey should include a minimum of twelve radiographs: ten periapical and two bitewing exposures. Periapical radiographs are exposed in each of the four molar and canine regions and in the two incisor regions (Figure 26-2).

Between 12 and 14 years of age, all the permanent teeth except the third molars have usually erupted. It is during this adolescent period that growth is rapid and metabolic changes occur that heighten the possibility of dental caries and increase the need for preventive oral hygiene care. The full mouth survey recommended for the adolescent is the same as that required for the adult patient, usually fourteen periapical and four bitewing radiographs. (See Chapters 14, 15, and 16.)

Extraoral Radiographs

The evidence-based selection criteria guidelines discussed in Chapter 6 (see Table 6-1) indicate the value of an extraoral technique called a **panoramic radiograph** (see Chapter 30) for assessing growth and development for the child in mixed dentition and for evaluating third molars in adolescents. Panoramic radiographs are often prescribed to supplement intraoral exposures. In addition, a panoramic radiograph may be an acceptable substitute when intraoral radiographs cannot be tolerated by the patient. Panoramic radiographs do not image structures with the clarity of intraoral radiographs and, therefore, do not reveal details such

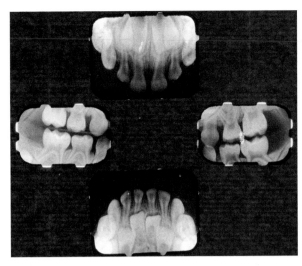

FIGURE 26-1 **Radiographic survey of primary dentition.** One anterior occlusal radiograph in each arch and one posterior bitewing radiograph on each side. (Courtesy DP Gutz, DDS, University Nebraska Medical Center, College of Dentistry, Lincoln, NE.)

as early carious lesions. However, these large radiographs are ideal for imaging overall jaw development and the eruption pattern of the teeth (Figure 26-3). The panoramic procedure is usually well tolerated by the child patient. However, the child must be able to hold still for the duration of the exposure (most panoramic machines have a 15- to 20-second exposure cycle), and the child must be able to understand and cooperate with the positioning requirements necessary for a diagnostic image (see Chapter 30).

Although largely replaced by the availability of panoramic machines in general practice, the **lateral jaw projection** (also called a mandibular oblique lateral projection; see Chapter 29) has been especially valuable to use with children (Figure 26-4). The lateral jaw radiograph is used to examine the posterior region

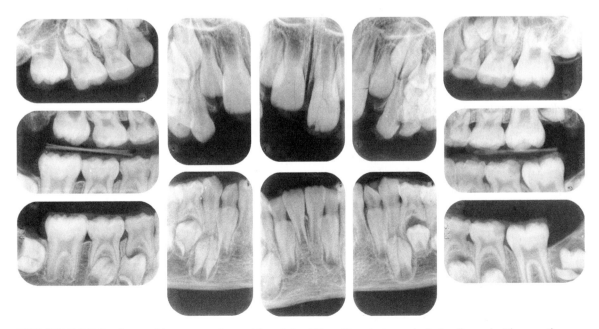

FIGURE 26-2 **Radiographic survey of transitional dentition.** Six anterior periapical radiographs (three on the maxilla and three on the mandible), one posterior periapical radiograph in each quadrant, and one posterior bitewing radiograph on each side.

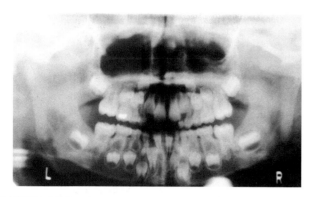

FIGURE 26-3 Panoramic radiograph of a child with transitional dentition. Note the overall jaw development and eruption pattern of the teeth.

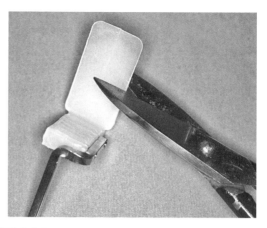

FIGURE 26-5 Modifying an image receptor holder biteblock for use with the child patient. (Thomson, E. M. (1993). Dental radiographs for the child patient. *Dental Hygiene News*, 6(4), 24, with permission from Procter & Gamble Company.)

of the mandible with patients who are unable to tolerate intraoral image receptor placement. The lateral jaw technique is described in Chapter 28.

Suggested Radiographic Techniques

Methods for exposing radiographs on children are essentially the same as those for adults. Although either the paralleling or bisecting technique can be used, the characteristics children present with usually require a slight variation in the vertical angulation. A smaller oral cavity and lowered palatal vault; the tendency toward an exaggerated gag reflex and lack of tongue and muscle control; and sensitive oral mucosa due to growth and the **exfoliation** (shedding) of primary teeth and the eruption of permanent teeth require that the radiographer be creative in improvising on the basic techniques in a manner that will produce diagnostic-quality images in the presence of these challenges.

The paralleling method is preferred for use on all patients because of its ability to produce accurate images with little distortion. The greatest challenge of using the paralleling technique with children is placing the image receptor parallel to the long axes of the teeth of interest. Switching to a smaller-sized image receptor may help with this placement. Often, it is the size and weight of the image receptor holder that the child has

difficultly tolerating. Switching to a smaller, lighter image receptor holder, modifying an adult image receptor holder, or designing a custom holder may help the child patient tolerate placement (Figures 26-5 and 26-6).

Once the image receptor is positioned, the vertical angulation may still need to be increased slightly (no more than 10 degrees) over the setting used for adult patients. Due to a shallow palatal vault, the image receptor will most likely lay flatter in position. Slightly increasing the vertical angulation over perpendicular will help to image the root apices and the unerupted developing permanent teeth (Figure 26-7).

The bisecting technique produces images with more distortion and magnification than the paralleling technique, but its greatest advantage is the ability to produce reasonably acceptable images when parallel image receptor positioning is not possible. The bisecting technique with its image receptor placement (see Chapter 15) is ideal for use with the child patient.

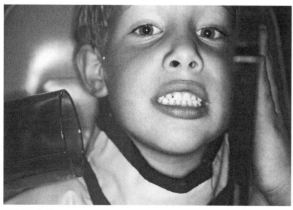

FIGURE 26-4 Lateral jaw extraoral radiograph being exposed on a child. The child holds the cassette that contains the extraoral film against the side to be imaged. The PID directs the x-ray beam under the chin up toward the cassette/film.

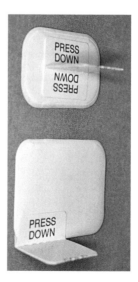

FIGURE 26-6 Adaptation of film holders for use with the child patient. Using a bitewing bitetab as a periapical film holder. (Thomson, E. M. (1993). Dental radiographs for the child patient. *Dental Hygiene News*, 6(4), 24, with permission from Procter & Gamble Company.)

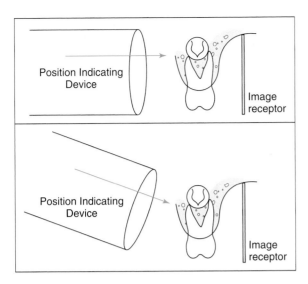

FIGURE 26-7 **Slightly increasing the vertical angulation** will image more of the unerupted developing permanent teeth and compensate for the child's lower palatal vault.

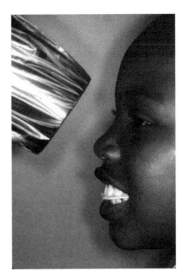

FIGURE 26-8 **Occlusal technique.** Using a size #2 film to expose a maxillary occlusal radiograph.

When the child patient cannot tolerate image receptor placement in either the parallel or the bisecting relationships, the radiographer can often use the occlusal technique to achieve reasonably acceptable images. Where an image receptor size #4 is utilized for occlusal radiographs for adults, an intraoral film size #2 or the equivalent sized digital sensor or phosphor plate can be used with children (Figure 26-8). The flat image receptor placement is usually readily accepted by the child patient. The angulation used for the occlusal technique for children differs slightly from the angles used for adults (Table 26-1).

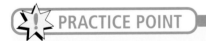

PRACTICE POINT

Children can easily understand the directive to bite on the image receptor as if it were a graham cracker. Occluding on the flat positioning of a size #2 image receptor placed for an occlusal projection is readily accepted by the child patient. It will be up to the radiographer to have the knowledge and skills to align the x-ray beam to produce an acceptable quality radiograph.

ALARA Radiation Protection

The child's smaller size places radiation-sensitive tissues closer to the path of the primary beam of radiation. It is imperative that a lead/lead equivalent apron and thyroid collar be placed over all patients, including children. Child-sized lead/lead-equivalent protective barriers are available commercially; some are decorated with cartoon figures, making these especially child-friendly. Other **ALARA** (as low as reasonably achievable; see

Chapter 6) protocols that apply to adult patients also apply to children. These include the use of fast film or digital image receptors, x-ray beam filtration and collimating devices, and appropriate exposure settings.

As the bone structure of a child is smaller and less dense than that of an adult, less radiation is required to produce an acceptable image. The amount of radiation required for most intraoral exposures can be reduced by about one-third to one-half of that required for the same exposure on an adult patient. Reducing the mA setting (amount of radiation) or the exposure time by one-half of that used for adult exposures is appropriate for children under 10 years of age. Exposures on children between the ages of 10 and 15 years can be reduced by approximately one-third. Once the adolescent reaches 15 or 16 years of age, the exposure settings should be the same as for an adult patient.

Patient Management

Obtaining quality radiographs on children can be challenging. The radiographer must be able to communicate and explain the procedure so that the child understands what is expected. The child must be able to follow directions and cooperate with the procedure. The patient management skills of the radiographer should bring out the child's natural curiosity and eagerness to participate.

First impressions are always important and lasting. The child's first experience should be pleasant and informative. Usually it is best to greet and take the child from the reception room to the x-ray room without the parents. The child should be a willing participant in the process. Only in emergencies should a child be forced to undergo dental treatment. If necessary, it is better to postpone taking radiographs until the next visit than to cause an unpleasant experience for the child. The child can be told that they will "be bigger" next time and that the procedure will be easier now that they have "practiced" for it. Planting a positive thought is better than risking instilling a fear of dentistry.

TABLE 26-1 Recommended Techniques for the Child Patient if Radiographic Need Is Assessed

DENTITION CATEGORY	TYPE AND REGION	IMAGE RECEPTOR SIZE	NUMBER OF IMAGE RECEPTORS	IMAGE RECEPTOR PLACEMENT	VERTICAL ANGULATION	HORIZONTAL ANGULATION	POINT OF ENTRY	EXPOSURE
Primary dentition (3 to 6 years of age)	Bitewing posterior	#0 or #1	1 on each side	Align the anterior edge of image receptor to line up behind the distal half of the primary maxillary or mandibular canine; choose the most mesially located canine	+5 to +10 degrees	Direct the central rays perpendicularly through the primary first and second molar embrasure	A spot on the occlusal plane between the primary maxillary and mandibular first molars	Reduce exposure to 1/2 the exposure used for this projection on an adult
Primary dentition (3 to 6 years of age)	Occlusal anterior	#2	1 on each arch	Place long dimension of image receptor across the mouth (buccal to buccal; Figures 26-9 and 26-10)	*Maxilla:* Direct the central rays perpendicular to the imaginary bisector approximately +60 degrees. *Mandible:* Direct the central rays perpendicular to the imaginary bisector approximately −30 degrees	Direct the central rays perpendicular to patient's midsagittal plane	*Maxilla:* Through a point at the tip of the nose toward the center of the image receptor. *Mandible:* Through a point in the middle of the chin toward the center of the image receptor	Reduce exposure to 1/2 the exposure used for this projection on an adult
Transitional dentition (7 to 12 years of age)	Bitewing posterior	*Prior to eruption of the permanent second molar:* #1 or #2	*Prior to eruption of the permanent second molar:* 1 on each side	*Prior to eruption of the permanent second molar:* Align the anterior edge of image receptor to line up behind the distal half of the primary or permanent maxillary or mandibular canine; choose the most mesially located canine (Figure 26-11)		*Prior to eruption of the permanent second molar:* Direct the central rays perpendicularly through the primary first and second molar embrasure or, if erupted, the first and second premolar embrasure	A spot on the occlusal plane between the primary maxillary and mandibular first molars or, if erupted, the first and second premolars to center the image receptor within the x-ray beam	Reduce exposure to 1/2 the exposure used for this projection on an adult

		After eruption of the permanent second molar: #2	*After eruption of the permanent second molar: 2 on each side (1 premolar bitewing and 1 molar bitewing)*		+10 degrees	*After eruption of the permanent second molar: Use the same criteria as for the adult patient (see Table 16-3)*	*After eruption of the permanent second molar: Use the same criteria as the adult patient (see Table 16-3)*	Reduce exposure by 1/3 to 1/2 the exposure used for this projection on an adult
Transitional dentition (7 to 12 years of age)	Anterior periapical	#0 or #1	3 on each arch (1 central-lateral, 1 right canine, and 1 left canine)	*Maxillary central-lateral incisors:* Center the image receptor to line up behind the primary or, if erupted, permanent central and lateral incisors (Figure 26-12) *Mandibular central-lateral incisors:* Center the image receptor to line up behind the primary or, if erupted, permanent central and lateral incisors (Figure 26-13)	*Maxillary central-lateral incisors:* *Paralleling technique—*Direct the central rays toward the image receptor or perpendicularly in the vertical dimension. *Bisecting technique—*Direct the central rays toward the imaginary bisector approximately +45 to +50 degrees *Mandibular central-lateral incisors:* *Paralleling technique—*Direct the central rays toward the image receptor or perpendicularly in the vertical dimension. *Bisecting technique:* Direct the central rays toward the imaginary bisector approximately −20 to −25 degrees	*Maxillary central-lateral incisors:* Direct the central rays perpendicularly through the maxillary left and right primary or, if erupted, permanent central incisor embrasure *Mandibular central-lateral incisors:* Direct the central rays perpendicularly through the mandibular left and right primary or, if erupted, permanent central incisor embrasure	*Maxillary central-lateral incisors:* At the root tips of the central incisors to center the image receptor within the x-ray beam *Mandibular central-lateral incisors:* At the root tips of the central incisors to center the image receptor within the x-ray beam	Reduce exposure by 1/3 to 1/2 the exposure used for this projection on an adult

(Continued)

TABLE 26-1 (Continued)

DENTITION CATEGORY	TYPE AND REGION	IMAGE RECEPTOR SIZE	NUMBER OF IMAGE RECEPTORS	IMAGE RECEPTOR PLACEMENT	VERTICAL ANGULATION	HORIZONTAL ANGULATION	POINT OF ENTRY	EXPOSURE
				Maxillary canine: Center the image receptor to line up behind the primary or, if erupted, permanent canine (Figure 26-14)	*Maxillary canine: Paralleling technique*—Direct the central rays toward the image receptor perpendicularly in the vertical dimension. *Bisecting technique*—Direct the central rays toward the imaginary bisector approximately +55 to +60 degrees	*Maxillary canine:* Direct the central rays perpendicularly at the center of the canine	*Maxillary canine:* At the root tip of the canine to center the image receptor within the x-ray beam	
				Mandibular canine: Center the image receptor to line up behind the primary canine, or, if erupted, the permanent canine (Figure 26-15)	*Mandibular canine: Paralleling technique*—Direct the central rays toward the image receptor or perpendicularly in the vertical dimension. *Bisecting technique:* Direct the central rays toward the imaginary bisector approximately −25 to −30 degrees	*Mandibular canine:* Direct the central rays perpendicularly at the center of the canine	*Mandibular canine:* At the root tip of the canine to center the image receptor within the x-ray beam	
Transitional dentition (7 to 12 years of age)	Posterior periapical	#1 or #2	*Prior to eruption of the permanent second molar:* 1 in each quadrant (4 molar periapicals)	*Prior to eruption of the permanent second molars:* Maxillary molar—Align the anterior edge of image receptor to line up behind the distal half of the primary or, if erupted, permanent maxillary canine (Figure 26-16)	*Prior to eruption of the permanent second molars:* *Maxillary molar: Paralleling technique*—Direct the central rays toward the image receptor or perpendicularly in the vertical dimension *Bisecting technique*—Direct the central rays toward the imaginary bisector approximately +30 to +55 degrees	*Prior to eruption of the permanent second molars:* *Maxillary molar:* Direct the central rays perpendicularly through the primary first and second molar embrasure or, if erupted, the first and second premolar embrasure	*Prior to eruption of the permanent second molars:* *Maxillary molar:* At the root tip of the primary first molar, or if erupted, the root tip of first premolar to center the image receptor within the x-ray beam	Reduce exposure by 1/3 to 1/2 the exposure used for this projection on an adult

Mandibular molar—Align the anterior edge of image receptor to line up behind the distal half of the primary or, if erupted, permanent mandibular canine (Figure 26-17)

Mandibular molar:
Paralleling technique: Direct the central rays toward the image receptor perpendicularly in the vertical dimension
Bisecting technique: Direct the central rays toward the imaginary bisector approximately −15 to −20 degrees

Mandibular molar: Direct the central rays perpendicularly through the primary first and second molar embrasure or, if erupted, the first and second premolar embrasure

Mandibular molar: At the root tip of the primary first molar, or if erupted, the root tip of first premolar to center the image receptor within the x-ray beam

After eruption of the second permanent molar: 2 in each quadrant (4 premolar and 4 molar periapicals)

After eruption of the second permanent molar: Use the same criteria as the adult patient (see Table 13-1)

After eruption of the second permanent molar: Use the same criteria as the adult patient (see Table 13-1)

After eruption of the second permanent molar: Use the same criteria as the adult patient (see Table 13-1)

Most children react favorably to the authority of a confident, capable operator. Occasionally, a stubborn or frightened child proves difficult to manage. If such a child does not respond to firmness, a parent or older brother or sister may accompany the child into the x-ray room. In fact, if the child is too small to understand instructions or unable to hold the image receptor in place, a parent or accompanying adult may have to assist with holding the image receptor while it is being exposed. The parent or guardian should be protected with lead/lead equivalent barriers such as an apron or gloves when they are in the path of the x-ray beam. The radiographer must never hold the image receptor in the mouth of a patient during exposure.

Show-Tell-Do

The use of **Show-tell-do** (see Chapter 12) is especially useful with children. Children, and adults, can be naturally fearful of the unknown. Orienting the child patient to the radiographic equipment will help to alleviate fear and pique curiosity. The child can be given a film packet to feel and to handle. It may be unwrapped so that the child can see the film. Showing the child different image receptor sizes and then choosing the size that is "just right" for the child's mouth may assist with cooperation during placement intraorally. If an image receptor holder is to be used, the child can be allowed to examine and handle it. The entire procedure should be carefully explained and rehearsed. The terms used to describe the radiographic equipment should be on the level the patient understands. Young children can be told that the x-ray tube head is the "camera" used to take special x-ray pictures of the teeth.

Modeling

Modeling, where the child is given the opportunity to observe the procedure being performed on another patient, is another successful tool the radiographer may apply to alleviate fear of the unknown and gain cooperation. The child may observe an older sibling or parent undergoing the procedure. Of course, care should be taken to not subject the child to unnecessary radiation exposure. The child can accompany the radiographer to the protected location of the exposure button and assist in the exposure by watching for, and confirming, that the red exposure indicator lights up.

Communication

Honest communication and good interpersonal skills that are utilized to gain procedure acceptance and cooperation from the adult can also be applied to the child patient (see Chapter 12). Praising the child for his/her cooperation and successful completion of each step of the procedure will encourage more of the same behavior. A young child's attention span can be short, so repeated praise and instructions given again with each exposure is often necessary. Young children can be get fidgety and restless, so when the child is ready, image receptor placement and exposures should be made as rapidly as possible.

Giving the child a job to do, such as listening for the "beep" sound to be sure that the x-ray machine worked will allow the patient to be a willing participant in the process. Giving the child a sense of control over the procedure will often boost cooperation. However, the radiographer should be careful about which procedures to maintain authority over. Allowing the patient to hold and examine the image receptor holder device is reasonable; giving the child patient permission to place the holder intraorally where he/she wants to may lead to less cooperation.

Many strategies that apply to managing patients with special needs, presented in Chapter 27, will apply to the child patient as well. The easiest and most comfortable exposures, usually radiographs of the maxillary anterior teeth, can be exposed first to gain the child's confidence and to get the child accustomed to having the image receptor in the mouth. Distraction techniques such as telling the child a story during the procedure; asking the child to take a deep breath and hold it while you count down from five to zero, allowing time to make the exposure; and palpating the tissues with an index finger to massage and desensitize sensitive mucosa and familiarize the patient with where the image receptor will be placed are strategies that help make the radiographic experience a comfortable one.

Interpretation

The radiographer must possess a working knowledge of eruption patterns and tooth morphology to read radiographs that record primary and developing permanent teeth. Figure 26-9 through Figure 26-17 illustrates the teeth and structures most likely to be recorded on radiographs of children with primary and transitional (mixed primary and permanent) dentition.

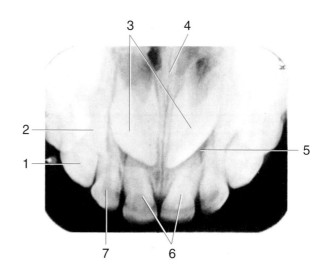

FIGURE 26-9 Maxillary anterior occlusal radiograph of primary dentition exposed with size #2 film. (**1**) Primary canine. (**2**) Unerupted permanent lateral incisor. (**3**) Unerupted permanent central incisors—note that root formation has not started yet. (**4**) Thin radiolucent line indicating the median palatine suture. (**5**) Partially resorbed root of primary central incisor. (**6**) Primary central incisors. (**7**) Primary lateral incisor.

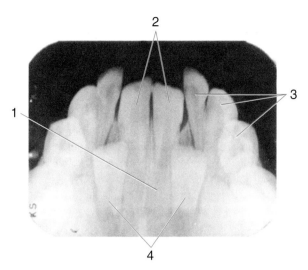

FIGURE 26-10 Mandibular anterior occlusal radiograph of primary dentition exposed with size #2 film. (**1**) Alveolar bone. (**2**) Partially erupted permanent central incisors. (**3**) Primary teeth. (**4**) Unerupted permanent lateral incisors.

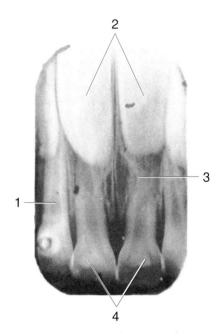

FIGURE 26-12 Maxillary central-lateral incisors periapical radiograph of transitional (mixed primary and permanent) dentition (**1**) Primary lateral incisor. (**2**) Unerupted permanent central incisors. (**3**) Roots of primary central incisors showing signs of physiological resorption. (**4**) Primary central incisors.

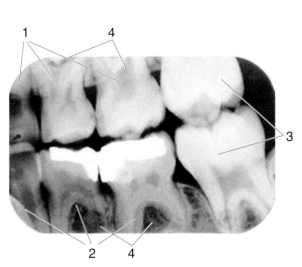

FIGURE 26-11 Posterior bitewing radiograph of transitional (mixed primary and permanent) dentition (**1**) Primary maxillary canine, first and second molars. (**2**) Primary mandibular canine, first and second molars. (**3**) Permanent maxillary and mandibular molars. (**4**) Note that this small size film does not adequately image the area of the developing premolars.

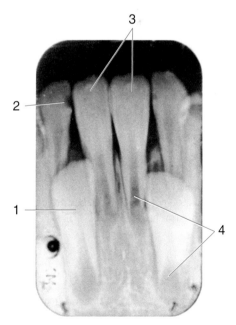

FIGURE 26-13 Mandibular central-lateral incisors periapical radiograph of transitional (mixed primary and permanent) dentition (**1**) Unerupted permanent lateral incisor. (**2**) Caries on mesial surface of primary lateral incisor. (**3**) Permanent central incisors. (**4**) Large open apex on all permanent teeth, indicating that root formation is still in progress. Root formation is generally not complete until about two or three years following tooth eruption.

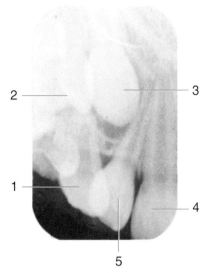

FIGURE 26-14 Maxillary canine periapical radiograph of transitional (mixed primary and permanent) dentition
(**1**) Primary canine. (**2**) Unerupted first premolar. (**3**) Unerupted permanent canine still in a follicle as indicated by radiolucency surrounding the crown. (**4**) Permanent central incisor. (**5**) Permanent lateral incisor, which appears to be tipped distally and overlapping with deciduous canine.

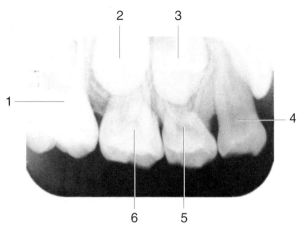

FIGURE 26-16 Maxillary molar periapical radiograph of transitional (mixed primary and permanent) dentition
(**1**) Permanent first molar. (**2**) Unerupted second premolar. (**3**) Unerupted first premolar. (**4**) Primary canine. (**5**) Primary first molar (note that the roots are almost completely resorbed). (**6**) Primary second molar.

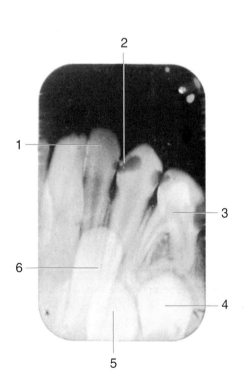

FIGURE 26-15 Mandibular canine periapical radiograph of transitional (mixed primary and permanent) dentition
(**1**) Primary lateral incisor. (**2**) Radiolucent areas on mesial and distal of primary canine. A visual examination is needed to determine if this indicates caries or restorative materials that mimic caries radiographically (see Chapter 21). (**3**) Primary first molar. (**4**) Unerupted first premolar. (**5**) Unerupted permanent canine. (**6**) Unerupted permanent lateral incisor.

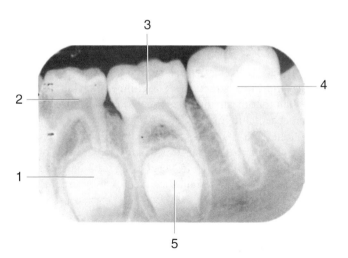

FIGURE 26-17 Mandibular molar periapical radiograph of transitional (mixed primary and permanent) dentition
(**1**) Unerupted first premolar. (**2**) Primary first molar with partial resorption of distal root. (**3**) Primary second molar. (**4**) Permanent first molar. (**5**) Unerupted second premolar.

REVIEW—Chapter summary

Children have the same basic needs for oral health care as do adults. Radiographic techniques and the types of projections used to image the oral cavity of the child patient do not differ significantly from those used for adult patients. The child patient presents with unique characteristics, such as a smaller oral cavity and special behavioral considerations that often require adaptation to standard procedures.

Radiographs for the child patient may be indicated for the detection of congenital dental abnormalities, to assess growth and development, and to detect and diagnose diseases and the effect of trauma. Selection criteria guidelines suggest that radiographs on children may not be necessary until all the primary teeth have erupted unless an emergency or suspected pathology exists. Once teeth have erupted in such a manner that the proximal surfaces of the teeth cannot be examined clinically for caries, radiographs may need to be exposed.

The number and size of image receptor used for radiographs for the child patient will depend on the child's age, size of the oral cavity, and cooperation level. Image receptor size #0 or #1 is usually used for bitewing radiographs for patients with primary dentition, prior to the eruption of the first permanent molars. Image receptor size #2 is usually used for patients with a transitional (mixed primary and permanent) dentition. Occlusal radiographs may be substituted for periapicals on children if necessary. After the eruption of the permanent second molars, the bitewing and full mouth surveys recommended for the child patient are the same as those recommended for an adult patient.

Evidence-based selection criteria recommend panoramic radiographs for the assessment of growth and development. Panoramic or lateral jaw (mandibular oblique lateral) extraoral radiographs may sometimes be acceptable substitutes for intraoral radiographs for the child patient who cannot tolerate intraoral image receptor placement.

As with the adult patient, the paralleling method is the technique of choice for use with children; however, image receptor placement may be easier with the bisecting method. Because the bone structure of a child is smaller and less dense than that of an adult, less radiation is required to produce an acceptable image. Exposure settings for radiographs on children under 10 years of age can be reduced by one-half of that used for adult exposures. Exposure settings for radiographs on children 10 to 15 years of age can be reduced by one-third of that used for adult exposures. Adolescents 15 or 16 years of age and older require the same exposure settings as an adult patient.

Show-tell-do and modeling are valuable patient management tools that can aid the radiographer in taking quality radiographic images. Orienting the child patient to the radiographic equipment will help alleviate fear of the unknown. Good communication and demonstration of authority are imperative when interacting with children. Most children react favorably to the authority of a confident, capable operator.

Sample illustrations are provided to assist with learning to interpret radiographs of children with primary and transitional (mixed primary and permenant) dentition.

RECALL—Study questions

1. List five conditions that would indicate the need for dental radiographs on the child patient.
   a. _____
   b. _____
   c. _____
   d. _____
   e. _____

2. Under which of these conditions would dental radiographs most likely NOT need to be exposed?
   a. When the child presents with poor self-care and suspected caries.
   b. When the child is under 12 years of age.
   c. When the proximal surfaces of the teeth are visible clinically.
   d. When the child has accidentally fallen, but there is no apparent damage to the primary teeth.

3. According to the evidence-based selection criteria guidelines listed in Table 6-1, which of these intervals is recommended for posterior bitewing radiographs on a 10-year-old child recall patient who presents with good self-care and no evidence of clinical caries?
   a. 6–12 months
   b. 12–24 months
   c. 18–36 months
   d. 24–36 months

4. Each of the following need to be considered when deciding what size image receptor to use on a child EXCEPT one. Which one is the EXCEPTION?
   a. Cooperation level
   b. Size of the dental arches
   c. Size of the mouth opening
   d. Amount of plaque present

5. Which image receptor size would be the easiest to position for a bitewing radiograph on a 5-year-old patient?
   a. #0
   b. #1
   c. #2
   d. #4

6. Which of the following is the best reason to use the largest size intraoral image receptor that the child will tolerate?
   a. So that a lesser number of image receptors will have to be exposed
   b. To be able to use the paralleling technique
   c. So that the radiation exposure can be reduced
   d. To image an increased amount of the tissues

7. Which of the following is the suggested number and size of projections to use for a 3-year-old patient with primary dentition?

   a. Two bitewing and two occlusal radiographs
   b. Two bitewing and two periapical radiographs
   c. Two bitewing and four periapical radiographs
   d. Four bitewing and 10 periapical radiographs

8. Which of the following is the suggested number and size of projections to use for a 10-year-old patient with transitional (mixed primary and permanent) dentition?

   a. Two bitewing and eight periapical radiographs
   b. Two bitewing and 10 periapical radiographs
   c. Four bitewing and 10 periapical radiographs
   d. Four bitewing and 14 periapical radiographs

9. Which of the following is the suggested number and size of projections to use for a 15-year-old patient with permanent dentition?

   a. Two bitewings and six periapical radiographs
   b. Four bitewing and eight periapical radiographs
   c. Four bitewing and 10 periapical radiographs
   d. Four bitewing and 14 periapical radiographs

10. When a child patient cannot tolerate intraoral placement of the image receptor for exposure of a periapical radiograph, which of the following may sometimes be an acceptable substitute?

    a. Bitewing
    b. Panoramic
    c. Lateral jaw
    d. Both b and c

11. If well tolerated, which of the following techniques will provide the best-quality images on the child patient?

    a. Panoramic
    b. Occlusal
    c. Paralleling
    d. Bisecting

12. What slight change in angulation is usually required when using the bisecting technique on a child patient?

    a. Increase the vertical angulation
    b. Decrease the vertical angulation
    c. Direct the horizontal angulation mesiodistally
    d. Direct the horizontal angulation distomesially

13. Which of the following image receptors is recommended for an occlusal radiograph on an 8-year-old patient?

    a. #0
    b. #2
    c. #3
    d. #4

14. The exposure settings for children under the age of 10 years should be

    a. reduced by one-half the exposure used for adults.
    b. reduced by one-third the exposure used for adults.
    c. three-fourths the exposure used for adults.
    d. the same exposure as used for adults.

15. The exposure settings for children between the ages of 10 and 15 years should be

    a. reduced by one-half the exposure used for adults.
    b. reduced by one-third the exposure used for adults.
    c. three-fourths the exposure used for adults.
    d. the same exposure as used for adults.

16. The exposure settings for children over the age of 16 years should be

    a. reduced by one-half the exposure used for adults.
    b. reduced by one-third the exposure used for adults.
    c. three-fourths the exposure used for adults.
    d. the same exposure as used for adults.

17. Allowing the child patient to observe a sibling or parent undergoing the radiographic procedure may help to alleviate fear of the unknown and promote cooperation. This patient management strategy is called modeling.

    a. The first statement is true. The second statement is false.
    b. The first statement is false. The second statement is true.
    c. Both statements are true.
    d. Both statements are false.

18. When taking a series of periapical radiographs on an 11-year-old patient, placing and exposing which of the following first will most likely aid in gaining the patient's confidence and cooperation?

    a. Mandibular molar
    b. Mandibular canine
    c. Maxillary molar
    d. Maxillary central-lateral incisors

REFLECT—Case study

The public health clinic where you have volunteered to work one day a week has just received funding to begin providing oral health care services to children. Currently the exposure times for radiographic projections posted near the x-ray unit control panels list only the following impulse times for adults. Based on what you learned in this chapter, design an exposure setting chart that lists the impulse timer settings that would be appropriate for children. Design your chart to include children of all ages: under age 10 and between the ages of 10 and 15. Current settings for adult patients are as follows:

Film speed:	F
PID length:	12 in. (30.5 cm)
mA:	7
kVp:	70

		Impulses	
Bitewings	Adult	Child (under 10 yrs)	Child (10–15 yrs)
Posterior	20	—	—
Anterior	16	—	—
Periapicals			
Maxillary anterior	18	—	—
Maxillary premolar	22	—	—
Maxillary molar	24	—	—
Mandibular anterior	16	—	—
Mandibular premolar	18	—	—
Mandibular molar	20	—	—

RELATE—Laboratory application

Observe the exposure charts that are used in your clinical facility. Write down the settings that are being recommended for use with adults and with children. How many categories of settings did you find? Are there parameters given for the settings? That is, are age, size of the patient, or dentition parameters listed to base the settings on? Compare and calculate the difference between the adult and child settings used at your facility. Do the differences match the recommendations presented in this chapter? What is the basis for the recommended settings at your facility? That is, why were they selected? After analyzing the settings and comparing them to the recommendations in this chapter, write a brief summary that would explain the use of different settings to a concerned parent.

REFERENCES

American Academy of Pediatric Dentistry. (2005). Guideline on prescribing dental radiographs for infants, children, adolescents, and persons with special health care needs. *Pediatric Dentistry, 27*(reference manual), 185–186.

Eastman Kodak Company. (2002). *Successful intraoral radiography.* N-418 CAT No. 103. Rochester, NY: Author.

Pinkham, J., Casamassimo, P., Fields, H. W., McTigue, D. J., & Nowak, A. J. (2005). *Pediatric dentistry: Infancy through adolescence* (4th ed.). St. Louis, MO: Elsevier Saunders.

Thomson, E. M. (1993). Dental radiographs for the child patient. *Dental Hygiene News, 6,* 19–20, 24.

Thomson, E. M. (2008). Panoramic radiographs and the pediatric patient. Part 1. *Dimensions of Dental Hygiene, 6*(2), 26–29.

White, S. C., & Pharoah, M. J. (2004). *Oral radiology: Principles and interpretation* (6th ed.). St. Louis, MO: Elsevier.

Managing Patients with Special Needs

CHAPTER OUTLINE

OBJECTIVES

Following successful completion of this chapter, you should be able to:

1. Define key words.
2. Discuss five actions for managing the apprehensive patient.
3. Identify the areas of the oral cavity that are most likely to initiate the gag reflex.
4. List the two stimuli that commonly initiate the gag reflex.
5. Describe five methods to reduce psychogenic stimuli to control the gag reflex.
6. Describe four methods to reduce tactile stimuli to control the gag reflex.
7. Discuss ways to manage radiographic procedures for the older adult patient.
8. Discuss ways to manage radiographic procedures for the patient with motor disorders and conditions of involuntary movement.
9. Discuss ways to manage radiographic procedures for the patient with disabilities.
10. Explain necessary radiographs for the cancer patient.
11. Explain necessary radiographs for the pregnant patient.
12. Value the need for cultural sensitivity.

KEY WORDS

Angular cheilitis
Apprehensive
Cultural barriers
Disability

Gag reflex
Hypersensitive gag reflex
Speech reading

Introduction

Each patient presents with unique characteristics. In addition to oral manifestations, the dental radiographer should be familiar with possible medical, physical, psychological, emotional, and cultural conditions that may require additional knowledge and skills to successfully produce diagnostic quality radiographs while practicing ALARA (as low as reasonably achievable; see Chapter 6).

The purpose of this chapter is to present some of these conditions that the radiographer must manage to produce quality radiographs. Recommendations based on current research for exposure of special conditions will be presented (Table 27-1).

TABLE 27-1	Conditions Prompting Alterations to Radiographic Procedures	
CONDITION	**ANTICIPATED PROBLEM**	**MANAGEMENT STRATEGY**
Apprehensive	Ability to tolerate placement of the image receptor	Develop a rapport Project confidence Maintain authority Be organized Reassure patient
Hypersensitive gag reflex	Ability to tolerate placement of the image receptor	Do not suggest gagging Empathize Use the power of suggestion Apply distraction techniques Give the patient breathing instructions Reduce tactile stimuli • Begin exposures in the anterior regions • Place image receptor firmly and expertly • Confuse the senses • Utilize special products Substitute extraoral radiographs as needed
Aging	Angular cheilitis (soft tissue cracking of lips) Decreased muscle function Unsteadiness, tremors Dementia (reduced attentiveness to instructions)	Smaller image receptor; lighter-weight image receptor holder; use of edge cushion products Set exposure to increase radiation and decrease exposure time Utilize caregiver as assistant to stabilize image receptor and/or patient Substitute extraoral radiographs
Motor disorders and conditions of involuntary movement	Ability to remain still throughout the exposure	Set exposure to increase radiation and decrease exposure time Utilize caregiver as assistant to stabilize image receptor and/or patient
Wheelchair-bound	Positioning patient within the range of the x-ray unit extension arm and tube head	Transfer the patient to the dental chair when possible
Visual impairment	Ability to communicate instructions to gain patient cooperation Ability to prevent apprehension of the unknown Patient personal eyewear may be in the path of the central ray	Explain each step of the procedure Use touch to explain equipment and procedures Announce when exiting and entering the room and explain why Allow the patient to wear their familiar eyewear whenever possible; explain the need to remove glasses; allow the patient to remove glasses
Hearing impairment	Ability to understand and follow directions	Be creative in finding alternate methods of communication
Cancer	Patient hesitant to undergo dental radiographic procedure	Explain the use of evidence-based selection criteria
Pregnancy	Patient hesitant to undergo dental radiographic procedure	Explain the use of evidence-based selection criteria Discuss necessary and elective radiographic procedures Explain the need for, and use lead/lead equivalent thyroid collar
Culturally diverse	Language, beliefs, traditions and familial influences can be barriers to care	Exhibit an accepting, nonjudgmental attitude Make an effort to understand the culture

The Apprehensive Patient

Apprehensive means to be anxious or fearful about the future. Apprehensive patients may consider the radiographic procedure to be unpleasant. These patients may have had a negative experience with a past procedure, which causes them to project those negative feelings onto the current radiographer. Therefore, it is important that the apprehensive patient's contact with the dental radiographer be pleasant and reassuring.

It is equally important that the radiographer not project his/her own negative feelings or experiences onto the patient. If the radiographer has personal views regarding the experience as uncomfortable or not necessary, he/she must not assume that the patient shares in those views. Most patients are not apprehensive about radiographic procedures, and the radiographer should not say or do anything that would prompt the patient to become anxious.

To reduce a patient's apprehension, the dental radiographer should

- **Develop a rapport.** Take the time to explain the procedure and allow the patient to ask questions. A conversation that demonstrates attentive listening and empathy can help relax the patient.
- **Project confidence.** A skilled radiographer who demonstrates confidence will gain the patient's trust and cooperation. A patient's apprehension is increased when the operator appears unsure of him/herself.
- **Maintain authority.** The radiographer should maintain control over the procedure. Be gentle, but firm. The patient who trusts in the radiographer's ability will be less anxious. For example, if placement of an intraoral image receptor is uncomfortable, and the radiographer allows the patient to tell the radiographer how it should be placed, instead of alleviating patient apprehensiveness, the operator may actually increase it. The patient may now feel responsible for directing the procedure and may become increasingly anxious that the radiographs may not come out right.
- **Be organized.** Progress through the procedure rapidly and accurately. For example, expose the easier maxillary anterior projections first, and then progress to the more difficult posterior areas.
- **Reassure the patient.** Compliment apprehensive patients on their cooperation. Thank them for their cooperation, even when the procedure may have been uncomfortable.

A Hypersensitive Gag Reflex

The **gag reflex** is a protective mechanism that serves to clear the airway of obstruction. The receptors for the gag reflex are located in the soft palate and lateral posterior third of the tongue. Two reactions occur prior to the gag reflex. The first is a cessation of respiration, and the second is a contraction of the muscles of the abdomen and the throat.

All patients have gag reflexes, but some are more sensitive than others. A **hypersensitive gag reflex** is probably the most troublesome problem the dental radiographer may encounter. Two stimuli that must be diminished or eliminated to reduce gagging are

1. **Psychogenic stimuli.** Originating in the mind; may result from the suggestion of gagging or as a result of a past experience of gagging.
2. **Tactile stimuli.** Originating from touch; a physical reaction to a feeling of the airway being blocked.

Reducing Psychogenic Stimuli

To help avoid a hypersensitive gag reflex that originates in the patient's mind, the radiographer should apply all the suggested behaviors just explained for alleviating patient apprehensiveness. If the patient reports a past experience with gagging during the radiographic procedure, or you suspect that a gagging reflex will occur, the following suggestions may help to prevent its occurrence:

- **Do not suggest gagging.** The dental radiographer should not ask the question, "Are you a gagger?" The power of suggestion is a strong psychogenic stimulus and can initiate the gag reflex. Unless the patient brings it up, do not mention it.
- **Empathize.** If the patient brings up the subject of gagging, do not dismiss their concern as "all in the mind." Instead, empathize with their response and explain that some tricks and techniques have been shown to help avoid stimulating the gag reflex and that you will individualize these to help them control their gag reflex.
- **Use the power of suggestion.** When applying these tricks and techniques, explain them to the patient. Letting the patient know that you are altering treatment to help them manage the gag reflex will increase the likelihood of success. The gagging patient will often be embarrassed by their involuntary reaction and most are willing to accept any methods you offer to help them regain control.
- **Apply distraction techniques.** There are many ways to divert the patient's attention away from the oral cavity. This can be done by maintaining an engaging dialogue or telling the patient to think of something pleasant, such as their favorite vacation. However, if the gag reflex has been identified, it may be better to tell the patient that you are going to give him/her a distraction task to perform. For example, the patient may be instructed to bite hard on the image receptor holder's biteblock; raise an arm or clench a fist; or press the head back against the head rest of the treatment chair. Anything that helps to divert the patient's attention from the oral cavity may lessen the likelihood of initiating the gag reflex (Figure 27-1).
- **Give the patient breathing instructions.** A gag reflex is often stimulated by a sense of not being able to breathe. Explain this to the patient and together, plan a breathing exercise that the patient can concentrate on during placement of the image receptor. For example, the patient may be coached to breathe deeply through the nose or the mouth; to hum a familiar song; or to hold the breath while counting to 10 slowly, by which time the radiographer should have completed the exposure.

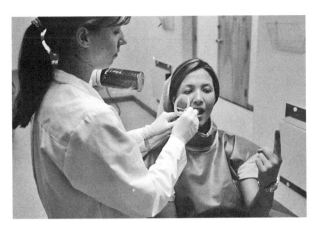

FIGURE 27-1 Distraction techniques. To help control a gag reflex, this patient has been given an exercise to bend and straighten her index finger. She has been instructed to keep a steady motion while continuing to watch her finger.

Reducing Tactile Stimuli

Some patients have an accentuated gag reflex because of hypersensitive pharyngeal tissues. Chronic sinus problems and postnasal drip can contribute to gagging as mucus and saliva accumulate into the nasopharygeal area. The dental radiographer can reduce tactile stimuli by use of the following techniques.

- **Begin exposures in the anterior regions first.** Anterior image receptor placements are less likely to initiate the gag reflex. Positioning the image receptor in the maxillary molar region is more likely to initiate the gag reflex. When exposing a series of bitewing radiographs, expose the premolar radiograph before the molar. It is often easier to prevent a gag reflex than to subdue it once excited. Placing the image receptor in the anterior regions first allows the patient to get used to the procedure, builds acceptance, and will usually permit the radiographer to proceed successfully to the more difficult posterior placements. Additionally, fears from psychic stimuli are most likely to have been forgotten by the time the maxillary molar exposure is made.

- **Place the image receptor firmly and expertly.** For all projections, carry the image receptor into the mouth parallel with the plane of occlusion. When in proper position, rotate into place against the appropriate structures. Retain in position without movement. Avoid sliding the image receptor across sensitive oral mucosa (soft tissue lining of the oral cavity).

- **Use the bisecting technique.** (See Chapter 15.) Because a gag reflex is sometimes excited by placement of the image receptor, using the bisecting technique may help prevent gagging. Placing the image receptor close to the lingual surface of the teeth and therefore not parallel to the long axes of the teeth may be less likely to stimulate a gag reflex on some patients.

- **Confuse the senses.** Stimulating the oral mucosa with digital palpation (rubbing with the finger) serves two purposes. When the radiographer places a finger in the area to simulate for the patient where the image receptor will be placed, the patient can experience what the actual placement will feel like. Second, palpation helps to massage and desensitize the soft tissue to make placement of the image receptor feel less foreign. Another technique that helps confuse the senses and lower the risk of gagging is to instruct the patient to rinse with cold water, ice cubes, or an antimicrobial oral rinse product just prior to image receptor placement. Placing table salt on the middle or tip of the patient's tongue has been shown to be effective at reducing the gag reflex. When introducing any of these agents, care must be taken to first be sure that there are no contraindications for their use. For example, the patient's teeth may be sensitive to cold; and the hypertensive patient (the patient with high blood pressure) may be on a salt-restricted diet.

- **Use special products.** A different image receptor holder may be successful at avoiding or managing a patient with a hypersensitive gag reflex. Different patients may find different image receptor holders more comfortable than others. Additionally, some products on the market, such as film packet edge protectors and plastic barriers for digital sensors, reduce the edge sharpness that some patients report stimulating a gag reflex (Figures 27-2 and 27-3).

Extreme Cases of the Gag Reflex

Occasionally, the radiographer will encounter a patient with a hypersensitive gag reflex that cannot be managed. The radiographer may be able to substitute a smaller-sized image receptor, such as a #1 or #0 for the standard #2 size. The radiographer should take as many intraoral radiographs as possible and then supplement these with extraoral radiographs.

In rare cases the dentist may prescribe the use of a topical anesthetic to numb the areas causing the patient to gag. However, some patients experience an increased anxiety as the result of this numbing sensation, especially in the soft palate and oral pharyngeal area. Additionally, the risks and contraindications of the topical anesthetic must be considered.

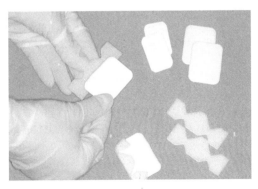

FIGURE 27-2 Edge protectors. Applying a commercial product to reduce the edge sharpness of the film packet.

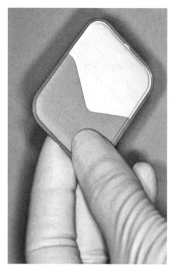

FIGURE 27-3 Edge protectors. Film is available with commercially applied edge softeners.

Aging

Normal changes in the body due to aging do not necessarily mean that all older adult patients will present with unique conditions that require alterations in the radiographic procedure. However, the dental radiographer should be aware of an increased incidence of conditions and diseases such as **angular cheilitis** (fissuring and cracking of the soft tissue at the corners of the mouth), missing teeth (see Chapter 28), hearing impairment, arthritis, stroke, and physical impairment that are seen increasingly with aging. Soft tissue changes in the lips may prevent accurate image receptor placement. Muscle function that diminishes with aging, resulting in unsteadiness and tremor, may present a barrier to holding still during exposures. Residual effects of stroke, such as paralysis, may involve the ability to move the tongue. Alzheimer's disease—which often results in inattentiveness to instructions, loss of coordination, and other motor abnormalities, including exaggerated reflexes—should be taken into consideration when planning to expose radiographs.

It is important to communicate with the older adult patient to ensure that they can follow instructions for a successful outcome to the radiographic procedure. Some of the alterations suggested earlier for managing the gag reflex will aid image receptor placement for the older adult patient. These include using a smaller, lighter-weight image receptor holder, using a smaller image receptor, and applying a commercial product that reduces image receptor edge sharpness.

To assist with possible patient movement that occurs as the result of slight tremors or unsteadiness, the exposure settings may be manipulated to provide the appropriate amount of radiation in the shortest period of time. This is discussed in detail in the next section. If the patient cannot hold still, a caregiver or family member may need to help steady the patient. The assistant must be offered protective barriers such as lead/lead-equivalent gloves, aprons, or shields. The dental radiographer must never hold the image receptor in the patient's mouth during the x-ray exposure.

Extraoral radiographs may prove to be an acceptable substitute if the patient's head can be stabilized throughout the duration of the exposure. Head stabilization may be possible with certain panoramic x-ray machines that have secure head positioner guides. It is important to note that in later stages of osteoporosis, the loss of stature and spinal deformity that creates a stooping posture will often make the use of the panoramic procedure difficult (see Chapter 30).

Motor Disorders and Conditions of Involuntary Movement

Many conditions present with unsteadiness and tremor that require careful consideration prior to exposing radiographs. In addition to the considerations listed earlier, patients who present with Parkinson's disease, Bell's palsy, cerebral palsy, multiple sclerosis, and myasthenia gravis (a neuromuscular disease characterized by weakened muscles, especially of the face and oral cavity) require careful assessment as to their ability to undergo a radiographic examination. If the possibility of movement during the exposure is identified, the exposure settings—the milliamperage (mA) and the exposure time—may be adjusted to decrease the time required for exposure by increasing the amount of radiation generated. As you will recall in Chapter 3, the mA setting controls the amount of radiation generated. By increasing the mA, the x-ray machine will generate more radiation. With this increase in radiation, the exposure time may be decreased (Table 27-2). The guidelines to adjust these settings are explained in Chapter 3.

Disabilities

A **disability** is defined as a physical or mental impairment that substantially limits one or more of an individual's major life activities. The dental radiographer must be prepared to accommodate patients with disabilities. When treating a patient with a disability

- **Talk directly to the patient.** Do not ask the patient's caregiver questions that should be directed to the patient. For

TABLE 27-2   Suggested Exposure Times When Changing the mA Setting* for Adult Patients

REGION TO BE RADIOGRAPHED	IMPULSE SETTING		
	7 mA	10 mA	15 mA
Maxillary anterior periapical	14	10	7
Maxillary posterior periapical	20	14	9
Mandibular anterior periapical	12	8	6
Mandibular posterior periapical	16	11	8
Anterior bitewing	12	8	6
Posterior bitewing	16	11	8

*F-speed film; 12 in. (20 cm) PID; 70 kVp.

example, do not say to the caregiver, "Can he (or she) stand up?" Instead, speak directly to the patient and say, "Can you stand up?"

- **Offer assistance to disabled patients.** Ask the patient how you can best assist them.
- **Do not ask personal questions about the patient's disability.**

The Patient Who Uses a Wheelchair

The difficulty encountered with the patient who uses a wheelchair is getting the patient into position close enough to the x-ray unit (Figure 27-4). Care should be taken to be sure that the extension arm can support the tube head in position without drifting. Unless the patient is in a total-support wheelchair, it may be best to transfer the patient to the dental chair.

Patients can be transferred from the wheelchair to the dental chair by use of the following techniques:

- **Patients who can temporarily support their weight** are transferred to the dental chair by placing the wheelchair alongside the dental chair. Set the brakes of the wheelchair and elevate the dental chair to the height of the wheelchair. Move the dental chair arm from between the chairs. Have the patient move or slide sideways into the dental chair with the caregiver and radiographer assisting.
- **If the patient is unable to support their weight,** the immobile patient may be transferred to the dental chair by radiographer and caregiver. With one taking a position behind the patient and the other facing the patient, the radiographer and caregiver may lift the patient from the wheelchair into the dental chair.

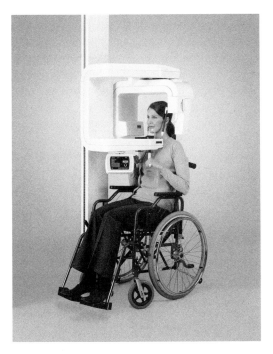

FIGURE 27-4 Panoramic unit that can accommodate wheelchair-bound patients. (Courtesy of Planmeca.)

The Patient with a Visual Impairment

The visually impaired or blind patient requires special consideration during the radiographic procedure. The radiographer must communicate using clear verbal explanations of each step of the procedure before performing it. When taking multiple exposures, it is important to maintain verbal contact to reorient the patient each time you must exit and reenter the oral cavity. Using touch, the radiographer can demonstrate placement of the image receptor and the feel of the receptor holder prior to its placement to help eliminate the feeling of anxiety when facing the unknown.

The personal eyewear worn by the patient with a visual impairment may have to be temporarily removed if the glasses will be positioned within the primary beam. Explain the need for this to the patient. Allow the patient to remove his/her own glasses. Immediately following the exposures, allow the patient to resume wearing their personal eyewear.

Maintain communication with the blind patient. Explain why you are leaving the room when you go to the darkroom to process the films. Immediately announce your return to the operatory by speaking directly to the patient.

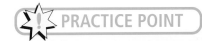

PRACTICE POINT

Never gesture to another person in the presence of a patient who is blind. Blind persons are sensitive to gesture communication and may feel you are "talking behind their back."

The Patient with a Hearing Impairment

Communication is vitally important to the success of all radiographic procedures. The radiographer must give the patient explicit detailed instructions before, during, and at the end of each placement and exposure. The production of quality radiographs depends on the patient's ability to understand and follow these instructions. Communication with the hearing-impaired patient requires that the radiographer be aware of what method of communication works best for the patient. The radiographer should always ask a hearing-impaired or deaf patient how he/she prefers to communicate. Several options are

- Use written instructions.
- Ask a relative or caregiver to act as an interpreter.
- Use gestures.

If the patient can use **speech reading** (reading lips), face the patient and speak slowly and clearly, allowing the patient to read your facial expressions and gestures. Because a face mask is recommended as PPE (personal protective equipment; see Chapter 10) during radiographic procedures, it is important that the patient and the radiographer agree on the meaning of certain gestures before beginning the procedure. In fact, the

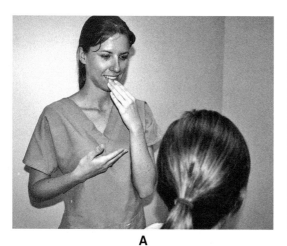
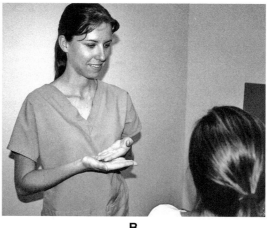

A   B

FIGURE 27-5 Example of signing. The radiographer is letting this hearing-impaired patient know that she is doing a good job cooperating with the radiographic procedure. (**A**) Right hand on chin. (**B**) Drops to left hand open palm. Communicating "Good patient."

hearing-impaired patient will appreciate the radiographer who takes the time to learn a few of the gestures or sign language he/she uses to communicate (Figure 27-5).

If the patient uses a hearing aid, it may have to be removed prior to the panoramic radiographic procedure (see Chapter 30). Explain the upcoming radiographic procedures before asking the patient to remove the hearing aid because communication will be diminished when it is removed.

Cancer

There is often a concern whenever the necessity arises to expose dental radiographs on any patient who is currently receiving or has recently undergone radiation therapy. The patient is often reluctant to receive additional radiation, no matter how minimal, and the dentist may be hesitant to prescribe dental radiographs. Likewise, the radiographer making the exposure may feel apprehensive about the procedure.

The patient should be told that the concerns for radiation safety are shared. Although the patient may already have received large therapeutic doses of radiation, this is not a contraindication to exposing dental radiographs, provided that they are determined to be necessary to make an oral diagnosis. The additional radiation that the patient would receive is minimal, and its use is justified if the patient benefits.

Pregnancy

Prior to a research report published by the American Medical Association (AMA) in 2004, the potential effects of dental radiation exposure centered on the possibility of exposure to the developing fetus. Then *JAMA* (*Journal of the American Medical Association*) published research that investigated the effect on pregnancy outcomes of radiation exposure of the hypothalamus and the pituitary and thyroid glands that suggests that dental radiation exposure is associated with full-term low-birth-weight infants. More research in this area

may lead to altered guidelines on dental radiographs for pregnant females. The American Dental Association (ADA) currently recommends that necessary dental radiographs that help the dentist diagnose and treat oral disease still be exposed on pregnant females; and that elective dental x-rays be postponed for the pregnant female until after delivery. The ADA strongly recommends the use of lead/lead-equivalent thyroid collars in conjuction with lead apron barriers for all patients, and especially for pregnant females and women of child-bearing age.

The Culturally Sensitive Radiographer

The diversity of culture in today's global society means that the radiographer is more and more likely to find him/herself performing radiographic examinations on patients of a variety of racial, ethnic, and cultural backgrounds. Educating these patients regarding the role radiographs play in the diagnosis and treatment of oral diseases requires that the radiographer be aware of possible **cultural barriers,** such as language, beliefs, traditions, and familial influences.

Because good communication is the foundation on which quality radiographs are produced, the radiographer should strive to develop a better understanding of the cultures most likely to be encountered in the community where the oral health care practice is located. To assist in developing cultural sensitivity the radiographer should take into consideration the patient's

- **Communication style.** Is eye contact considered respectful or a sign of rudeness? Does the patient consider discussing the oral cavity personal and private? Is the patient comfortable having a family member translate personal or sensitive information?

- **Comfortable personal space zone.** Does touch convey acceptance, or is it offensive? Is the patient uncomfortable being treated by a professional of the opposite gender? Does the patient wear certain articles of clothing or spiritual jewelry that they would be uncomfortable removing for the radiographic procedure?

- **Gestures and body language.** Does the hand gesture you use mean the same thing to the patient in his/her culture? Are there hand gestures that you need to use to convey instructions regarding the radiographic procedure considered obscene in another culture?

The dental radiographer who presents an accepting, non-judgmental attitude when presented with diverse cultures is more likely to gain the trust and cooperation of the patient.

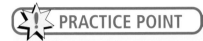

Do not confuse the terms "elective" and "unnecessary." The evidence-based selection guidelines (see Chapter 6) used by dentists to help with the decision to expose radiographs on all types of patients prevent the exposure of unnecessary radiographs. Unnecessary radiographs should never be exposed on any patient. When considering radiographs for the pregnant female, the ADA recommends that elective dental x-rays be postponed until after delivery. Although the ADA Council on Scientific Affairs publication, "The use of dental radiographics: update and recommendations" (*Journal of the American Dental Association, 137*(9), 1304–1312, 2006) does not define "elective" radiographs, this example is offered to help differentiate elective from unnecessary.

- Pregnant patient A presents for dental hygiene services after a one-year time frame. Bitewing radiographs were last taken three years ago. After the assessment it is determined that the patient has periodontal disease. According to the evidence-based selection criteria guidelines (see Table 6-1), this patient should be treatment planned for a set of vertical bitewing radiographs. These radiographs have been determined to be necessary to diagnose and treat this oral condition.

- Pregnant patient B presents for a dental consultation to replace a removal partial denture with a fixed bridge. To determine the health of the teeth and the periodontium that will support the bridge, periapical radiographs are necessary. However, the dentist would most likely assess this dental treatment and the need for radiographs as elective at this time and recommend postponement until after delivery.

REVIEW—Chapter summary

The dental radiographer must be competent in altering procedures to meet the needs of individual patients. To help manage apprehension, the dental radiographer should develop a rapport with the patient, project confidence, maintain authority, be organized, and reassure the patient throughout the procedure.

A hypersensitive gag reflex is probably the most troublesome problem the radiographer encounters. Psychogenic and tactile stimuli must be diminished or eliminated to reduce gagging.

The elderly sometimes present with conditions that require management to produce quality radiographs. Motor disorders and conditions of involuntary movement may be managed by increasing the amount of radiation (mA) and decreasing the exposure time (impulses).

A disability is a physical or mental impairment that substantially limits one or more of an individual's major life activities. The dental radiographer must be prepared to accommodate patients with disabilities.

Patients who have received radiation therapy should be reassured that necessary dental radiographs are justified if the patient benefits. The American Dental Association currently recommends that necessary dental radiographs that help the dentist diagnose and treat oral disease be exposed on pregnant females; and that elective dental x-rays be postponed for the pregnant female until after delivery.

The dental radiographer who presents an accepting, non-judgmental attitude when presented with diverse cultures is more likely to gain the trust and cooperation of the patient.

RECALL—Study questions

1. List five actions for managing the apprehensive patient.
   a. _____
   b. _____
   c. _____
   d. _____
   e. _____

2. A hypersensitive gag reflex that results from a physical reaction to a feeling of the airway being blocked is called a psychogenic stimulus.

   Eliminating psychogenic and tactile stimuli will assist with managing a hypersensitive gag reflex.
   a. The first statement is true. The second statement is false.
   b. The first statement is false. The second statement is true.
   c. Both statements are true.
   d. Both statements are false.

3. Dental radiographers who demonstrate confidence can lead to improved patient cooperation.

   A patient who is told that gagging is "all in their mind" will experience fewer gagging problems.
   a. The first statement is true. The second statement is false.
   b. The first statement is false. The second statement is true.
   c. Both statements are true.
   d. Both statements are false.

4. Each of the following suggestions help the radiographer avoid exciting a hypersensitive gag reflex EXCEPT one. Which one is the EXCEPTION?
   a. Ask the patient to breathe through the nose.
   b. Ask the patient to rinse the mouth with ice water prior to placement of the image receptor.
   c. Ask the patient if they have ever gagged during x-ray exposures.
   d. Ask the patient to press their head against the head-rest during the procedure.

5. Placement of the image receptor in which of these following regions is most likely to initiate a gag reflex?
   a. Maxillary premolar
   b. Maxillary molar
   c. Mandibular premolar
   d. Mandibular molar

6. The patient is less likely to gag
   a. the longer the image receptor stays in the mouth.
   b. if they concentrate on the image receptor placement.
   c. when the image receptor is slid into position over the oral mucosa.
   d. while performing a breathing exercise during image receptor placement.

7. Older adults who present with soft tissue degeneration that makes placement of the image receptor uncomfortable may benefit from each of the following EXCEPT one. Which one is the EXCEPTION?
   a. Increasing the exposure time
   b. Using a smaller-sized image receptor
   c. Using a lighter-weight image receptor holder
   d. Applying an edge protector to the image receptor

8. To compensate for slight movement that results from Parkinson's disease tremors, the radiographer can adjust the exposure settings to
   a. decrease the mA and decrease the impulses.
   b. increase the mA and increase the impulses.
   c. decrease the mA and increase the impulses.
   d. increase the mA and decrease the impulses.

9. When performing radiographic services for the patient with a disability, the radiographer should
   a. remove the patient's eyewear for them prior to exposures.
   b. offer to assist the patient in the manner that they want.
   c. communicate with the caregiver instead of talking directly to the patient.
   d. ask personal questions about the patient's disability.

10. Unnecessary radiographs may be taken on the cancer patient, *but* only elective radiographs may be taken on the pregnant female.
    a. The first part of the statement is true, the second part of the statement is false.
    b. The first part of the statement is false, the second part of the statement is true.
    c. Both parts of the statement are true.
    d. Both parts of the statement are false.

11. It is ethical practice to take unnecessary radiographs on
    a. the older adult.
    b. the pregnant female.
    c. the cancer patient.
    d. no one.

12. The dental radiographer should consider each of the following to develop sensitivity for the culturally diverse patient EXCEPT one. Which one is the EXCEPTION?
    a. Lowered mental capacities
    b. Personal space zone
    c. Communication style
    d. Culturally different meanings to hand gestures

REFLECT—Case study

You have just greeted your patient in the reception area, introduced yourself, and asked her to follow you to the operatory, where you will be taking a full mouth series of radiographs. Once seated, you notice that the patient appears apprehensive. As you get ready to begin the procedure, you engage her in a conversation to assess why she appears so nervous. The patient eventually tells you that her last experience taking radiographs could not be completed because she experienced a gagging problem. She states that she was so embarrassed by it that she never went back to that practice.

1. Explain how you would respond to this patient. Include how you would develop a rapport, project confidence, and maintain authority.
2. Prepare a conversation with this patient where your responses reassure her about your ability to perform the procedure; how the procedure today can be different than her past experience; and what techniques you have to help her control the gag reflex.
3. Answer the following questions:
   a. Why should you not tell this patient that gagging is all in her mind?
   b. What area of the oral cavity should you try placing the image receptor first, and why?
   c. What is the purpose of thanking and praising the patient for her cooperation with the procedure?
   d. What is the difference between psychogenic and tactile stimuli? Give an example of each.
   e. What is the purpose of asking the patient to do breathing exercises during radiographic exposures?
   f. What is the purpose of rinsing with ice water or placing salt on the tongue?
   g. If you use any of these tricks and techniques, why is it best to tell the patient what trick you are planning to use?

RELATE—Laboratory application

For a comprehensive laboratory practice exercise on this topic, see Thomson, E. M. (2012). *Exercises in oral radiography techniques: A laboratory manual* (3rd ed.). Upper Saddle

River, NJ: Pearson Education. Chapter 9, "Patient Management and student partner practice."

REFERENCES

American Dental Association. (2004, April 28). Statement on ante partum dental radiography and infant low birth weight. *JAMA*. Retrieved from www.da.org/public/media/releases/0404_release03.asp

American Dental Association Council on Scientific Affairs. (2006). The use of dental radiographs: Update and recommendations. *Journal of the American Dental Association, 137*, 1304–1312.

Darby, M. L., & Walsh, M. M. (2009). *Dental hygiene theory and practice* (3rd ed.). St. Louis, MO: Elsevier.

Hujoel, P. P., Bollen, A., Noonan, C. J., & del Aguila, M. A. (2004). Ante partum dental radiography and infant low birth weight. *JAMA, 291,* 16–1993.

Khan, F. M. (2009). *The physics of radiation therapy* (4th ed.). Philadelphia: Lippincott Williams & Wilkins.

Langland, O. E., Langlais, R. P., & Preece, J. (2002). *Principles of dental imaging* (2nd ed.). Philadelphia: Lippincott Williams & Wilkins.

White, S. C., & Pharoah, M. J. (2008). *Oral radiology: Principles and interpretation* (6th ed.). St. Louis, MO: Elsevier.

Wilkins, E. M. (2010). *Clinical practice of the dental hygienist* (10th ed.). Philadelphia: Lippincott Williams & Wilkins.

OBJECTIVES

Following successful completion of this chapter, you should be able to:

1. Define the key words.
2. Demonstrate the ability to adapt standard techniques when necessary.
3. Demonstrate appropriate adaptations in image receptor placement to avoid overlap.
4. Explain the need to alter vertical angulation in the presence of a shallow palatal vault.
5. Demonstrate knowledge of setting the exposure time based on patient characteristics.
6. Demonstrate the ability to place an intraoral image receptor in the presence of large maxillary or mandibular tori.
7. Discuss the procedures for image receptor placement in patients with edentulous areas.
8. Discuss the procedures for image receptor placement during endodontic procedures.
9. List three methods of localization.
10. Utilize the buccal-object rule to identify the location of a foreign object.
11. Describe the difference between a standard molar periapical radiograph and a disto-oblique periapical radiograph.
12. List four reasons to duplicate radiographs.
13. Demonstrate the step-by-step procedures for duplicating radiographs.

KEY WORDS

Buccal-object rule
Disto-oblique periapical radiographs
Duplicate radiograph
Duplicating film
Edentulous
Endodontic therapy
Film duplicator
Hemostat

Localization
Root canal treatment
SLOB rule
Tori
Torus mandibularis
Torus palatinus
Tube shift method
Working radiograph

Introduction

It is important that the dental radiographer possess a working knowledge of radiographic theory and techniques to produce diagnostic quality radiographs. However, each patient presents with unique characteristics, some of which may require that the dental radiographer have the knowledge and skills to adapt these ideal procedures to best suit the circumstances. What sets the skilled radiographer apart from the average is the ability to alter techniques and still produce diagnostic images.

The purpose of this chapter is to provide specific information on acceptable alterations of the ideal skills you have learned in this book.

Acceptable Variations in Technique

Anatomical limitations, such as rotation of the teeth, variations in the height of the palate, the presence of unerupted third molars, or excessive root lengths, may require that the radiographer apply acceptable variations in the radiographic technique. Such changes may occur in the horizontal or vertical angulations or in placement of the image receptor. Although image receptor holders with external aiming devices assist the radiographer in producing diagnostic radiographs some conditions may affect the ideal placement of these holders. If the image receptor holder cannot be placed precisely, the radiographer may be aligning the x-ray beam to the wrong place. The radiographer who possesses the skills necessary to evaluate image receptor placement for correctness may still produce a diagnostic quality radiograph by aligning the angles and points of entry to the image receptor itself, instead of relying on the external aiming device alone. The external aiming device on an image receptor holder is an indicator, but does not have to be the absolute "dictator" on where to line up the x-ray beam (Figure 28-1). The radiographer who can judge the accuracy of the image receptor placement can compensate when positioning is less than ideal.

Avoiding Overlap

MOLARS Because the interproximal surfaces of the molars are in a mesiodistal relationship to the patient's sagittal plane, conventional image receptor placement parallel to the buccal

surfaces may result in overlapping of the contact areas and closure of the embrasure spaces. To assist with avoiding the occurrence of overlap error, the image receptor should be positioned perpendicularly to the embrasures. To achieve this position, the image receptor should be placed slightly diagonal, with the front edge of the receptor a greater distance from the lingual surfaces of the teeth than the back edge (Figure 28-2).

CANINE-PREMOLAR The canine periapical and bitewing radiographs will almost always exhibit overlap between the distal of the canine and the mesial of the premolar. This overlap occurs because the curve of the arches in this region superimposes the lingual cusp of the premolar onto the distal edge of the canine. To help minimize this overlap, the horizontal angulation can be adjusted slightly to direct the central rays of the x-ray beam to intersect the image receptor from the distal. Shifting the PID slightly toward the posterior will help separate these two teeth on the resultant image (Figure 28-3).

Because the mesial portion of the premolar will often overlap the distal portion of the canine on canine periapical and bitewing radiographs, it is important that the distal portion of the canine be imaged clearly when exposing premolar periapical and bitewing radiographs when taking a series of radiographs.

Malaligned or Crowded Teeth

When teeth are malaligned or crowded, it may be necessary to take additional radiographs at various horizontal angles to image every interproximal area clearly, with no overlap (Figure 28-4). The image receptor should be positioned perpendicularly to the embrasures of each tooth as necessary.

Altering Vertical Angulation

Absolute parallelism between the image receptor and the long axes of the teeth is sometimes difficult to achieve. If the deviation from parallel does not exceed 15 degrees, the radiograph is generally acceptable (Figure 28-5). When the patient presents with a shallow palate that prevents the image receptor from being placed parallel to the teeth, the root apices may not be recorded on the radiograph. Increasing the vertical angulation by up to 15 degrees over what is indicated will image more of the apical region (see Figure 26-6 and Figure 28-7). It is important to

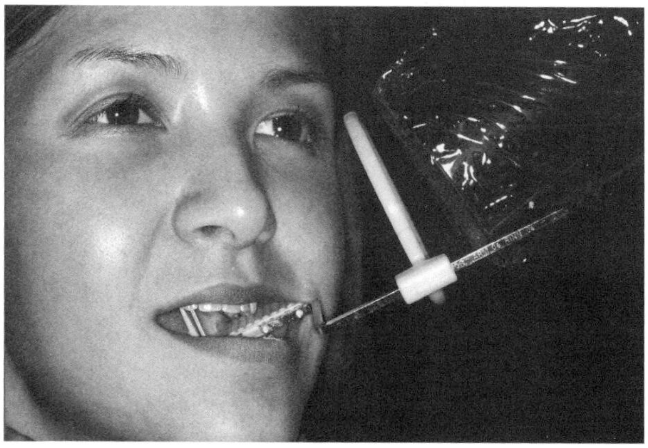

FIGURE 28-1 Indicator ring not a dictator. The radiographer has chosen to increase the vertical angulation to increase the periapical coverage on the resultant image.

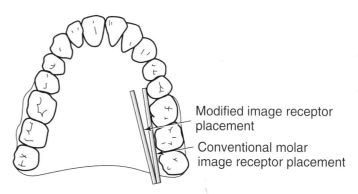

FIGURE 28-2 Image receptor position to avoid molar overlap. The anterior portion of the image receptor is placed a greater distance away from the lingual surfaces of the teeth.

Modified image receptor placement

Conventional molar image receptor placement

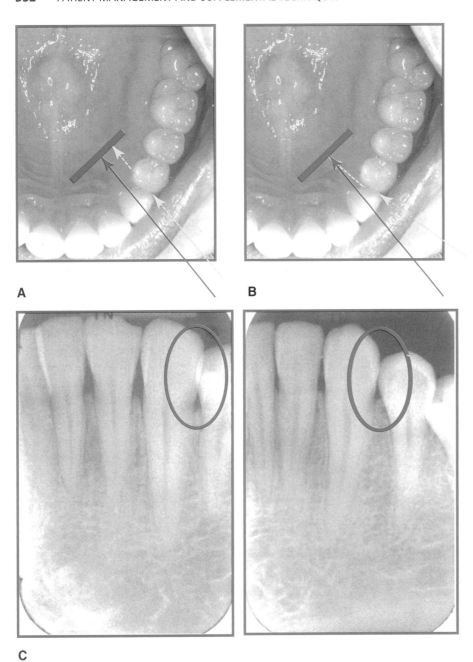

A

B

C

FIGURE 28-3 Minimize canine and premolar overlap. (A) The curve of the arches in this region superimposes the lingual cusp of the premolar onto the distal edge of the canine. (B) Shifting the horizontal angulation slightly to direct the x-ray beam to intersect the image receptor from the distal will help avoid overlap of these two teeth. (C) Note the elimination of overlap error in the radiograph on the right.

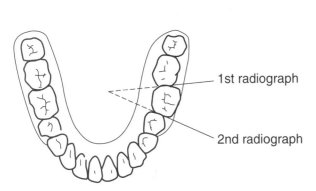

FIGURE 28-4 Different horizontal sangluation is required when teeth are malaligned.

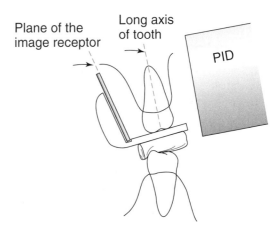

FIGURE 28-5 Shallow palate. The tissue edge of the image receptor is shown tipped away from the teeth. When the lack of parallelism is less than 15 degrees, the resultant radiograph will generally be acceptable.

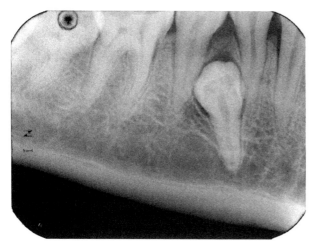

FIGURE 28-6 Increased vertical angulation recorded more of the apical region imaging this supernumerary (extra) impacted premolar, while cutting off a portion of the occlusal region of the teeth.

remember that varying the vertical angulation must be slight, no more than 15 degrees, or noticeable distortion will result.

Exposure Factors

Bone and tissue density vary with the age and physical structure of the patient. In most patients the bone structures are thinner in the mandibular incisor region and denser in the maxillary molar region, making it desirable to alter the exposure time or milliamperage to produce radiographs of ideal density. Making changes in the exposure settings customizes the radiation dose the patient receives. We learned in Chapter 26 that the exposure settings for a child patient, whose bone structures are less dense, should be less than the setting for an adult patient. In addition, patients who present with **edentulous** regions would require less radiation for those areas with missing teeth. Exposure recommendations depend on the characteristics of the patient and the film speed and the type of x-ray equipment in use. Because these exposure recommendations vary widely, recommended settings for all patients and all regions of the oral cavity should be posted next to the x-ray unit control panel for easy reference.

Anatomical Variations

The dental radiographer should be familiar with anatomical variations patients may present with. In addition to a shallow palate, patients may present with bony outgrowths on the palate and the lingual surfaces of the mandible, called tori.

Tori

Tori (torus, singular) are commonly seen in the oral cavity. A maxillary torus, called **torus palatinus,** is a benign outgrowth of bone along the midline of the hard palate. A mandibular torus, called **torus mandibularis** or lingual torus, is a benign outgrowth of bone along the lingual aspect of the mandible in the canine-premolar area.

A large torus palatinus or torus mandibularis may interfere with placement of the image receptor. Care should be taken when

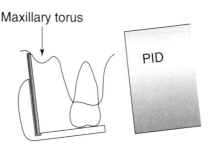

FIGURE 28-7 Maxillary torus. Image receptor placed on the far side of the torus away from the teeth.

placing the image receptor in the presence of tori. In addition to its intrusion into the oral cavity, the oral mucosa covering the tori can be thin and sensitive. The edge of the image receptor should not be placed directly on top of the tori, as this would result in only a partial image of the roots of the teeth. Instead, the image receptor should be placed on the far side of the torus (Figure 28-7). When placing the image receptor in the presence of mandibular tori, place the image receptor between the torus and the tongue (Figure 28-8). This recommended placement may prove difficult when bitewing tab holders are used. Positioning the image receptor away from the teeth requires that the patient bite on the very end of the bitewing tab. To aid with proper placement in such cases, the bite tab would need to be lengthened (see Figure 16-7).

The Edentulous Patient

Preventive radiography is often beneficial to the fully and partially edentulous patient because the normal appearance of the dental ridges may conceal problems underneath. Radiographs benefit the edentulous patient for the following reasons:

- To detect the presence of retained roots, impacted teeth, foreign bodies, cysts, and other pathological lesions.
- To establish the position of the mental foramen before constructing dentures.
- To establish the position of the mandibular canal before implant surgery.
- To determine the condition and extent of alveolar bone present.

Periapical radiographs may be taken of edentulous areas using either the paralleling or the bisecting technique with minor modifications. Normally, the teeth serve as landmarks to guide

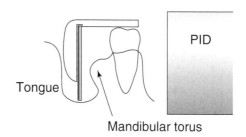

FIGURE 28-8 Mandibular torus. Image receptor placed between the torus and the tongue.

placement of the image receptor. Because these landmarks are not present in the edentulous patient, one must estimate the best positions. Additionally, visualizing and establishing horizontal and vertical planes is more difficult, particularly when the bisecting technique is used. However, in the totally edentulous patient a fair amount of leeway in horizontal angulation is permissible because the absence of teeth eliminates the problem of overlapping tooth images. The focus of interest is no longer the teeth but the bone structure of the edentulous ridge.

Because it produces the best diagnostic images, the paralleling technique should be the radiographer's first choice. Radiographic detail is improved and dimensional distortion is minimized when the image receptor holder can be properly supported with cotton rolls or polystyrene blocks to position the image receptor parallel to the long axis of the edentulous ridge (Figures 28-9 and 28-10). The central rays of the x-ray beam are

then directed horizontally and vertically toward the center of the image receptor perpendicular to the mean tangent of the facial side of the ridge and to the plane of the image receptor.

If parallel placement of the image receptor remains difficult in an edentulous area, it is better to try using the bisecting technique than to risk taking a poor-quality radiograph that would need to be retaken. When using the bisecting technique, the image receptor is placed against the lingual surface of the edentulous ridge. The vertical angulation is determined by bisecting the angle formed between the recording plane of the image receptor and an imaginary line through the ridge that substitutes for the long axes of the teeth (Figure 28-11). This position often results in some dimensional distortion. However, acceptable radiographs can still be produced.

Because the edentulous region is less dense, the amount of radiation needed to produce an acceptable radiographic image

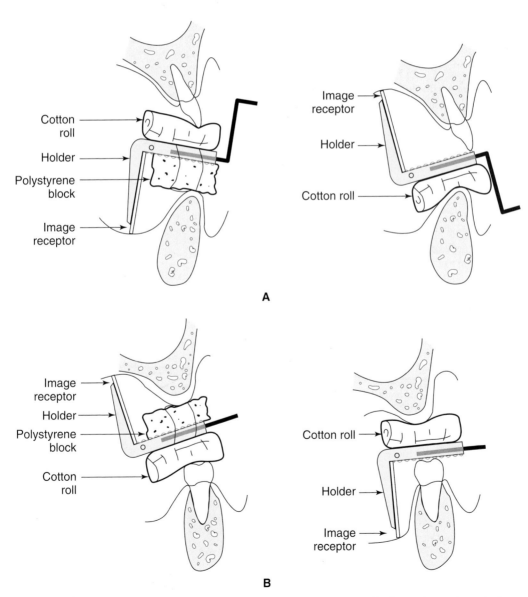

A

B

FIGURE 28-9 Partially edentulous mouth. Cotton rolls or polystyrene blocks can be used to substitute for missing teeth to help hold the image receptor holder in place. (**A**) Edentulous mandibular anterior region. (**B**) Edentulous maxillary posterior region.

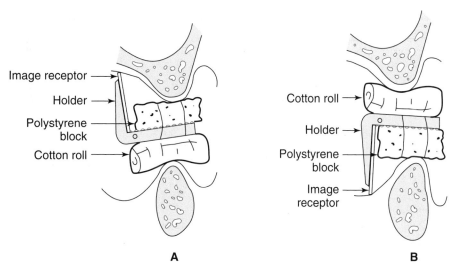

FIGURE 28-10 Totally edentulous mouth. When all teeth are missing, cotton rolls, polystyrene blocks, or a combination of both can be used as substitutes for the crowns of the teeth. These will allow the patient to bite and stabilize the image receptor holder. The thickness of the cotton rolls or blocks will determine the amount of edentulous ridge recorded. (**A**) Maxillary anterior region. (**B**) Mandibular posterior region.

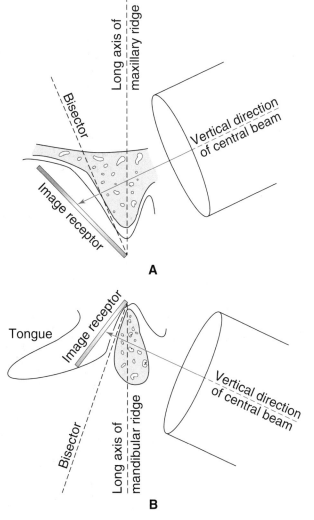

FIGURE 28-11 Illustration of the bisecting technique for an edentulous patient. The central ray is directed perpendicular to the bisector, an imaginary line estimated to be halfway between the plane of the image receptor and a line drawn vertically through the ridge to substitute for the long axes of the teeth. (**A**) Maxillary edentulous ridge, (**B**) Mandibular edentulous ridge.

is less. Exposure settings for edentulous regions should be reduced by about one-fifth less than the exposure required for an area where teeth are present.

Endodontic Techniques

Endodontic therapy involves the treatment of the tooth by removing the nerves and tissues of the pulp cavity and replacing them with filling material. Successful endodontic therapy or **root canal treatment** depends on the use of radiographs. A series of radiographs on the same tooth is needed to evaluate various stages of endodontic treatment. The initial radiograph is exposed to determine the preoperative condition and to make a diagnosis. Additional radiographs are made as the work progresses to determine the length of the root; the position of a reamer, broach, or file in the canal; or the position of the sealer and point or points (the tooth may have several canals). And finally, a posttreatment radiograph is needed to make sure that the canal or canals are closed satisfactorily.

Once again, the paralleling technique is the technique of choice. Standard periapical radiographic procedures can be applied in endodontic radiographic exposures; however, there are some differences. The materials used in endodontic treatment—such as a rubber dam, reamers, broaches, files, or silver or gutta-percha points—often hinder placement of the image receptor. The presence of these materials, which must be left in place during radiographic exposures, makes it impossible for the patient to bite down on the biteblock of an image receptor holder to hold it in place. Avoiding distortion and magnification of the image is a major concern in endodontic treatment because the length of each canal must be accurately measured. Therefore the paralleling technique, which consistently produces the least distortion, should be used whenever possible. Although preoperative and postoperative radiographs are made in the usual manner, some technique modifications are required for the **working radiographs** that are exposed with the rubber dam and instruments in place.

The ideal image receptor holder is one specifically designed for exposure of working radiographs (Figure 28-12). Other types of holders may be modified to accommodate retention of the image receptor during endodontic therapy (Figure 28-13). However, it may become necessary to use methods of image receptor retention that rely on visual alignment of the PID. Image

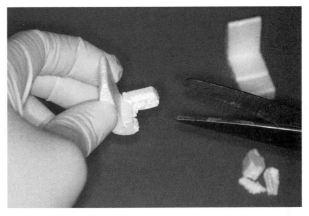

FIGURE 28-13 Modifying a film holder for use in endodontic therapy. Removing a portion of this disposable polystyrene image receptor holder will allow the endodontic materials placed in the tooth to remain in place during the exposure.

receptor holders such as the Rinn Snap-A-Ray (Figure 28-14) or the employment of a dental instrumental called a **hemostat** (Figure 28-15) or a tongue depressor as a custom-made holder will allow the patient to help stabilize the image receptor in the correct position (Figure 28-16).

When imaging multirooted teeth, such as the maxillary premolars and molars, the buccal and lingual root canals will often

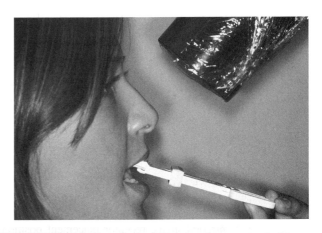

FIGURE 28-14 Rinn Snap-A-Ray image receptor holder.

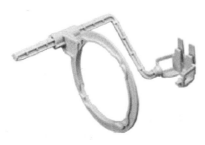

FIGURE 28-12 Endodontic film holder. (Courtesy of Dentsply Rinn.)

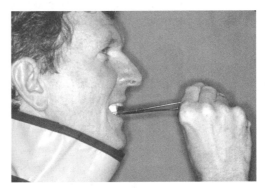

FIGURE 28-15 Hemostat as a film holder for endodontic procedures eliminates the need to occlude on on a biteblock.

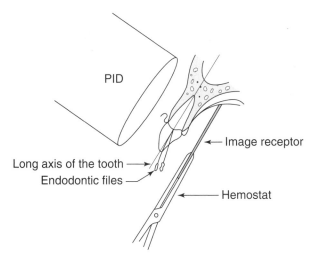

FIGURE 28-16 Hemostat facilitates holding the image receptor in a parallel position to the long axis of the tooth.

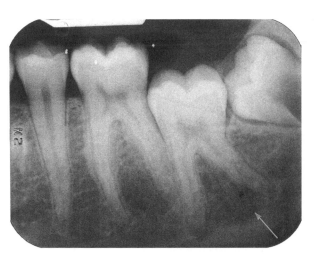

FIGURE 28-17 **Definitive method of localization.** Note the barely visible supernumerary (extra) root on this first molar. Applying the definitive method of localization, it is most likely a buccal root. The buccal position would place this root a greater distance away from the image receptor, resulting in its magnified and less distinctly defined appearance.

appear superimposed. The ability to separate the buccal and lingual roots on the image increases the radiograph's value during endodontic procedures. The radiographer can accomplish this through the use of tube head shifting called **localization.**

Methods of Localization

Radiographs are a two-dimensional picture of three-dimensional objects. To get that third dimension from a radiographic image, the dental radiographer should be skilled in reading the images. Localization methods help the radiographer determine whether a structure such as a root canal or a foreign object embedded within the maxilla or mandible is in front of (facial or buccal) or behind (lingual) the teeth. There are three methods of localization.

Definitive Evaluation Method

The definitive method of localization is based on the shadow casting principles explained in Chapter 4. The principle that an object positioned farther away from the image receptor will be magnified and less clearly imaged is applied with the definitive method. Because intraoral image receptor placement positions the receptor close to the lingual surface of the teeth, those objects on the lingual are more likely to appear distinctly defined on the resultant radiograph. Those objects positioned more toward the buccal or facial surface will be farther away from the image receptor and therefore are more likely to appear magnified and less clearly imaged on the resultant radiograph (Figure 28-17). Although true in principle, the definitive method of localization is not consistantly reliable.

Right-angle Method

Once identified on a periapical radiograph, a better way to determine whether or not a foreign object or structure, such as an impacted tooth, is located on the buccal or the lingual is to take an occlusal radiograph. A cross-sectional occlusal radiograph, described in Chapter 17, places the image receptor at a right

angle to the tooth. In this position the occlusal radiograph will image the object clearly on the buccal or lingual (Figure 28-18).

Tube Shift Method (Buccal-object Rule)

The **tube shift method,** also called the **buccal-object rule,** is the most versatile method of localization. To apply the tube shift method, two radiographs are needed. The two radiographs must have been exposed using either a different horizontal or a different vertical angulation. If a full mouth series of periapicals or a complete set of bitewing radiographs, or a combination of both, are available and the object in question is imaged in more than one radiograph, it is possible to apply the tube shift method when reading the radiographs to determine the buccal or lingual location of the object.

The principle behind the tube shift method is that if the structure or object in question appears to have moved in the same direction as the horizontal (Figure 28-19) or vertical (Figure 28-20) shift of the tube, then the structure or object is located on the lingual. Conversely, if the move is in the opposite direction of the shift of the tube, the structure or object is located on the buccal or facial. The tube shift method is summarized as the **SLOB Rule,** which stands for same on lingual–opposite on buccal.

Disto-oblique Periapical Radiographs

Shifting the tube (the PID and tube head) has another useful application. **Disto-oblique periapical radiographs** utilize a tube shift to help image posterior objects such as impacted third molars, especially when the patient cannot tolerate posterior image receptor placement. Standard vertical and horizontal angulation utilized when exposing periapicals may be altered slightly (no more than 15 degrees) to project posterior objects forward or anteriorly onto the image receptor (Procedure Box 28-1).

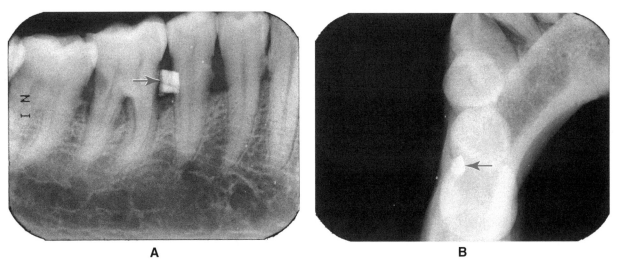

FIGURE 28-18 Right angle method of localization. (**A**) A foreign object appears in the periodontal pocket between the second premolar and the first molar. It is impossible to tell from this periapical radiograph whether the object is located toward the buccal or the lingual. (**B**) The occlusal radiograph, placed at a right angle position to the tooth, clearly images the object on the buccal side of the pocket.

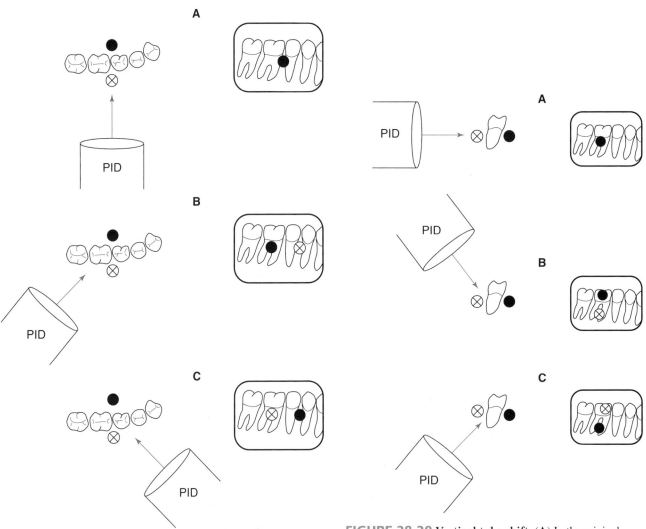

FIGURE 28-19 Horizontal tube shift. (**A**) In the original radiograph, buccal and lingual objects are superimposed. (**B**) When the tube head is moved distally, the buccal object appears to move mesially, whereas the lingual object appears to move distally. (**C**) When the tube head is moved mesially, the buccal object appears to move distally, whereas the lingual object appears to move mesially.

FIGURE 28-20 Vertical tube shift. (**A**) In the original radiograph, buccal and lingual objects are superimposed. (**B**) When the tube head is moved superiorly, the buccal object appears to move inferiorally, whereas the lingual object appears to move superiorly. (**C**) When the tube head is moved inferiorly, the buccal object appears to move superiorly, whereas the lingual object appears to have moved inferiorally.

PROCEDURE 28-1
Disto-oblique periapical radiographs

1. Perform infection control procedures (see Procedure 10-2).

2. Prepare unit, patient, and supplies needed according to the procedure for exposing periapical radiographs (see Procedure 13-1).

3. Place the image receptor into the holding device. (If using film, place such that the embossed dot will be positioned toward the occlusal/incisal edge–dot in the slot).

Maxillary Disto-oblique Periapical Radiographs

1. Position the image receptor and align the horizontal and vertical angulations for a standard maxillary molar periapical radiograph.

2. From this standard alignment, shift the tubehead and PID to direct the central rays of the x-ray beam to intersect the image receptor obliquely from the distal by 10 degrees.

3. Increase the vertical angulation by 5 degrees.

4. Check that the image receptor is centered in the middle of the x-ray beam.

5. Increase the recommended exposure setting for the standard periapical radiograph to the next higher impulse or timer setting.

Mandibular Periapical Radiograph

1. Position the image receptor and align the horizontal and vertical angulations for a standard mandibular molar periapical radiograph.

2. From this standard alignment shift the tube to direct the central rays of the x-ray beam to intersect the image receptor obliquely from the distal by 10 degrees.

3. Check that the image receptor is centered in the middle of the x-ray beam.

4. No change is made to the standard vertical angulation.

5. No change is made to the standard recommended exposure setting.

For example, if an impacted third molar is positioned so far posterior in the oral cavity that the standard image receptor placement is not likely to record it, the PID and tube head can be moved to project the impacted tooth forward onto the image receptor (Figure 28-21). By directing the x-ray beam mesially, the posterior object will be projected anteriorly. Because the central rays will intersect the plane of the image receptor at an oblique angle, there will be slight overlap and distortion of the image (Figure 28-22). However, the focus of disto-oblique periapical radiographs is on recording an object or structure that may not be in standard periapical radiographs, so this distortion is tolerated.

The maxillary disto-oblique periapical radiograph requires three changes to the standard maxillary molar periapical radiograph. The first and most important step is to shift the horizontal angulation so that the posterior object will be projected forward. Second is to increase the vertical angulation.

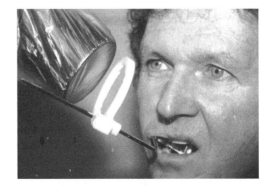

FIGURE 28-21 Disto-oblique periapical technique. The horizontal angulation is shifted 10 degrees from the distal, and the vertical angulation is increased 5 degrees.

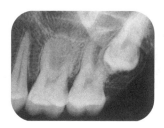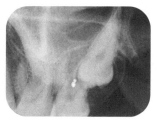

FIGURE 28-22 Comparision of standard and disto-oblique periapical radiographs. (A) Standard periapical radiograph images a portion of the impacted third molar. **(B)** Disto-oblique periapical radiograph images more of the impacted third molar. Note that shifting the tube horizontally causes overlap error, and shifting the tube head vertically causes the crowns to be cut off the the image.

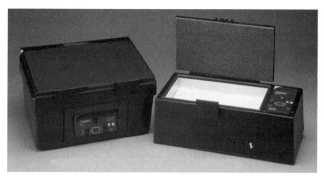

FIGURE 28-23 Radiograph duplicating machines. Contain a built-in ultraviolet fluorescent light source and a timer to permit variations in density. These x-ray film duplicators accommodate duplication of multiple films at a time, with room for a full mouth series, or a panoramic radiograph. (Courtesy of Densply Rinn.)

Most impactions, or foreign objects in the posterior region of the maxilla, will be located farther superior than the erupted teeth. As discussed at the beginning of this chapter, increasing the vertical angulation will increase the periapical coverage of the image. And finally, the exposure setting for a maxillary disto-oblique radiograph must be increased to the next higher timer setting. The oblique angle of the x-ray beam will require a longer passage through the patient's tissues. The increased vertical angulation will most likely direct the x-ray beam through the zygomatic arch. These two changes, in the horizontal and the vertical angulations, necessitate more radiation to produce adequate radiographic image density.

The mandibular disto-oblique periapical radiograph requires only the change to the horizontal angulation, to project the impaction or object forward. Most impactions of the posterior mandible will be located at the level of, or higher than, the erupted teeth so no change is required in the vertical angulation. There are no thick bony structures, like the zygoma, to penetrate, so the exposure time does not have to be increased.

Film Duplicating Procedure

Original radiographs should remain a part of the patient's permanent record, so there are times when a duplicate radiograph is needed. These include copies for third-party payment (insurance companies), when referring the patient to a specialist, when the patient changes dentists or moves, for consultations with other professionals, for publications in professional journals or for use in professional study clubs, to accompany biopsies of pathological conditions, and for evidence in legal cases. A **duplicate radiograph** is an identical copy of the original radiograph and may be obtained through the use of two-film intraoral film packets. If a double film packet is not available or the film is an extraoral film, the use of a film duplicator will produce a copy of the original radiograph. Radiographs can be duplicated as often as necessary without additional patient exposure.

Equipment

Duplicating radiographs requires **duplicating film** and a duplicator.

DUPLICATING FILM Duplicating film is available in sheet form in a variety of sizes. The film is emulsion-coated on one side only. Under a safelight, the emulsion side looks dull or lighter, whereas the side without the emulsion coating looks shiny or darker (see Chapter 7). It is possible to duplicate either a single radiograph or a full mouth series at a single printing.

FILM DUPLICATOR A **film duplicator** is a device that provides a diffused light source (usually ultraviolet) that evenly exposes the duplicating film. There are different size film duplicator models available commercially (Figure 28-23). Large duplicators accommodate all film sizes, whereas small duplicators may be used only for #2 film and smaller (Figure 28-24).

PROCEDURES FOR FILM DUPLICATION Flm duplicators come with manufacturer's instructions for use. All duplication must be done in the darkroom under a safelight (Procedure Box 28-2).

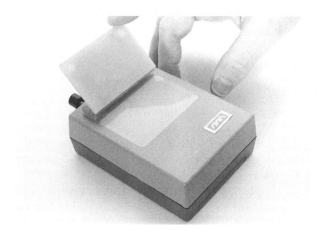

FIGURE 28-24 Small radiograph duplicator accommodates film sizes #0, #1, and #2.

PROCEDURE 28-2
Film duplication

1. Select radiographs for duplication (referrals, third-party payment, consultations).

2. Prepare duplicator. Raise cover and wipe glass surface with glass cleaner if necessary.

3. Place duplicator mode switch in the VIEW position to turn on the view box as necessary to arrange original radiographs into position for duplicating.

4. Remove the original radiographs from the film mounts prior to duplication. (Leaving the original radiographs in the film mount will prevent close contact between the originals and the duplicating film, resulting in the fuzzy appearance of the duplicate radiograph.)

5. Place original radiographs on the duplicator glass surface with the embossed dots concave (dimple). Placing the "down dot" on the duplicator surface will allow for close contact between the original radiographs and the duplicating films.

6. Place the radiographs near the L or R on the duplicator glass surface to identify the left or right sides respectively on the duplicate images.

7. Turn the duplicator mode switch to the DUPLICATE position to turn off the view box light. Be sure to turn off this view box light prior to opening the box of duplicating film.

8. Set the timer to the desired exposure time. See the manufacturer's recommendations. If a darker duplicate is desired, decrease the exposure time; if a lighter duplicate is desired, increase the exposure time. (Increasing and decreasing the exposure time from the duplicator light has the opposite effect on the resulting image than increasing and decreasing the x-ray exposure.)

9. Obtain a box of duplicating film.

10. Under safelight conditions, remove a sheet of duplicating film from the box. When duplicating individual films, use scissors to cut duplicating film to the approximate size needed.

11. Place the duplicating film emulsion (light) side down on top of the originals.

12. Close the duplicator cover and secure the latch tightly. (Failure to secure the latch will result in a loss of contact between the originals and the duplicating film, resulting in the fuzzy appearance of the duplicate image.)

13. Depress the exposure button to activate exposure.

14. When the indicator light goes off at the end of exposure cycle, unlatch and raise the cover, remove the duplicating film, and process the duplicating film either automatically or manually.

15. Remount the original radiographs and return to the patient's permanent record.

16. Clean the darkroom and replace materials.

17. When the duplicate film exits the processor, label it with the patient's name, date, and any other information necessary. Ensure that the right and left sides of the image are identified appropriately.

REVIEW—Chapter summary

Anatomical conditions such as malaligned or crowded teeth, a shallow palatal vault, the presence of tori, and endentulous regions may require alterations in radiographic technique. A skilled radiographer can apply acceptable variations in aligning the horizontal and vertical angulations and still produce diagnostic quality radiographs. The radiographer should possess the skills necessary to evaluate image receptor placement for correctness, align horizontal and vertical angluations, and determine points of entry when using an image receptor holder with and without an external aiming device.

Exposure times should be adjusted based on the patient's characteristics and the area of the oral cavity to be imaged. Edentulous regions require one-fifth the dose of radiation required in regions with teeth present. The paralleling technique is preferred, however, periapical radiographs may be exposed in edentulous regions using the paralleling or the bisecting technique. Cotton rolls and/or polystyrene blocks may be used to help stabilize the image receptor to a position parallel to the edentulous ridge.

Image receptor holders are available commercially or may be altered by the radiographer to produce working radiographs during endodontic therapy.

Localization methods add a third dimension to two-dimensional radiographs. Definitive method is the least reliable method of localization. The right angle method of localization uses a periapical radiograph and a cross-sectional occlusal radiograph. With the tube shift method of localization, the object in question is located on the lingual if it moves in the same direction as the horizontal or vertical shift of the tube and on the buccal if it moves in the opposite direction as the horizontal or vertical shift of the tube. The tube shift method, or buccal object rule, is summarized as the SLOB (same on lingual–opposite on buccal) rule.

Disto-oblique periapical radiographs are useful when the patient cannot tolerate posterior placement of the image receptor. Disto-oblique periapical radiographs allow the radiographer to shift the PID and tube head to project posterior objects and structures anteriorly onto the image receptor.

Copies of radiographs are used to send to insurance companies or to another oral health care practice; for use in referrals, consultations with other professionals, or publication in professional journals; or when needed in litigation. Duplicate radiographs are made using a commercially made duplicator and special duplicating film.

RECALL—Study questions

1. To help avoid molar overlap, the radiographer should place the image receptor
   a. parallel to the buccal surfaces of the molars.
   b. perpendicular to the buccal surfaces of the molars.
   c. parallel to the molar embrasures.
   d. perpendicular to the molar embrasures.

2. To minimize canine-premolar overlap, the radiographer should direct the x-ray beam toward the image receptor slightly obliquely from the
   a. mesial.
   b. distal.
   c. occlusal.
   d. apical.

3. To compensate for a shallow palatal vault, the vertical angulation may be adjusted to
   a. increase by up to15 degrees.
   b. decrease by up to 15 degrees.
   c. increase by up to 25 degrees.
   d. decrease by up to 25 degrees.

4. Which area of the oral cavity would require the highest exposure setting?
   a. Maxillary anterior region
   b. Maxillary posterior region
   c. Mandibular anterior region
   d. Mandibular posterior region

5. The presence of a large mandibular torus may make which of these difficult?
   a. Aligning the correct horizontal angulation
   b. Determining the accurate vertical angulation
   c. Placing the image receptor precisely
   d. Directing the central ray of the x-ray beam at the center of the image receptor

6. The best image receptor placement for a patient with a torus palatinus is
   a. between the torus and the tongue.
   b. on the top of the torus.
   c. near the front of the torus.
   d. behind the torus.

7. The paralleling technique is the best technique for imaging edentulous areas.
   The bisecting technique is the best technique when imaging endodontic treatment.
   a. The first statement is true. The second statement is false.
   b. The first statement is false. The second statement is true.
   c. Both statements are true.
   d. Both statements are false.

8. Which of the following radiographs would be the least beneficial for the totally edentulous patient?
   a. Bitewing
   b. Periapical
   c. Panoramic
   d. Occlusal

9. The exposure setting for edentulous regions should be decreased from the exposure time for the same region with teeth by
   a. one-half.
   b. one-third.
   c. one-fourth.
   d. one-fifth.

10. Which of the following would be the BEST image receptor holder for exposing working radiographs during a root canal procedure?
   a. Rinn XCP^R
   b. Rinn Snap-A-Ray^R
   c. Commercially made endodontic holder
   d. Polystyrene block

11. Localization adds which of the following dimensions to two-dimensional radiographs?
   a. Anterior-posterior
   b. Buccal-lingual
   c. Mesial-distal
   d. Inferior-superior

12. Which of the following methods of localization utilizes a cross-sectional occlusal radiograph?
   a. Definitive method
   b. Right-angle method
   c. Tube shift method
   d. Buccal-object rule

13. If the tube shifts to the mesial and the object in question shifts to the distal, the object is located on the lingual. This is an example of the definitive method of localization.

    a. The first statement is true. The second statement is false.

    b. The first statement is false. The second statement is true.

    c. Both statements are true.

    d. Both statements are false.

14. When exposing a disto-oblique periapical radiograph of the maxilla, which of the following changes should be made to the standard periapical radiograph?

    a. 5-degree shift in the vertical angulation

    b. 10-degree shift in the horizontal angulation

    c. An increase in the time/impulse setting

    d. All of the above

15. To project an impacted mandibular third molar anteriorly onto the image receptor, a mandibular disto-oblique periapical radiograph requires a

    a. 5-degree shift in the vertical angulation.

    b. 10-degree shift in the horizontal angulation.

    c. An increase in the time/implulse setting.

    d. All of the above.

16. List four reasons to duplicate radiographs.

    a. _____

    b. _____

    c. _____

    d. _____

REFLECT—Case study

A patient has presented at your practice today for a consult regarding extensive dental work. This patient has several areas of missing teeth and has expressed an interest in dentures. The dentist has prescribed a full mouth series of radiographs, and you are preparing to take the exposures. After performing a cursory exam of the patient's oral cavity, you note the following:

Several missing and/or broken down teeth

Malaligned and crowded teeth

Partially erupted third molars

Large torus palatinus and bilateral torus mandibularis

A shallow palatal vault

Consider the following and write out your answers:

1. Describe the alterations in technique you will apply to obtain radiographs in the edentulous areas.

2. Describe the alterations in technique you will apply to avoid overlap error in the areas of malaligned and crowded teeth.

3. Identify and describe the technique you will use to best image the partially erupted third molars.

4. Describe the problems you anticipate facing with the presence of large tori and a shallow palatal vault.

5. Identify alterations in techniques that will help you overcome these obstacles.

6. If broken root tips or other foreign objects are identified on the radiographs, describe how the interpretation of these can reveal whether or not the objects in question are located on the buccal or the lingual.

7. Describe other methods of localization that can aid in making this determination.

8. Identify reasons why this patient's radiographs may need to be duplicated.

RELATE—Laboratory application

For a comprehensive laboratory practice exercise on this topic, see Thomson, E. M. (2012). *Exercises in oral radiography techniques: A laboratory manual* (3rd ed.). Upper Saddle River, NJ: Pearson Education. Chapter 11, "Supplemental Radiographic Techniques and Tips"

REFERENCES

Del Rio, C. E., Canales, M. L., & Preece, J. W. (1982). *Radiographic technique for endodontics.* San Antonio: University of Texas Health Science Center.

Rinn Corporation. (1983). *Intraoral radiography with Rinn XCP/BAS instruments.* Elgin, IL: Dentsply/Rinn Corporation.

Thomson, E. M. (2010). *Exercises in oral radiography techniques: A laboratory manual* (3rd ed.). Upper Saddle River, NJ: Pearson Education.

Extraoral Radiography and Alternate Imaging Modalities

CHAPTER OUTLINE

OBJECTIVES

Following successful completion of this chapter you should be able to:

1. Define the key words.
2. Describe the purpose and use of extraoral radiographs.
3. List seven extraoral radiographs that contribute to the treatment of dental patients.
4. Explain the need for proper extraoral film handling.
5. Explain the role intensifying screens play in producing a radiographic image.
6. Match blue- and green-light sensitive film with the appropriate intensifying screen.
7. Explain the role of the extraoral film cassette.
8. Describe how extraoral radiographs are labeled.
9. Explain the need for proper care and cleaning of cassettes and intensifying screens.
10. Explain the role grids play in extraoral radiography.
11. Explain tomography and describe its role in oral health care.
12. Explain cone beam computed tomography and describe its role in oral health care.

KEY WORDS

Ankylosis
Artifacts
Calcium tungstate
Cassette
Cephalostat
Computed tomography (CT)
Cone beam computed tomography (CBCT)
Cone beam volumetric imaging (CBVI)
Grid
Intensifying screens
Lateral cephalometric radiograph (lateral skull)

Lateral jaw radiograph (mandibular oblique lateral)
Maxillofacial
Occult disease
Panoramic radiograph
Phosphors
Pixel (picture element)
Posteroanterior (PA) cephalometric radiograph
Rare-earth phosphors
Reverse Towne radiograph
Screen film

Submentovertex radiograph

Temporomandibular disorder (TMD)

Temporomandibular joint (TMJ)

Tomograph

Tomography

Transcranial radiograph (TMJ)

Voxel (volume element)

Waters radiograph

Introduction

Extraoral radiographs and alternate imaging modalities such as computed tomography record large areas of the dental arches, supporting facial structures, and skull using image receptors that are positioned outside the mouth. Most of these extraoral imaging techniques require special equipment not readily available in the general practice dental office (Figure 29-1). Even though dental assistants and hygienists may not routinely perform these services, a base knowledge in types of extraoral radiographs and alternate imaging modalities; an understanding of what conditions will most likely benefit from which type of examination; and the ability to recognize the different images are valuable skills. Patients may need to be referred to an oral surgeon or to a medical imaging center for examination of a condition affecting the maxillofacial region. The dental assistant and dental hygienist may be called on to educate the patient regarding the procedure or may need to assist with scheduling the patient's appointment for the referral. Oral radiographers should be able to communicate professionally with other health care professionals.

The purpose of this chapter is to provide an overview of the types of extraoral radiographs that contribute to the treatment of dental patients and identify the equipment and image receptors required and to introduce cutting-edge alternate imaging modalities that have developed from digital and computer technological advances.

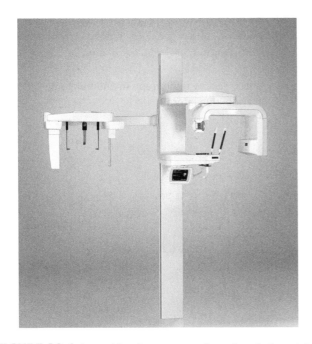

FIGURE 29-1 A combination panoramic and cephalometric dental x-ray unit. (Courtesy of Planmeca.)

Purpose and Use of Extraoral Imaging Modalities

The purpose of extraoral imaging modalities is to examine structures of the oral cavity and the **maxillofacial** region that includes the maxilla and mandible, the facial bones and sinuses, and the temporomandibular joint. Extraoral radiographs are used to

- Examine large areas of the dental arches and skull
- Study growth and development of bone and teeth
- Detect fractures and evaluate trauma
- Detect pathological lesions and diseases of the jaws
- Detect and evaluate impacted teeth
- Evaluate **temporomandibular disorder (TMD)**
- Plan treatment for dental implants and prosthetic appliances

Extraoral radiographs may also be substituted for intraoral radiographs when patients cannot or will not open the mouth. Handicapped patients or patients with trismus or TMD may not be able to tolerate the placement of intraoral image receptor. Extraoral radiographs can be used alone or in conjunction with intraoral radiographs. For example, it is common to expose both a panoramic radiograph (see Chapter 30) and intraoral bitewing radiographs on the same patient.

The general practitioner is most likely to limit the use of extraoral radiographs to panoramic imaging, discussed in detail in Chapter 30. The practitioner who specializes in dental implants will increasingly rely on **cone beam computed tomography,** introduced later in this chapter. Othodontists, prosthodontists, and oral surgeons are more frequent users of extraoral imaging modalities for diagnosing and treating conditions of the oral cavity and head and facial regions.

- **Orthodontists** use facial profile radiographs, produced with **cephalostat** headplates ("cephalometric," meaning measuring the head) to record, measure, and compare changes in growth and development of the bones and the teeth.
- **Prosthodontists** use facial profile radiographs to record the contour of the lips and face and the relationship of the teeth before removal to help in constructing prosthetic appliances that look natural (Figure 29-2).
- **Oral surgeons** use extraoral radiographs extensively to evaluate trauma, to determine the location and extent of fractures; to locate impacted teeth, abnormalities, and malignancies; and to evaluate injuries to the temporomandibular joint.

Extraoral Radiographs Useful in Oral Health Care

There are many techniques for exposing radiographs of the oral cavity and the maxillofacial region. It is not within the scope of this book to describe every available technique. The seven

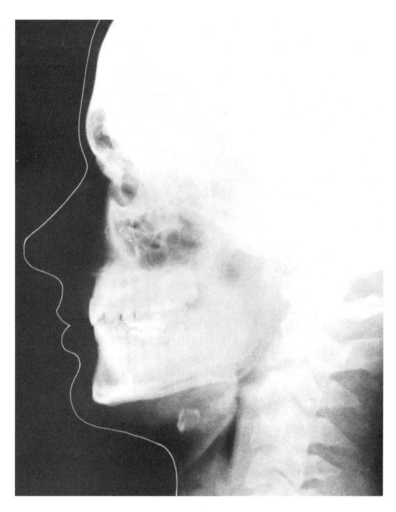

FIGURE 29-2 **Cephalometric radiograph** produced with a filter placed between the tube and patient to remove some of the x-rays to record outlines of the soft tissue profile.

projections presented in Table 29-1 are the most common extraoral radiographs in which the x-ray source and the image receptor remain still and in position during exposure. The **panoramic radiograph,** which requires movement of the x-ray source and the image receptor during exposure, is discussed in Chapter 30.

Extraoral Image Receptors

Traditional Film

To produce a diagnostic quality radiograph while maintaining a low radiation dose for the patient, extraoral **screen film** (see Chapter 7) must be used in conjunction with a pair of intensifying screens housed within a light-tight cassette. Because they are extremely light sensitive and not packaged in a protective sealed wrapper like intraoral films, extraoral films must be carefully loaded into a cassette under darkroom safelight illumination (Figure 29-3 and Procedure Box 29-1).

Extraoral films are generally packaged 25, 50, or 100 to a box, so care should be taken to ensure that overhead white light is turned off when removing the box cover. Darkroom safelight filter color and bulb wattage must be appropriate for use with extraoral film (see Chapter 8). Because extraoral film is more sensitive than intraoral film, filters that are safe for intraoral film handling may not be safe for extraoral film handling. The type of safelight required for extraoral film can usually be found written on the film package or by checking with the manufacturer.

Extraoral films should be removed from the box with clean, dry hands. Latex or vinyl treatment gloves should be avoided. Treatment gloves and plastic overgloves increase the risk of generating static electricity. A static charge results in a white light spark that will expose the film, leaving radiolucent **artifacts** (black lines or smudges) on the resultant image (Figure 29-6). Glove powder residue on films will also cause radiolucent artifacts.

Handle films by the edges only. Remove each sheet of film from the box slowly to avoid generating static electricity that will create artifacts on the films inside the box as well as the

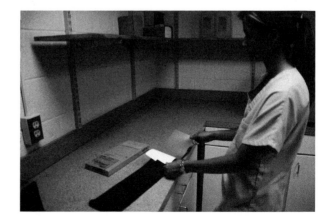

FIGURE 29-3 **Loading film into a flexible cassette under safelight conditions.**

TABLE 29-1 Extraoral Radiographs of the Maxillofacial Region

TYPE OF RADIOGRAPH	AREA OF INTEREST	PURPOSE	POSITIONING
Lateral jaw (mandibular oblique lateral)	Body or ramus of mandible; coronoid process; condyle	To examine posterior region of the mandible, third molars, especially when panoramic machine not available; when children or patients who have fractures or swelling are unable to tolerate placement or hold intraoral image receptor in place	Sagittal plane / Image receptor / Central ray
Lateral cephalometric (lateral skull)	Entire skull from the side (lateral); sinus cavities	Prior to orthodontic intervention, at various stages of treatment, on completion of treatment; to evaluate growth/development, trauma, pathology, developmental abnormalities; can reveal facial soft tissue profile when a filter is placed between the tube and patient to remove some of the x-rays; to establish pre-/posttreatment records	Image receptor / Central ray / X-ray beam
Posteroanterior (PA) cephalometric (posterior skull)	Entire skull in the posteroanterior plane; orbit; frontal sinus	To examine facial growth/development, disease, trauma, developmental abnormalities. Used to supplement lateral survey because the right and left sides of the facial structures are not superimposed on each other	Image receptor / Central ray / X-ray beam
Waters	Middle third of the face to include zygoma, coronoid process, sinuses	To evaluate maxillary, frontal, ethmoid sinuses	Tip of nose $\frac{3}{4}$" from image receptor / X-ray beam / Central ray / Image receptor

(Continued)

TABLE 29-1 (Continued)

TYPE OF RADIOGRAPH	AREA OF INTEREST	PURPOSE	POSITIONING
Reverse Towne	Condyles	To examine fractures of the condylar neck	X-ray beam · Central ray · Image receptor · Mouth open, head tipped down
Submentovertex	Base of the skull; condyles; sphenoid sinus; zygoma	To evaluate the position/orientation of the condyles; fractures of the zygomatic arch	Frankfort line · X-ray beam · Central ray · Floor · Image receptor
Transcranial	Head of condyle; glenoid fossa; temporal bone; temporomandibular joint in open, closed and at rest positions	Aids in diagnosing **ankylosis** (a stiffening of the temporomandibular joint); malignancies, fractures, and tissue changes caused by arthritis	Sagittal plane · Image receptor · Central ray 25°

one being removed. Try to place the film into the cassette without sliding it across the intensifying screens, again to prevent a static discharge. Film should be loaded into the cassette just prior to use. Storing film inside cassettes may increase the likelihood of generating artifacts. Only one film should be loaded into the cassette at a time unless special film made for exposing two films at once is used.

Intensifying Screens

Intensifying screens transfer x-ray energy into visible light. This visible light, in turn, exposes the film. The image produced on an extraoral film results from exposure to this fluorescent light instead of directly from the x-rays. As the name implies, intensifying screens "intensify" the effect of x-rays on film. The use of intensifying screens allows the amount of radiation required to expose the film to be reduced and therefore reduces the amount of radiation the patient is exposed to.

Intensifying screens work in pairs. An intensifying screen is a smooth cardboard or plastic sheet coated with minute fluorescent crystals mixed into a suitable binding medium. Intensifying screens are based on the principle that crystals of certain salts—**calcium tungstate,** barium strontium sulfate, or **rare-earth phosphors** [lanthanum (La) and gadolinium (Gd)]—will fluoresce and emit energy in the form of blue or green light when they absorb x-rays. Each of these fluorescent crystals, also called **phosphors,** gives off blue or green light that varies in intensity

PROCEDURE 29-1
Loading an extraoral cassette

1. Obtain the cassette and box of film. Ensure that the film sensitivity matches the intensifying screens used.

2. Open the cassette and inspect to ensure that the hinge and snaps are working. Examine the intensifying screens for debris or scratches. Clean with solution recommended by the manufacturer if necessary.

3. Turn off overhead white light and turn on safelight.

4. Open the package containing the film and slowly pull out one film.

5. Handle the film by the edges only with clean, dry hands. Place film inside cassette (rigid) (Figure 29-4). When loading film into a flexible plastic sleeve cassette, pull the screens part way out of the cassette to separate the pair. Slowly slide the film between the folded screens (Figure 29-5). Make sure that the film is seated all the way down to the fold in the screen.

6. Close the cassette and ensure that the hinge is secured (rigid). Close the snaps or Velcro® closures on the flexible cassette. When the cassette is not tightly closed, the film and screen contact is not tight, and it causes the radiograph to be blurry.

7. Replace the cover on the film box to protect from white light.

8. Turn on the overhead white light and exit the darkroom.

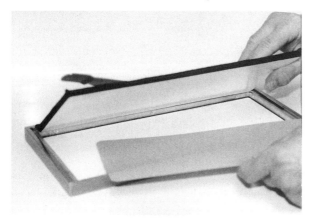

FIGURE 29-4 Loading a rigid cassette.

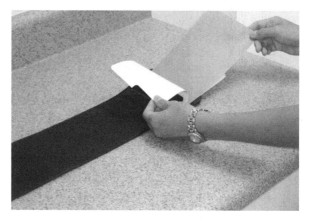

FIGURE 29-5 Film is placed between the intensifying screens.

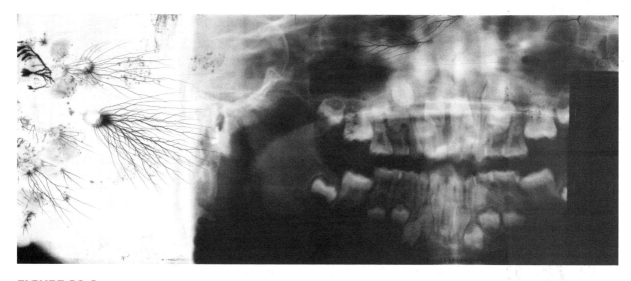

FIGURE 29-6 **Static electricity artifacts.** Blank area on a panoramic film showing static electricity artifacts.

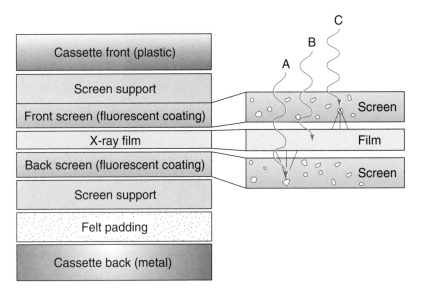

FIGURE 29-7 Cross-section of cassette showing the effect of x-ray and fluorescent light on the film. X-ray A strikes a crystal in the screen behind the film, producing light that then forms latent images in the silver halide crystal of the film. **X-ray B** strikes a silver halide crystal in the film, forming a latent image. **X-ray C** strikes a crystal in the screen in front of the film, producing light, which then forms latent images in the silver halide crystals of the film.

according to the x-rays in that part of the image. Screen film is more sensitive to this type of fluorescent light than to radiation. When the film is sandwiched tightly between a pair of two intensifying screens, the x-rays cause the crystals on the screens to fluoresce and return the emitted light to the film emulsion to produce the radiographic image (Figure 29-7).

Rare earth screens emit green light when energized by x-rays and must be paired with green-light–sensitive film. Calcium tungstate screens give off a blue to violet fluorescent light and must be paired with blue-light–sensitive film. Inappropriately interchanging green- or blue-light–sensitive films between calcium tungstate and rare earth screens produces undiagnostic radiographic images.

The use of intensifying screens decreases the amount of radiation required to produce an image. However, the sharpness of the radiographic image also is reduced over the images produced on intraoral films. The sensitivity and image sharpness of different types of intensifying screens varies and depends on the:

- **Size of the crystals.** The larger the crystal size, the less radiation required to produce an image. Larger crystals produce a less sharp image.
- **Thickness of the emulsion.** The thicker the emulsion, the faster the speed of the screen, requiring less radiation to produce an image. Thicker emulsion results in a less sharp image.
- **Type of phosphor used.** Rare earth screens produce a latent image on the film with less radiation exposure than calcium tungstate screens.

Although varying speeds of screens are available, the American Dental Association and the American Association of Oral and Maxillofacial Radiology recommend that the fastest speed screen–film combination be used to reduce the amount of radiation exposure to the patient. While reducing the radiation

required to produce an image, a large crystal size and a thick emulsion will produce a less sharp radiographic image. The slight reduction in image clarity produced by fast speed screen–film combinations is considered acceptable to reduce the radiation dose to the patient.

Cassettes

The purpose of the **cassette** is to hold the intensifying screens in close contact with the film and to protect the film from white light exposure. Cassettes are available in a variety of shapes and sizes, depending on the intended use. Cassettes are available as a rigid box or case that may be flat or curved. Rigid cassettes are usually 5 × 7 in. (13 × 18 cm) or 8 × 10 in. (20 × 25 cm). A typical rigid cassette has a front and back cover joined together with a hinge (Figure 29-8). The front cover is constructed of plastic to permit the passage of the x-ray

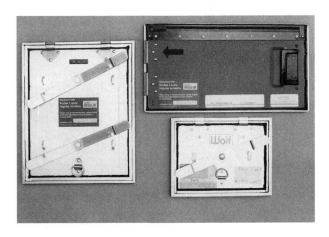

FIGURE 29-8 The back side of three rigid cassettes of various sizes.

beam and must be positioned so that it faces the patient. The back cover is constructed of heavy metal to absorb remnant x-rays. A pair of intensifying screens lines the inside of the front and back covers of the cassette.

Flexible plastic sleeve cassettes are most often used for exposing panoramic radiographs (see Figure 30-11). Flexible cassettes measure 5 or 6 × 12 in. (13 or 15 × 30 cm) and are composed of a plastic sleeve with intensifying screens inside. The paired intensifying screens are usually joined together at one end, so that a film may be inserted in between (Figure 29-5). Snaps or Velcro® closures seal the cassette to prevent white light from leaking in.

Film Identification

Extraoral films do not have the embossed identification dot that intraoral films have to aid in identifying the left and right sides of the image. Extraoral films are best identified by fastening an identification letter or plate to one of the corners of the front of the cassette. Special lettering sets, made of lead, are available for this purpose. The letters R (for right) and L (for left) can be placed on the front of the cassette prior to exposure. These identifications become visible on the processed radiograph. Identification plates can be used to record the patient's name and date of exposure directly onto the radiograph. Commercial film identification imprinters are available that permanently image pertinent data on the processed radiograph (Figure 29-9).

Care of Cassettes and Intensifying Screens

Extraoral cassettes and intensifying screens should be inspected periodically. Rigid and flexible cassette hinges and snaps should be checked to ensure light tightness to prevent film fog. Cassettes should be checked for warping to ensure close screen–film contact. Poor screen–film contact results in an image of reduced sharpness (blurry image). Defective cassettes should be repaired or replaced.

Intensifying screens should be examined for cleanliness and scratches. Debris present on the screens will block the light given off by the crystals and result in radiopaque artifacts on the resultant radiographic image. Screens may be carefully cleaned as needed with solutions recommended by the manufacturer. However, overuse of chemical cleaning may cause scratches and should be avoided. A scratched or damaged screen will not produce the light needed to expose the film and will result in radiopaque artifacts.

Grids

Grids are sometimes used in extraoral radiography to absorb scattered x-rays that contribute to film fog that reduces image contrast (Figure 29-10). Radiation that strikes the patient's tissues has the potential to be deflected back toward the film, reexposing it. A **grid** is a mechanical device composed of thin strips of lead alternating with a radiolucent material (usually plastic). The grid is placed between the patient and the film to absorb scattered x-rays and reduce film fog to improve image contrast. However, the use of a grid requires an increased dose of radiation, usually double the dose of radiation required when not using a grid. The use of a grid with its increased radiation dose to the patient must be carefully weighed against the diagnostic benefits. For example, when exposing radiographs to assess growth and development, a grid may be contraindicated. However, when evaluating the extent of a tumor, the increased image contrast obtained by using a grid may be justified.

Exposure Factors

The exposure factors for extraoral techniques vary considerably. The settings depend largely on the intensifying screen–film combination, which plays a similar role to intraoral film speed in determining appropriate exposure settings and the use of digital extraoral radiographic equipment. The patient's size and tissue density and the target–image receptor distance also must be considered. Refer to the x-ray equipment and film and screen manufacturers' recommendations to determine appropriate mA, kVp, and impulse settings.

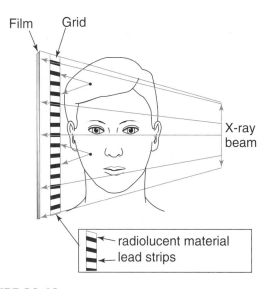

FIGURE 29-10 Grid used to absorb back scattered radiation is placed between the patient and the film to absorb scattered x-rays to reduce film fog.

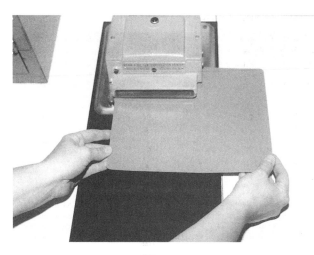

FIGURE 29-9 Film identification printer for imprinting permanent identification information on the radiographic image.

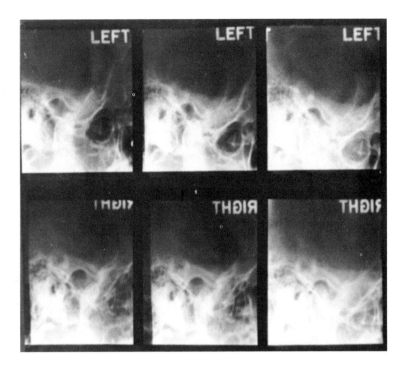

FIGURE 29-11 **Serial radiographs produced by tomography of the temporomandibular joint** showing the head of the condyle in the glenoid fossa with the mouth closed, in the at-rest position, and with the mouth open. (Courtesy of McCormack Dental X-ray Laboratory.)

Tomography, Computed Tomography, Cone Beam Computed Tomography

Radiographs are taken with a stationary x-ray source and image receptor. Structures such as the teeth and the supporting bone that lie along the same path travelled by the x-ray beam will be superimposed on the radiograph, limiting radiographs to distinctly separate structures. In addition, there are oral conditions, such as the need for an orthodontic evaluation or implant dentistry when the diagnosis and treatment planning would be enhanced by three-dimensional imaging. **Tomography** is a special radiographic technique that uses simultaneous movement of the x-ray source and the image receptor to record images of structures located within a selected plane of tissue, while blurring structures outside the selected plane. Tomography produces images by utilizing a narrow beam of x-rays to image a curved layer or slice of tissue. Tomography has been a valuable tool in imaging the **temporomandibular joint (TMJ)** (Figure 29-11). Panoramic radiography, discussed in Chapter 30, is also based on tomography. In fact, panoramic x-ray machines are available with multiple functions, allowing the operator to produce not only panoramic radiographs, but TMJ **tomographs** as well (Figure 29-12).

With digital technological advances, modern-day tomography now uses complex computer systems and multiple image receptors to produce enhanced two-dimensional and three-dimensional images out of the slices of tissue recorded with no superimposed blurring of the structures that lie outside the selected plane. A familiar medical use of this technology is a CT scan or **computed tomography.** Patients undergoing a CT scan of the maxillofacial region lie on a table with the head positioned inside the scanner (Figure 29-13). The scanner emits a narrow, fan-shaped x-ray beam that rotates 360 degrees around the patient's head while up to 2,000 image receptors receive the data. The table supporting the patient moves as the x-rays focus on each new layer or slice of tissue. Most CT systems have imaging software programs for dental implant treatment planning. These programs translate the data received by the image receptors into workable cases the practitioner can use to formulate decisions regarding implant size, orientation, and placement.

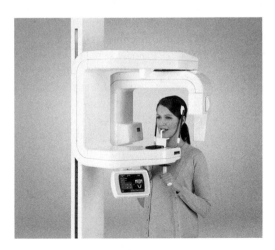

FIGURE 29-12 **A combination panoramic and TMJ tomography imaging dental x-ray unit.** (Courtesy of Planmeca.)

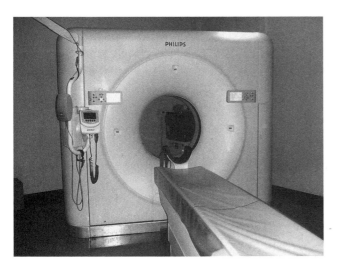

FIGURE 29-13 CT scanner.

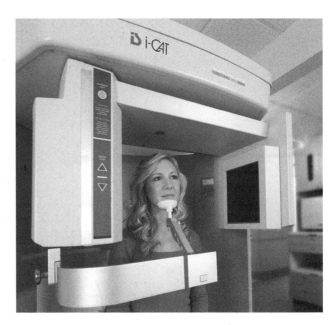

FIGURE 29-14 Cone beam volumetric imaging machine.
Designed for the oral health care practice, can also produce panoramic radiographs. (Courtesy of Gendex Dental Systems/Imaging Sciences Intl.)

Computed tomography is a highly regarded, accurate method of choice for imaging bone height, density, and the shape and contours of the edentulous ridges prior to dental implant surgery. However, the radiation dose to the patient from computed tomography is high, so this method of imaging must be balanced with the benefits it will provide. Although the actual radiation dose to the patient depends on many factors, the effective dose from a CT scan of the maxilla is estimated to be between 240 and 1200 μSv and between 480 and 3324 μSv for a scan of the mandible. You will recall from Chapter 5 that the effective dose from a panoramic radiograph is approximately 7 μSv. (See Table 5-3.)

In the desire to use computed tomography technology for dental applications while limiting the radiation dose to the patient, CT scanners are now available that are dedicated for maxillofacial use. **Cone beam computed tomography (CBCT),** also called **cone beam volumetric imaging (CBVI),** provides accurate, multiplanar images with no superimposed blurring with lower radiation doses (approximately 42 μSv for a scan of the maxilla and 75 μSv for a scan of the mandible). The technology of these lower-dose CT scanners is specifically targeted at imaging the maxillofacial region for oral health care applications. In fact, some machines allow the operator to switch from CBCT or CBVI mode to panoramic radiography, making this technology increasingly accessible for adoption by the oral health care practice (Figure 29-14).

The patient position for exposure is seated or standing upright, similar to the positioning for producing a panoramic radiograph. The cone-shaped x-ray beam is collimated to control radiation exposure to record only a limited region around the dental arches in one rotation around the head, reducing the radiation dose over CT scans. Whereas digital sensors used in intraoral radiography use pixels to produce the image (see Chapter 9), CBCT utilize voxels. A **pixel,** or **picture element,** is essentially a square with two sides. A **voxel,** or **volume element,** adds a third side to this square, making a cubed area for capturing more data. The computer software then converts this data into an image that can be

read on a computer monitor. The images can be interpreted and studied from not only the sagittal plane, as film-based and digital radiographic images are, but also from the coronal and axial planes and as a three-dimension reconstructed image (Figure 29-15).

At this point in time, CBCT has not been widely taught or practiced by oral health care professionals and is considered new technology for dental applications, although widely accepted in the medical community. Currently most patients who would benefit from this technology can be referred to a medical imaging center for the procedure. An expert dental or medical professional at these centers would be responsible for interpreting the images and providing a report or summary to the referring dentist. When the CBCT scanning equipment is available in an oral health care practice, it is usually a specialty practice such as an orthodontist, periodontist, or specialist in dental implantology. Even in these practices, unless he or she has been trained and is comfortable making the final diagnosis, the dentist will often have the images interpreted by a medical expert, especially because these images are likely to reveal information beyond the teeth and oral cavity. Although the dentist may be an expert at determining conditions of the teeth and the supporting structures, conditions beyond the oral cavity such as the oral and nasal airways, paranasal sinuses, and other tissues outside the maxillofacial region must be examined for potential **occult diseases** (diseases that were not apparent clinically).

Cone beam **computed tomography** will continue to play an increasingly valuable role in oral health care treatment, especially as technology finds ways to reduce the radiation dose to the patient. Some experts in the field of dentistry predict that CBCT will become the standard of care in implant dentistry in the near future.

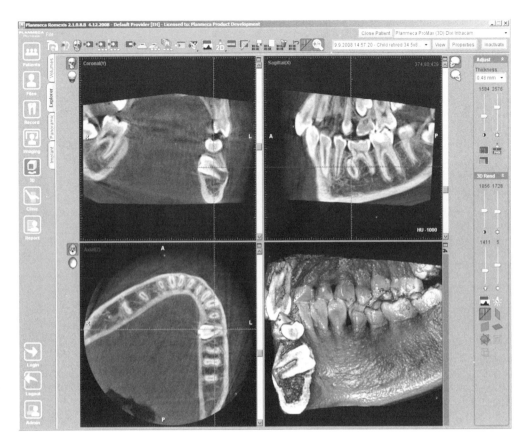

FIGURE 29-15 Image produced by CBCT and reconstructed software. Note the images produced from different planes and the reconstructed 3D image of the teeth in the arches. (Courtesy of Planmeca.)

REVIEW—Chapter summary

Extraoral radiographs image large areas of the head and facial regions. Extraoral radiographs are useful in examination of large areas of the dental arches and skull; to study growth and development of bone and teeth; in the detection of fractures, pathological lesions, and diseases of the jaws; in assessment of impacted teeth; in evaluation of temporomandibular disorders (TMD); and in treatment planning for dental implants and prosthetics. Orthodontists, prosthodontists, and oral surgeons are major users of extraoral imaging modalities.

The purpose of exposing the following extraoral radiographs was presented: lateral jaw, lateral cephalometric, posteroanterior (PA) cephalometric, Waters, Reverse Towne, submentovertex, and transcranial.

Extraoral screen film is used in conjunction with a pair of intensifying screens housed in a light-tight cassette. Extraoral film is more sensitive than intraoral film. Careful handling is needed to avoid static electricity and glove powder artifacts. Intensifying screens transfer x-ray energy into visible light that in turn exposes screen film to produce an image. Intensifying screens intensify the effect of x-rays on the film, resulting in a reduced dose of radiation required to produce an image. Faster speed intensifying screens have larger sized fluorescent crystals (phosphors) and thicker emulsion, but produce a slightly less sharp image. Rare earth phosphor screens are faster than calcium tungstate screens. Rare earth screens emit green light and

must be paired with green-light–sensitive film. Calcium tungstate screens emit blue light and must be paired with blue-light–sensitive film. The use of fast-speed screen–film combinations is recommended to produce acceptable images at a reduced radiation dose to the patient.

Special lettering sets or commercial film imprinters are used to label and identify extraoral film. Cassettes hold the intensifying screens in close contact with the film in a light-tight rigid case or a flexible plastic sleeve. Cassettes and intensifying screens should be examined periodically to ensure optimum performance. Dirty or scratched screens will result in radiopaque artifacts that compromise diagnosis.

Grids are devices used to absorb scatter radiation that would fog the film and compromise image contrast. The use of grids requires increased radiation exposure and so they are not usually recommended unless a fine detail contrasting image is required for accurate diagnosis.

Exposure settings for extraoral techniques depend on the intensifying screen–film combination used, the patient's size and tissue density, and the target–image receptor distance.

Radiographs are produced with a stationary x-ray source and image receptor. Tomography employs a simultaneously moving x-ray source and image receptor to produce an image within a selected plane while blurring objects outside the selected layer. Computed tomography (CT) utilizes complex digital x-ray systems and multiple image receptors to produce images within a slice of tissue without blurred superimposition of objects outside the layer of interest. CT scans provide accurate images of bone height, density, and shape and contours of edentulous ridges prior to dental implant surgery. Radiation doses from computed tomography are significantly higher than extraoral radiography.

Cone beam computed tomography (CBCT), also called cone beam volumetric imaging (CBVI), focused on maxillofacial imaging with oral health care applications provides accurate, multiplanar images with no superimposed blurring with lower radiation doses than CT scans. Some CBCT machines can produce panoramic radiographs. The practitioner must be skilled in interpreting images obtained by CBCT, which uses voxels to reconstruct data received by the image receptor that can be interpreted and studied from the sagittal, coronal, and axial planes. CBCT technology will continue to increase in value as an imaging modality in oral health care treatment.

RECALL—Study questions

1. For which of these purposes are extraoral radiographs least suitable?
   a. Detection of interproximal caries
   b. Locating impacted teeth
   c. Viewing the sinuses
   d. Determining the extent of a fracture

2. Which of these radiographs is most frequently prescribed by the orthodontist?
   a. Transcranial
   b. Lateral cephalometric
   c. Waters
   d. Reverse Towne

3. The general practitioner is most likely to use which of these extraoral radiographs?
   a. Posteroanterior cephalometric
   b. Reverse Towne
   c. Panoramic
   d. Submentovertex

4. Which of these radiographs would best image the maxillary sinus?
   a. Transcranial
   b. Waters
   c. Periapical
   d. Posteroanterior cephalometric

5. What size film is generally used to produce a cephalometric radiograph?
   a. 5 × 7 in. (13 × 18 cm)
   b. 8 × 10 in. (20 × 25 cm)
   c. 5 × 12 in. (13 × 30 cm)
   d. 6 × 12 in. (15 × 30 mm)

6. Black artifacts on extraoral radiographs may result from each of the following EXCEPT one. Which one is the EXCEPTION?
   a. Static electricity
   b. Glove powder residue
   c. Rapidly removing films from the packaging
   d. Scratched intensifying screens

7. Intensifying screens will
   a. increase x-ray intensity.
   b. increase image detail.
   c. reduce exposure time.
   d. decrease processing time.

8. What term describes the crystals used in the emulsion of intensifying screens?
   a. Phosphors
   b. Halides
   c. Sulfates
   d. Bromides

9. Fast intensifying screens have _____ sized crystals and _____ thickness of emulsion.
   a. large; decreased
   b. large; increased
   c. small; decreased
   d. small; increased

10. Rare-earth intensifying screens require less radiation to produce a quality image.

    Rare-earth intensifying screens emit blue light when energized by x-radiation.
    a. The first statement is correct. The second statement is incorrect.
    b. The first statement is incorrect. The second statement is correct.
    c. Both statements are correct.
    d. Both statements are incorrect.

11. Which of these is NOT a way to identify extraoral radiographs?
    a. Embossed identification dot
    b. Commercial identification printer
    c. Lead letters "R" and "L"
    d. Lead plates affixed to the cassette

12. Unsharp (blurry) images result from which of the following?
    a. Film and screens not in close contact
    b. Faulty (not tight) hinge on rigid cassette
    c. Not closing the cassette tightly
    d. All of the above

13. Which of the following is used to help reduce film fog during exposure of extraoral radiographs?
    a. Voxel
    b. Cephalostat
    c. Grid
    d. Phosphors

14. Which of the following is true regarding tomography when compared to extraoral radiography?
    a. Requires less radiation to produce an image of the maxillofacial region.
    b. Utilizes a moving x-ray source and moving image receptor.
    c. Superimposes structures in the path of the x-ray beam on the image.
    d. Less likely to exhibit film fog.

15. Cone beam computed tomography plays a valuable role in which of the following?
    a. Assessing growth and development of the orthodontic patient.
    b. Imaging the height and contour of edentulous ridges.
    c. Treatment planning for dental implants
    d. All of the above.

REFLECT—Case study

Consider the following patients and conditions. Which of the seven extraoral radiographs described in this chapter might be the *best* recommendation for these cases? (*Note:* Radiographs of the skull are difficult to interpret due to the numerous structures that exist in a very small area. These structures often appear superimposed over each other, requiring multiple views to obtain a good diagnosis. Therefore, in some of these cases, although there is usually a *best* answer, there may be more than one correct answer.)

1. A 20-year-old patient presents with pain and swelling from an impacted third molar. The patient can open only 10 mm. No panoramic unit is available. What is an alternate extraoral projection type that can be used to assist with diagnosis for this patient?
2. A 13-year-old patient presents for an orthodontic consultation. Occlusal (teeth) and facial disharmonies (soft tissue relationships) need to be assessed prior to treatment intervention.
3. A difficult extraction case presents with a severely decayed maxillary molar. During the extraction procedure, the root tip fractures and is possibly lost in the sinus cavity.
4. A medically compromised patient suffered a seizure and fell. A fractured mandibular condyle is suspected.
5. A 69-year-old patient presents with a history of degenerative joint disease that may be affecting the temporal mandibular joint. An examination for the purpose of diagnosing ankylosis (a stiffening of the TMJ) is planned.
6. A patient presents for extraction of several badly decayed teeth, following which the prosthodontist will construct a maxillary full denture and a mandibular partial denture.

RELATE—Laboratory application

Because intensifying screens fluoresce visible light when energized by x-radiation, you can perform this experiment to confirm what types of intensifying screens are available for use at your facility:

Open the cassette to expose the intensifying screens and place on the counter or operatory chair, face up. No film is needed. Place the tube head of the intraoral dental x-ray machine directly over the opened cassette and aim the PID so that x-rays will strike the exposed intensifying screens. Set the exposure timer to the maximum setting, a full second, for example. Stand at least six feet away from the tube head at a 90- to 135-degree angle (see Figure 6-15) or remain behind a barrier that allows visual contact with the screens during the exposure (see Figure 3-7). Depress the exposure button and observe the intensifying screens. Make note of the color, either blue or green, of the light emitted during exposure. Match the color observed with what you learned about calcium tungstate and rare-earth screens.

Next, perform an inventory on the extraoral films available for use at your facility. Does the film, either blue-light–sensitive or green-light–sensitive, match the screens? Use the information learned in this chapter to explain why this is important.

REFERENCES

Chau, A. C. M., & Fung K. (2009). Comparison of radiation dose for implant imaging using conventional spiral tomography, computed tomography, and cone-beam computed tomography. *Oral Surgery, Oral Medicine, Oral Pathology, Oral Radiology, and Endodontology, 107,* 559–565.

Farman, A. G., Nortje, C. J., & Wood, R. E. (1993). *Oral and maxillofacial diagnostic imaging.* St. Louis, MO: Mosby.

Horner, K., Drage, N., & Brettle, D. (2008). *21st century imaging.* London: Quintessence Publishing Co.

Miles, D. A. (2008). *Color atlas of cone beam volumetric imaging for dental applications.* Chicago: Quintessence Publishing Co.

White, S. C., & Pharoah, M. J. (2004). *Oral radiology: Principles and interpretation* (5th ed.). St. Louis, MO: Elsevier.

Panoramic Radiography

OBJECTIVES

Following successful completion of this chapter, you should be able to:

1. Define the key words.
2. List uses of panoramic radiography.
3. Compare the advantages and limitations of panoramic versus intraoral radiographs.
4. Explain how the panoramic technique relates to the principles of tomography.
5. Identify the three dimensions of the focal trough.
6. List the components of a panoramic x-ray machine.
7. Explain how to use each of the head positioner guides found on a panoramic x-ray machine.
8. Identify the planes used to position the dental arches correctly within the focal trough.
9. Explain the use of a cape-style lead/lead equivalent barrier or the use of an apron without an attached thyroid collar.
10. List patient preparation errors and describe how these will affect the appearance of the panoramic radiograph.
11. Match the patient-positioning errors with the characteristic affect on the appearance of the panoramic radiograph.
12. List exposure and image receptor handling errors and describe how these will affect the appearance of the panoramic radiograph.
13. List and identify the anatomic landmarks of the maxilla and surrounding tissues as viewed on a panoramic radiograph.
14. List and identify the anatomic landmarks of the mandible and surrounding tissues as viewed on a panoramic radiograph.
15. List and identify soft tissue images as viewed on a panoramic radiograph.
16. List and identify three air space images as viewed on a panoramic radiograph.
17. List and identify machine part artifacts as viewed on a panoramic radiograph.
18. List and identify ghost image artifacts as viewed on a panoramic radiograph.
19. Identify in sequence the basic steps in the panoramic radiographic procedure.

Introduction

The panoramic radiograph is probably the most common extraoral projection used in general oral health care practice. **Panoramic radiography** refers to a technique for producing a broad view image of the entire dentition of both the maxilla and mandible with the surrounding alveolar bone, the sinuses, and the temporomandibular joints on a single radiograph (Figure 30-1). The purpose of this chapter is to explain the fundamental concepts of panoramic radiography and to interpret normal anatomy and other structures that will be recorded on these images.

Purpose and Use

The term **panoramic** means "wide view." Panoramic radiography is descriptive of the wide view of the maxilla and mandible produced on a single radiograph. Panoramic radiographs play a valuable role in:

- Examining large areas of the face and jaws
- Locating impacted teeth or retained root tips
- Evaluating trauma, lesions, and diseases of the jaws
- Assessing growth and development

Panoramic image quality, especially with the introduction of digital imaging, continues to improve, suggesting that panoramic radiographs may also aid in the evaluation of large caries and moderate periodontal diseases. However, panoramic imagery is not as sharp and detailed as the images produced by intraoral radiographs. When specific conditions or diseases are suspected, intraoral radiographs are often prescribed in conjunction with panoramic radiographs (see Table 6-1).

Advantages and Limitations

The greatest advantage of panoramic radiographs is that they image a greater area and provide an increased amount of diagnostic information when compared to a full mouth series of individual radiographs with a reduced amount of radiation dose to the patient (Box 30-1). In addition, the broad image produced by a panoramic radiograph is easy for patients to understand, aiding in the explanation of the diagnosis and the proposed treatment plan in a manner that is clear and understandable. Panoramic procedures are relatively easy to perform, requiring less time than a full mouth series. The simple procedure demands less patient cooperation, and because the image receptor is not placed intraorally, there is less discomfort, making the panoramic procedure an acceptable substitute, under certain conditions, for patients who cannot tolerate intraoral procedures. Because of the relative ease with which a panoramic radiograph may be obtained, there may be a tendency to overuse this diagnostic tool. It is important to note that research on the use of panoramic radiographs cautions against using panoramic images as a screening film for **occult disease** (diseases that may exist without signs or symptoms).

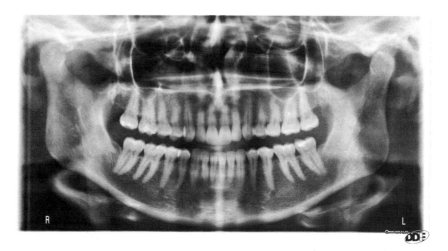

FIGURE 30-1 Panoramic radiograph. Provides a broad view of the dental arches. Note, however, the inherent image distortion as the panoramic view broadens the arches.
(Courtesy of Gendex Dental Systems/Imaging Sciences Intl.)

BOX 30-1   Advantages and Limitations of Panoramic Radiographs

Advantages

- Increased coverage of supporting structures of the oral cavity.
- Reduced patient radiation dose over a film-based intraoral full mouth series of radiographs.
- Can be performed in less time than the exposure of a full mouth series of radiographs.
- Simple procedure to perform.
- May be performed on patients who cannot, or will not tolerate placement of an intraoral image receptor.
- Requires minimal patient instruction and cooperation.
- Infection control protocol minimized.
- Mounting time is eliminated.
- Aids in explaining treatment plan to patients.

Limitations

- Increased image distortion. The amount of vertical and horizontal distortion is not constant—it varies from one part of the radiograph to another
- Reduced image sharpness.
- Increased occurrence of overlapping of the proximal contact areas, especially in the premolar region.
- Focal trough size and shape limits imaging only those structures that "fit" into the image layer. Teeth with labial or lingual tilting may not image well.
- The size and shape of the focal trough is predetermined by the manufacturer, therefore not all patients' arches will be recorded equally well.
- Superimposition of structures (e.g., the spinal column) may make interpretation difficult.
- Soft tissue shadows present on the resulting image may mimic pathology.
- Ghost images present on the resulting image may hide pathology.
- Not useful in detecting incipient carious lesions or early periodontal changes.
- Simple procedure may be overused inappropriately.
- Length of exposure time may limit its use on young children and other patients who cannot remain still throughout the exposure cycle.
- Cost of panoramic machine is significant.

The greatest limitation of panoramic radiographs is image quality. Magnification, distortion, and poor definition are inherent with panoramic techniques. **Ghost images, negative shadows,** and other artifacts can make interpreting panoramic images difficult. Further compromising the ability to obtain quality images is the difficulty associated with positioning the patient within the **focal trough** (area of image sharpness). Manufacturers design panoramic x-ray machines to be able to image the average patient. However, it may be difficult to record all structures with relative clarity when a patient's dental arches do not fall into this average range.

Fundamentals of Panoramic Radiography

Panoramic radiography is based on the principle of tomography. As discussed in Chapter 29, **tomography** is a special radiographic technique used to record images of structures located within a selected plane of tissue, while blurring structures outside the selected plane. During panoramic imaging as during tomography, the x-ray source and image receptor move in relationship to each other. Panoramic x-ray machines operate with the patient positioned between the x-ray tube head and the cassette that holds the image receptor. The exposure is made as the tube head and cassette rotate slowly around the patient's head during the operational cycle (usually about 15 to 20 seconds). The cassette with image receptor and the x-ray tube head move in directions opposite each other while the patient stands or is seated in a stationary position (Figure 30-2). The x-ray tube head moves around the back of the patient while the cassette with image receptor moves

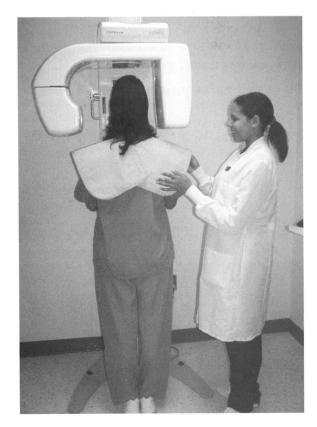

FIGURE 30-2 **Panoramic x-ray machine.** Radiographer positions the patient between the image receptor and the x-ray tube head of this digital panoramic dental x-ray machine.

Moving x-ray source

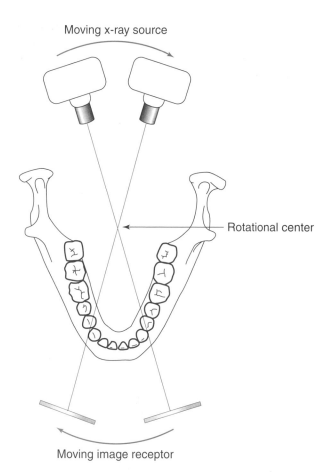

Rotational center

Moving image receptor

FIGURE 30-3 Panoramic radiography. The moving x-ray source passes through the center of rotation in a horizontal plane toward the path of the moving image receptor. As the beam scans the object (the dental arches), a continuous image is recorded on the moving image receptor.

around the front. The x-ray beam strikes the patient's tissues from the back of the head.

Through the use of a series of rotational points or centers (differing according to the unit manufacturer), the x-ray beam is directed toward the moving image receptor to record a select plane of dental anatomy (Figure 30-3). The **rotational center,** which is defined as the axis on which the x-ray tube head and the cassette rotate, is the functional focus of the projection. Most panoramic machines available today utilize a continuous moving rotational center to refocus the x-ray beam during movement to produce an image (Figure 30-4). This type of rotational center will keep the inherent horizontal and vertical magnification of the image relatively constant. All panoramic images have between 10 and 30 percent image magnification, depending on where the structures are located in relationship to the center of the slice of tissue being focused on. It is desirable to keep the inherent magnification even throughout the image. The elliptical pattern made by the rotational center in Figure 30-4 very closely matches the arc of the teeth and jaws and is likely to keep image magnification relatively constant.

Unlike the concentric or rectangular beam of x-radiation of intraoral radiography, the x-rays emerge from a narrow vertical slit opening in the tube head and are constricted to form a narrow band. This narrow opening collimates (constricts) the x-ray

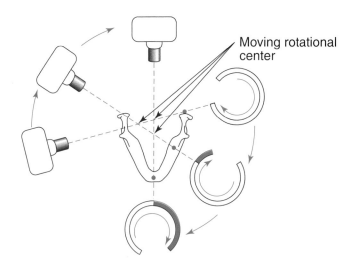

Moving rotational center

FIGURE 30-4 Moving rotational center allows the x-ray beam to continuously focus as the tube head and the image receptor simultaneously move.

beam so that a limited amount of tissue is irradiated. The narrow vertical beam of radiation then passes through the patient and through a secondary collimator vertical slit in the cassette holder to expose the image receptor that is moving or rotating in the opposite direction (Figure 30-5).

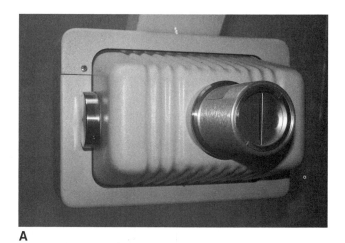

A

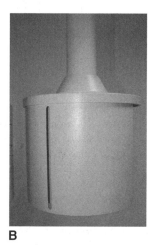

B

FIGURE 30-5 Slit collimator (A) and slit opening **(B)** to the image receptor.

Concept of the Focal Trough

The **focal trough** or **focal layer** is where the dental arches should be positioned to achieve the sharpest image. The focal trough is that area between the x-ray source and the image receptor that will be imaged distinctly on the panoramic radiograph (Figure 30-6). Objects located at various distances from the center of the focal trough become less sharp the farther away they are located.

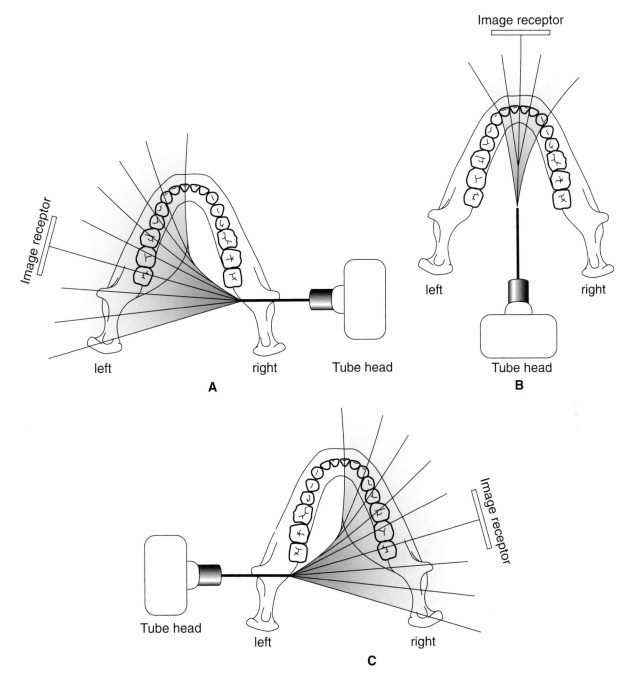

FIGURE 30-6 Plane of focus within the focal trough. The x-ray beam is focused on imaging the structures that are positioned closest to the image receptor. As the tube head and image receptor rotate, the x-ray beam is refocused to image the next section of anatomy. (**A**) Illustrated here is one moment in the continuous exposure. At this precise moment, the tube head is positioned on the right side, allowing the x-ray beam to penetrate the right side, then continue on to penetrate the left side and carry the images of the structures penetrated to the receptor. At this moment the right side is farther from the image receptor than the left side. At this moment in the exposure sequence, the left side will be recorded on the image, while the right side will be blurred out as a ghost image. (**B**) As the tube head and image receptor rotate, the x-ray beam now penetrates the back of head (and the cervical vertebrae), then continues on to penetrate the anterior teeth. Because the anterior teeth at this moment are closer to the image receptor, the cervical vertebrae will most likely appear magnified and blurred out as a ghost image, while the anterior teeth will be more distinctly recorded onto the image. (**C**) As the tube head and image receptor continue to rotate to the opposite side, the x-ray beam now penetrates the left side first, blurring it out of the image. The right side is now closer to the image receptor, so it will be imaged more clearly.

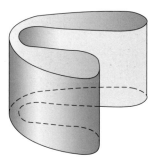

FIGURE 30-7 Diagram of the focal trough.

The focal trough is three-dimensional, and its actual shape varies depending on the equipment used (Figure 30-7). The three-dimensions of the focal trough are (1) anterior–posterior, (2) lateral or left–right, and (3) superior–inferior or up–down.

The panoramic x-ray machine's moving center rotation system results in a focal trough that is wider in the posterior regions and narrower in the anterior regions, making it imperative that the anterior teeth be positioned precisely to be imaged correctly. It is important to note that a mistake in positioning the arches in the anterior region of the focal trough by as little as 3 or 4 mm will make a significant difference in the degree of magnification on the resultant radiograph.

Components of the Panoramic X-Ray Machine

Although considerable differences exist in the size and configuration of panoramic x-ray machines, the operational procedures are similar and relatively simple (Procedure Box 30-1). Many machines require that the patient stand during the exposure; others operate with the patient seated. The machine's design will determine whether the patient is positioned to face the radiographer and away from the machine or to face the machine with their back to the radiographer. Film-based panoramic radiographs require the use of either a rigid or flexible cassette with intensifying screens (Figure 30-8; see Chapter 29); phosphor plates utilize a rigid or flexible cassette without intensifying screens (Figure 30-9); and the image receptor, usually a CCD (see Chapter 9), is built into digital panoramic x-ray machines (Figure 30-10).

All panoramic x-ray machines have four basic components:

1. Rotational x-ray tube head
2. Cassette holder (for film or phosphor plate) or digital image receptor
3. Head positioner guides
4. Exposure control panel

The x-ray tube used in panoramic x-ray machines generates electrons to produce x-ray energy similar to x-ray units used for intraoral exposures. The panoramic tube head is in a fixed vertical position with the short PID pointing up slightly, about negative 8 degrees. Film-based panoramic machines require that the film be loaded into a cassette that is then attached to the **cassette holder** so that it will rotate in relation with the tube head. Each machine manufacturer provides specific instructions for attaching the cassette to the unit (Figure 30-11).

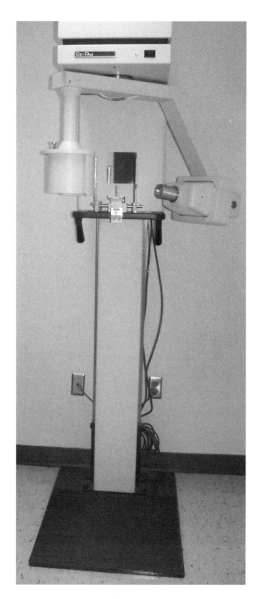

FIGURE 30-8 Film-based panoramic x-ray machine.

FIGURE 30-9 Phosphor plates used for indirect digital panoramic x-ray machine. (Courtesy of Air Techniques.)

PROCEDURE 30-1
*Panoramic radiographic procedure**

Cassette and film preparation

1. Examine cassette for proper function. Check hinge for wear. Check for light-tight seal.
2. Examine intensifying screens (if film-based) or phosphor plates for quality. Check for scratches and need of cleaning.
3. Obtain a box of extraoral film. Ensure that the film sensitivity matches the screen type used (see Chapter 29). The image receptor is built in to digital panoramic machines and will already be in place.
4. Turn off white overhead light and turn on safelight. (Ensure that safelight color filter recommended by the film manufacturer is in use.)
5. Remove the cover from the box of film and carefully, with clean, dry hands, remove one film from the box. Remove slowly to avoid generating static electricity.
6. Handling the film by the edges only, load into the cassette. (When using a flexible cassette, ensure that the film is inserted between the screens and is seated all the way down to the fold). Close tightly, securing the hinge (rigid cassette) or snaps (flexible cassette). Replace the cover on the box of film prior to turning on overhead white light and leaving the darkroom.

Unit preparation

1. Clean and disinfect with appropriate disinfectant all surfaces that will come in contact either directly or indirectly with the patient, such as the:
   a. Forehead rest
   b. Chin rest
   c. Side head positioner guides
   d. Patient support handles
   e. Chair (sit-down units)
2. Select sterile or disposable biteblock or cotton roll.
3. Attach the cassette onto the cassette holder of the unit according to the manufacturer's instructions. Ensure that the cassette is placed so that the exposure will begin at the appropriate edge of the film.
4. Turn on the machine. Raise or lower the overhead assembly to the approximate height of the patient, and move to the patient-entry position or move out of the way (if necessary) so that the way is clear for the patient to get into position.

Patient preparation

1. Inform patient of the need for the panoramic radiograph. Explain the procedure, answer patient concerns/questions regarding the procedure, and obtain patient's consent.
2. Request that the patient remove eyeglasses, necklaces, hair barrettes, facial jewelry (tongue, lip piercing adornments), removable dental appliances and any other material that may interfere with the radiographic procedure such as chewing gum or a thick hooded sweatshirt.
3. Place the lead/lead-equivalent cape or apron without a thyroid collar over the patient. Ensure that the lead apron will not impede the rotation of the cassette or image receptor holder.

*The procedures for taking panoramic radiographs are similar on most panoramic machines. As the complexity of the controls and head holder adjustments varies from unit to unit, the radiographer should read the manufacturer's instructions carefully before attempting to operate an unfamiliar machine.

(Continued)

PROCEDURE 30-1
Panoramic radiographic procedure (continued)*

Patient positioning

1. To position the arches into the focal trough's anterior/posterior dimension, instruct the patient to bite on the bite guide with the anterior teeth occluding edge to edge, or to place the chin completely forward into the chin rest or against the forehead rest. If available, align the laser light beam at the interproximal space recommended by the machine manufacturer.

2. To position the arches into the focal trough's lateral (right–left) dimension, close the head positioner guides or instruct the patient to view reflection in the mirror (on some units) and align the midsaggital plane perpendicular to the floor. Utilize unit light beams if available.

3. To position the arches into the focal trough's superior–inferior dimension, adjust the patient's chin up or down until the Frankfort plane is parallel to the floor or until the ala–tragus line is approximately positive 5 degrees to the floor. (Some panoramic x-ray units have indicator lines scribed on the head positioner guides or projected as a beam of light from the unit to align either the Frankfort plane or the ala–tragus line to obtain correct superior–inferior patient positioning in the focal trough.)

Exposure

1. Select the appropriate kVp and mA for the patient. Refer to posted exposure settings or use the manufacturer's recommendations.

2. Instruct the patient to place the tongue up against the hard palate and to close the lips around the bite guide or cotton roll. (Asking the patient to swallow or suck in the cheeks will assist with correct placement of the tongue and lips.)

3. Instruct the patient to remain still throughout the exposure cycle.

4. Take a position behind a protective barrier or an adequate distance away from the x-ray source and depress the exposure button for the duration of the cycle. You should be able to watch the procedure during the exposure from a protected location (see Figure 3-7) to ensure that the patient does not move and that the rotation of the unit continues unhindered. If patient movement occurs or the unit contacts the patient or protective barrier cape, release the exposure button to stop the process. The cassette should be removed from the unit and the procedure should start over, beginning with a new film.

5. When the exposure cycle is complete, move the overhead assembly to the patient-exit position or move out of the way (if necessary) so that the way is clear for the patient to be released. Remove the protective barrier cape. Return glasses, earrings, appliances, or other personal belongings to the patient.

6. Return the head positioner and overhead assembly to the closed position and turn off the machine. Discard the disposable bite guide or prepare autoclavable bite guide for sterilization. Clean and disinfect with appropriate disinfectant all surfaces that came in contact either directly or indirectly with the patient. (See Step 1.)

Processing

1. Remove the cassette from the cassette holder.

2. Proceed to the darkroom. Turn off the overhead white light and turn on the safelight. Open the cassette and remove the film from between the intensifying screens. Handle the film with clean, dry hands by the edges only. Use care to avoid sliding the film across the screens in such a manner that would generate static electricity or scratch the screens or the film.

3. Manually or automatically process the film according to the manufacturer's instructions.**

**Prior to processing, a film identification printer may be utilized to permanently label the film with the patient's name, the date of exposure and other information (see Figure 29-9).

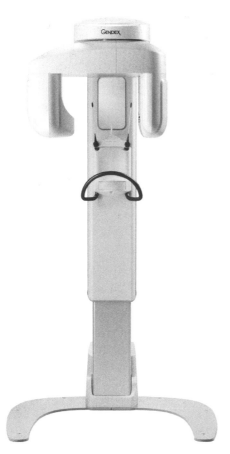

FIGURE 30-10 **Digital panoramic x-ray machine.** (Courtesy of Gendex Dental Systems/Imaging Sciences Intl.)

Because the focal trough is determined and set by the machine manufacturer, **head positioner guides** will assist the radiographer in positioning the patient correctly. Most panoramic machines are equipped with a biteblock or forehead rest that allows the radiographer to correctly determine how far forward or back the patient should be positioned, side positioner guides or a mirror for determining the correct side-to-side or right–left or lateral alignment, and a chin rest

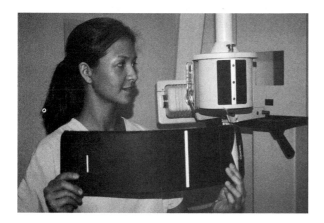

FIGURE 30-11 **Radiographer preparing to attach flexible cassette to the cassette holder carriage.** Note the markings on the outside of the cassette that indicate the correct direction for attaching the cassette to the unit.

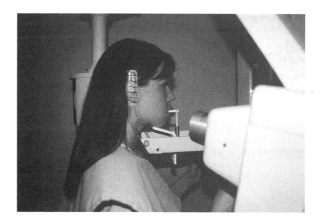

FIGURE 30-12 **Head positioner guides.** A biteblock aids the radiographer in locating the correct forward and back dimension of the focal trough; side positioner guides aid with locating the correct left and right dimension; and a chin rest aids with locating the correct up and down dimension. Note the cape-style lead/lead equivalent apron without a thyroid collar for use with panoramic exposures.

to correctly locate how far up or down the arches should be positioned (Figure 30-12). Some panoramic machines have beams of light that when turned on to shine on the patient's face will guide the operator to find each of these three dimensions (Figure 30-13).

The exposure control panel will usually allow the radiographer to select the mA and kVp as recommended by the manufacturer (Figure 30-14). The size of the patient and density of the tissues to be imaged will determine what settings are used.

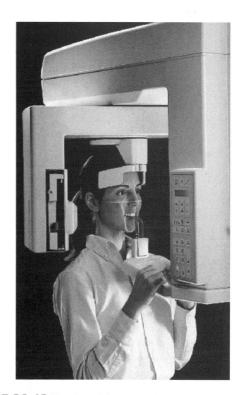

FIGURE 30-13 **Head positioner guides.** Beams of light shine on the patient's face to aid the radiographer in positioning the arches in the focal trough. (Courtesy of Gendex Dental Corporation.)

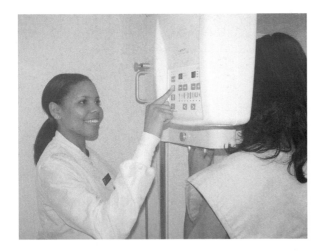

FIGURE 30-14 The radiographer uses the control panel to set the exposure.

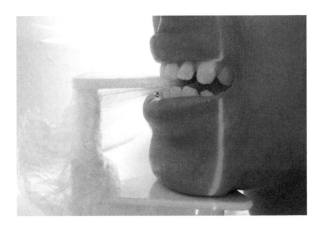

FIGURE 30-15 **Aligning the correct anterior–posterior position** with the light beam guide illuminated over the interproximal space of the canine and the premolar.

The kVp controls the penetrating ability of the beam, so it is often adjusted up when exposing larger patients or denser tissues and adjusted down when exposing children and edentulous patients. The exposure time is preset by the manufacturer and varies from 15 to 20 seconds to complete the cycle. To activate the exposure, the radiographer must depress the exposure button and hold for the duration of the cycle.

Importance of Correct Patient Positioning

Positioning the patient's head and dental arches within the focal trough is necessary for producing diagnostic images. Correct positioning will vary, depending on whether the area of interest is in the region of the temporomandibular joints, the sinuses, or the teeth and their supporting structures. Because the focal trough is predetermined by the panoramic machine manufacturer, the radiographer must refer to the manufacturer's instructions when positioning the patient. Each manufacturer provides an instruction manual that must be carefully read and followed. It is the radiographer's responsibility to position the patient's dental arches in relation to the focal trough to avoid images that are magnified, diminished, or blurred.

As discussed previously, most panoramic x-ray machines have guides such as a head positioner, chin rest, or beams of light that shine on the patient's face to aid the radiographer in positioning the patient within the focal trough (Figures 30-12 and 30-13). Because the focal trough or area of image sharpness is three dimensional (Figure 30-7), the patient's dental arches must be positioned in the correct: anterior–posterior (forward or back) position; lateral (left or right) position; and superior–inferior (up or down) position. Directing the patient to occlude the anterior teeth in the correct position on the bite-block of the panoramic machine will align the correct anterior–posterior position. Some panoramic x-ray machines have a light beam guide, that when illuminated can be used to align with a specific tooth or interproximal space as determined by the manufacturer. For example, Figure 30-15 illustrates a vertical positioning light that has been aligned with the interproximal space of the canine and the premolar. To correctly align the dental arches within the other two dimensions of the focal

trough, the radiographer must be able to determine the location of three facial landmarks. (1) The **midsaggital plane** (see Figure 13-13) that divides the patient's head into a right and left side must be positioned perpendicular to the floor for the correct lateral (left–right) position. (2) The **ala–tragus line**—an imaginary plane or line from the **ala** (a winglike projection at the side of the nose) to the **tragus** (the cartilaginous portion in front of the acoustic meatus of the ear)—must be positioned approximately 5 degrees down toward the floor. (3) When the ala–tragus line is positioned correctly, the **Frankfort plane**—an imaginary plane or line from the orbital ridge (under the eye) to the acoustic meatus of the ear—will be parallel to the floor. Some panoramic machines utilize guides that aid the radiographer in locating the ala–tragus line, whereas others focus on the Frankfort plane. The radiographer should be able to utilize either landmark (Figure 30-16).

When the arches are correctly positioned within the focal trough, all teeth and supporting structures are recorded and there is less unequal magnification and unsharpness over all parts of the radiographic image (Figure 30-17). If the patient has been positioned incorrectly, the resultant radiographic image will exhibit unique errors that are characteristic of the positioning mistake made. It is important that the radiographer be able to identify the causes of common panoramic image errors to be able to apply the appropriate corrective actions.

Patients should be protected with a lead/lead equivalent barrier when undergoing the panoramic exam. The thyroid collar must be removed from the apron for use during a panoramic exposure. Due to the position of the tube head and PID, the thyroid collar would get in the way of the primary beam and block the radiation from reaching the tissues. Lead/lead equivalent aprons are available without a thyroid collar, and there are cape-style aprons made especially for panoramic use (see Figures 6-12 and 30-12).

Panoramic Imaging Errors

Panoramic imaging errors may result from incorrectly preparing the patient for the procedure; incorrectly positioning the patient and dental arches in the focal trough; and incorrectly handling, exposing, and processing the image

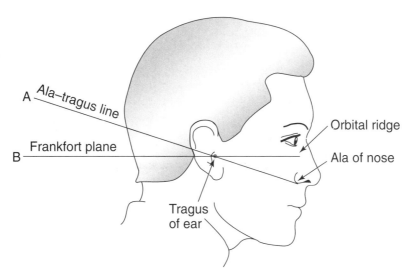

FIGURE 30-16 Landmarks used to position the patient. (A) When the ala–tragus line is positioned 5 degrees down, **(B)** the Frankfort plane will be in a position parallel to the floor.

receptor. The radiographer should possess a working knowledge of the characteristic appearance of errors made in these steps to avoid producing undiagnostic radiographic images and to better implement appropriate corrective actions.

Patient Preparation Errors

It is important to remember that the x-ray beam rotates around the patient from behind. Any objects made of metal or other dense material located here, such as a necklace, earrings, or hair adornments will be in the path of the primary beam and result in radiopaque artifacts. These items, along with the patient's glasses, dental appliances, patient napkin chain, oral piercings and other facial jewelry, must be removed prior to exposure. As already discussed, the thyroid collar must be removed from the lead/lead equivalent apron for panoramic exposures. There are occasions when the clothing the patient is wearing may interfere with the rotation of the tube head. Thickly padded shoulders of clothing and hooded sweatshirts need to be assessed to ensure that they won't impede the movement of the cassette and tube head during the rotational cycle.

Patient understanding of the procedure and cooperation are necessary to produce quality images. The patient must hold still, in position, throughout the exposure. The patient should be requested to rest the tongue against the palate and close the lips around the bite guide. The open air space between the tongue and the roof of the mouth (palatoglossal

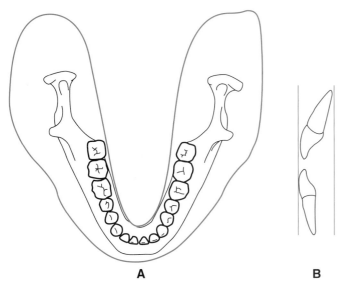

FIGURE 30-17 Correct positioning. The arches are positioned correctly within the focal trough in all three dimensions: **(A)** Anterior–posterior and left–right; and **(B)** superior–inferior (up-down).

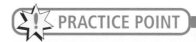

PRACTICE POINT

When asked to place the tongue against the roof of the mouth to reduce the radiolucency caused by the palatoglossal air space, the patient will sometimes incorrectly touch only the tip of the tongue to the palate. To assist with placing the entire dorsal surface of the tongue flat against the palate, ask the patient to swallow and note the position of the tongue. Another method used to get the tongue into the correct position is to ask the patient to suck in the cheeks, which automatically raises the tongue into a position flat against the palate. This directive works especially well when communicating with the child patient.

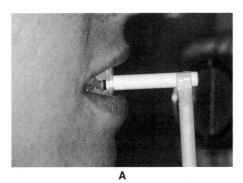 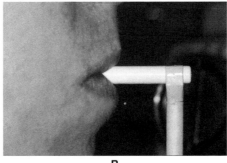

A   **B**

FIGURE 30-18 **Positioning of lips on the biteblock.** (**A**) The lips incorrectly open on the biteblock. (**B**) The lips correctly positioned closed around the biteblock.

air space) will create a large radiolucency on the image that will obscure the root apices of the maxillary teeth. Raising the flat, dorsal surface of the tongue to the palate utilizes the soft tissue image of the tongue to "fill in" this airspace and create a more even density to the image. Closing the lips together around the biteblock will avoid recording an image of the lip line across the anterior teeth. Open lips will create an image that can mimic caries of the anterior teeth (Figure 30-18).

Positioning Errors

Positioning the patient too far forward in the focal trough results in all of the anterior teeth appearing blurred and narrowed in width (Figure 30-19). Consequently, when the patient is too far back toward the tube head, the anterior teeth will appear blurred and magnified (Figure 30-19). Most panoramic machines have a relatively narrow focal trough in the anterior region, requiring precision in locating the forward and backward dimension of image sharpness. Panoramic machines will have a forehead rest or may require the patient to bite on a biteblock to position the arches correctly in this dimension. When using a biteblock the radiographer should request that the patient bring both maxillary and mandibular central incisors into an edge-to-edge position on the biteblock. When using a machine with laser light beams, follow the manufacturer's recommendation for aiming the lateral or vertical beam of light at a predetermined interproximal space.

If the midsaggital plane is not positioned perpendicular to the floor, the patient's head will be rotated, turned, or tipped to the left or to the right. This rotation of the dental arches will cause the anatomy of condyles, sinus, and teeth on the side closer to the image receptor to appear narrowed, whereas these anatomical landmarks on the side closer to the x-ray tube head will appear magnified and widened (Figure 30-20). When the patient is positioned too far to the left, the anatomy and teeth on the right appear magnified and widened. When the patient is positioned too far to the right, the anatomy on the left appears

magnified and widened. Depending on the angle that the patient is tipped, the condyles can appear higher on one side than the other.

If the patient's chin is tipped too low (Frankfort plane angled downward and ala–tragus line angled downward greater than 5 degrees), the resultant image will appear as an exaggerated smile (Figure 30-21). The mandibular condyles slant inward and the nasopharyngeal air space appears larger and darker, reducing the quality of the image. The appearance of a reversed smile (frown) results when the patient's chin is raised too high (Figure 30-21). Tipping the chin up causes the bottom of the nasal cavity and the hard palate to widen into a radiopaque band that obscures the apices of the maxillary teeth. Tipping the chin up or down will also cause the anterior teeth to be positioned outside the focal trough, often resulting in the appearance of root resorption.

If the patient is not standing or sitting up straight, or is slumped over, the radiation (which strikes the patient from behind) is attenuated by the compressed vertebrae, resulting in a wide radiopacity superimposed over the anterior teeth (Figure 30-22).

Exposure and Film Handling Errors

Careful attention to exposure settings and film handling will avoid errors that result in undiagnostic radiographs. Consideration should be given to the following. Exposure settings should be posted near the control panel to avoid over- or underexposures. Extraoral film requires careful handling to avoid static electricity artifacts (see Figure 29-6). Darkroom safelighting must be appropriate for light-sensitive extraoral film. Cassettes should be inspected to ensure a tight contact between film and intensifying screens. Blurry images result when the film and screens are not in tight contact. Intensifying screens must be free of scratches that would result in a loss of image and radiopaque artifacts.

Careful loading of flexible plastic sleeve cassettes must ensure that the film is seated all the way down at the fold in

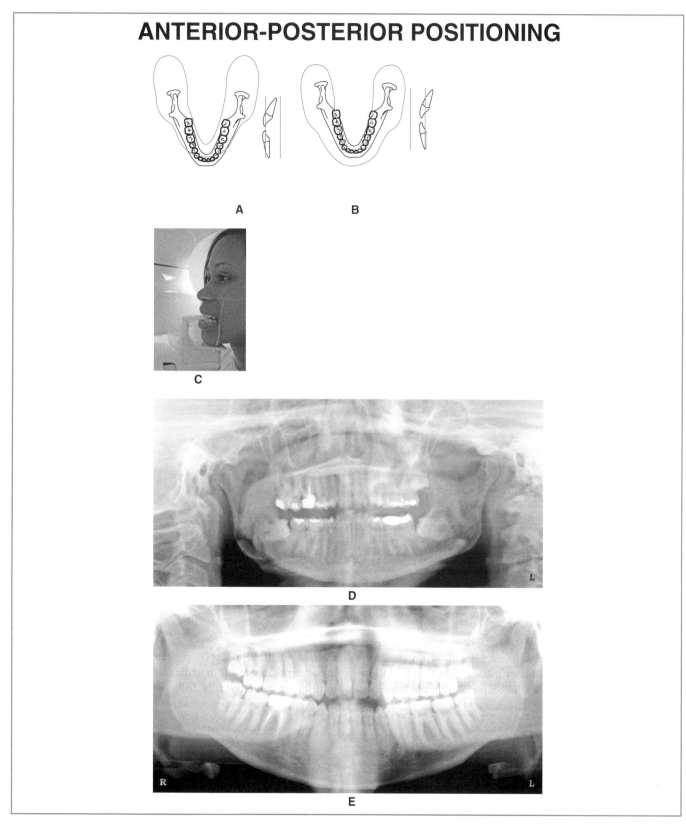

FIGURE 30-19 Incorrect positioning. (A) Arches too far forward, causing the anterior teeth to be positioned outside and forward from the center of the focal trough. (B) Arches too far backward, causing the anterior teeth to be positioned outside and backward from the center of the focal trough. (C) Patient positioned too far forward. Note the incorrect position of the laser light beam. Compare with the correct position in Figure 30-15. (D) Radiographic image resulting from positioning the arches too far forward. Note the blurred and magnified anterior teeth and the prominent imaging of the spinal column on both sides. (E) Radiographic image resulting from positioning the arches too far backward. Note the widened and magnified anterior teeth.

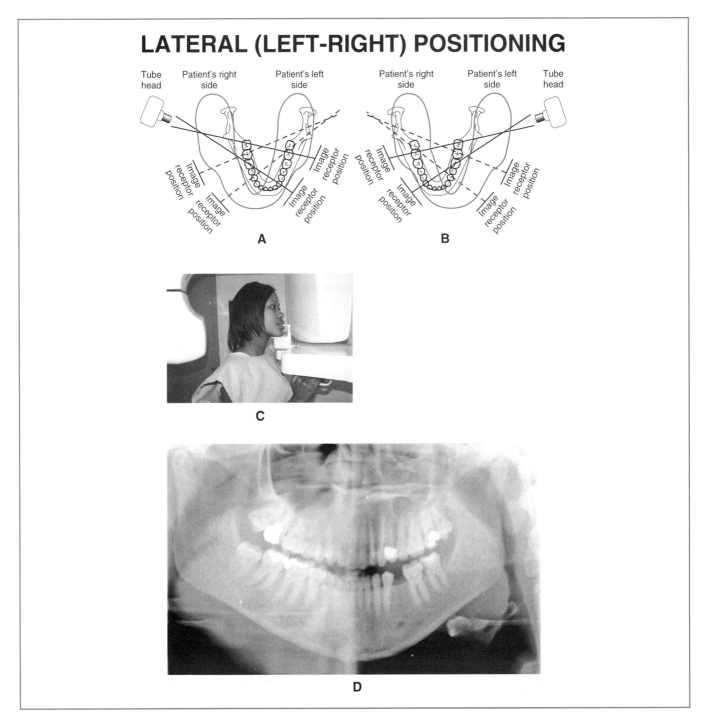

LATERAL (LEFT-RIGHT) POSITIONING

FIGURE 30-20 Incorrect positioning: patient's head is rotated. Midsaggital plane rotated to position the **(A)** left side of the arches closer to the image receptor and right side farther away from the x-ray tube head or **(B)** right side closer to the image receptor and left side farther away from the x-ray tube head. Diminution is apparent on the side malpositioned closer to the image receptor and magnification is apparent on the side malpositioned farther away from the x-ray tube head. **(C)** Patient positioned with the midsaggital plane rotated to the left. **(D)** Radiographic image resulting from a position rotated to the left. Note the arches, condyles, sinus, and teeth on the left appear narrowed, and these anatomical landmarks and teeth on the right appear widened and magnified. Note the higher position of the left condyle.

SUPERIOR-INFERIOR (UP-DOWN) POSITIONING

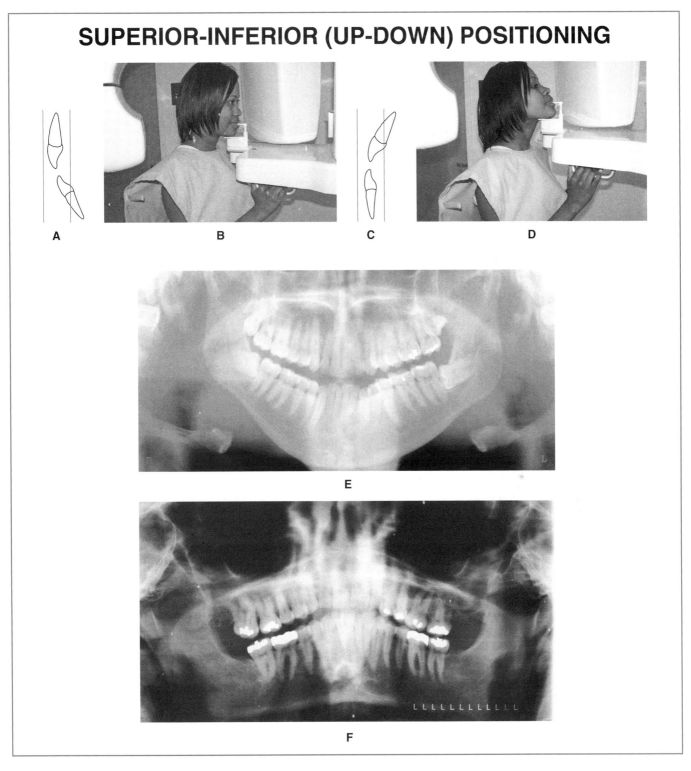

FIGURE 30-21 Incorrect positioning. (A) Patient's chin too low. The root apices of the mandibular anterior teeth slant out of the focal trough. **(B)** Frankfort plane/ala–tragus line incorrectly aligned to position the chin too low. **(C)** Patient's chin too high. The root apices of the maxillary anterior teeth slant out of the focal trough. **(D)** Frankfort plane/ala–tragus line incorrectly aligned to position the chin too high. **(E)** Radiograph with the characteristic exaggerated "smile" appearance. **(F)** Radiograph with the characteristic exaggerated "frown" appearance.

ACHIEVING CORRECT POSTURE POSITIONING

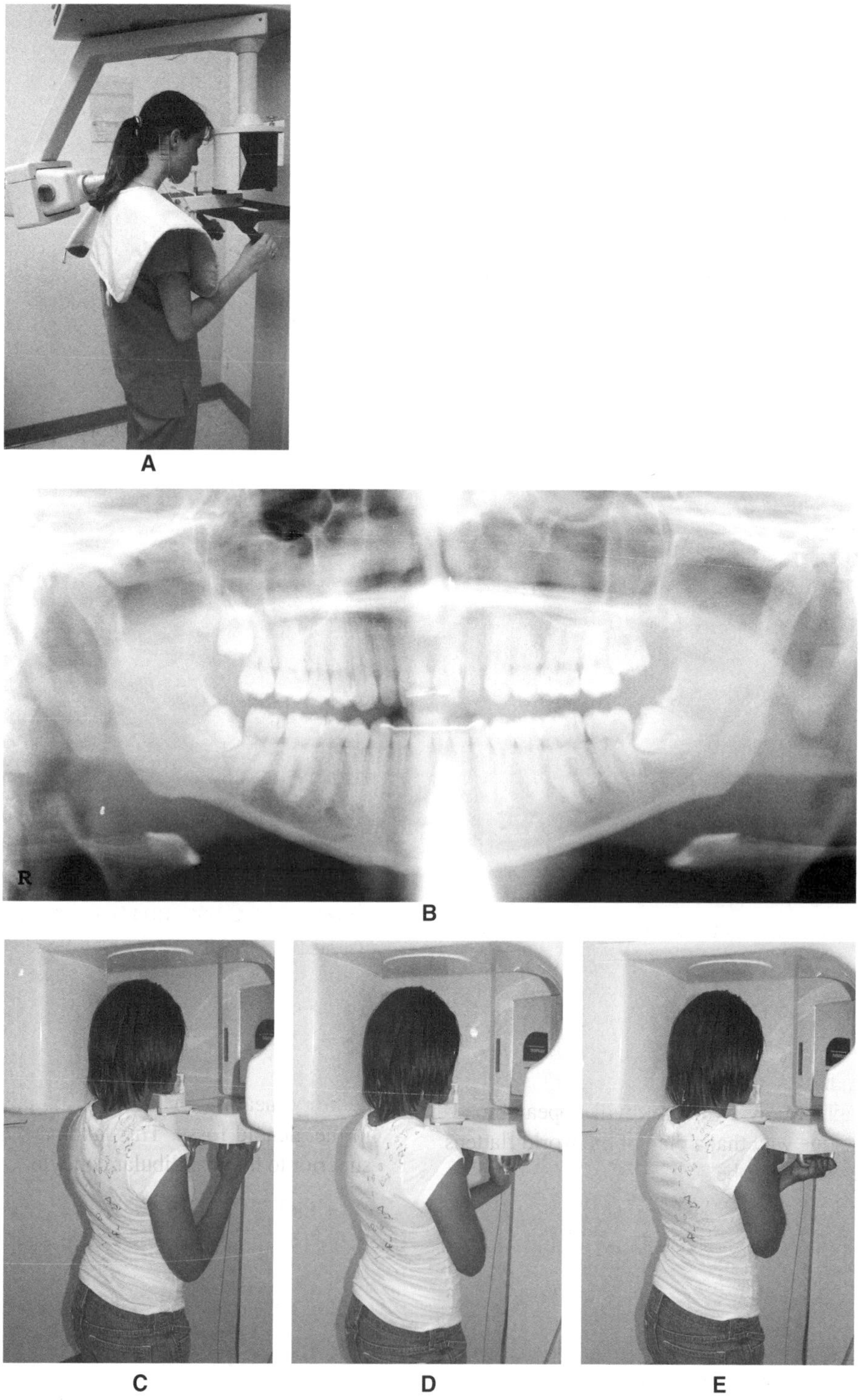

FIGURE 30-22 Incorrect patient positioning (A) Patient not standing up straight. Compare with the correct straight posture illustrated in Figures 30-12 and 30-13. **(B)** Radiograph with wide radiopacity representing the compressed vertebrae superimposed over the anterior teeth. **(C)** Normal hand position on machine handles. **(D)** Altered hand position with arms crossed, left hand holding the right handle and right hand holding the left handle. **(E)** Altered hand position with arms crossed, left hand holding the right handle with palm facing up and right hand holding the left handle with palm facing up.

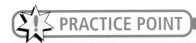

PRACTICE POINT

When standing straight is compromised due to the patient's stature or build/size, direct the patient to hold on to the handles of the machine with the arms crossed. Holding on to the right handle with the left hand and to the left handle with the right hand will bring the patient's shoulders in and usually out of the way of the machine rotation. For patients with a very short neck, or short distance between the shoulders and chin, crossing the arms and holding on to the handles with the palms up will further round the shoulders in and out of the way during the rotational cycle of the exposure (Figure 30-22).

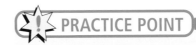

PRACTICE POINT

The panoramic radiograph records more structures of the maxillofacial region than the dentition and the surrounding supporting bone. Although the oral health care professional is primarily concerned with the oral cavity, panoramic radiographs must be interpreted by the dentist for all deviations from normal anatomy. Research has indicated that it is possible to identify carotid arterial plaques on some panoramic radiographs. This serious medical condition known as carotid artery stenosis can lead to a stroke, called a cerebrovascular accident (CVA). When suspected carotid artery calcifications are recorded on a panoramic radiograph, the dentist must immediately refer the patient to a physician for further evaluation.

the pair of intensifying screens. Failure to correctly load the film into the cassette will result in a loss of part of the image.

All panoramic machines have special instructions on how to load the film cassette onto the rotational arm of the unit. The manufacturer's instructions must be followed to avoid positioning the film so that only a portion gets exposed (see Figure 29-6).

Normal Panoramic Anatomical Landmarks

The principles of panoramic radiography result in the formation of a unique image. The superimposition of anatomical structures and the broadening of the arches produces unusual anatomical relationships in the panoramic image not seen in intraoral radiographs. In the panoramic radiograph, the mandible and maxilla as well as the spine are imaged as if they were split vertically in half down the midsagittal plane, with each half folded outward. The split cervical spine appears twice, beyond the mandibular rami at the extreme right and left edges of the radiograph. Many structures will appear broadened and wider in the same way that a map of the world flattens and broadens the images of a globe.

To develop the skills needed to recognize normal anatomic structures viewed on the panoramic radiograph, the radiographer should build on his/her knowledge of how normal anatomy appears on intraoral radiographs and transfer this knowledge to the panoramic image. For example, when viewing the maxillary posterior area on a panoramic image, the radiographer can visualize a periapical radiograph taken in this same area. Because the radiographer would be able to identify anatomical landmarks most likely to be imaged here (e.g., the zygomatic arch and maxillary sinus) on an intraoral radiograph, he/she can expect to see these landmarks here on the panoramic image as well. Of course the panoramic radiograph will image more structures of the maxillofacial regions than intraoral radiographs. The structures listed here are those anatomical landmarks that commonly appear on the panoramic image.

Anatomic Landmarks of the Maxilla and Surrounding Tissues (Figures 30-23 and 30-24)

Mastoid process of the temporal bone is located posterior and inferior to the temporomandibular joint (TMJ), appears as a rounded radiopacity.

Styloid process appears as a long, narrow radiopaque spine that extends downward, from the inferior surface of the temporal bone, just anterior to the mastoid process.

External auditory meatus (external acoustic meatus), a round opening in the temporal bone located anterior and superior to the mastoid process, appears as a round radiolucency.

Glenoid fossa (mandibular fossa) is a concave, depressed area of the temporal bone located anterior to the external auditory meatus. The head of the mandibular condyle rests in the glenoid fossa. This landmark appears as a concavity superior to the mandibular condyle.

Articular eminence appears as a rounded projection of the temporal bone just anterior to the glenoid fossa.

Lateral pterygoid plate appears as a radiopaque winglike bony projection of the sphenoid bone located posterior to the maxillary tuberosity.

Maxillary tuberosity appears as a radiopaque rounded prominence distal to the third molar region.

Infraorbital foramen, a small round opening in the maxilla, appears as a round radiolucency inferior to the border of the orbit.

Orbit, the bony cavity of the eye socket, appears as a large round radiolucency with radiopaque borders superior to the maxillary sinuses. Often, only the inferior border of the orbit is visible as a radiopaque line.

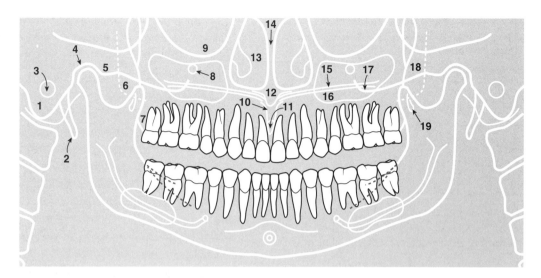

FIGURE 30-23 Drawing of panoramic radiograph showing the maxilla and surrounding normal anatomic landmarks. (**1**) Mastoid process, (**2**) styloid process, (**3**) external auditory meatus, (**4**) glenoid fossa, (**5**) articular eminence, (**6**) lateral pterygoid plate, (**7**) maxillary tuberosity, (**8**) infraorbital foramen, (**9**) orbit of the eye, (**10**) incisive canal, (**11**) incisive foramen, (**12**) anterior nasal spine, (**13**) nasal cavity, (**14**) nasal septum, (**15**) hard palate, (**16**) maxillary sinus, (**17**) zygomatic process of the zygoma, (**18**) zygoma, and (**19**) hamulus.

Incisive canal (nasopalatine canal) is a Y-shaped passageway that extends from the floor of the nose to the hard palate lingual to the central incisors. This landmark appears as a tunnel-like radiolucency with radiopaque borders located between the maxillary central incisors.

Incisive foramen (nasopalatine foramen), an opening in bone located in the anterior midline of the hard palate directly posterior to the maxillary central incisors, appears as a round or oval radiolucency between the roots of the maxillary central incisors.

Anterior nasal spine, a pointed bony projection of the maxilla located at the most anterior point of the floor of the nasal cavity, appears as a V-shaped radiopacity located at the intersection of the floor of the nasal cavity and the nasal septum.

Nasal cavity (nasal fossa), a pear-shaped compartment of bone located superior to the maxilla, appears as a large radiolucency above the maxillary incisors.

Nasal septum, a vertical bony wall that separates the right and left nasal fossae, appears as a vertical radiopacity that divides the nasal cavity into two parts.

Hard palate, a bony wall that separates the oral cavity from the nasal cavity, appears as a horizontal thick radiopaque band superior to the maxillary teeth.

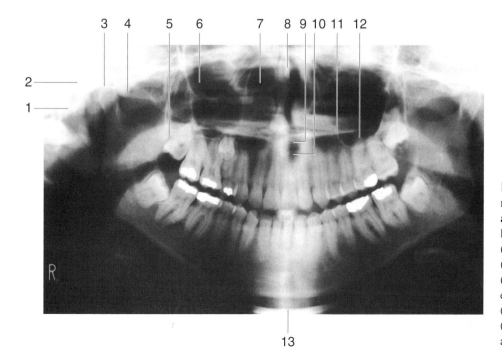

FIGURE 30-24 Panoramic radiograph showing the maxilla and surrounding normal anatomic landmarks. (**1**) Mastoid process, (**2**) external auditory meatus, (**3**) glenoid fossa, (**4**) articular eminence, (**5**) maxillary tuberosity, (**6**) orbit of the eye, (**7**) nasal cavity, (**8**) nasal septum, (**9**) incisive canal, (**10**) incisive foramen, (**11**) hard palate, (**12**) maxillary sinus, and (**13**) chin rest (machine part artifact).

Maxillary sinus consists of two paired cavities that appear radiolucent, located within the maxilla apical to the maxillary posterior teeth.

Zygomatic process of the maxilla is a bony process of the maxilla that extends laterally to articulate with the zygoma and appears as a J- or U-shaped radiopacity located apically to the maxillary first molar.

Zygoma is the cheekbone that articulates with the zygomatic process of the maxilla. This structure appears as a thick radiopaque band that extends posteriorly from the zygomatic process of the maxilla.

Hamulus (hamular process) appears as a very small radiopaque hooklike process of bone that extends downward and slightly backward from the medial pterygoid plate of the sphenoid bone.

Anatomic Landmarks of the Mandible and Surrounding Tissues (Figures 30-25 and 30-26)

Mandibular condyle appears as a radiopaque rounded bony process extending from the posterior superior border of the ramus of the mandible that articulates with the glenoid fossa of the temporal bone.

Mandibular notch appears as a concavity of bone located posterior to the coronoid process on the superior border of the ramus of the mandible.

Coronoid process appears as a large radiopaque triangular prominence of bone located on the anterior superior ramus of the mandible.

Mandibular foramen, an ovoid opening in the bone on the lingual aspect of the ramus of the mandible, appears as a round radiolucency located in the center of the ramus of the mandible.

Lingula (meaning "little tongue") is a small tongue-shaped projection of bone located anterior and adjacent to the mandibular foramen. This landmark appears as a small radiopacity anterior to the mandibular foramen.

Mandibular canal, a long tunnel-like passageway extending from the mandibular foramen on the medial aspect of the ramus of the mandible to the mental foramen on the lateral aspect of the body of the mandible, appears as a radiolucent tube outlined by two thin radiopaque lines representing the walls of the canal.

Mental foramen, an opening through which the mental nerve and related blood vessels emerge on the lateral aspect of the body of the mandible, appears as a small round radiolucent area near the roots of the mandibular premolars.

Mental ridge, appears as a thick radiopaque band representing the prominence of bone located on the external surface of the mandible and extends anteriorly from the premolar area to the midline.

Mental fossa appears as a radiolucent depressed area of bone in the region of the roots of the mandibular incisor teeth.

Lingual foramen, a very small round opening located in the center of the genial tubercles on the lingual side of midline of the mandible, appears as a small round radiolucency located inferior to the apices of the mandibular incisor teeth.

Genial tubercles The genial tubercles, four small projections of bone located on the lingual surface of the midline of the mandible, appear as a radiopaque donut-shaped circle surrounding the lingual foramen.

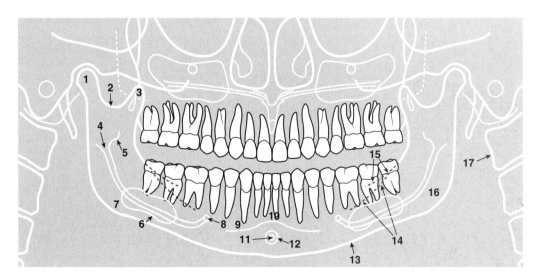

FIGURE 30-25 Drawing of panoramic radiograph showing the mandible and surrounding normal anatomic landmarks. (**1**) Mandibular condyle, (**2**) mandibular notch, (**3**) coronoid process, (**4**) mandibular foramen, (**5**) lingula, (**6**) submandibular fossa, (**7**) mandibular canal, (**8**) mental foramen, (**9**) mental ridge, (**10**) mental fossa, (**11**) lingual foramen, (**12**) genial tubercles, (**13**) inferior border of the mandible, (**14**) mylohyoid ridge, (**15**) oblique ridge, (**16**) angle of the mandible, (**17**) cervical vertabrae.

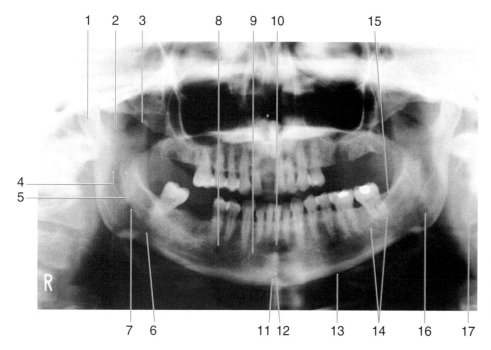

FIGURE 30-26 Panoramic radiograph showing the mandible and surrounding normal anatomic landmarks. (**1**) Mandibular condyle, (**2**) mandibular notch, (**3**) coronoid process, (**4**) mandibular foramen, (**5**) lingula, (**6**) submandibular fossa, (**7**) mandibular canal, (**8**) mental foramen, (**9**) mental ridge, (**10**) mental fossa, (**11**) lingual foramen, (**12**) genial tubercles, (**13**) inferior border of the mandible, (**14**) mylohyoid ridge, (**15**) oblique ridge, (**16**) angle of the mandible, (**17**) cervical vertabrae.

Inferior border of the mandible, composed of the thick cortical bone that outlines the lower border of the mandible, appears as a dense radiopaque band.

Mylohyoid ridge, a ridge of bone running diagonally downward and forward on the lingual aspect of the ramus of the mandible to near the apices of the molar roots, appears as a dense radiopaque band.

Submandibular fossa, a concavity in the mandible where the salivary glands are located, appears as a diffuse radiolucenct area below the mylohyoid ridge and the roots of the mandibular molars.

Oblique ridge, a diagonal ridge of bone on the lateral aspect of the mandible that runs downward and forward from the anterior border of the ramus to the level of the cervical portion of the molar and premolar roots, appears as a dense radiopaque band.

Angle of the mandible is the area at the posterior and inferior corners of the mandible, where the body of the mandible meets and joins the ascending ramus of the mandible.

Cervical spine radiopaque vertebrae appear beyond the rami of the mandible at the extreme right and left edges of the radiograph.

Soft Tissue Images Viewed on the Panoramic Radiograph (Figures 30-27 and 30-28)

The panoramic radiograph is unique in that some soft tissue structures (e.g., tongue, soft palate, lipline, and ear) attenuate the beam of radiation enough to become visible on the radiograph.

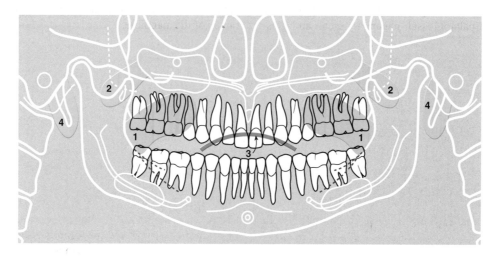

FIGURE 30-27 Drawing of panoramic radiograph showing soft tissue images. (**1**) Tongue, (**2**) soft palate, (**3**) lipline, and (**4**) ear.

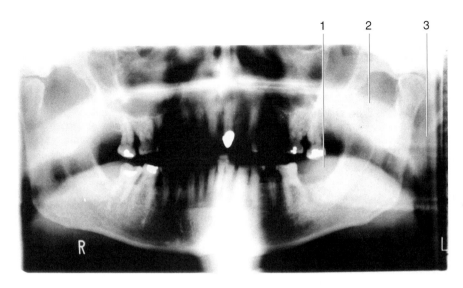

FIGURE 30-28 Panoramic radiograph showing soft tissue images. (**1**) Tongue, (**2**) soft palate, and (**3**) ear.

Tongue, when positioned correctly, resting on the palate, allows the soft tissue image of the tongue to be minimally visible. When visible, the radiopaque dorsal side of the tongue appears superimposed over the ramus. Remember that the panoramic view of the tongue will be broadened and much wider than it appears clinically.

Soft palate, located posterior to the hard palate, separating the oral cavity from the nasal cavity, appears as a diagonal radiopaque structure above and posterior to the maxillary tuberosity.

Lipline image can be avoided if the patient is instructed to close the lips together around the bite guide (Figure 30-18). When imaged, the outline of the patient's lips appears as a radiopacity superimposed over the anterior teeth.

Ear appears radiopaque and superimposed over the styloid process, anterior and inferior to the mastoid process.

Air Space Images Viewed on the Panoramic Radiograph (Figures 30-29 and 30-30)

Air does not attenuate the beam of radiation as much as hard or soft tissue. For this reason, air spaces appear radiolucent (black) on a panoramic radiograph. Air spaces that may be recorded include the palatoglossal, nasopharyngeal, and glos-

sopharyngeal air spaces. The radiolucencies produced by these landmarks often are so dark that they may obscure other structures, compromising the diagnostic ability of the panoramic radiograph. Careful positioning of the patient into the focal trough will help minimize the appearance of these negative shadows. The term *negative shadow* implies to these radiolucencies because they are shadows of "nothing."

Palatoglossal air space appears as a radiolucency between the palate and the tongue. When the patient is instructed to rest the tongue against the hard palate, the palatoglossal air space negative shadow is minimized. If the tongue is not correctly positioned against the palate during exposure, the radiolucency appears superimposed on or above the apices of the maxillary teeth.

Nasopharyngeal air space is the radiolulcency located posterior to the nasal cavity. The negative shadow it creates on the image often appears as a radiolucent diagonal streak located superior to the radiopaque soft palate. This negative shadow is emphasized when the patient's chin is incorrectly tipped down.

Glossopharyngeal air space is the portion of the pharynx located posterior to the tongue and oral cavity (the oropharyngeal region). The negative shadow it creates on the image appears as a vertical radiolucent band superimposed over the ramus of the mandible.

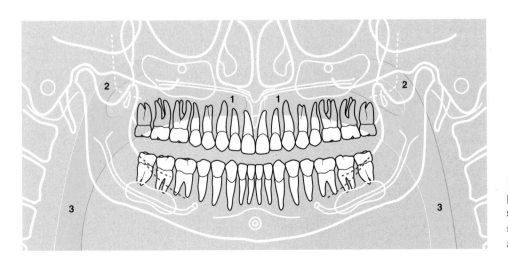

FIGURE 30-29 Drawing of panoramic radiograph showing air space images. (**1**) Palatoglossal air space, (**2**) nasopharyngeal air space, and (**3**) glossopharyngeal air space.

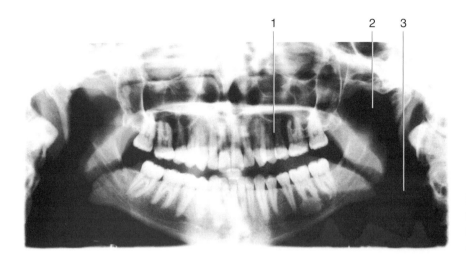

FIGURE 30-30 Panoramic radiograph showing air space images. (**1**) Palatoglossal air space, (**2**) nasopharyngeal air space, and (**3**) glossopharyngeal air space.

Images of Machine Parts Viewed on the Panoramic Radiograph (Figures 30-31 and 30-32)

The chin rest, side head positioner guides, and biteblock are often recorded on a panoramic radiograph. Care should be taken to identify these artifacts so that they are not confused with normal anatomical landmarks or the presence of disease.

Ghost Images Viewed on the Panoramic Radiograph (Figures 30-33 and 30-34)

The rotation of the panoramic tube head and the use of a focal trough to isolate slices or layers of the image creates ghost images on the resultant panoramic radiograph. Ghost images are mirror or second images of structures that are penetrated by the x-ray beam twice. Consider that when the x-ray tube

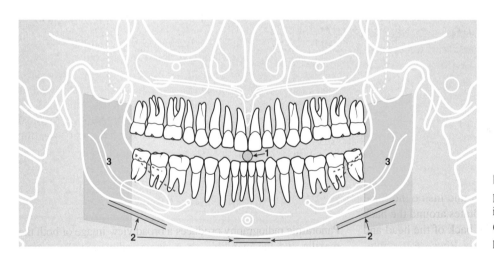

FIGURE 30-31 Drawing of panoramic radiograph showing images of machine parts. (**1**) Biteblock, (**2**) chin rest, (**3**) side positioner guides.

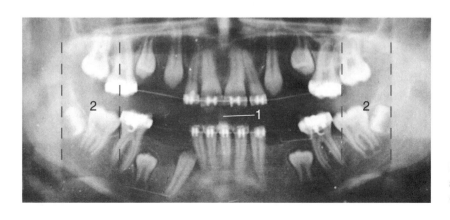

FIGURE 30-32 Panoramic radiograph showing images of machine parts. (**1**) Biteblock, (**2**) side positioner guides.

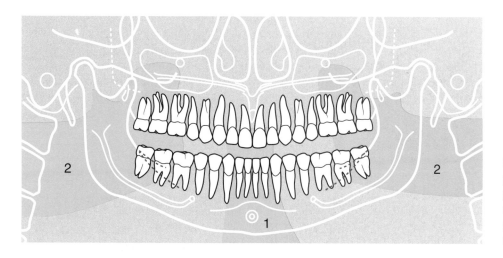

FIGURE 30-33 Drawing of panoramic radiograph showing ghost images. (**1**) Ghost image of the spinal column (cervical vertebrae), (**2**) ghost image of the opposite side mandible.

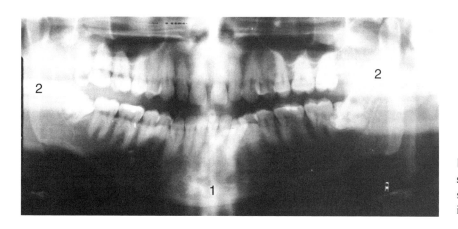

FIGURE 30-34 Panoramic radiograph showing ghost images. (**1**) Ghost image of the spinal column (cervical vertebrae), (**2**) ghost image of the opposite side mandible.

head is on the patient's right side, the x-ray beam penetrates the right side first. Because this right side is closer to the x-ray source and farther from the image receptor, the structures here are blurred almost completely out of the image. The beam continues through the patient to the left side, which is at that moment closer to the image receptor and inside the focal trough (Figure 30-6). As the tube head rotates around the back of the patient, the x-ray beam enters the back of the head and "refocuses" on imaging the anterior teeth. Because the anterior teeth at that moment are closer to the image receptor, and in the focal layer, they are being imaged onto the radiograph and the back of the skull is being blurred out. As the beam continues around the patient to the left side, the blurring out and refocusing continues along the predetermined focal layer. In principle those structures outside the focal trough will not be imaged on the radiograph. However, a magnified, unsharp image called a **ghost image** often appears. For example, when viewing a panoramic image of the patient's right mandible, a ghost image of the left mandible can be observed superimposed over the actual right mandible, as a mirror image (Figures 30-33 and 30-34). Ghost images appear on the opposite side of the image than the actual structure and will often appear larger (more magnified) and higher (due to the slight

negative vertical angulation of the PID). Being aware of ghost images will assist the radiographer in interpreting panoramic radiographs.

REVIEW—Chapter summary

Panoramic radiography produces a broad view image of both the maxilla and the mandible on a single radiograph. Panoramic radiographs are valuable in examining large areas of the maxillofacial region; locating impacted teeth or retained root tips; evaluating trauma, lesions, and diseases of the jaws; and assessing growth and development.

The greatest advantage of the panoramic radiograph is that it can image a large region of structures and provide an increased amount of diagnostic information when compared to a full mouth series of intraoral radiographs. The greatest limitation of the panoramic radiograph is the image magnification and distortion that make interpreting the image difficult.

Panoramic imagery is based on tomography where a slice or layer of tissue is imaged with relative clarity, while blurring out other structures not of interest. During the panoramic exposure, the image receptor and x-ray tube head move slowly (about 15–20 seconds cycle) in opposite directions of each other around the patient's head. The patient remains still during the exposure, either in a standing or seated position (depending on the machine type). Through the use of a series of rotational points or centers, the x-ray beam is directed toward the moving cassette to record a select plane of dental anatomy. The rotational center is defined as the axis on which the tube head and the cassette rotate. Most modern panoramic machines use a moving-center rotation.

The focal trough is the area between the x-ray source and the image receptor where structures will be imaged clearly on the radiograph. Structures positioned outside the focal trough will be blurred out of the image. The focal trough is three-dimensional, and the size and shape is determined by the machine manufacturer. Each manufacturer provides instructions and head positioner guides to assit the radiographer in positioning the patient within the focal trough.

All panoramic units have (1) a rotational x-ray tube head; (2) a cassette holder for film or phosphor plate or a built-in digital sensor; (3) head positioner guides; and (4) an exposure control panel. The PID is collimated to a narrow slit opening, allowing the x-ray beam to fan out to expose a narrow slice of tissue as the tube head rotates around the patient's head. The x-ray beam penetrates the patient from the back of the head.

Positioning the patient's head within the focal trough is key to producing a diagnostic image. Most panoramic units have a forehead rest, chin rest, or biteblock to aid the radiographer in positioning the arches in the correct anterior–posterior dimension; side head positioner guides, a mirror, or beams of light that shine on the patient's face to determine the correct left–right dimension; and a chin rest or light beams to aid in locating the ala–tragus line or Frankfort plane to determine the correct superior–inferior dimension of the focal trough.

Artifacts that compromise diagnostic quality result when metal or dense material objects, such as a necklace, earrings, oral piercings, and other facial jewelry, are not removed prior to exposure. The patient must be instructed to rest the tongue against the palate and to close the lips around the biteblock during the exposure to minimize the appearance of these structures on the radiograph. Accurate exposure settings and careful film handling will avoid errors that result in undiagnostic radiographs.

Positioning errors result in characteristic image appearances. Positioning the arches too far forward in the focal trough produces blurred and narrowed anterior teeth; positioning the arches too far back in the focal trough produces blurred and widened anterior teeth. Positioning the arches too far to the lateral (tipping or turning the head to the right or left) results in narrowed teeth on the side closer to the image receptor and magnified teeth on the side closer to the x-ray tube head. Positioning the patient's chin too far down results in an image with an exaggerated "smile." Positioning the patient's chin too far up results in an image with an exaggerated "frown."

The skilled radiographer should be able to identify normal radiographic anatomy of the maxilla and the mandible, including soft tissue images and air spaces that appear on a panoramic radiograph. The radiographer should be able to distinguish normal radiographic anatomy from artifacts such as machine parts and ghost images that appear on the radiograph.

RECALL—Review questions

1. A panoramic radiograph is valuable when diagnosing each of the following EXCEPT one. Which one is the EXCEPTION?
   a. A cyst
   b. An impacted molar
   c. Recurrent caries
   d. A supernumerary tooth

2. Which of these is an advantage of a panoramic radiograph when compared to an intraoral radiograph?
   a. A larger region is recorded.
   b. The image is magnified.
   c. Distortion is eliminated.
   d. Definition is improved.

3. Which of these is a limitation of a panoramic radiograph when compared to an intraoral radiograph?
   a. Larger radiation dose to the patient.
   b. Increased time required for exposure.
   c. Superimposition of structures may make interpretation difficult.
   d. Requires an increase in patient instruction and cooperation with the procedure.

4. What is the term given to the technique where a slice of tissue is exposed distinctly, whereas structures outside the designated area are blurred out of the image?
   a. Ghost image
   b. Artifact
   c. Focal trough
   d. Tomography

5. All panoramic radiographs have 10 to 30 percent magnification.
   It is desirable to keep the magnification less in the anterior region and greater in the posterior region.
   a. The first statement is true. The second statement is false.
   b. The first statement is false. The second statement is true.
   c. Both statements are true.
   d. Both statements are false.

6. The panoramic PID is collimated to what shape?
   a. Round
   b. Rectangular
   c. Narrow slit

7. What term is given to the area where structures will be imaged with relative clarity, whereas structures outside this area are blurred out of the image?

    a. Ghost image
    b. Artifact
    c. Focal trough
    d. Tomography

8. Each of the following is a component of the panoramic x-ray machine EXCEPT one. Which one is the EXCEPTION?

    a. Rotational x-ray tube head
    b. Cassette holder or built-in digital sensor
    c. Head positioner guides
    d. Variable exposure timer

9. Which dimension of the focal trough does the biteblock of the panoramic x-ray machine assist the operator with positioning?

    a. Anterior–posterior
    b. Lateral (left–right)
    c. Superior–inferior

10. Which of the following planes is used to position the patient correctly within the superior–inferior (up–down) dimension?

    a. Ala–tragus line
    b. Frankfort plane
    c. Midsaggital plane
    d. Both (a) and (b)

11. Which of the following positioning errors results in anterior teeth that are blurry and narrowed in size?

    a. Too far forward in the focal trough
    b. Too far backward in the focal trough
    c. Too far to the left in the focal trough
    d. Too far to the right in the focal trough

12. When the dental arches are rotated to the left, the teeth on the right side will be positioned closer to the image receptor.

    The teeth closer to the image receptor will appear blurry and magnified.

    a. The first statement is true. The second statement is false.
    b. The first statement is false. The second statement is true.
    c. Both statements are true.
    d. Both statements are false.

13. Which of the following positioning errors results in an exaggerated "smile" appearance of the arches?

    a. Midsaggital plane tipped to the left
    b. Midsaggital plane tipped to the right
    c. Chin tipped too far up
    d. Chin tipped too far down

14. The appearance of a large radiolucency that obscures the maxillary teeth apices results when

    a. the lips are not closed around the biteblock during exposure.
    b. the tongue is not resting on the palate during exposure.
    c. the lead thyroid collar gets in the way of the primary beam.
    d. facial jewelry (e.g., oral piercing) is not removed prior to exposure.

15. Which of the following appears radiolucent on a panoramic radiograph?

    a. Nasal cavity
    b. Nasal septum
    c. Nasal spine
    d. Hard palate

16. Which of the following appears radiopaque on the panoramic radiograph?

    a. External auditory meatus
    b. Zygomatic process of the maxilla
    c. Mental fossa
    d. Mandibular foramen

17. Which of the following could be called a negative shadow?

    a. Tongue
    b. Ghost image
    c. Glossopharyngeal air space
    d. Biteblock

18. List three air spaces that may be recorded on panoramic radiographs.

    a. _____
    b. _____
    c. _____

19. List three machine parts that may be recorded on panoramic radiographs.

    a. _____
    b. _____
    c. _____

20. What is the term given to a structure that is recorded a second time, with less sharpness, and on the opposite side?

    a. Ghost image
    b. Focal trough
    c. Split image
    d. Tomograph

REFLECT—Case study

You have to expose a panoramic radiograph on the following patients today. Each of these patients presents with a characteristic that will make positioning the patient for the procedure a challenge. Carefully review each of the patient descriptions and answer the following questions:

1. What patient positioning step do you anticipate having a problem with?
2. What error is most likely to occur?
3. What will the image look like?
4. How can you prevent this error from occurring or minimize the result on the image?
5. Write out the specific steps you plan to take to produce a diagnostic quality image.

Case A

A hyperactive 10-year-old child who seems to be having difficulty paying attention to your directions.

Case B

A young adult with multiple facial piercings, including a tongue ring and several earrings.

Case C

A young woman with fashionable hair extensions gathered into a large ponytail.

Case D

A middle-aged man who wears partial dentures that when removed reveal missing anterior teeth.

Case E

An older woman with osteoporosis who exhibits a pronounced stooped posture as a result of collapsed vertebrae.

RELATE—Laboratory application

For a comprehensive laboratory practice exercise on this topic, see Thomson, E. M. (2012). *Exercises in oral radiography techniques: A laboratory manual* 3rd ed.). Upper Saddle River, NJ: Pearson. Chapter 12, "Panoramic radiographic technique."

REFERENCES

Eastman Kodak. (2000). *Successful Panoramic Radiography.* Rochester, NY: Eastman Kodak.

Farman, A. G., Nortje, C. J., & Wood, R. E. (1993). *Oral and maxillofacial diagnostic imaging.* St. Louis, MO: Mosby.

Ferrús-Torres, E., Gargallo-Albiol, J., Berini-Aytés, L., & Gay-Escoda, C. (2009). Diagnostic predictability of digital versus conventional panoramic radiographs in the presurgical evaluation of impacted mandibular third molars. *International Journal of Oral Maxillofacial Surgery, 38,* 1184–1187.

Horner, K., Drage, N., & Brettle, D. (2008). *21st century imaging.* London: Quintessence Publishing Co.

Langland, O. E., Langlais, R. P., McDavid, W. D., et al. (1989). *Panoramic radiology* (2nd ed.). Philadelphia: Lea & Febiger.

Rushton, V. E., Horner, K., & Worthington, H. V. (1999). The quality of panoramic radiographs in a sample of general dental practices. *British Dental Journal, 26, 186*(12), 630-633.

Rushton, V. E., & Rout, J. (2006). *Panoramic radiography.* London: Quintessence Publishing Co.

Serman, N., Horrell, B. M., & Singer, S. (2003). High-quality panoramic radiographs. Tips and tricks. *Dentistry Today, 22*(1), 70–73.

Thomson, E. M. (2009). Focusing on the image. How to produce error-free radiographic images for the pediatric patient. *Dimensions of Dental Hygiene, 7*(2), 24–26, 27.

White, S. C., & Pharoah, M. J. (2008). *Oral radiology: Principles and interpretation* (6th ed.). St. Louis, MO: Elsevier.

Answers to Study Questions

Chapter 1
1. c
2. a
3. d
4. e
5. b
6. d
7. c
8. b
9. c
10. a
11. a
12. b
13. d
14. Use Box 1-1 to list uses

Chapter 2
1. a
2. Use chapter information and Figure 2-1 to draw diagram
3. d
4. c
5. b
6. b
7. a
8. d
9. b
10. d
11. Use chapter information to list properties
12. a
13. c
14. d
15. b
16. a
17. Use chapter information to list sources
18. c

Chapter 3
1. c
2. a
3. d
4. 0.5, 0.75, 20, 6
5. a
6. b
7. d
8. Use chapter information to list conditions
9. Use chapter information and Figure 3-8 to draw and label diagram
10. c
11. b
12. d
13. a
14. a
15. c
16. c
17. a

Chapter 4
1. Use chapter information to list criteria
2. d
3. c
4. b
5. d
6. a
7. d
8. d
9. a
10. d
11. b
12. c
13. d
14. a
15. a

Chapter 5
1. a
2. c
3. a
4. d
5. c
6. b
7. b
8. d
9. As low as reasonably achievable
10. Use chapter information to list responses
11. c
12. a
13. b
14. d
15. c
16. d
17. d
18. c
19. d
20. b

Chapter 6
1. d
2. d
3. b
4. c
5. b
6. c
7. d
8. c
9. d
10. a
11. b
12. c
13. c
14. b
15. Use Table 6-3 to list organizations.

Chapter 7
1. a
2. d
3. c
4. b
5. b
6. c
7. c
8. b
9. a
10. d
11. a
12. a

Chapter 8
1. b
2. c
3. a
4. a
5. c
6. d
7. b
8. d
9. a
10. c
11. b
12. b
13. b
14. a
15. c
16. b
17. c
18. b
19. a
20. d
21. c

Chapter 9
1. d
2. e
3. c
4. a
5. b
6. c
7. d
8. d
9. d
10. c
11. d
12. e
13. d
14. Use chapter information to list features
15. c
16. c
17. a
18. b

Chapter 10
1. d
2. a
3. b
4. a
5. Use chapter information to list items
6. c
7. b
8. c
9. c
10. b
11. d
12. d
13. b
14. d
15. a
16. c
17. c

Chapter 11
1. d
2. a
3. d
4. b
5. Use chapter information to list aspects
6. c
7. Use chapter information to list items
8. c
9. a
10. d
11. b
12. d
13. c
14. a

Chapter 12
1. d
2. Use chapter information to list aspects
3. a
4. a
5. c
6. d
7. b
8. a
9. d
10. c
11. b
12. Use chapter information to complete list.

Chapter 13
1. c
2. a
3. b
4. a
5. a
6. c
7. b
8. d
9. a
10. a
11. b
12. d
13. c

14. d
15. Use chapter information to list contraindications
16. d
17. a
18. b

Chapter 14
1. d
2. a
3. d
4. c
5. b
6. a
7. d
8. c
9. a
10. c
11. b
12. d

Chapter 15
1. b
2. b
3. d
4. b
5. a
6. a
7. d
8. c
9. d
10. d
11. b
12. b
13. d
14. d
15. d
16. a
17. c

Chapter 16
1. c
2. b
3. b
4. d
5. c
6. b
7. c
8. a
9. d
10. c
11. a
12. d
13. c
14. d
15. d

Chapter 17
1. a
2. d
3. d
4. b
5. c

6. a
7. b
8. a
9. c
10. d

Chapter 18
1. d
2. d
3. c
4. a
5. c
6. c
7. b
8. c
9. a
10. d
11. a
12. c
13. d
14. d
15. c

Chapter 19
1. c
2. c
3. Use chapter information to list objectives
4. d
5. b
6. a
7. d
8. b
9. d

Chapter 20
1. Use chapter information to list agencies
2. b
3. a
4. d
5. Use chapter information to list wastes
6. c
7. a
8. d
9. b
10. c
11. c

Chapter 21
1. Use chapter information to list advantages
2. d
3. d
4. b
5. d
6. c
7. a
8. d
9. b
10. c
11. a
12. d
13. b
14. d

Chapter 22
1. c
2. d
3. b
4. b
5. a
6. d
7. a
8. c
9. d
10. b
11. a
12. c
13. b
14. d
15. c
16. b
17. a

Chapter 23
1. b
2. a
3. d
4. d
5. c
6. c
7. b
8. a
9. b
10. c
11. d
12. c
13. a

Chapter 24
1. b
2. d
3. a
4. b
5. c
6. a
7. a
8. c
9. b
10. d
11. c
12. a
13. b
14. b

Chapter 25
1. b
2. Use Box 25-1 to list uses

3. c
4. d
5. c
6. a
7. b
8. Use chapter information to list limitations
9. d
10. c
11. a
12. b

Chapter 26
1. Use chapter information to list conditions
2. c
3. b
4. d
5. a
6. d
7. a
8. b
9. d
10. d
11. c
12. a
13. b
14. a
15. b
16. d
17. c
18. d

Chapter 27
1. Use chapter information to list actions
2. b
3. a
4. c
5. b
6. d
7. a
8. d
9. b
10. d
11. d
12. a

Chapter 28
1. d
2. b
3. a
4. b

5. c
6. d
7. a
8. a
9. d
10. c
11. b
12. b
13. d
14. d
15. b
16. Use chapter information to list reasons.

Chapter 29
1. a
2. b
3. c
4. b
5. b
6. d
7. c
8. a
9. b
10. a
11. a
12. d
13. c
14. b
15. d

Chapter 30
1. c
2. a
3. c
4. d
5. a
6. c
7. c
8. d
9. a
10. d
11. a
12. d
13. d
14. b
15. a
16. b
17. c
18. Use chapter information to list air spaces
19. Use chapter information to list machine parts
20. a

Glossary

Abscess: A localized pus formation often accompanied by swelling and pain. When involving an infected tooth, an abscess is usually located near the apex of the roots. May be chronic or acute. Appears radiolucent when large enough to be visible on a radiograph.

Absorbed dose: The amount of energy deposited in any form of matter, such as teeth, soft tissues, treatment chair, air, and so forth, by any type of radiation (alpha or beta particles, x- or gamma rays, etc.). The units for measuring the absorbed dose are the gray (Gy) and the rad (radiation absorbed dose).

Absorption: The process through which radiation imparts some or all of its energy to any material through which it passes.

Acetic acid: A chemical in the fixer solution that provides the acid medium to stop further development by neutralizing the alkali of the developer.

Acidifier: A chemical (acetic acid) in the fixer solution that neutralizes the alkali in the developer solution and stops further action of the developer.

Acquired immune deficiency syndrome (AIDS): The end stage of an infection with the human immunodeficiency virus (HIV). A complex disease that interferes with the body's immune system.

Activator: A chemical (usually sodium carbonate) in the developer solution that causes the emulsion on the radiographic film to swell. Initiates the reducing action of the developing agents. Sodium carbonate makes the developer alkaline.

Acute radiation syndrome: Symptoms of the short-term radiation effects after a massive dose of ionizing radiation.

Added filtration: Added to the inherent filtration built into the x-ray machine. Added filtration is in the form of thin disks of pure aluminum, which can be inserted between the x-ray tube and the lead collimator when the inherent filtration is not sufficient to meet modern radiation safety requirements.

Advanced caries: A classification of proximal surface caries. Category where caries has progressed all the way through the enamel, to or through the dentinoenamel junction (DEJ) but less than halfway through the dentin toward the pulp

AIDS: *See* Acquired immune deficiency syndrome..

Ala: The wing of the nose. The depression at which the nostril connects with the cheek. Used as a facial landmark in dental radiography.

ALARA: As low as reasonably achievable. Adopted as a culture and attitude by professionals who work with ionizing radiation to minimize radiation exposure and risks.

Ala–tragus line: An imaginary plane or line from the ala of the nose (a winglike projection at the side of the nose) to the tragus of the ear (the cartilaginous projection in front of the acoustic meatus of the ear). Important in determining the correct position of the patient's head.

Alkaline: Having a pH greater than 7. Less than 7 is acidic, 7 is neutral.

Alpha particle: A common form of particulate (corpuscular) radiation. Alpha particles contain two protons and two neutrons and are positively charged.

Alternating current (AC): A flow of electrons in one direction, followed by a flow in the opposite direction.

Aluminum equivalent: The thickness of aluminum affording the same degree of attenuation, under specified conditions, as the material in question.

Alveolar (crestal) bone: That portion of the maxillary or mandibular bone that immediately surrounds and supports the roots of the dentition.

Alveolar process: The most coronal portion of the alveolar bone. Appears radiopaque when visible on a radiograph.

Alveolus: In dentistry, that part of the alveolar bone that forms the bony socket in which the roots of the tooth are held in position by fibers of the periodontal ligament.

Amalgam: Metallic restorative material.

Amalgam tattoo: The bluish-purple color of the gingival tissue caused by fragments of amalgam under the tissue.

Ameloblastoma: An odontogenic tumor of enamel origin that does not undergo differentiation to the point of enamel formation.

American Dental Assistants Association (ADAA): Professional organization for the purpose of promoting the dental assisting profession in ways that enhance the delivery of quality oral health care to the public.

American Dental Association (ADA): Professional organization of dentists committed to the public's oral health through professional advancement, research, education, and the development of standards of care.

American Dental Hygienists' Association (ADHA): Professional organization for the purpose of advancing the art and science of dental hygiene by ensuring access to quality oral health care and increasing awareness of the cost-effective benefits of prevention.

Amperage: The strength of an electric current measured in amperes.

Ampere (A): The unit of intensity of an electric current produced by 1 volt acting through a resistance of 1 ohm.

Analog: Relating to the mechanism in which data is represented by continuously variable physical quantities.

Anatomical order: The order in which the teeth are arranged in the dental arches.

Angle of mandible: The area at the posterior and inferior corners of the mandible, where the body of the mandible meets and joins the ascending ramus of the mandible.

Angstrom: A unit of measurement that describes the wavelengths of certain high-frequency radiation. One angstrom unit (AU or Å) measures 1/100,000,000 of a centimeter. Most wavelengths used in dentistry vary from about 0.1 AU to a maximum of 1.0 AU.

Angular chelitis: Fissuring and ulcerations at the corners of the mouth.

Angulation: The direction in which the central ray and the PID of the x-ray machine are directed toward the teeth and the image receptor. *See* Horizontal angulation, Negative angulation, Positive angulation, and Vertical angulation.

Ankylosis: A stiffening of a joint, such as the TMJ, caused by a fibrous or bony union. In dentistry the term can also apply to a union of the tooth to the alveolus caused by mineralization and hardening of the fibers of the periodontal ligament.

Anode: The positive electrode (terminal) in the x-ray tube. Tungsten block, normally set at a 20-degree angle facing the cathode, imbedded in the copper portion of the terminal.

Anodontia: A congenital absence of teeth. Any tooth in the dental arch may fail to develop. The teeth most frequently absent are the third molars, the premolars, and the maxillary lateral incisors.

Anomaly: A deviation from the normal.

Anterior nasal spine: V-shaped projection from the floor of the nasal fossa in the midline. Appears as a triangle-shaped radiopacity.

Antihalation coating: A dye added to the nonemulsion side of duplicating film to prevent backscattered ultraviolet light from coming through the films and creating an unsharp image.

Antiseptic: Refers to agents used on living tissues to destroy or stop the growth of bacteria.

Apical foramen: The opening to the pulp canal at the apex (terminal end) of the root of the tooth. A three-rooted tooth would have three apical foramina.

Appearance: Outward impression of self that the radiographer presents to the patient.

Apprehensive: To be anxious or fearful about the future.

Area monitoring: The routine monitoring of the level of radiation in an area such as a room, building, space around radiation-emitting equipment, or outdoor space.

Arrested caries: Caries that are no longer progressing.

Artifacts: Images other than anatomy or pathology that do not contribute to a diagnosis of the patient's condition.

Artificial intelligence: Ability of a computer to perform decision making similar to a human being.

Asepsis: The absence of septic matter, or freedom from infection.

Atom: The smallest particle of an element that has the properties of that element. Atoms are extremely minute and are composed of a number of subatomic particles. *See* Proton, Electron, and Neutron.

Atomic number (also called Z number): The total number of protons in the nucleus of an atom.

Atomic weight (also called A number or mass number): The total number of protons and neutrons in the nucleus of an atom.

Attitude: The position assumed by the body in connection with a feeling or mood.

Automatic processor: A machine that develops, fixes, washes, and dries radiographic film.

Autotransformer: A special single-coil transformer that corrects fluctuations in the current flowing through the x-ray machine.

Background radiation: Ionizing radiation that is always present. Consists of cosmic rays from outer space, naturally occurring radiation from the earth, and radiation from radioactive materials.

Barrier envelope: Plastic sheaths used to seal intraoral film packets, phosphor plates, and digital sensors to protect from contact with fluids in the oral cavity during exposure.

Base material: A thick layer of cement used as a cavity preparation under a restoration. Base material often appears slightly more radiopaque than dentin.

Beam indicating device (BID): *See* Positioning indicating device (PID).

Benign: Noncancerous. Not usually an immediate threat to overall health.

Beta particle: A form of particulate radiation. High-speed negative electrons.

BID: Beam indicating device. *See* Positioning indicating device (PID).

Binding energy: The internal energy within the atom that holds its components together.

Biodegradable: Capable of being broken down into harmless products by living organisms such as those found in a wastewater treatment facility.

Bisecting technique (bisecting-angle or short-cone technique): An exposure technique in which the central beam of radiation is directed perpendicular to an imaginary line that bisects the angle formed by the recording plane of the image receptor and the long axes of the teeth.

Bisector: The imaginary line that bisects the angle formed by the image receptor and teeth. *See* Bisecting technique.

Biteblock: A plastic or polystyrene device that functions to hold the image receptor in position while it is being exposed. The patient occludes and holds the image receptor in place by biting on the biteblock.

Bite extension: That portion of the biteblock that allows the patient to occlude in such a way that image receptor will be positioned parallel to the long axes of the teeth.

Bitetab: An extension, made out of heavy paper or plastic, that is attached at the center of the image receptor and on which the patient bites to stabilize the image receptor during a bitewing exposure.

Bitewing radiograph: An intraoral radiograph that shows the crowns of both the upper and lower teeth.

Bremsstrahlung radiation: *See* General radiation.

Buccal caries: Caries that involves the buccal surface of a tooth.

Buccal-object rule: Principle that structures portrayed in two or more radiographs exposed at different angles will appear to shift positions.

Calcium tungstate: Barium strontium sulfate salt crystals that are used in intensifying screens. When x-rays are absorbed, the crystals fluoresce and emit energy in the form of blue light.

Calculus: Calcified microbial plaque.

Cancellous bone: *See* Trabecular bone.

Canthus: The angle at either end of the slit that separates the eyelids. The inner canthus is nearest the nose. The outer canthus is farthest from the nose.

Carcinoma: Malignant growth of epithelial cells. A form of cancer.

Caries: Disease of the calcified tissues of the teeth. The inorganic portion is demineralized and the organic tissues are destroyed.

Cassette: A rigid or flexible extraoral film or phosphor plate (indirect digital technology) holder. Cassettes contain a pair of intensifying screens.

Cassette holder: That part of a panoramic x-ray machine where the cassette is positioned for exposure.

Cathode: The negative electrode (terminal) in the x-ray tube. The cathode consists of a tungsten filament wire that is set in a molybdenum focusing cup that directs the cathode stream toward the target on the anode.

Caustic: Capable of burning biological tissues.

Cemental (root) caries: Caries that develops on the roots of teeth between the enamel border and the free margin of the gingiva.

Cementoenamel junction (CEJ): The area where the enamel covering of the tooth crown meets the cementum covering of the tooth root.

Cementum: One of the four basic tooth structures. The thin layer of dense tissue that covers the root of a tooth. Because the cementum layer is thin, it is generally radiographically indistinguishable from dentin. When the condition of hypercementosis presents, the overgrowth of cementum will appear radiopaque and bulbous.

Central ray: The central portion of the primary beam of radiation.

Cephalostat: A device used to stabilize the patient's head in a plane that is parallel to the image receptor and at right angles to the central rays of the x-ray beam. Ear rods that can be placed into the openings of the acoustic meatus of the ear help to accomplish this.

Cervical burnout: A radiolucency often observed on the mesial and distal root surfaces near the cementoenamel junction. The radiolucent appearance is caused by the concave shape of the root at the cervical line and may be mistaken for caries.

Chairside manner: Refers to the conduct of the dental radiographer while working at the patient's chairside.

Chairside processing: *See* Rapid processing

Characteristic radiation: A form of radiation originating from an atom following removal of an electron or excitation of the atom. The wavelength of the emitted radiation is specific for the element and the particular energy levels involved.

Charge-coupled device (CCD): A CCD is a solid-state detector used in many electronic devices such as video cameras and fax machines. A CCD is used as the image receptor found in digital sensors. Converts x-rays to electrons that are sent to a computer via a wire, or wirelessly via radio frequency.

Code of ethics: A professional organization's principles to assist members in achieving a high standard of ethical practice.

Coherent scattering: Radiation that is scattered when a low-energy x-ray passes near an atom's outer electron. Approximately 8 percent of interactions of matter with the dental x-ray beam are the result of coherent scattering.

Coin test: Quality control test used to determine the adequacy of safelighting in the darkroom.

Collimation: The restriction of the useful beam to an appropriate size. Intraoral beam diameter is collimated to 2 3/4 in. (7 cm) at the skin surface.

Collimator: A diaphragm, usually lead, designed to restrict the dimensions of the useful beam.

Communication: The process by which information is exchanged between two or more persons.

Complementary metal oxide semiconductor (CMOS): A solid-state integrated circuit similar to the CCD. Used in digital radiography as an image receptor in the intraoral sensor. Converts x-rays to electrons that are sent to a computer via a wire, or wirelessly via radio frequency.

Composite (composite resin): Tooth-colored material used for restorations.

Compton effect (Compton scattering): An attenuation (absorption) process for x- and gamma radiation in which a photon interacts with an orbital electron or an atom to form a displaced electron and a scattered photon (x-ray) of reduced energy.

Computed tomography (CT): Radiographic imaging technique that images an isolated "slice" of tissue while blurring out other structures.

Condensing osteitis: Term used to describe the formation of compact sclerotic bone. Such areas of hardened bone are frequently seen on dental radiographs and appear more radiopaque than the surrounding bone areas. Such areas are generally irregular in shape or location.

Condyle: A rounded knob or projection on a bone, usually where that bone articulates (joins) with another bone. The condyle of the mandible articulates with the glenoid fossa (depression) of the temporal bone.

Cone: Older term used to describe the positioning indicating device (PID) or beam indicating device (BID).

Cone beam computed tomography (CBCT): Computed tomography (CT) scanning that is designed specifically for maxillofacial use. Patient radiation dose is significantly less when compared with conventional CT exposure of the maxillofacial region.

Cone beam volumetric imaging (CBVI): *See* Cone beam computed tomography (CBCT).

Conecut error: A term used to describe a technique error in which the central beam is not directed toward the center of the image receptor, resulting in a blank area in that part of the radiograph that was not reached by the radiation.

Confidentiality: Private information, such as dental records, that is protected by law from being shared with nonprivileged individuals.

Consumer-Patient Health Act: Action that sought to establish minimum standards for personnel who administer radiation in medical and dental radiographic procedures. Passed and signed into law to protect patients from unnecessary radiation.

Contact point: The area of a tooth surface that touches another tooth. This generally refers to the mesial surface of one tooth making contact with the distal surface of the tooth adjacent to it in the dental arch. The spot where the teeth actually touch is the contact point, and the area between the contact point and the gingiva (gum) is called the embrasure.

Contamination: The soiling by contact or mixing.

Contrast: The visual differences between shades ranging from black to white in adjacent areas of the radiograph. A radiograph that shows few shades has a short-scale or high contrast. A radiograph that shows many variations in shade has a long-scale or low contrast. High kilovoltage produces a radiograph with long-scale contrast. Low kilovoltage produces a radiograph with short-scale contrast. Digital software can be used to adjust the contrast of digital images.

Control panel: That portion of the x-ray machine that houses the major controls. Includes the line switch, timer, milliamperage and kilovoltage selectors, and the exposure button.

Coronoid process of the mandible: The pointed, anterior process on the upper border of the mandible.

Cortical bone: The solid, outer portion of the dense, compact bone. Appears very radiopaque on radiographs.

Coulombs per kilogram (C/kg): Système Internationale unit for measuring exposure. A coulomb is a unit of electrical charge (equal to 6.25×10^{18} electrons). The unit C/kg measures electrical charges (ion pairs) in a kilogram of air.

Cross-contamination: To contaminate from one place or person to another place or person.

Cross-sectional technique: An occlusal radiographic technique in which the central ray is directed perpendicular to the image receptor.

Crown: That portion of the tooth covered with enamel. "Clinical crown" refers to the entire portion of a tooth that is visible in the oral cavity. May also refer to a metallic or porcelain or combination of metal and porcelain restoration.

Crystal: Term used to refer to the silver halide combinations that are present in the film emulsion. Larger crystals require less radiation exposure to produce an image. However, larger crystal size may result in slightly less image resolution.

Cultural barriers: When language, beliefs, traditions, and familial influences become obstacles to the patient achieving optimal oral health.

Cumulative effect: The theory that radiation-exposed tissues accrue damage and may function at a diminished capacity with each repeated exposure.

Cyst: An epithelium-lined sac containing fluid or other fibrous or solid materials that appear radiolucent. Common cysts observed on dental radiographs are dentigerous, follicular, radicular (apical or periapical), and residual.

Darkroom: A light-tight room with special safelighting where x-ray film is handled and processed.

Daylight loader: A light-shielded compartment attached to an automatic processor so films can be unwrapped in a room with white light.

"Dead-man" switch: A switch so constructed that a circuit-closing contact can only be maintained by continuous pressure by the operator.

Dead pixel: Term given to a damaged pixel that does not respond to x-radiation exposure. A dead pixel will not record radiographic information.

Decay: The radioactive disintegration of the nucleus of an unstable atom by the emission of particles, photons of energy, or both.

Definition: Sharpness and clarity of the outline of the structures in a radiographic image. Poor definition is generally caused by movement of the patient, image receptor, or the tube head during exposure.

Dens in dente: A developmental anomaly in which the enamel invaginates within the body of the tooth.

Density: The overall darkening or blackening of the radiographic image. Increasing or decreasing the milliamperage and exposure time (milliampere/second) affects density. Digital software can be used to adjust the density of digital images.

Dentigerous cyst: A cyst derived from the enamel organ and always associated with the crown of a tooth.

Dentin: One of the four basic tooth structures. The chief tissue of the tooth that surrounds the pulp. Dentin is covered by enamel on the crown of the tooth and by cementum on the root. Appears slightly less radiopaque than enamel.

Dentinoenamel junction (DEJ): The junction between the dentin and enamel of a tooth.

Dentition: Teeth. The term dentulous refers to areas of the jaws having teeth.

Deterministic (nonstochastic): Observable adverse biological effects caused by radiation exposure. The severity of change in tissues depends on the radiation dose.

Developer: The chemical solution used in film processing that makes the latent image visible.

Developing agent: Elon and hydroquinone, substances that reduce the halides in the film emulsion to metallic silver. Elon brings out the details, and hydroquinone brings out the contrast in the film.

Diagnosis: The art of differentiating and determining the nature of a problem or disease.

Digital image: Radiographic image that exists as bits of information in a computer file. Special computer software constructs an image on a monitor for viewing.

Digital imaging: A method of producing a filmless radiographic image using a sensor (instead of film) and transmitting the electronic information directly into a computer, which serves to acquire, process, store, retrieve, and display the radiographic image. The terms *digital imaging* and *digital radiography* are often used interchangeably.

Digital Imaging and Communications in Medicine (DICOM): A joint committee formed in 1983 by the American College of Radiology and the National Electrical Manufacturers Association to create a standard method for electronic transmissions of digital images, the goal of which is to achieve compatibility and ease exchange of electronic information between digital image systems.

Digital radiograph: *See* Digital image.

Digital subtraction: Using a computer to superimpose two standardized radiographic images, causing the like areas of the image to "cancel" each other out, leaving only the changes visible.

Digitize: To convert an image into a digital form that can be processed by a computer.

Dilaceration: A sharp bend in the tooth root.

Direct current (DC): Electric current that flows continuously in one direction. Similar to current produced in batteries. Ideal for use with digital imaging.

Direct digital imaging: A method of directly obtaining a digital image by exposing an intraoral sensor to x-rays to produce an image that can be viewed on a computer monitor.

Direct supervision: Means the dentist is present in the office when the radiographs are taken on patients.

Direct theory: States that cell damage results when ionizing radiation directly hits critical areas within the cell.

DIS (direct ion storage) monitor: A personnel radiation monitoring device that uses a miniature ion chamber to absorb radiation. Exposure is determined through digital processing.

Disability: A physical or mental impairment that substantially limits one or more of an individual's major life activities.

Disclosure: The process of informing the patient about the risks and benefits of a treatment procedure.

Disinfect: Chemical applications that reduce disease-producing microorganisms to an acceptable level.

Distomesial overlap: When the projection angle of the x-ray beam is directed from distal to mesial, resulting in overlapping error.

Disto-oblique periapical radiographs: Periapical radiographs that utilize a tube shift to help image posterior objects such as impacted third molars. Shifting the tube to the distal, causing the x-rays to be directed from the distal aspect, will project the posterior object forward onto the image receptor.

Distortion: The variation in the true size and shape of the object being radiographed.

Dosage: The radiation absorbed in a specified area of the body measured in grays (Gy) or rads.

Dose: The amount of absorbed radiation in grays or rads at any given point. Dose may refer to absorbed dose, depth of the dose, entrance dose, or surface dose.

Dose equivalent: Compares the biological effects of various types of radiation. Dose equivalent is defined as the product of the absorbed dose times a biological effect qualifying factor. Because the qualifying factor for x-rays is one, the absorbed dose and the dose equivalent are equal. The units for measuring the dose equivalent are the sievert (Sv) and the rem.

Dose-response curve: Graph produced when radiation dose and the resultant biological response are plotted.

Dosimeter: A radiation measuring device.

Double exposure: Using the same image receptor to expose two radiographs. Results in an overexposed, double-image error.

Duplicate radiograph: A copy made of a radiograph. Useful in referrals, consultations, and for submitting to insurance companies for payment of dental treatment.

Duplicating film: A photographic film similar to x-ray film. Duplicating film is exposed by the action of infrared and ultraviolet light rather than by x-rays. Used to duplicate x-ray films in a contact-printer-type x-ray duplicating unit.

Edentulous: Without teeth. Areas of the jaws with no teeth.

Effective dose equivalent: Aids in making more accurate comparisons between different radiographic exposures. Compensates for the differences in area exposed and the tissues that may be in the path of the x-ray beam. Measured in microsieverts (μSv).

Electric current: The flow of electrons through a conductor.

Electrical circuit: A path of electrical current.

Electrode: Either of two terminals of an electric source. In the x-ray tube, either the anode or the cathode.

Electromagnetic radiation: Forms of energy propelled by wave motion as photons. This is a combination of electric and magnetic energy. Has no charge, mass, or weight and travels at the speed of light. Differs in wavelength, frequency, and properties. For convenience, electromagnetic radiations are arranged in diagrammatic form as the electromagnetic spectrum.

Electromagnetic spectrum: Types of electromagnetic energies arranged in diagrammatic form on a chart. Include radio and television waves, infrared waves, visible light, ultraviolet waves, x-rays, gamma rays, and cosmic radiations. The longer wavelengths are measured in meters and the shorter ones in centimeters or angstroms.

Electron: A small, negatively charged particle of the atom containing much energy and little mass.

Electron cloud: A mass of free electrons that hovers around the filament wire of the cathode when it is heated to incandescence. The number of free electrons increases as the milliamperage is increased.

Electronic noise: The digital equivalent to film fog. An electrical disturbance that clutters the digital image reducing image clarity and contrast.

Element: In chemistry, a simple substance that cannot be decomposed by chemical means.

Elon: Developer reducing agent that converts exposed silver halide crystals to black metallic silver. Builds up gray tones in the image.

Elongated image : Refers to a distortion of the radiographic image in which the tooth structures appear longer than the anatomical size. Often caused by insufficient vertical angulation of the central beam.

Elongation: *See* Elongated image.

Embrasure: The space between the sloping proximal surfaces of the teeth. The space may diverge facially, lingually, occlusally, or apically. The interdental papillae normally fill most of the apical embrasures.

Empathy: The ability to share in another's emotions or feelings.

Emulsion: The gelatinous coating on radiographic film containing silver halide crystals.

Enamel: One of the four basic tooth structures. The dense, hard substance that covers the dentin of the crown of the teeth. Appears very radiopaque on the radiograph.

Endodontic therapy: The treatment of the tooth by removing the nerves and tissues of the pulp cavity and replacing them with filling material.

Energy: The ability to do work and overcome resistance.

Energy levels (electron shells or orbits): A term used in chemistry and physics to denote spherical levels containing the electrons of the atom.

Ethics: A sense of moral obligation regarding right and wrong behavior.

Exfoliation: Shedding of primary teeth.

Exostosis: A bony growth projecting outward from the surface of a bone or tooth. Occasionally encountered on the palate or the lingual surface of the mandible as tori.

Exposure: A measure of ionization produced in air by x- or gamma radiation. The units of exposure are coulombs per kilogram (C/kg) and the roentgen (R).

Exposure button: Keypad or switch that activates the x-ray production process.

Exposure chart: A chart listing the exposure factors (milliamperage, exposure time, and kilovoltage) for each radiographic procedure.

Exposure factors: Settings for milliamperage (mA), exposure time, and kilovoltage (kVp).

Exposure time: The time interval, expressed in seconds or impulses, that x-rays are produced.

Extension arm: Flexible arm from which the tube head of the x-ray machine is suspended.

External aiming device (indicator ring): An indicating component of some image receptor holders that is used to aid in aligning the x-ray beam to the image receptor.

External auditory meatus (foramen): An opening in the temporal bone located superior and anterior to the mastoid process.

External resorption: Tooth structure lost through a resorptive process. Characterized by tooth roots that appear shorter than normal, but can also occur anywhere along the tooth root. Resorption of the roots of primary teeth in response to the erupting permanent teeth is considered normal. Pathologic external resorption may be associated with an impacted or unerupted tooth, a tumor, or trauma. Often the cause is idiopathic (unknown).

Extraoral film: Designed for use outside the mouth.

Extraoral radiography: Radiographic examinations made of the head and facial region using image receptors positioned outside the mouth. Extraoral film requires the use of a cassette and intensifying screens.

Eyewash station: Sink with faucets designed for the purpose of flushing the eyes with copious amounts of water in an accidental chemical contamination.

FAQs: Stands for frequently asked questions.

Federal Performance Act of 1974: Requires that all x-ray equipment manufactured or sold in the United States meet federal performance standards.

Filament: The spiral tungsten coil in the focusing cup of the cathode of the x-ray tube.

Film badge: A monitoring device containing a special type of film which, when properly developed and interpreted, gives a measurement of the exposure received during the time the badge was worn.

Film contrast: *See* Contrast.

Film duplicator: A device that provides a diffused light source (usually ultraviolet) that evenly exposes the duplicating film.

Film feed slot: Opening in an automatic film processor where the film is inserted for processing.

Film fog: An overall darkening of the radiograph caused by old or contaminated processing solutions, exposure to chemical fumes, faulty safelight, or scatter radiation.

Film hanger: A stainless steel hanger equipped with clips used to hold films during manual processing.

Film holder/Image receptor holder: Device used to hold and stabilize an intraoral film packet or digital sensor or phosphor plate in the mouth.

Film loop (bitewing loop): Cardboard or plastic loop used as an image receptor holder in bitewing radiography. The patient bites on the tab portion to hold the image receptor in position during exposure.

Film mount: Plastic or cardboard holder with frames or windows that display films for viewing.

Film mounting: The placement of dental radiographs in a film mount for viewing and interpretation.

Film packet: Intraoral film packaged in a moisture-proof outer plastic or paper wrap. May contain one or two films, wrapped in dark protective paper on either side, and a thin sheet of lead foil on the back side of the film(s).

Film recovery slot: Opening in an automatic film processing unit where the finished radiograph exits at the completion of the processing cycle.

Film speed: The sensitivity of the film to radiation exposure. Fast-film speed requires less radiation to produce an image. Slow film speed requires more radiation to produce an image.

Filter: Absorbing material, usually aluminum, placed in the path of the beam of radiation to remove a high percentage of the low energy (longer wavelength) x-rays.

Filtration: The use of absorbers for selectively absorbing or screening out low-energy x-rays from the primary beam. *See* Added filtration, Inherent filtration, and Total filtration.

Fixer: A solution of chemicals that stops the action of the developer and makes the image permanently visible.

Fixing agent: Sodium thiosulfate, also known as "hypo" or hyposulfite of sodium. It is one of several chemical ingredients in the fixer solution and functions to remove all unexposed and any remaining undeveloped silver bromide grains from the emulsion.

Focal spot: Small area on the target on the anode toward which the electrons from the focusing cup of the cathode are directed. X-rays originate at the focal spot.

Focal trough: That area between the x-ray source and the image receptor that will be imaged distinctly on the panoramic radiograph. The size and shape of the focal trough vary with each panoramic x-ray machine.

Focusing cup: A curved device around the cathode wire filament that is designed to focus the free electrons toward the tungsten target of the anode.

Follicular (eruptive) cyst: A cyst associated with the enamel follicle.

Foreign body: Any object or material not normally found in the area.

Foreshortened image: Distortion of the radiographic image in which the tooth structures appear shorter than their actual anatomical size. Most often caused by excessive vertical angulation of the central beam.

Foreshortening: *See* Foreshortened image.

Fracture line: A break in a bone or a tooth. Appears radiolucent radiographically.

Frankfort plane: An imaginary plane or line from the orbital ridge (under the eye) to the acoustic meatus of the ear.

Frequency: The number of crests of a wavelength passing a given point per second.

Fresh film test: Quality control test used to monitor the quality of each new box of film.

Frontal bone: Cranial bone that forms the forehead.

Full mouth series (survey): The complete radiographic examination of the arches in which all teeth are imaged at least once, usually consists of 14 to 22 periapical and bitewing radiographs.

Furcation involvement: Bone loss between the roots of multi-rooted teeth.

Fusion: A condition where the dentin and one other dental tissue of adjacent teeth are united.

Gag reflex: A protective mechanism that serves to clear the airway of obstruction.

Gamma rays: A form of electromagnetic radiation with properties identical to x-rays. Usually produced spontaneously in the form of emission from radioactive substances.

Gelatin: Component of the film emulsion in which the halide crystals are suspended.

Gemination: A single tooth bud that divides and forms two teeth.

General radiation: Also called bremsstrahlung (which means "braking" in German) radiation. The stopping or slowing of the electrons of the cathode stream as they collide with the nuclei of the target atoms.

Generalized bone loss: Bone loss that occurs throughout the dental arches.

Genetic cells: The cells contained within the testes and ovaries, containing the genes.

Genetic effect: Radiation effect that is passed on to future generations.

Genetic mutation: Change in the genetic material of a cell that passes from one generation to another.

Genial tubercles: Anatomical landmark situated near the midline on the lingual surface of the mandible about halfway between the alveolar crest and the inferior border of the mandible. Appear radiographically as a small doughnut-shaped, radiopaque ring. The lingual foramen is located in the center of this ring.

Geometric factors: Factors that relate to the relationships of angles, lines, points, or surfaces that contribute to the quality of radiographic image definition.

Ghost image: Mirror or second image of a structure that is penetrated twice by the x-ray beam observed on panoramic radiographs.

Gingivitis: Inflammation of the gingiva.

Globulomaxillary cyst: Type of nonodontogenic cyst arising between the maxillary lateral incisor and the canine.

Glossopharyngeal air space: Open space posterior to the tongue that continues into the oral-pharyngeal (throat) region. Appears as a radiolucent negative shadow on a panoramic radiograph.

Granuloma: A tumor or neoplasm made up of granulation tissue. Often follows an abscess. Usually round or oval and surrounded by a fibrous capsule. Appears radiolucent on a radiograph.

Gray (Gy): Système Internationale unit for measuring absorbed dose. One Gy equals 100 rads; 1,000 milligrays equals 1 Gy.

Gray scale: Refers to the total number of shades of gray visible in an image.

Gray value: Number that corresponds to the amount of radiation received by a pixel within a digital sensor. The computer uses this value to determine the shade of gray displayed on the computer monitor.

Grid: A device used in extraoral radiography to prevent scatter radiation from fogging the image.

Gutta percha: Endodontic filling material.

Halide: Part of a halogen compound such as bromine and iodine that together with silver make up radiographic film emulsion.

Half-value layer (HVL): Thickness of a specified material that, when introduced into the path of a given beam of radiation, reduces the exposure rate by half.

Hamulus (hamular process): A very small hooklike process of bone that extends downward and slightly backward from the sphenoid bone. Appears radiopaque and can occasionally be seen posterior to the maxillary tuberosity.

Hard radiation: Rays of high energy and extremely short wavelengths. Essential for dental radiography.

Hardening agent (hardener): Potassium alum, one of the chemicals of the fixing solution. Functions to shrink and harden the wet emulsion.

Hazardous waste: Waste materials that present a threat to community health or the environment.

Head positioner guides: Device used on panoramic and cephalometric x-ray machines to stabilize the patient's head in the correct position.

Health Insurance Portability and Accountability Act of 1996 (HIPAA): Federal law designed to provide patients with more control over how their personal health information is used and disclosed. A patient will usually be asked to sign a notice that indicates how their radiographs may be used and their privacy rights under this law.

Hemostat: A clamplike dental instrumental. Can be used as forceps to grasp a film packet.

Hepatitis B (HBV): Form of viral hepatitis. May be transferred between patient and oral health care professionals via contact with blood. Hepatitis B vaccine in a series of three doses is recommended to achieve immunity.

Herringbone error (also called tire-track pattern): Image produced on a radiograph when the film packet is placed in the mouth backwards. The embossed pattern in the lead foil produces this image when the x-ray beam passes through the reversed film packet.

HIV: *See* Human immunodeficiency virus.

Horizontal angulation: Direction of the central beam in a horizontal plane. Incorrect horizontal angulation results in overlapping the proximal structures.

Horizontal bitewing radiograph: Bitewing radiograph placed in the oral cavity with the long dimension of the image receptor positioned horizontally. Considered the traditional placement for most patients.

Horizontal bone loss: Bone loss that occurs in a plane parallel to the cementoenamel junctions of adjacent teeth.

Human immunodeficiency virus (HIV): A type of retrovirus that causes AIDS (acquired immunodeficiency syndrome).

Hydroquinone: Reduces (converts) exposed silver halide crystals to black metallic silver. Slowly builds up black tones and contrast.

Hypercementosis: An excessive development of cementum that makes the tooth root appear bulbous. Most frequently observed on premolars. Appears radiopaque.

Hypersensitive gag reflex: Exaggerated gag response that is overly sensitive.

Identification dot: Small circular embossed mark on the corner of intraoral x-ray film. Used to determine the patient's right or left side when viewing radiographs.

Idiopathic resorption: Of unknown original. *See* External resorption and Internal resorption.

Image receptor holder (positioner): See film holder.

Immunization: Method, such as vaccines, of inducing resistance to an infectious disease.

Impacted tooth (impaction): A tooth embedded in alveolar bone in such a manner that its eruption is prevented. An impaction may be partial or total.

Impulse: Measure of exposure time. There are 60 impulses per second.

Incandescence: Stage when the tungsten filament in the cathode becomes red hot and glows. Free electrons are liberated and swarm around the glowing wire to form the electron cloud.

Incipient (enamel) caries: The earliest stage of the caries process.

Incisive canal cyst: A type of nonodontogenic cyst arising in the incisive canal.

Incisive (anterior palatine) foramen: Maxillary landmark situated at the midline of the palate immediately behind the central incisors from which the nasopalatine nerve and vessels emerge. Shape varies but is usually observed as a round pea-shaped radiolucency. Incorrect horizontal angulation superimposes the incisive foramen over the apex of the root of the central incisor where it may then be mistaken for an abscess or a cyst.

Indicator ring: *See* External aiming device.

Indirect digital imaging: Photostimuable phosphor (PSP) plate sensor technology. Method of obtaining a digital image in which an exposed phosphor plate is placed into a scanner and then converted into a digital image.

Indirect theory: States that cell damage results indirectly when x-rays cause the formation of toxins in the cell such as hydrogen peroxide. Toxins in turn cause the cell damage.

Infection control: The prevention and reduction of disease-causing (pathogenic) microorganisms.

Inferior border of the mandible: Dense layer of cortical bone that forms the lower portion of the body of the mandible. Appears very radiopaque on the radiograph.

Informed consent: Permission given by a patient after being informed of the details of a treatment procedure.

Inherent filtration: Filtration built into the x-ray machine by the manufacturer. This includes the glass x-ray tube envelope, the insulating materials of the tube head, and the materials that seal the port.

Intensifying screen: Plastic sheet coated with calcium tungstate or rare earth fluorescent salt crystals. Positioned in a cassette. When exposed to radiation, the fluorescent salts glow, giving off a blue (calcium tungstate) or green (rare earth) light. Produces a latent image faster than is possible when radiation alone is used.

Intensity: The total energy of the x-ray beam. The product of the number of x-rays (quantity) and energy of each x-ray (quality) per unit of area per time of exposure.

Interdental septa: Alveolar bone between adjacent teeth.

Internal resorption: Tooth structure lost through a resorptive process. Typically appears as a radiolucent widening of the root canal, representing the resorption process taking place from the inside out. Often the cause is idiopathic (unknown).

Interpersonal skills: Techniques that increase successful communication with others.

Interpretation: The ability to read and explain what is revealed by the radiograph.

Interproximal: Between two adjacent tooth surfaces.

Interproximal caries: *See* Proximal caries

Interproximal radiograph: *See* Bitewing radiograph.

Intraoral: Inside the mouth.

Intraoral dental film: Film that is placed in the oral cavity for exposure.

Intraoral film: *See* Intraoral dental film.

Intraoral radiography: Radiographic examinations where the image receptor is placed inside the mouth.

Inverse square law: States that the intensity of radiation is inversely proportional to the square of the distance from the source of the radiation to the point of measurement.

Inverted Y: Radiographic landmark made up of the lateral wall of the nasal fossa and the anterior-medial wall of the maxillary sinus often observed near the canine-premolar region.

Ion: An electrically charged particle, either negative or positive.

Ion pair: A pair of ions, one positive and one negative.

Ionization: The formation of ion pairs.

Ionizing radiation: Radiation that is capable of producing ions.

Irradiation: The exposure of an object or a person to radiation. Term can be applied to radiations of various wavelengths, such as infrared rays, ultraviolet rays, x-rays, and gamma rays.

Irreparable injury: Following exposure to radiation, injury that results in damage that is not repaired during the recovery period. May give rise to later long-term effects of radiation exposure.

Isosceles triangle: A triangle with two sides equal in length and two identical angles opposite these two equal sides.

Isotope: Alternate form of an element, having the same number of protons but a different number of neutrons inside the nucleus. Many isotopes are radioactive.

Kilovolt (kV): A unit of electromotive force, equal to 1,000 volts. High kilovoltage is essential for the production of dental x-rays.

Kilovolt peak (kVp): The crest value in kilovolts of the potential difference of a pulsating generator.

Kinetic energy: Energy possessed by a mass because of its motion.

Labial mounting method: Radiographs mounted so that the embossed dot is convex. The viewer is reading the radiograph as if standing in front of, and facing, the patient. Recommended by the American Dental Association and the American Academy of Oral and Maxillofacial Radiology over the lingual mounting method.

Lamina dura: A thin, hard layer of cortical bone that lines the dental alveolus. Appears as a thin, radiopaque line around the roots of the teeth on dental radiographs.

Latent image: The invisible image produced when the film is exposed to x-ray photons. Image remains invisible until the film is processed.

Latent period: The time between exposure to radiation and the first clinically observable symptoms. Latent means hidden.

Lateral cephalometric radiograph: Extraoral radiograph of the side of the skull often used by orthodontists at various stages of treatment. Made by placing the patient's head in a cephalostat. Also called a lateral skull projection.

Lateral fossa: Slight decreased thickness (concavity) in bone between the maxillary lateral incisor and the maxillary canine.

Lateral jaw (mandibular oblique lateral) radiograph: Extraoral radiograph of the posterior mandible. Also called mandibular oblique lateral projection.

Lateral skull projection: *See* Lateral cephalometric radiograph.

Law of B and T (Bergonie and Tribondeau): States that the radiosensitivity of cells and tissues is directly proportional to their reproductive capacity and inversely proportional to their degree of differentiation.

Lead apron: Protective barrier made of lead or lead-equivalent materials. Shields patients' gonadal areas from radiation during dental x-ray exposures.

Lead equivalent: The thickness of a material that affords the same degree of attenuation (absorption) to radiation as a specified thickness of lead.

LED (light-emitting diode): A semiconductor device that emits light when electrical current passes through it. Used for safelighting the darkroom.

Lethal dose: The amount of radiation that is sufficient to cause the death of an organism.

Liable: To be legally obligated to make good any loss or damage that may occur.

Light-tight: Securing an area against all sources of white light. Characteristic of a darkroom.

Line pair: Refers to the number of paired lines visible in 1 mm of an image. The more line pairs visible, the better the spatial resolution in an image.

Line switch: Toggle switch that is used to turn the x-ray machine on or off.

Lingual caries: Caries that involves the lingual surface of a tooth.

Lingual foramen: A very small opening through which a branch of the incisive artery emerges. Located in the center of the genial tubercles on the lingual side of the mandible. *See* Genial tubercles.

Lingual mounting method: Radiographs are mounted so that the embossed dot is concave. The viewer is reading the radiograph as if standing behind the patient.

Local contributing factor: Amalgam overhangs, poorly contoured crown margins, and calculus deposits that act as food traps and lead to the buildup of bacterial deposits that cause periodontal disease.

Localization: Methods to provide a third dimension to two-dimensional radiographs. Assists the radiographer in determining whether an object is located on the facial (buccal) or lingual.

Localized bone loss: Bone loss that occurs in isolated areas.

Long-scale contrast: Low-contrast image. A radiographic image with many shades of gray. Produced with high kilovoltage.

Mach band effect: An optical illusion that mimics the appearance of decay. Often occurs along boundaries of sharp contrast, especially around areas of slight overlapping between adjacent teeth.

Magnification (enlargement): Enlargement of the structures imaged on a radiograph over the actual size. Enlargement is greatest when the target of an x-ray machine is closer to the structures of interest and is decreased when distance is greater.

Malignant: Tendency to progress in virulence and spread. Condition that may result in death.

Malpractice: Improper practice. Malpractice results when one is negligent.

Mandible: Lower arch (jaw).

Mandibular canal: Long canal extending from the mandibular foramen on the medial aspect of the ramus of the mandible to the mental foramen on the lateral aspect. Carries nerves and blood vessels that supply most of the teeth in the mandible. Appears radiolucent, with thin radiopaque lines above and below outlining the cortical bone that lines the canal.

Mandibular foramen: Small opening on the lateral side of the body of the mandible. Usually observed near the apices of the premolars.

Mandibular notch: Notch between the condyle and coronoid process of the mandible. Also called the sigmoid notch.

Mandibular oblique lateral projection: *See* Lateral jaw projection.

Mastoid process: Large rounded protuberance of the temporal bone located behind the ear.

Material Safety and Data sheets (MSDS): Documentation available from the manufacturers of chemical products that provide the oral health care professional with information regarding the properties and the potential health effects of the product.

Maxilla: Upper arch. The maxillae are actually two bones, a right and left maxilla.

Maxillary sinus: Large radiolucent cavity observed within the maxilla apical to the maxillary posterior teeth.

Maxillary tuberosity: A radiopaque prominence of bone on the distal portion of the maxillary alveolar ridge.

Maxillofacial: Pertaining to the dental arches (maxilla and mandible) and other supporting facial structures of the head and neck region.

Maximum permissible dose (MPD): The maximum accumulated dose that persons who are occupationally exposed may have at any given time of their life. It is the dose of ionizing radiation that, in the light of present knowledge, is not expected to cause detectable body damage. Currently established at 0.05 Sv per year (5 rem/year) whole body.

Mean tangent: Average point where several curved surfaces touch if a ruler is held against them. The labial or buccal surfaces of all teeth have their most prominent point toward the lips or the cheeks and curve toward the mesial or distal. A mean tangent would be established by using a small ruler or any straight edge (such as a tongue depressor) and attempting to align as many of the teeth as possible. Occasionally, four or even five of the posterior teeth will touch the ruler at some point. Used to establish correct horizontal angulation, which requires that the central ray of the x-ray beam be directed at right angles to the mean tangent.

Median palatine suture: An irregular line formed by the junction of the palatine processes of the right and left maxillae. Appears as a thin radiolucent line running vertically between the roots of the maxillary incisors.

Mental foramen: An opening through which the mental nerve and related blood vessels emerge on the lateral aspect of the body of the mandible; exact location varies. When imaged on radiographs, appears as a small round radiolucent area near the roots of the mandibular premolars. Should not be mistaken for an abscess, cyst, or other pathological condition.

Mental fossa: A depression on the labial aspect of the mandibular incisor area.

Mental ridge: Raised ridge of bone located in the anterior region on the lateral surface of the mandible.

Mesiodens: A supernumerary tooth located in the maxillary midline.

Mesiodistal overlap: When the projection angle of the x-ray beam is directed from mesial to distal resulting in overlapping error.

Microbial aerosol: Suspension of microorganisms that may be capable of causing disease produced during normal breathing and speaking

Microsievert (μSv): One millionth of a seivert. *See* Seivert.

Midsagittal plane (midsagittal line): An imaginary vertical line or plane passing through the center of the body that divides it into a right and left half. Important orientation line in determining the ideal position of the patient's head during radiographic exposures.

Milliampere (mA): One thousandth of an ampere. Milliamperage determines the number of electrons available at the filament. *See* Ampere.

Milliampere second (mAs): The relationship between the milliamperage and the exposure time in seconds. When one is increased, the other must be correspondingly decreased to maintain film density.

Modeling: Technique used to orient patients, especially children, to the radiographic procedure. Child is given the opportunity to observe procedure being performed on another, such as a sibling or parent. May help to alleviate fear of the unknown and gain patient cooperation.

Moderate caries: A classification of proximal surface caries. Category where caries penetrate over halfway through the enamel toward the dentinoenamel junction (DEJ), but do not reach the DEJ.

Molecule: Chemical combination of two or more atoms that forms the smallest particle of a substance that retains the properties of that substance.

Monitoring: Use of any of several devices to determine whether an area is within safe radiation limits or whether a person's exposure is within permissible limits. *See* Area monitoring and Personnel monitoring.

Motion: Movement of the image receptor, patient, or tube head during radiographic exposure that results in a less sharp image.

MPD: *See* Maximum permissible dose.

Mylohyoid ridge: Raised ridge of bone running diagonally downward and forward on the medial aspect of the ramus of the mandible to near the apices of the molar roots. Parallels the (external) oblique ridge, but on the lingual surface and about 1/4 in (6 mm) lower. Appears radiopaque when observed on a radiograph.

Nasal bones: Bones that make up the upper bridge of the nose.

Nasal conchae: Thin bony extensions of the nasal wall.

Nasal fossa (cavity): Large air space divided into two paired radiolucencies by the radiopaque nasal septum. Visible above the roots of the maxillary incisors.

Nasal septum: Dense cartilage that separates the right nasal fossa from the left. Appears as a vertical radiopaque line separating the paired radiolucencies of the nasal cavity

Nasopharyngeal air space: Open space superior to the soft palate. Appears as a radiolucent negative shadow on a panoramic radiograph.

Negative angulation (negative vertical angulation): Achieved by pointing the tip or end of the PID upward from a horizontal plane.

Negative shadows: Term given to the radiolucencies produced on a panoramic radiograph as a result of more radiation reaching the image receptor in the areas of air spaces. Negative shadows are shadows of "nothing."

Negligence: Failure to use a reasonable amount of care that results in injury or damage to another.

Neoprene gloves: Synthetic rubber utility gloves that provide increased protection for handling potentially damaging or hazardous chemicals.

Neutron: One form of particulate (corpuscular) radiation or subatomic particle. A neutron has no electric charge and has about the same mass as a proton.

Nitrile gloves: Synthetic latex utility gloves that provide increased protection for handling potentially damaging or hazardous chemicals

Noise: *See* Electronic noise

Nonmetallic restoration: Restoration containing no metal. May appear radiolucent, or radiopaque when radiopaque fillers have been added to the restorative material.

Nonodontogenic cyst: Cyst that arises from epithelium other than that associated with tooth formation.

Nonthreshold dose response curve: A graph showing the relationship between the dose of exposure and the response of the tissues, indicating that any amount of radiation, no matter how small, has the potential to cause a biological response.

Nonverbal communication: Communication achieved without words. Includes gestures, facial expressions, body movement, and listening.

Nutrient canal: Small tubelike passageway through bone that contains blood vessels and nerves. Appears radiolucent in radiographs.

Nutrient foramen: Occasionally imaged on a radiograph as a tiny radiolucent dot indicating the small opening in the tubelike passageway of a nutrient canal.

Object-image receptor distance: Distance between the object being recorded and the image receptor.

Oblique ridge: Diagonal ridge of bone on the lateral aspect of the mandible that runs downward and forward from the anterior border of the ramus to the level of the cervical portion of the molar and premolar roots. Sometimes referred to as the external oblique ridge. The internal oblique ridge appears faintly parallel to the external oblique ridge. The internal oblique ridge is not identified as an anatomical structure, but as a landmark only.

Occipital bone: Forms the posterior part of the skull.

Occlusal caries: Caries found on the occlusal (chewing) surface of posterior teeth.

Occlusal plane: Plane between the maxillary and the mandibular teeth.

Occlusal radiograph: Radiograph produced by placing the image receptor against the incisal or occlusal plane. The patient stabilizes the image receptor by biting down on it. In addition to the teeth, occlusal radiographs may show surrounding maxillary or mandibular structures. Depending on the placement of the image receptor and angle of exposure, cross-sectional or topographic radiographs are produced. *See* Cross-sectional technique and Topographical technique.

Occlusal trauma: Excessive or repetitive force against the teeth that results in a response.

Occult disease: The presence of disease that is not apparent clinically, but can only be detected via a diagnostic test, such as a radiograph.

Odontogenic cyst: A cyst that arises from epithelial cells associated with the development of a tooth.

Odontoma: A tumor of odontogenic origin in which enamel and dentin are formed. May contain soft tissues that appear radiolucent and a hard calcified mass, sometimes resembling a tooth, which appears radiopaque. Compound odontoma refers to odontogenic tissues that resemble teeth. Complex odontoma denotes odontogenic tissues arranged in a haphazard manner with no resemblance to tooth formation. Compound-complex odontoma is a mixture of the two types.

Oral radiography: Procedures that pertain to producing radiographs of the teeth and/or the oral cavity.

OSL (optically stimulated luminescence) monitor: A personnel radiation monitor that absorbs radiation similar to TLD, but crystals release energy during optical stimulation instead of heat.

Ossification: The pathological or abnormal conversion of soft tissues into bone.

Osteosclerosis: Abnormal increase in bone density. Appears as in increased radiopacity on a radiograph.

Overdevelopment: Leaving the film in the developer solution too long or using developer that is too warm. Overdevelopment results in a dark image.

Overexposure: Exposing the image receptor too long or subjecting the image receptor to an inappropriately increased kVp or mA setting. Overexposure results in a dark image.

Overhang: A restoration that is not contoured to the tooth properly.

Overlap: Term used to refer to a distortion of the tooth image in which the structures of one tooth are superimposed over the structures of the adjacent tooth. Caused by incorrect horizontal angulation of the central beam and/or incorrect positioning of the image receptor in relationship to the teeth of interest.

Oxidation: The process during which the chemicals of the developing and fixing solutions combine with oxygen and lose their strength.

Palatoglossal air space: Open space between the tongue and palate. Appears as a radiolucent negative shadow on a panoramic radiograph.

Panoramic radiograph: Generic term pertaining to the radiographic image produced by a panoramic x-ray machine. Images all the teeth and supporting structures of the maxilla and mandible.

Panoramic radiography: Procedure performed with a special-purpose x-ray machine that uses a stationary patient and a simultaneously moving x-ray source and image receptor to produce an image of the entire dentition and surrounding structures.

Paralleling technique: Intraoral technique that places the image receptor positioned parallel to the long axes of the teeth while the central beam of radiation is directed perpendicularly (at right angles) toward both the teeth and the image receptor.

Particulate radiation (corpuscular radiation): Minute subatomic particles such as protons, electrons, and neutrons; also alpha and beta particles. These particles occupy space; have mass and weight; and, with the exception of neutrons, have an electrical charge.

Pathogen: A disease-causing microorganism.

Patient education: Informing patients about the benefits of oral health and preventive oral hygiene. Providing the patient with necessary information that explains the value of dental radiographs and demonstrates radiation safety measures employed in the practice.

Patient relations: Establishment of the relationship between the patient and the oral health care professional.

Pediatric dentistry: Branch of dentistry that specializes in providing comprehensive preventive and therapeutic oral health care for children.

Pedodontic image receptor: Any smaller-sized film packet, phosphor plate, or digital sensor used for radiographs of children's teeth.

Penumbra: Partial shadow or fuzzy outline around the image.

Periapical cemental dysplasia (PCD): Sometimes referred to as cementoma. A tumor derived from the periodontal ligament of a fully developed and erupted tooth, usually a mandibular incisor. Early PCD is radiolucent and appears identical to radicular cysts. In the later stages of development, calcification occurs that appears as radiopaque masses surrounded by a radiolucent line. The teeth are vital and need no treatment.

Periapical radiograph: Image that shows the entire tooth or teeth and surrounding tissues. Peri means "around" and apical is the root end of the tooth.

Period of injury: Radiation-induced changes that follow the latent period.

Periodontal diseases: Diseases that affect the supporting tissues of the teeth.

Periodontal ligament (PDL) space: The space between the root of a tooth and the lamina dura where the thin but dense and strong fibrous tissues of the periodontal ligament are located. Radiographically, the periodontal ligament appears as a thin radiolucent line between the lamina dura and the root.

Periodontitis: Inflammation of the periodontium.

Periodontium: Tissues that invest and support the teeth (gingiva and alveolar bone).

Permanent teeth: Teeth that erupt after the primary teeth have been exfoliated (shed). Consists of 32 teeth—8 incisors, 4 canines, 8 premolars, and 12 molars.

Personal protective equipment (PPE): Clothing, masks, eyewear, and gloves worn by dental personnel as a protective barrier that prevents the transmission of infective microorganisms between oral health care practitioners and patients.

Personnel monitoring: The occasional or routine measuring of the amount of radiation to which a person working around radiation has been exposed during a given period of time.

Personnel monitoring device: Device (film badge, thermoluminescent dosimeter [TLD], direct ion storage [DIS] dosimeter and optically stimulated luminescent [OSL] dosimeter) worn by a radiation worker to measure the amount of radiation received in a given period of time.

pH: Chemical symbol used with a number from 0 to 14 to designate the relative acidity or alkalinity of a solution. Under 7 is acidic, over 7 is alkaline, 7 is neutral, neither acidic or alkaline.

Phleboliths: Calcified masses that are observed as round or oval bodies in the soft tissues of the cheeks.

Phosphors: Fluorescent crystals, calcium tungstate or rare earth, used in the emulsion that coats intensifying screens. Give off light when subjected to radiation.

Photoelectric effect: An attenuation process for x- and gamma radiation in which a photon interacts with an orbital electron of an atom. All of the energy of the photon is absorbed by the displaced electron in the form of kinetic energy.

Photon (x-ray photon): A quantum of energy. Both x-rays and gamma rays are photons.

Photostimuable phosphors (PSP): Digital imaging sensors that use rare earth phosphor (barium europium fluorohalide) coated plates. When exposed to x-rays, the PSP sensor or plate "stores" the x-ray energy until stimulated by a laser beam to produce a digital image.

PID: *See* Position indicating device.

Pixel: Small, discrete units of digital information that together constitute an image. Pixel is a term shortened from the words "picture" and "element" (pix = plural of picture; el = element).

Point of entry: Spot on the surface of the face toward which the central beam of radiation is directed when aligning the PID for intraoral exposures.

Polychromatic: A term derived from the Greek meaning "having many colors." Used in dental radiography to describe the x-ray beam because it is composed of many different wavelengths.

Port: Opening in the tube head that is covered with a permanent seal of glass, beryllium, or aluminum through which the x-rays exit. The port is opposite the window in the x-ray tube and is the place where the PID attaches to the tube head.

Position indicating device (PID): Also called beam indicating device (BID). An open-ended, cylindrical or rectangular device attached to the tube head at the aperture to direct the useful beam of radiation. PIDs are available in different lengths.

Positive angulation (positive vertical angulation): Angulation achieved by pointing the end of the PID downward from a horizontal plane.

Post and core: Metal restorative material used in an endodontically treated tooth when support for a crown is needed. Appears radiopaque.

Posteroanterior cephalometric radiograph: Extraoral radiograph of the entire skull in the posteroanterior plane. Also called a posterioranterior projection (PA).

Posteroanterior projection (PA): *See* Posterioanterior cephalometric radiograph.

Potassium alum: One of the components of fixer solution. Shrinks and hardens the gelatin emulsion.

Potassium bromide: Restrains the developing agents from developing the unexposed silver halide crystals.

PPE: *See* Personal protective equipment.

Preservative: One of the chemicals (sodium sulfite) used in both the developer and fixer solutions to slow down the rate of oxidation and prevent spoilage of the solution.

Primary beam (primary radiation or useful beam): The original undeflected useful beam of radiation that emanates at the focal spot of the x-ray tube and emerges through the aperture of the tube head.

Primary teeth: Teeth that fall out or are exfoliated naturally. Consists of 20 teeth—8 incisors, 4 canines, and 8 molars.

Processing: The act of bringing out the latent image and making it permanently visible. Includes the following darkroom procedures: developing, rinsing, fixing, washing, and drying.

Processing tank: Stainless steel receptacle divided into compartments for developer solution, water rinse, and fixer solution. Used to process radiographs.

Protective barrier: Shield of radiation-absorbing material used to protect against radiation exposure.

Proton: A subatomic particle of the atom. The proton is contained in the nucleus and has a positive electrical charge. The proton has mass and weight. The number of protons determines the chemical element.

Proximal caries: Caries found on the proximal surfaces (mesial and distal) of teeth.

Proximal surface: Where adjacent teeth contact each other in the arch. The mesial and distal surfaces are proximal surfaces.

Pterygoid plates: Extensions of the sphenoid bone.

Pulp chamber (cavity): Noncalcified tooth tissue containing blood vessels and nerves. Appears radiolucent, as this soft tissue offers only minimal resistance to the passage of x-rays.

Pulp stone: Calcification that appears in the pulp chamber of the teeth, caused by an abnormal disposition of calcium salts. Often described as nodules or denticles. Seen on radiographs as one or more small radiopaque, irregularly shaped, rounded masses within the pulp chamber.

Quality: Term used when describing the intensity of the x-ray beam. Refers to the energy strength or penetrating ability of the x-ray beam.

Quality assurance: The planning, implementation, and evaluation of procedures used to produce high-quality radiographs with maximum diagnostic information while minimizing radiation exposure.

Quality control: A series of tests to ensure that the radiographic system is functioning properly and that the radiographs produced are of an acceptable level of quality.

Quantity: Term used when describing the intensity of the x-ray beam. Refers to the number of x-rays in the beam.

Rad: Traditional unit for measuring absorbed dose. 100 rads equals one gray (Gy). One rad equals 0.01 Gy. 1,000 millirads equals 1 rad.

Radiation: The emission and propagation of energy through space or through a material medium in the form of electromagnetic waves, corpuscular emissions such as alpha and beta particles, or rays of mixed and unknown types such as cosmic rays. Most radiations used in dentistry are capable of producing ions directly or indirectly by interaction with matter.

Radiation leakage: Refers to the x-rays that escape out of the tube head at places other than the port.

Radiation worker: A radiographer or professional who works with or around ionizing radiation or equipment that produces ionizing radiation.

Radiator: A large mass of copper just outside the x-ray tube and connected to the anode terminal. The radiator functions to carry off the excess heat produced in the energy exchange that takes place when the electrons of the cathode stream are converted into about 1% x-rays and 99% heat. The radiator conducts the heat away from the target and cools the tube.

Radicular cyst: A cyst around the apex of a tooth. Generally observed as a small radiolucent circular area that extends away from the apical portions of the root. The sac of the cyst has a distinct wall or capsule that surrounds it and can be distinguished as a faint radiopaque thin line.

Radioactivity: The process whereby certain unstable elements undergo spontaneous disintegration (decay). The process is accompanied by emissions of one or more types of radiation and generally results in the formation of a new isotope.

Radiograph: An image produced on photosensitive film by exposure to x-rays. Developing the film produces a negative image that can be viewed and interpreted.

Radiographic contrast: *See* Contrast.

Radiography (roentgenography): The making of radiographs by exposing and processing x-ray film.

Radiology: That branch of medical science that deals with the use of radiant energy in the diagnosis and treatment of disease.

Radiolucent: That portion of the radiograph that is dark. Structures that lack density permit the passage of x-rays with little or no resistance. These structures appear dark on the image.

Radiolysis of water: Ionization can dissociate water within a cell into hydrogen and hydroxyl radicals that have the potential to recombine into new chemicals such as hydrogen peroxide. These new chemicals act as toxins (poisons) to the body, causing cellular dysfunction. Considered an indirect effect of radiation exposure.

Radiopaque: That portion of the radiograph that appears light. Dense structures resist the passage of radiation. These structures appear light on the image.

Radioresistant: Refers to a substance or tissue that is not easily injured by ionizing radiation.

Radiosensitive: Refers to a substance or tissue that is relatively susceptible to injury by ionizing radiation.

Rampant caries: Severe, unchecked caries that affect multiple teeth.

Ramus: The ascending portion of each end of the mandible.

Rapid (chairside) processing: The use of a chairside darkroom (a light-tight box with a filter cover) and concentrated and/or heated developer to quickly process working films, such as those used during endodontic procedures.

Rare-earth phosphors: Salt crystals, usually lanthanum (La) and gadolinium (Gd), used to coat intensifying screens. When these absorb x-rays, they fluoresce and emit energy in the form of green light.

Recovery period: Period following exposure to radiation, where some healing can take place.

Recurrent (secondary) caries: Caries that occurs under a restoration or around its margins.

Reference film: A radiograph processed under ideal conditions and then used to compare periodically subsequent films. Quality control procedure to monitor processing solution quality.

Rem (roentgen equivalent in man): Traditional unit for measuring dose equivalent. Used to compare the biological effects of the various types of radiation. One rem equals 1 rad times a biological effect weighting factor. Because the weighting factor for x- and gamma radiation equals 1, the number of rems is identical to the absorbed dose in rads for these radiations. 100 rem equals one sievert (Sv); one rem equals 0.01 Sv; 1,000 millirems equal 1 rem.

Replenisher: A superconcentrated solution of developer or fixer that is added daily, or as indicated, to the developer or fixer in the processing tank to compensate for loss of volume and loss of strength from oxidation. The act of adding replenisher to the processing solutions is known as replenishment.

Residual cyst: Cyst that remains in the jaw after the tooth that caused it to form is extracted or exfoliated. May remain within the bone, becoming encapsulated with an epithelial lining, or may undergo considerable growth. Appears radiolucent, and the lining of the cyst appears as a thin radiopaque line.

Resorption: Refers to a loss of bone or tooth structure. May originate from natural causes such as the gradual reduction of size of the roots of primary teeth, or may be idiopathic (the result of unknown causes).

Restrainer: Potassium bromide in the developer solution that slows down the action of the elon and hydroquinone and inhibits the tendency of the solution to chemically fog the films.

Retained root: Root remaining after the tooth has been extracted.

Retake radiograph: A radiograph that has been taken after the first image is deemed undiagnostic.

Retention pin: Metal pin used to support a restoration.

Reverse Towne radiograph: Extraoral projection used to view the condylar neck of the mandible. Also called open mouth projection.

Rhinoliths: Calcifications within the maxillary sinuses.

Risk: The chance or likelihood of adverse effects or death resulting from exposure to a hazard.

Risk management: Policies and procedures to be followed by the radiographer to reduce the chances that a patient will file legal action against the dentist and oral health care team.

Roentgen (R): Traditional unit measurement of exposure to radiation. Measured in air. A simplified definition of the roentgen is the amount of x-radiation or gamma radiation required to ionize 1 cc of air at standard conditions of pressure and temperature (2.083 billion ion pairs).

Roentgen ray: *See* X-ray.

Roentgenograph: *See* Radiograph.

Roller transport system: Moves films through the developer, fixer, water, and drying compartments of an automatic processor. Motor-driven gears or belts propel the roller transport system.

Root canal treatment: *See* Endodontic therapy.

Root surface caries: *See* Cemental caries.

Rotational center: The axis on which the panoramic tube head and the drum rotate. Based on tomographic radiography principles.

Rule of isometry: Geometric theorem stating that two triangles with two equal angles and a common side are equal (isosceles) triangles. This theorem is the basis of the bisecting technique.

Safelight: Special filtered light that can be left on in the darkroom while films are processed.

Safelight filter: Removes short wavelengths in the blue-green region of visible light. The longer wavelength red-orange light is allowed to pass through the filter, illuminating the darkroom without fogging the film.

Sarcoma: Malignant tumor of connective tissue origin.

Scatter radiation: Radiation that has been deflected from its path by impact during its passage through matter. This form of secondary radiation is scattered in all directions by the tissues of the patient's head.

Sclerotic bone: A hardening of the bone as a result of inflammation or excessive growth of fibrous tissue and deposition of mineral salts. *See* Condensing osteitis.

Screen film: Extraoral film for use in cassettes with intensifying screens. Emulsion is more sensitive to green, blue, and violet light, emitted when the radiation strikes the phosphors in the intensifying screens than to the x-radiation.

Secondary radiation: Given off by any matter irradiated with x-rays. Created at the instant the primary beam interacts with matter and gives off some of its energy, forming new and less powerful wavelengths. Often referred to as scatter radiation.

Selection criteria: Guidelines developed by an expert panel of health care professionals to assist in deciding when, what type, and how many radiographs should be taken.

Selective reduction: Chemical change that takes place within the film emulsion during development. During this change, the nonmetallic elements are separated from the silver halide of the exposed crystals, leaving a coating of metallic silver on the film emulsion while the bromide is removed. The process is called selective because the unexposed grains are not reduced.

Self-determination: The legal right of an individual to make choices concerning health care treatment.

Sensor: For use in digital imaging. An electronic or specially coated plate that is sensitive to x-rays. Placed intraorally to capture a radiographic image when exposed to x-rays.

Sepsis: Infection, or the presence of septic matter.

Septum: Thin wall of bone that acts as a partition to separate the nasal cavity or the maxillary sinuses. Appears radiopaque.

Severe caries: A classification of proximal surface caries. Category where caries has penetrated over halfway through the dentin toward the pulp.

Shadow casting: Principle that x-rays cast shadows of images onto the image receptor, producing a radiographic image of the teeth and supporting structures.

Sharpness (See Definition): The distinct outlines of structures observed on a radiograph.

Short-scale contrast: High-contrast image. A radiograph that exhibits black and white with few shades. Produced with low kilovoltage.

"Show-tell-do": Technique used to orient the patient, especially children, to the radiographic procedure. Showing the radiographic equipment—image receptor and holder, x-ray machine—to the patient while explaining their use may help to alleviate fear of the unknown and gain patient cooperation.

Sialolith: A salivary calculus or hardened, stonelike mass that forms within the passage of the salivary ducts. If sufficiently large, such masses appear slightly radiopaque on the radiograph.

Sievert (Sv): Système Internationale unit for measuring the dose equivalent. The sievert is used to compare the biological effects of various types of radiation. One sievert equals one gray times a biological effect weighting (qualifying) factor. Because the weighting factor for x- and gamma radiation equals 1, the number of sieverts is identical to the absorbed dose in grays for these radiations. One sievert equals 100 rem. *See* Microsievert.

Silver halide crystals: Compounds of a halogen (either bromine or iodine) with silver. Dental film emulsion is approximately 90 to 99 percent silver bromide and 1 to 10 percent silver iodide. Silver halide crystals are sensitive to radiation. It is the silver halide crystals that, when exposed to x-rays, retain the latent image.

Silver thiosulphate complex: A very stable compound found in used fixer of dental radiographic processors following the interaction of sodium thiosulphate with the silver ions in the emulsion of film.

Silver point: Endodontic filling material.

Sinus projection: *See* Waters radiograph.

SLOB rule: Stands for same on lingual, opposite on buccal. Used in localization techniques to determine the facial (buccal) or lingual position of objects. The tube shift method of localization states that if the structure or object in question appears to move in the same direction as the horizontal or vertical shift of the tube, then the structure or object is located on the lingual. Conversely, if the move is in the opposite direction of the shift of the tube, the object is located on the buccal (facial).

Sodium carbonate: Provides required alkalinity of the developer solution to activate developing agents.

Sodium sulfite: Chemical of the developing solution that prevents rapid oxidation of the developing agents.

Sodium thiosulfate: Chemical of the fixer solution that together with the ammonium thiosulfate removes the unexposed and any remaining undeveloped silver halide crystals.

Soft radiation: Longest wavelength of the x-rays. Removed from the polychromatic beam by filtration because soft radiation (Grenz rays) have no value in producing dental radiographs.

Solarized emulsion: Used for duplicating film. Produces a duplicate image that gets lighter the longer the film is exposed to light. Darker images result from shorter exposure times.

Solid state: Specifically means, no moving parts. Refers to digital image sensors, usually CCD or CMOS technology.

Somatic cells: Any body cells except the reproductive cells.

Somatic effect: When radiation affects all body cells except the reproductive cells.

Spatial resolution: The discernable separation of closely adjacent image details that contributes to image sharpness. The greater the spatial resolution, the sharper the image appears. When referring to a digital image, sharpness is determined by the number and size of pixels and measured in line pairs. When the number of pixels is low, the image appears to have jagged edges and becomes difficult to see.

Spatter: A heavier concentration of microbial aerosols such as visible particles from a cough or sneeze.

Speech reading: Method of lip reading used by the hearing impaired.

Sphenoid bone: Cranial bone bordered by the frontal and ethmoid bones.

Standard precautions: A practice of care to protect persons from pathogens spread via blood or any other body fluid, excretion, or secretion (except sweat). All-inclusive term that has replaced universal precautions, where the focus was on blood-borne pathogens.

Static electricity: A white-light spark that creates a radiolucent artifact on the film.

Statute of limitations: Time period during which a person may bring a malpractice action against another person.

Step-down transformer (low-voltage transformer): Device consisting of two metal cores and coils so positioned within the circuitry of the tube head to decrease the line voltage to between 3 and 12 volts. Low voltage is required in the cathode to warm up the filament wire.

Step-up transformer (high-voltage transformer): Device consisting of two metal cores and coils positioned within the circuitry of the tube head to increase the potential of the line current to the high kilovoltage required to produce x-radiation.

Step-wedge (penetrometer): A device consisting of increasing increments of an absorbing material. A radiographic exposure made with a step-wedge is used to determine the amount of radiation reaching the image receptor through each of the increments. Measurements of radiographic image density may be used to evaluate the intensity and penetrative power of the radiation.

Sterilize: Aseptic treatment, autoclaving or dry heat processes, that results in the total destruction of spores and disease-producing microorganisms.

Stochastic effect: When a biological response is based on the probability of occurrence rather than the severity of the change.

Storage phosphor: Usually composed of europium activated barium fluorohalide, coating on a photostimulable phosphor plate used in indirect digital imaging. The storage phosphor "stores" the x-ray energy similar to the way silver halide crystals within film emulsion store a latent image. A scanning device is used to release the stored energy to be converted to a radiographic image on a computer monitor.

Structural shielding: The protection afforded by building materials found in walls, partitions, and cabinetry, present in most buildings where dental radiographs are exposed.

Styloid process: Long, narrow spine that extends downward, from the inferior surface of the temporal bone, just anterior to the mastoid process.

Subject contrast: The difference in densities of a radiographic image caused by the differing thicknesses of the tissues or objects penetrated by the x-ray beam.

Submandibular fossa: Irregular depression in the bone near the angle on the lingual of the mandible. Usually observed radiographically below the roots of the molars and extending forward as far as the premolar region. Thin and offering little resistance to the passage of the x-rays, it appears radiolucent.

Submentovertex projection: Extraoral projection showing the base of the skull, the position of the mandibular condyles, and the zygomatic arches. Also called a base projection.

Supernumerary teeth: Extra teeth not normally a part of the dentition. May resemble normal teeth, only smaller with conical crowns, or bear no resemblance to a normal tooth. Often malpositioned or unerupted.

Suture: A line of union of adjacent cranial or facial bones that appears radiolucent on radiographs.

Symphysis: Prominent bone where the right and left sides of the mandible fuse at the midline.

Système Internationale (SI): A metric system of units of that measures radiation quantities. The Système Internationale units are coulombs per kilogram (C/kg), gray (Gy), and sievert (Sv).

Target: Small block of tungsten imbedded in the face of the anode, bombarded by the electrons streaming from the cathode. The focal spot is located on the target.

Target–image receptor distance (source–image receptor distance): Distance between the focal spot on the target and the recording plane of the image receptor.

Target–object distance (source–object distance): Distance between the focal spot on the target and the object being radiographed.

Target–surface distance (source–surface distance): Distance between the focal spot on the target and the skin surface of the patient.

Taurodontia: Teeth characterized by very large pulp chambers and very short roots.

Temporal bone: Cranial bone the makes up the temple, or side of the face. Contains the ear structures, including the auditory meatus.

Temporomandibular disorders (TMD): Term used to describe the collection of symptoms and diseases that are generally found involving the temporomandibular joint.

Temporomandibular joint (TMJ): One of two joints connecting the mandible to the temporal bone.

Temporomandibular joint projection: *See* Transcranial radiograph.

Thermionic emission: The release of electrons when a material such as tungsten is heated to incandescence. Electrons are boiled off from the cathode filament in the x-ray tube when electric current is passed through it.

Thermoluminescent dosimeter (TLD): Monitoring device containing certain crystalline compounds (usually lithium fluoride) that store energy when struck by x-rays. When heated, the crystals give off light in proportion to the amount of radiation exposure.

Threshold dose response curve: A graph showing the relationship between the dose of exposure and the response of the tissues, indicating that there is a "threshold" amount of radiation, below which no biological response would be expected.

Thyroid collar: An attached or detachable supplement to the lead apron. Contains 0.25 mm lead or lead-equivalent materials to protect the radiosensitive thyroid gland in the neck region during the exposure of intraoral radiographs.

Timer: A mechanical, electrical, or electronic device that can be set to predetermine the duration of the interval that current flows through the x-ray machine to produce x-rays.

Time–temperature: Principle of film processing. The length of time the film spends in the developer is based on the temperature of the developer solution. When the temperature is cool, processing time is increased. When the temperature is warm, processing time is decreased. Film manufacturer will usually recommend an ideal temperature and time that will produce quality images.

TLD: *See* Thermoluminescent dosimeter.

Tomograph: A radiograph made using the tomography technique.

Tomography: A radiographic technique used to show detailed images of structures located within a predetermined plane of tissue while eliminating or blurring those structures in the planes not selected.

Topographical technique: Occlusal radiography technique that follows the rules of bisecting. The central rays of the x-ray beam are directed through the apices of the teeth perpendicularly toward the bisector to produce an image.

Torus (tori-plural): Form of benign tumor. Outgrowth of bone called exostosis.

Torus mandibularis (lingual torus): Hard, bony protuberance on the lingual surface of the mandible. Usually located above the mylohyoid line near the premolars. Often bilateral.

Torus palatinus: Hard, bony protuberance on the midline of the maxilla.

Total filtration: The combination of inherent and added filtration in an x-ray machine. Many states require a total filtration of 2.5 mm of aluminum equivalent for x-ray machines operating at or above 70 kVp.

Trabeculae: Tiny bars or plates of bone that form a network of various-sized compartments that account for the honeycomb appearance of bone.

Trabecular bone (cancellous bone): The softer spongy bone that makes up the bulk of the inside portion of most bones. The cells of trabecular bone vary in size and density.

Tragus: Small cartilaginous prominence of tissues located near the center and in front of the acoustic meatus (outer ear opening).

Transcranial projection: Extraoral projection used to image the temporomandibular joint (TMJ) in both an open and closed position. Also called a TMJ projection.

Transformer: One of several types of electrical devices capable of increasing or decreasing the voltage of an alternating current by mutual induction between primary and secondary coils or windings on cores of metal. *See* High-voltage transformer and Low-voltage transformer.

Transitional (mixed) dentition: Having both primary and permanent teeth present in the oral cavity. Usually exists between 6 and 12 years of age.

Triangulation: Widening of the periodontal ligament space at the crest of the interproximal bone.

Tube head (tube housing): Protective metal covering that contains the x-ray tube, the high-voltage and low-voltage transformers, and insulating oil. Attached to the flexible extension arm by a yoke. The PID attaches to the tube head at the port.

Tube shift method: Method of localization. *See* Buccal-object rule.

Tube side: Describes the side of an intraoral film packet, phosphor plate, digital sensor, and extraoral film or phosphor plate cassette that must face the source of x-rays coming from the x-ray tube.

Tuberosity: Broad eminence on a bone.

Tumor: Swelling or a growth of tissue.

Tungsten (Wolfram): Element with an atomic number of 74. High melting point makes this metal ideal for use as the cathode filament and as the anode target.

Underdevelopment: Not leaving the film in the developer solution long enough or using developer that is too cool or an old, weak solution. Underdevelopment results in a light image.

Underexposure: Not exposing the image receptor long enough or using an inappropriately decreased kVp or mA setting. Underexposure results in a light image.

Universal precautions: A method of infection control in which blood and certain body fluids are treated as if known to be infectious for HIV, HBV, and other blood-borne pathogens. The all-inclusive term standard precautions has replaced universal precautions, where the focus is on blood-borne pathogens.

Useful beam (useful radiation): That part of the primary beam that is permitted to emerge from the tube head and limited by the port, collimator, and lead-lined PID.

Velocity: Property exhibited by electromagnetic radiation. Refers to the speed of the wave as it travels through space. In a vacuum, all electromagnetic radiations travel at the speed of light (186,000 miles/sec or 3×10^8 m/sec).

Verbal communication: Using words to exchange information between two or more persons.

Vertical angulation: The direction of the central beam in an up or down direction achieved by directing the tip of the PID upward or downward. *See* Negative angulation and Positive angulation.

Vertical (angular) bone loss: Occurs in a vertical direction. Alveolar crest is reduced in a manner that creates angular defects.

Vertical bitewing radiograph: Bitewing radiograph placed in the oral cavity with the long dimension of the image receptor positioned vertically. Covers an increased area in the vertical dimension, resulting in more information regarding the periodontium being recorded.

Vertical bitewing series: A set of 4 to 7 vertical bitewings. May include both posterior and anterior images.

View box: Device used to view dental radiographs. Consists of a light source illuminator behind an opaque glass.

Volt: Unit of electromotive force or potential that is sufficient to cause a current of l ampere (A) to flow through a resistance of 1 ohm (W).

Voltage: Electrical pressure or force that drives the electric current through the circuit of the x-ray machine. *See* Kilovolt and Kilovolt peak.

Voltmeter: Device for measuring the electromotive force (the difference in potential or voltage) across the x-ray tube.

Voxel (volume element): Similar to a pixel, but adds a third dimension of digital data that together constitute an image. Used in computed tomography imaging. Voxel is a term shortened from the words "volume" and "element" (similar to the shortened term for pixel where pix = plural of picture and el = element)

Waste stream: The collective flow of waste materials beginning at the point of discard, through waste treatments, to the final disposition of the material.

Waters radiograph: Also called the sinus projection. Similar to the posteroanterior cephalometric radiograph except that the center of interest is focused on the middle third of the face.

Wavelength: In radiography, the length in angstrom units or centimeters of the electromagnetic radiations produced in the x-ray machine. The distance from the crest, or top of one wave to the crest of the next, determines the wavelength—hence its penetration ability.

Weighting factor (qualifying factor): Used to convert absorbed dose to dose equivalent. Takes into consideration the difference in biological effectiveness of various types of radiation (x-, gamma, alpha, beta, etc). Some radiations (such as alpha particles) cause more biological damage than others (such as x-rays). The qualifying factor for dental x-rays is 1; for alpha particles it is 10.

Wet reading: Viewing a radiograph under white light conditions after only two or three minutes of fixation. Used when a diagnosis from the radiograph is needed quickly. Following the wet reading, the film must be returned to the fixer to complete processing.

Working radiograph: A film that is rapidly processed when information is needed quickly. Often used during endodontic procedures. However, short developing and fixing times, combined with minimal washing, result in a substandard radiograph.

x-coordinate: One of two values assigned to dimensions of a pixel that tell the computer where the pixel is located. Computer software uses the *x*-coordinate along with the *y*-coordinate to reconstruct digital data captured by a sensor or photostimuable plate into a radiographic image displayed on a monitor.

X-ray (roentgen ray): Radiant energy of short wavelength that has the power to penetrate substances and to record shadow images on photographic film, phosphor plates, and digital sensors.

X-ray film: *See* Radiograph and Film packet.

X-ray tube: Electronic tube located in the tube head that generates x-rays.

y-coordinate: One of two values assigned to dimensions of a pixel that tell the computer where the pixel is located. Computer software uses the *y*-coordinate along with the *x*- coordinate to reconstruct digital data captured by a sensor or photostimuable plate into a radiographic image displayed on a monitor..

Yoke: Curved portion of the x-ray machine that is connected to the extension arm. The tube head is suspended within the yoke and can be rotated vertically and horizontally within it.

Zygoma: Cheek bone. Attaches to the zygomatic process of the temporal bone to form the zygomatic arch.

Zygomatic arch: Arch formed by the temporal process of the zygomatic bone and the zygomatic process of the temporal bone. Forms the outer margin of the cheek prominence.

Zygomatic process: Process of the temporal bone that attaches to the zygoma to form the zygomatic arch.

Index